Acute Respiratory Care *of the* Neonate

• Second Edition •

A Self-Study Course

Edited by
Debbie Fraser Askin, RNC, MN

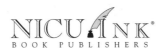
NICU Ink®
BOOK PUBLISHERS

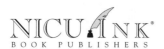

1304 Southpoint Blvd., Suite 280
Petaluma, CA 94954-6861
(707) 762-2646

COPYRIGHT © 1997 BY NICU INK BOOK PUBLISHERS

Trademarks: Throughout this book we use trademarked names. Instead of using a trademark symbol with each occurrence, we state that we are using the names in an editorial fashion to the benefit of the trademark owner, with no intention of infringement of the trademark.

Editor-in-Chief: Charles Rait, RN, MSEd, PNC

Managing Editor: Suzanne G. Rait, RN

Editorial Coordinator: Tabitha Parker

Reviewers: Terri Erdman, RN, MS, NNP
Debbie O'Banion, RNC, MSN, NNP

Editors: Judith K. Jenna, MA, BSN
Marlys Ulyshen, RNC, MSN, MPH, NNP
Sylvia Stein Wright, BA

Proofreader: Jane Holly Love, MA

Indexer: Eleanor Lindheimer

Book design and composition by
Marsha Godfrey Graphics

LIBRARY OF CONGRESS CATALOGING-IN-PUBLICATION DATA
Acute respiratory care of the neonate : a self-study course / edited by Debbie Fraser Askin.—2nd ed.
     p.   cm.
    Includes bibliographical references and index.
    ISBN 1-887571-01-9
    1. Respiratory therapy for newborn infants. 2. Respiratory distress syndrome—Nursing.
I. Askin, Debbie Fraser, 1959–   .
    [DNLM: 1. Respiratory Distress Syndrome—nursing. 2. Intensive Care, Neonatal—methods. WY 157.3 A189 1997]
RJ312.A28 1997
618.92'200428—dc21
DNLM/DLC
for Library of Congress   97-17399
                                                          CIP

ISBN: 1-887571-01-9   Library of Congress catalog number 97-17399

TABLE OF CONTENTS

CONTRIBUTING AUTHORS

Steven H. Abman, MD
The Children's Hospital
University of Colorado School of Medicine
Denver, Colorado

Debbie Fraser Askin, RNC, MN
St. Boniface General Hospital
Winnipeg, Manitoba
Canada

V. L. Cassani III, RNC, MSN, MSNA, NNP, CRNA
Georgetown University School of Medicine
Division of Neonatology
Washington, DC
Pediatric Anesthesia Associates of Dayton, Ohio
The Children's Medical Center
Dayton, Ohio

James A. Cullen, RN
Thomas Jefferson Medical College
Philadelphia, Pennsylvania

Diane Deveau, MS, RNC
Columbia-Presbyterian Medical Center
New York City, New York

Jay S. Greenspan, MD
Thomas Jefferson Medical College
Philadelphia, Pennsylvania

Debra Bingham Jones, MS, RN,C
St. Luke's-Roosevelt Hospital
New York, New York

Tracy Karp, RNC, MS, NNP
Primary Children's Medical Center
Salt Lake City, Utah

John P. Kinsella, MD
The Children's Hospital
University of Colorado School of Medicine
Denver, Colorado

Kathleen Koszarek, RNC, MSN
Ochsner Foundation Hospital
New Orleans, Louisiana

Donna Lee Loper, RN, MS, CNS
San Francisco General Hospital
San Francisco, California

Gerry Matranga, RNC, MN, NNP
Ochsner Foundation Hospital
New Orleans, Louisiana

Barbara Nightengale, RNC, MSN, NNP
West Virginia University
Department of Pediatrics
Morgantown, West Virginia

Jan Nugent, RNC, MSN, MD
Louisiana State University Medical School
New Orleans, Louisiana

Roxanne Geidel Oellrich, RNC, MSN
Winthrop-University Hospital
Mineola, New York

Susan Orlando, RNC, MS
Ochsner Foundation Hospital
New Orleans, Louisiana

Judith D. Polak, RNC, MSN, NNP
West Virginia University Hospitals
Morgantown, West Virginia

Susan S. Spinner, MSN, RN
Thomas Jefferson Medical College
Philadelphia, Pennsylvania

Barbara S. Turner, RN, DNSc, FAAN
Duke University
Durham, North Carolina

Todd L. Wandstrat, PharmD
West Virginia University
Charleston, West Virginia

Acknowledgment

I would like to acknowledge and thank the following people for their help and support:

the dedicated authors whose wealth of experience enrich the pages of this book; my colleagues at St. Boniface Hospital, especially Dr. Maria Davi, Dr. Gerada Cronin, Bill Petranick, Joe Millar for their review and suggestions and Laura-Lee Bouchard for secretarial support; Chuck and Suzanne Rait, and Tabitha Parker for making this book possible; and special thanks to my husband Tom and daughters Cayly and Nicole.

Dedicated to the NICU babies and their families from whom we've all learned.

Introduction

Since the first edition of "ARC" came off the press in 1991, newborn respiratory care has continued to evolve. The second edition of this text has added information on new technologies such as synchronized and volume ventilation, nitric oxide, pulmonary function testing and liquid ventilation. Other additions include chapters on respiratory pharmacology, blood gas interpretation, and CPAP. The remaining chapters have been updated and revised to reflect the continued growth in our understanding of the impact of respiratory disease on the newborn infant.

This text continues its commitment to provide that blend of the nursing art and science so critical to the care of high risk infants. As never before, the challenge of providing care to our future leaders and their families lies before us. This book is dedicated to helping those that accept that challenge.

Debbie Fraser Askin, RNC, MN
Neonatal Nurse Practitioner
St. Boniface General Hospital

1 Physiologic Principles of the Respiratory System

Donna Lee Loper, RN, MS, CNS

In order to provide effective and appropriate nursing interventions to sick neonates, it is necessary to understand the disease process and its usual course as well as to appreciate the various treatment modalities. The foundation for this understanding and awareness is a strong knowledge base of the normal growth, development, and function of the fetus and neonate. This chapter provides the basis for this foundation. It discusses the embryologic development of the lung and the role of lung fluid and fetal breathing movements in development as well as surfactant synthesis and secretion. First breath events and the concomitant changes in pulmonary perfusion are presented, along with a discussion of lung physiology. These provide the basis for understanding the chapters that follow.

EMBRYOLOGIC DEVELOPMENT

ANATOMY

Prenatal lung growth occurs in four stages: embryonic, pseudoglandular, canalicular, and terminal air sac (Figure 1-1). After birth, the numbers of alveoli continue to increase for approximately eight years.

Prenatal Lung Growth

Embryonic Stage. This stage begins at conception and ends at the fifth week of gestation. Around day 24, a ventral diverticulum (outpouching) known as the laryngotracheal groove can be seen developing from the foregut. This groove extends downward and is gradually separated from the future esophagus by a septum. Failure of the septum to develop completely results in a tracheoesophageal fistula. Table 1-1 describes other congenital anomalies of the respiratory system.

Between two and four days later, the first dichotomous branches of the lung (bronchial) buds can be seen. At the end of this stage, three divisions are evident on the right and two on the left (lobar and segmental bronchi). While these buds are dividing, the trachea is forming through the elongation of the upper portion of the lung bud.

Pseudoglandular Stage. From 5 to 17 weeks, a tree of narrow tubules forms. New airway branches arise through a mixture of cell multiplication and necrosis.[1] These tubules have thick epithelial walls made of columnar or cuboidal cells. This morphology, along with the loose mesenchymal tissue surrounding the

FIGURE 1-1 ▲ Fetal lung development from four weeks (A to C) to five weeks (D and E) to six weeks (F) to eight weeks (G).

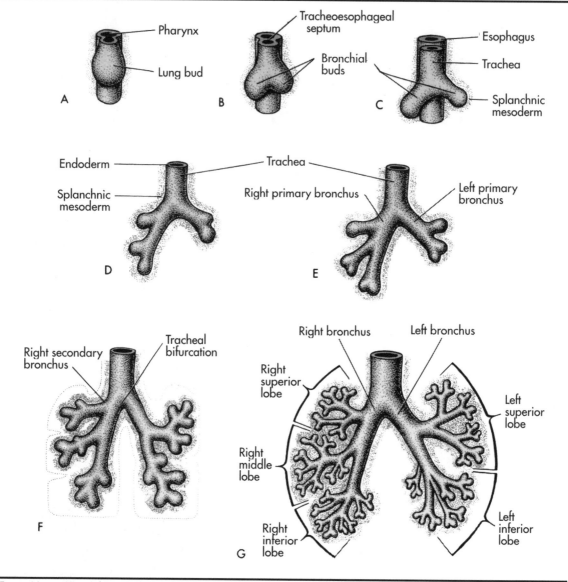

From: Moore KL, and Persaud TVN. 1993. The respiratory system. In *The Developing Human,* 5th ed. Philadelphia: WB Saunders, 230. Reprinted by permission.

tree, give the lungs a glandular appearance, hence the name "pseudoglandular stage."

By 16 weeks, branching of the conduction portion of the tracheobronchial tree (trachea to terminal bronchioles) is established. These preacinar airways can from this point forward increase only in length and diameter, not in number.[2,3] Toward the end of the pseudoglan-

dular period, rudimentary forms of cartilage, connective tissue, muscle, blood vessels, and lymphatics can be identified.[4]

Canalicular Stage. The epithelial cells of the distal air spaces (future alveolar lining) flatten sometime between weeks 13 and 25, signaling the beginning of the canalicular stage.[5] A rich vascular supply begins to proliferate, and

TABLE 1-1 ▲ **Congenital Anomalies of the Respiratory System**

Anomaly	Origin	Time Frame/Incidence
Pulmonary atresia (single lung or lobe)	Failure of primitive foregut branches to develop	Four to six weeks
Tracheoesophageal fistula	Failure of foregut (tracheoesophageal) septum to completely divide the esophagus and trachea	Four to five weeks Incidence: 1 in 2,500 births
Tracheal stenosis/atresia	Unequal division of foregut into trachea and esophagus	Four to five weeks Incidence: Rare
Diaphragmatic hernia	Failure of fusion of the septum transversum, pleuroperitoneal membranes, lateral body wall, and dorsal mesentery of esophagus	Six to ten weeks Incidence: 1 in 2,000 births

with the changes in mesenchymal tissue, the capillaries are brought closer to the airway epithelium. Primitive respiratory bronchioles begin to form during this stage, delineating the acinus (gas-exchanging) section from the conducting portion of the lung.

Terminal Air Sac Stage. At 24 weeks gestation, terminal air sacs appear as outpouchings of the terminal bronchioles. As the weeks progress, the number of terminal sacs increases, forming multiple pouches off a common chamber (the alveolar duct). The surface epithelium thins considerably as vessels proliferate. The vessels stretch, thinning the epithelium that covers them even more, bringing the capillaries into close proximity to the developing airways.[2]

Eventually this leads to fusion of the basement membrane between the endothelium and epithelium, thus creating the future blood-gas barrier (Figure 1-2).[1] Near term, shallow indentations in the saccule walls can be detected. These primitive alveoli will deepen and multiply postnatally.

Pulmonary Vasculature

Pulmonary vessel development occurs in conjunction with the branching of the bronchial tree.[6-8] The arteries have more branches than the airways, and the veins develop more tribu-

taries. The preacinar region has an arterial branch (conventional artery) that runs along each conducting airway branch; supernumerary arteries feed the adjacent alveoli. The preacinar arteries are all present by 16 weeks gestation. If for any reason there is a decrease in the number of airways, there is a concomitant decrease in conventional and supernumerary arteries.[1,7] From 16 weeks on, the preacinar vessels increase in length and diameter only.[4]

As development progresses into the canalicular and terminal air sac stages, intra-acinar arteries appear and will continue their development during the postnatal period.[4,7,8] The conventional arteries continue their development for the first 18 months of life. Supernumerary

FIGURE 1-2 ▲ **Blood-gas barrier of the respiratory membrane.**

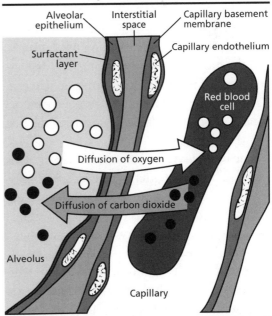

From: Chaffee EE, and Lytle IM. 1980. *Basic Physiology and Anatomy*, 4th ed. Philadelphia: JB Lippincott, 395. Reprinted by permission.

arteries continue to be laid down for the first eight years.[1,8] These latter vessels are smaller and more numerous, servicing the alveoli directly.[9] If blood flow is reduced or blocked through the conventional arteries, the supernumerary arteries may serve as collateral circulation, thereby maintaining lung function during periods of ischemia or increased pulmonary vascular resistance.[10] Postnatally, the intra-acinar vessels multiply rapidly as alveoli appear.[4]

The pulmonary veins develop more slowly. By 20 weeks, however, preacinar veins are present.[8] The structural development of the veins parallels that of the arteries and conducting airways, although supernumerary veins outnumber supernumerary arteries. Interestingly, both types of veins appear simultaneously.[4] The development of additional veins, as well as the lengthening of existing veins, continues postnatally.

Further development of the pulmonary circulation is related to changes in muscle wall thickness and muscle extension into arterial walls. The pulmonary artery wall is quite thick at birth, as a result of the low oxygen tension encountered in the intrauterine environment. The wall thins as oxygen tension rises at birth, and the medial layer elastic fibrils become less organized. The pulmonary vein is deficient in elastic fibers at birth and progressively incorporates muscle and elastic tissue during the first two years of life.[8]

The intrapulmonary arteries have thick walls as well. The smaller arteries have increased muscularity and dilate actively with the postnatal increase in oxygen tension.[7] There is a concomitant fall in pulmonary vascular resistance.[4] Between 3 and 28 days postnatally, these vessels achieve their adult ratio of wall thickness to external diameter. The larger arteries take longer, achieving adult levels between 4 and 18 months.[8]

The systemic arteries of the fetus are also more muscular than those of the adult or child.

The ratio between muscle thickness and external diameter decreases postnatally.[4] Muscle distribution changes following birth (with the muscle extending peripherally) and continues changing during the first 19 years of life.

Lung structures and cells are differentiated to the point that extrauterine life can be supported around 24 weeks. Although the normal number of air spaces has not developed, the epithelium has thinned enough and the vascular bed has proliferated to the point that oxygen exchange can occur.

Cell Structure

The respiratory portion of the lung has a continuous epithelial lining composed mainly of two cell types: Type I and Type II pneumocytes. The Type I pneumocyte (squamous pneumocyte) covers approximately 95 percent of the alveolar surface via its long cytoplasmic extensions.[11,12] The thinnest area of the alveolus is composed of these extensions, and gas exchange occurs here most rapidly.

The Type II pneumocyte (granular pneumocyte), although more numerous than the Type I, occupies less than 5 percent of the alveolar surface.[11] Osmiophilic, lamellated bodies are characteristic of these cells, and it is here that surfactant is thought to be produced and secreted. The first Type II cells are seen during the terminal sac stage, between 20 and 24 weeks. Surfactant secretion is detectable between 25 and 30 weeks gestation, although the potential for alveolar stability does not occur until later, between 33 and 36 weeks.[10,13]

PHYSIOLOGY

The functional development of the lung revolves around the biochemistry of surfactant. The lung does, however, secrete other substances and has its own particular macrophage function.

Large particles (bacteria) not swept away by ciliary action are thought to be removed and

TABLE 1-2 ▲ Surfactant Composition

Composition by Weight (Percent)		
Phospholipids		85
Saturated phosphatidylcholine	60	
Unsaturated phosphatidylcholine	20	
Phosphatidylglycerol	8	
Phosphatidylinositol	2	
Phosphatidylethanolamine	5	
Sphingomyelin	2	
Others	3	
Neutral lipids and cholesterol		5
Proteins		10
Contaminating serum proteins	8	
Surfactant protein 35 (32–36,000 daltons)	~1	
Lipophilic proteins (6–12,000 daltons)	~1	

From: Jobe A. 1987. Questions about surfactant for respiratory distress syndrome (RDS). In *Mead Johnson Symposium on Perinatal and Developmental Medicine.* Evansville, Indiana: Mead Johnson, 43. Reprinted by permission.

destroyed by pulmonary macrophages. Foreign material, once identified, is engulfed by the macrophage. Lysosomes then release enzymes which destroy the particle. These cells are critical to the health and continued function of the lung because they contribute to maintaining the sterility of the environment. They are most likely involved in removing surfactant from the alveolar surface as well.

Surfactant Synthesis

Surfactant is of major importance to the adequate functioning of the lung. Table 1-2 lists the composition of pulmonary surfactant, a lipoprotein with 90 percent of its dry weight composed of lipid.[14] The majority of the lipid is saturated phosphatidylcholine (PC), of which dipalmitoylphosphatidylcholine (DPPC) is the most abundant. The latter is the component responsible for decreasing the surface tension to almost zero when compressed at the surface during inspiration.

Phosphatidylglycerol (PG) accounts for another 8 percent of the phospholipids in surfactant. This is a substantial quantity and is unique to lung cells. PG is the last phospolipid to develop in surfactant. Because fetal lung fluid flows into the amniotic cavity, the presence of PG in amniotic fluid is a good marker for the presence of surfactant and hence, lung maturity. The rest of the compound is involved in intracellular transport, storage, exocytosis, adsorption, and clearance at the alveolar lining.[11,14,15]

Surfactant synthesis involves a series of biochemical events that include synthesis and integration of surfactant components in the membranes of the smooth and rough endoplasmic reticulum and multivesicular bodies of the Type II pneumocyte.[11,14] Once assembled, surfactant is transported intracellularly to the Golgi apparatus and then on to the lamellar bodies.[16] The biosynthesis of surfactant is discussed in detail in several publications.[11,14] See also Chapter 9.

FIGURE 1-3 ▲ Pathways for phosphatidylcholine synthesis.

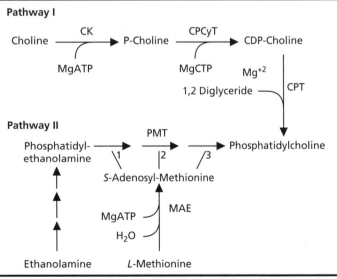

From: Farrell PM, and Ulane RE. 1981. The regulation of lung phospholipid metabolism. In *Physiological and Biochemical Basis for Perinatal Medicine,* Monset-Couchard M, and Minkowski A, eds. Basel, Switzerland: S. Karger AG, 31. Reprinted by permission.

FIGURE 1-4 ▲ Biosynthesis of phospholipids.

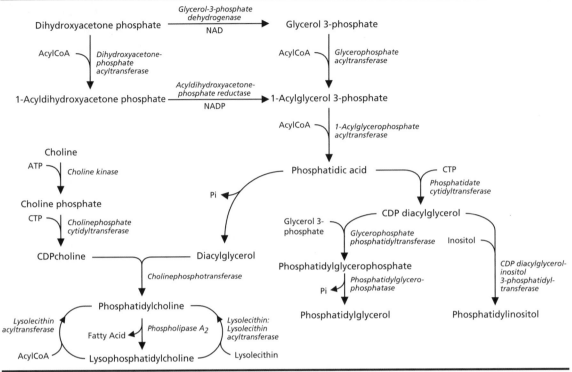

From: Jobe A. 1987. Questions about surfactant for respiratory distress syndrome (RDS). In *Mead Johnson Symposium on Perinatal and Developmental Medicine*. Evansville, Indiana: Mead Johnson, 13. Reprinted by permission.

Prior to being physiologically functional, surfactant undergoes a chemical change, becoming a lattice-shaped structure known as tubular myelin. This structural change enhances spreadability and adsorption. Once surfactant is synthesized and transformed, it is stored in the lamellar body. Secretion occurs by exocytosis; however, surfactant must migrate to the surface of the liquid layer in order to be physiologically functional.[11,16,17]

There are two major pathways for phosphatidylcholine synthesis (Figure 1-3). Key precursors for PC synthesis include glycerol, fatty acids, choline, glucose, and ethanolamine.[15] The major pathway is the cytidine diphosphate choline system, which provides the biochemical maturity necessary for alveolar structural integrity and stability.

The other pathway—the methyltransferase system—leads to phosphatidylethanolamine formation. This pathway has minor significance in the adult lung and seems to play a relatively insignificant role in fetal lung development.[15]

Figure 1-4 depicts the biosynthesis of phosphatidylcholine, phosphatidylinositol, and phosphatidylglycerol and demonstrates the dependency of the system upon the biosynthesis of phosphatidic acid. The increased production of phospholipids seen in late gestation depends on the increased synthesis of this acid. The majority of phospholipid produced is PC; Figure 1-5 represents the biosynthesis and remodeling of this critical phospholipid.[14,15]

Figure 1-5 also demonstrates the interaction of the choline pathway and the diglyceride synthesis mechanisms that yield increased PC synthesis during late gestation. Although this interaction yields increased quantities of PC, it is not the highly saturated version identified in the final surfactant compound. The remodeling

FIGURE 1-5 ▲ Biosyntheses and remodeling of phosphatidylcholine.

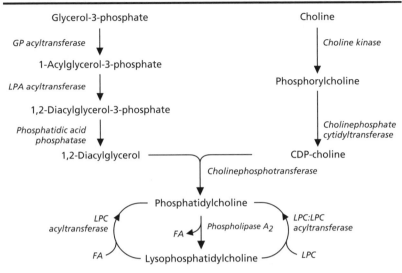

From: Farrell PM, and Ulane RE. 1981. The regulation of lung phospholipid metabolism. In *Physiological and Biochemical Basis for Perinatal Medicine*, Monset-Couchard M, and Minkowski A, eds. Basel, Switzerland: S. Karger AG, 33. Reprinted by permission.

of PC that occurs in the phosphatidylcholine-lysophosphatidylcholine cycle provides the dipalmitoyl-PC required for surfactant.[15]

As gestation advances, phospholipid content increases, as does the level of saturation. This is accompanied by an increase in osmiophilic inclusion bodies within the Type II pneumocytes. Choline incorporation, which is low in early gestation, has been reported to increase abruptly in rhesus monkeys when 90 percent of gestation is completed.[5] This suggests that pathway regulatory mechanisms are modified/enhanced in order to meet postnatal needs. Figure 1-6 demonstrates the changes in glycerophospholipids in response to system maturation during gestation.

Enzymatic changes in the phospholipid synthesis pathway are discussed in several review articles.[14,15,18] The correlation of these changes with the surge in saturated PC and increase in phosphatidylglycerol and the concomitant decrease in phosphatidylinositol (Figure 1-6) is not yet understood. Whether it is a change in concentration of enzyme or substrate, adjustment

in catalytic efficiency, change in substrate affinity, or activation of latent enzymes is not known.

Hormonal Influences

In addition to enzymes, hormones regulate surfactant biosynthesis and secretion. Those hormones that have been implicated include glucocorticoids, adrenocorticotropic hormone, thyroid hormone, estrogens, prolactin, thyrotropin-releasing hormone, catecholamines, insulin, fibroblast pneumocyte factor, prostaglandins, and epidermal growth factor. Only glucocorticoids, thyroid hormones, insulin, and catecholamines are reviewed here.

Glucocorticoids. These are probably the best known of the hormones affecting surfactant. Liggins's observations in 1969 set off a flurry of research in the area of hormonal control of fetal lung development that has continued to the present.[19] Glucocorticoids accelerate the normal pattern of fetal lung development by increasing the rate of glycogen depletion and phospholipid biosynthesis.

The depletion in glycogen leads to direct anatomic changes of the alveolar structures, thinning the interalveolar septa while increasing the size of the alveoli (air space). Morphologic changes include increases in the numbers of Type II pneumocytes and lamellar bodies within those cells. This occurs in conjunction with a functional maturation of these cells, leading to an accelerated synthesis of surfactant phospholipid.[14,20–23]

Glucocorticoids act by binding to specific receptors within the cytoplasm. This complex interacts with deoxyribonucleic acid (DNA) to

FIGURE 1-6 ▲ Changes in glycerophospholipids during gestation.

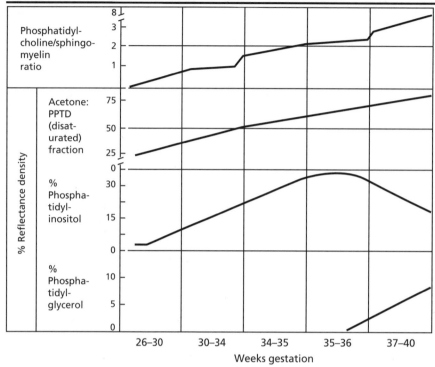

From: Merritt TA. 1984. Respiratory distress. In *Assessment of the Newborn: A Guide for the Practitioner*, Ziai M, Clarke TA, and Merritt TA, eds. Boston: Little, Brown, 177. Reprinted by permission.

produce a specific messenger ribonucleic acid (RNA) that translates its protein code to the ribosomes. The identity of these proteins is currently unknown. Dexamethasone and betamethasone have a higher affinity for the glucocorticoid receptor than do the natural corticoids (cortisol and cortisone), which explains the use of betamethasone to enhance lung maturation during preterm labor.[22]

The question of whether the triggering of protein synthesis mechanisms accounts for the increase in fatty acid synthetase, phosphatidic acid phosphatase, and choline-phosphate cytidyltransferase activity is yet to be answered. Conflicting evidence suggests that glucocorticoids could promote the synthesis of an enzyme activator that may influence the production of the heavier of the surfactant apoproteins.[24–28]

Several other questions have yet to be answered as well. It is evident that glucocorticoid action is centered on synthesis, not secretion, and that it affects more than surfactant synthesis. Acting directly on lung tissue, glucocorticoids increase the number of β-adrenergic receptors and enhance elastin and collagen production, which improves lung compliance.[29]

What is not evident is whether glucocorticoids directly affect Type II pneumocytes or mediate their action through other lung cells (fibroblasts). Smith suggests that rather than having a direct impact on Type II cells, glucocorticoids may act on fibroblasts (increasing the production of fibroblast pneumocyte factor), which then affect surfactant production.[30] Of course, it may not be strictly one or the other but some combination of these actions.

Thyroid Hormones. The idea that hormones may work in conjunction with other compounds or hormones is reinforced by observations of the actions of thyroid hormones. Thyroxine (T_4) and tri-iodothyronine (T_3) have been shown to increase the rate of phospholipid synthesis.[14,27,31,32] Thyroid hormones, like glucocorticoids, enhance production of phosphatidylcholine through choline incorporation. They do not, however, increase phosphatidylglycerol synthesis or stimulate the production of surfactant-specific proteins.[20,33] Although glucocorticoids increase fatty acid synthetase activity, thyroid hormone seems to decrease it.[34] These differences suggest different sites of action for these hormones as well as the need for action in conjunction with other hormones.[20]

Low T_3 and T_4 levels have been associated with respiratory distress syndrome, although exact mechanisms are unclear.[15,17,21,35] Ballard, Hovey, and Gonzales have shown that the effects of thyroid hormones are mediated by a specific thyroid receptor that is a potent phospholipid synthesis stimulator and to which T_3 has a higher affinity.[36]

Clinical application of this information is aimed at maximizing beneficial effects through the delivery of hormones or hormone-activating substances that cross the placenta. Naturally occurring thyroid hormones do not readily cross the placenta unless concentrations far exceeding normal levels are achieved. However, thyrotropin-releasing hormone does cross the placenta and stimulates the fetal pituitary gland to produce thyroid-stimulating hormone, resulting in increased production of PC.[21,37]

Continued investigation of the precise mechanisms of thyroid hormone action is essential. There seems to be little doubt that synergistic interaction between glucocorticoids and thyroid hormones occurs, apparently at the level of messenger RNA.[20] Significant increase in PC production occurs in a shorter period of time when these two hormones are used together.[31,32,36] These findings may have significant clinical implications and modify future therapeutic interventions.

Catecholamines. While glucocorticoids and thyroid hormones play a role in enhancing the synthesis of phospholipids, catecholamines stimulate the secretion of surfactant into the alveolar space. This appears to be a direct action of adrenergic compounds on Type II cells.[38] The

response is prompt, occurring in less than an hour.

Research has shown that catecholamines increase surfactant and saturated phosphatidylcholine in the lung fluid and improve lung stability. This is demonstrated in an increased ratio of lecithin to sphingomyelin. An added benefit is the inhibition of fetal lung fluid within the alveoli at the time of delivery. These two effects (increase in surfactant and decrease in lung fluid) work together to prepare the fetus for respiratory conversion.[21,38–41]

Insulin. Surfactant development appears to be inhibited in neonates born to diabetic mothers whose blood sugar levels are not well controlled. Whether this is caused by hyperglycemia, hyperinsulinemia, or both is unclear, and research continues to provide conflicting answers. Maturation of surfactant synthesis occurs at the same time glycogen is depleted from the lungs. Insulin inhibits glycogen breakdown, thereby decreasing the substrate available for PC synthesis as well as altering the natural anatomic changes that occur with glycogen depletion.[14,20] These alterations affect the ability of the lungs to perform respiratory functions.

Smith found that the effect of cortisol on choline incorporation was reduced by insulin, even though the cortisol effects on cell growth were not.[42] Gross and coworkers documented no insulin influence and no antagonistic action on the usual dexamethasone response.[43] Mendelson and associates reported a synergistic effect when cortisol and insulin were combined.[9]

It remains unclear whether the increased insulin levels or the increased serum glucose is the problem in diabetic pregnancies.[42–44] Insulin may antagonize glucocorticoids at the fibroblast level, affecting the production of the fibroblast pneumocyte factor.[45] Clinically, the incidence of respiratory distress syndrome has decreased as the need for stricter control of maternal glucose levels has been recognized and monitoring has been made easier.

At present, there seems to be a complex interaction of several hormones and factors that control surfactant synthesis. There continues to be much to learn about surfactant, its synthesis and removal. However, normal lung function seems to depend on the presence of surfactant, which permits a decrease in surface tension at end expiration and an increase in surface tension during lung expansion. This prevents atelectasis at end-expiration and facilitates elastic recoil on inspiration. Surfactant provides the lung with the stability required to maintain homeostatic blood gas pressures while decreasing the work of breathing.

Lung Fluid

Lung fluid is secreted from the beginning of the canalicular stage. This fluid is thought to be derived from alveolar epithelial secretions, but the site and specific formation mechanism are unclear. It is known that lung fluid is not an ultrafiltrate of plasma or amniotic fluid, nor is it a mixture of the two. Active transport is required to achieve the ion concentrations encountered: therefore, fluid is probably derived from the active transport of chloride, with sodium following passively. The water flux can be attributed to the osmotic force of sodium chloride.[46]

Osmolarity, sodium, and chloride levels are lower in amniotic fluid than in tracheal fluid; pH, glucose, and protein are higher.[47] The secretion rate is approximately 5 ml/kg/hour in lambs, which in term infants is equal to approximately 250 ml/day.[48]

Some lung fluid is swallowed, and some moves into the amniotic fluid, although the contribution to the latter is not significant when compared to the volume secreted by the kidneys. The fluid volume is approximately equal to the functional residual capacity and must be either expelled or absorbed at birth.[49,51]

The alveolar fluid is continually secreted and completely turned over every ten hours in the lamb at term.[47] Although its functional importance is not entirely known, lung fluid does play an important part in cell maturation and development, as well as determining the formation, size, and shape of the developing air space. Alterations in fluid dynamics affect pulmonary cell proliferation and differentiation.

Alcorn and associates demonstrated (based on the assessment of Type II cells) that fetuses whose tracheas were ligated had relatively large but immature lungs. Fetuses whose lungs were drained had thick alveolar walls, smaller lungs, and more abundant Type II cells.[52] This was confirmed by Perlman, Williams, and Hirsch, who found reduced numbers of alveoli in human infants who experienced amniotic fluid leakage.[53]

Therefore, reduced lung fluid production or leakage of amniotic fluid places the fetus at risk for lung hypoplasia.[13] Chronic tracheal obstruction leads to hyperplasia with an increase in the number of alveoli, although they are functionally immature.[10]

At the time of birth, the lungs must move from secretion to absorption of lung fluid, or the infant will rapidly succumb, drowning in his own secretions. Normally, secretion ends with birth, and ventilation of the lungs leads to liquid dispersion across the pulmonary epithelium during the absorptive period. At this time, the pulmonary epithelium undergoes a reversible increase in solute permeability, leading to a rapid transfer of lung liquid solutes.[50] This is confirmed clinically as the interstitial spaces and lymphatics become distended during the first five to six hours of life, and pulmonary lymph flow increases.[54]

Along with this increase in absorption, there seems to be a decrease in the rate of secretion.

The administration of epinephrine to lambs leads to a decrease in fluid secretion. This effect is mediated by β-adrenergic receptors in the alveolar epithelium and may either suppress the chloride pump or activate a second pump that triggers the absorption process.[50,55] Avery, Fletcher, and Williams suggest that resorption depends on the sodium pump because an amiloride infusion can modify the process.[56] This supports the second pump theory.

The absorption rate is known to increase as gestation progresses, and this can be correlated with an increase in catecholamine levels.[57] During gestation the fetal adrenal glands are probably not stimulated to produce sufficient amounts of catecholamines to trigger the absorption process; labor, however, provides sufficient stimulus to release enough epinephrine to stimulate the switch from secretion to absorption.[50] The catecholamine surge that occurs at delivery is probably the final mechanism to assure that this change is completed.[47]

The drop in pulmonary vascular resistance with aeration and the rise in oxygen tension increase the number of alveolar capillaries perfused, resulting in an increase in blood removal capacity. Between the increased lymphatic flow and the dramatic change in the pulmonary blood flow, lung fluid is dispersed within the first few hours following delivery.

Fetal Breathing Movements

Fetal breathing movements can be seen on ultrasound as early as 11 weeks gestation.[58] They are rapid (80–120 breaths per minute) and irregular, occurring intermittently early in gestation. As gestation progresses, their strength and frequency increase, until they occur between 40 and 80 percent of the time, at a rate of 30–70 breaths per minute.[47,58–60] Large movements (gasping) occur 5 percent of the total breathing time, one to four times per minute.[58]

This respiratory activity may contribute to lung fluid regulation, thereby influencing lung growth. The diaphragm seems to be the major structure involved, with minimal chest wall excursion (4–8 mm change in transverse diameter).[61] Movement of the diaphragm is necessary for the chest wall muscles and diaphragm to gain adequate strength for the initial breath.[60]

Diaphragm movement also influences the course of lung cell differentiation and proliferation. Bilateral phrenectomy results in altered lung morphology, with an increase in Type II over Type I cells.[52] Presumably, the innervated diaphragm increases the size of the thorax and thereby increases tissue stress, affecting morphology. Beyond this, however, hypoplastic lungs are found in those situations in which fetal breathing movements do not occur.[62]

Fetal breathing movements vary significantly from fetus to fetus. Initially, they are infrequent, increasing with gestational age and becoming more organized and vigorous.[47] Even with these gestational changes, tracheal fluid shifts are negligible, the pressure generated being no more than 25 mmHg.[62] Fetal maturation leads to the appearance of cycles, with an increase in fetal breathing movements during daytime hours.[58,63] Patrick and associates report that fetal breathing movements peak in late evening and reach their nadir in the early morning hours.[64]

Abnormal breathing patterns can be seen during periods of hypoxia. Mild hypoxemia decreases the incidence of fetal breathing movements; severe hypoxemia may lead to their cessation for several hours. The onset of asphyxia leads to gasping that persists until death.[65] Interestingly, the onset of mild hypoxemia (as with umbilical artery occlusion of short duration) may lead to quiet sleep, which for the fetus decreases activity, energy expenditure, and oxygen consumption.[58] Although paradoxical in nature, this conservation mechanism may save the fetus while cardiac output is redistributed toward the placenta.

A reduction of fetal breathing movements prior to delivery coincides with the increase in prostaglandin E concentrations seen during the last days of gestation. These factors play a role in respiratory conversion at birth.[66] Why irregular fetal breathing movements lead to the sustained respirations of postnatal life remains unknown.

TRANSITIONAL EVENTS

RESPIRATORY CONVERSION

At term, the acinar portion of the lung is well established, although "true" alveoli are only now beginning to develop. The pulmonary blood vessels are narrow; only 5–10 percent of the fetal cardiac output perfuses the lungs to meet cellular nutrition needs. This low-volume circulation is in part due to the high pulmonary vascular resistance created by constricted arterioles.

At term, the lung holds approximately 20 ml/kg of fluid.[48] Lung aeration is complete when the liquid is replaced with an equal volume of air, and a functional residual capacity (FRC) is established. A substantial amount of air is retained with the early breaths. Within an hour of birth, 80–90 percent of the FRC is created. The retention of air is due to surfactant and a decrease in surface tension. Surfactant decreases the tendency toward atelectasis, promotes capillary circulation by increasing alveolar size (which indirectly dilates precapillary vessels), improves alveolar fluid clearance, and protects the airway.[11] Therefore, the concentration and adsorption properties of surfactant must be sufficient to react during the short first breath (one to ten seconds). Exactly how all this happens is not known.[50,51]

The gas tension levels that characterize the fetal state would result in significant hyperventilation postnatally; this indicates a dimin-ished respiratory center responsiveness to chemical stimuli in the blood during intrauterine life. Postnatal breathing is responsive to stimuli from arterial and central chemoreceptors (oxygen and carbon dioxide tension in the blood), chest wall and lungs, musculoskeletal system, and skin, as well as emotions and behavior. The changes that take place at birth and the increase in aerobic metabolism are not only rapid but irreversible. Within a few hours of birth, the neonate is responsive to hypoxia and hypercapnia in much the same manner as an adult.[50]

The actual mechanics of respiratory conversion begin with the passage of the fetus through the birth canal. The thorax is markedly squeezed during this passage, with external pressures of 160–200 cm H_2O being generated.[47,67–69] When the infant's face or nares are exposed to atmospheric pressure, variable amounts of lung fluid are expressed.[68] As much as 28 ml of fluid have been expelled during the second stage of labor, leading to the creation of a potential air space.[47] Recoil of the chest to predelivery proportions allows for passive "inspiration" of variable amounts of air. This initial step helps reduce viscous forces that must be overcome in order to establish an air-liquid interface in the alveoli.[68]

The forces that must be overcome during the first breaths include the viscosity of the lung fluid column, the tissue resistive forces (compliance), and the surface tension forces at the air-liquid interfaces. Surface tension results when the intermolecular attraction among liquid molecules exceeds the attraction between air and liquid, and plays a major part in the lung's retractive forces. The viscosity of lung fluid which provides resistance to movement of fluid in the airways is at its maximum at the beginning of the first breath. The greatest displacement of fluid with first breath occurs in the trachea.[68,70] The dissipation of tracheal fluid during the vaginal squeeze reduces the amount of pressure that must be generated to push the liquid column down the conducting airways.

As the column progresses down the conducting branches, the total surface area of the air-liquid interface increases as the bronchiole diameter is progressively reduced. The surface tension, however, increases.[47] The surface tension forces are the hardest to overcome during first breath events. Maximal forces are encountered where the airways are smallest (terminal bronchioles) and pressure is inversely proportional to the radius of the curvature in the airway.[47,68] In this vicinity, the intraluminal pressure must be at its peak in order to prevent closure by tension in the intraluminal walls (Laplace relationship).[13] If the airways were filled with fluid only (no air-liquid interface), the inspiratory pressures needed to move from liquid to air-filled would be considerably less. But this would make alveolar expansion more difficult because surface tension forces would be extremely high and moving columns of fluid is extremely difficult. Surface tension forces drop again once air enters the terminal air sacs.[47]

Tissue-resistive forces are unknown at birth. However, the small amount of fluid within the terminal air sacs enhances air introduction, possibly by modifying the configuration of the smaller units of the lung. The fluid enlarges the radius of the alveolar ducts and terminal air sac, thereby facilitating expansion (LaPlace relationship). The lung fluid also reduces the possibility of cellular debris obstructing the small ducts.

The first diaphragmatic inspiration has been reported to begin within nine seconds of delivery and to generate very large negative intrathoracic pressures (mean of 70 cm H_2O). Air enters as soon as the intrathoracic pressure begins to drop, with mean inspiratory pressures of 30–35 cm H_2O.[2,47,71]

The large transpulmonary pressure generated by the diaphragm lasts only 0.5–1 second, pulling in 10–70 ml of air.[72] The layer of fluid at the alveolar lining becomes established after the first breath, allowing the molecules of surfactant to reduce the surface tension during expiration.[68] The first expiration is also active, leaving behind a residual volume of up to 30 ml. The magnitude of the expiratory pressure contributes to FRC formation, even distribution of air, and elimination of lung fluid.[47] The second and third breaths are similar to the first but require less pressure because the small airways are open, and surface-active forces are diminished.[68] Lung expansion augments surfactant secretion, providing alveolar stability and FRC formation.

By 10 minutes of age, an infant's FRC is equal to 17 ml/kg; at 30 minutes, it is 25–35 ml/kg.[73] The relative hypoxia of birth results in a decrease in muscle tone; as muscle tone returns after the first breath, chest wall stability improves and helps to maintain FRC.[47,67]

Lung compliance increases by four to five times in the first 24 hours of extrauterine life and continues to increase gradually over the first week of life. Flow resistance decreases by one-half to one-fourth during this time, and the distribution of ventilation is as even after day 1 as it is on day 3 or 4.[47]

PULMONARY VASCULAR CHANGES

According to Haworth and Hislop, postnatal structural changes in the pulmonary circulation occur in three overlapping phases:[74]

1. Recruitment (progressive opening of arterial beds) of nonmuscular and partially muscular arteries occurs in the first 24 hours of life. The external diameter of these vessels increases, and the swollen endothelial lining cells flatten. These endothelial cells may play a role in the relaxation of smooth muscle by metabolizing substances such as acetylcholine.

FIGURE 1-7 ▲ Fetal circulation.

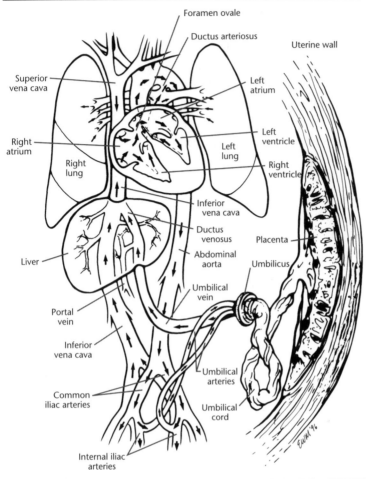

In utero: Oxygenated blood flows from the placenta via the umbilical vein through the ductus venosus in the liver and into the inferior vena cava (IVC). Upon entering the heart, much of the oxygenated blood is shunted across the foramen ovale to the left atrium, left ventricle, and into the aorta. Venous blood from the head and lower extremities flows predominantly into the right ventricle where it mixes with a small amount of oxygenated blood coming from the IVC. The majority of this blood shunts across the ductus arteriosus into the aorta. A small amount of this mixed blood moves into the pulmonary arteries and perfuses the lung tissue.

2. Reduced muscularity occurs during the first two weeks of life. During this time, partially muscular and wholly muscular vessels become nonmuscular and partially muscular, respectively.
3. A growth phase begins after the first two weeks. Muscle tissue begins to reappear in the acinus and continues to develop slowly during childhood. The initial phases allow for the functional adaptation necessary for extrauterine life, and the third phase brings about structural remodeling. This growth creates the relationships seen in the mature system between the external vessel diameter and muscle wall thickness.

In conjunction with the local vascular changes in the pulmonary bed, there are major reorganizational changes within the cardiovascular system. The breath events and cardiovascular events cannot be separated; they are interdependent, and both must occur for transition to be successful.

CARDIOVASCULAR CONVERSION

In the fetus, oxygenated blood returns from the placenta via the umbilical vein with an arterial oxygen tension (PaO_2) of 35 mmHg. The blood enters the liver, where a small percentage feeds the liver microcirculation, and ends up in the inferior vena cava. The major portion of the returning blood is shunted directly into the inferior vena cava via the ductus venosus.

The inferior vena cava enters the right atrium, where the majority of its blood flow (approximately 60 percent) is deflected across the right atrium and through the foramen ovale into the left atrium. Here it mixes with the unoxygenated blood returning from the fetal lungs, drops into the left ventricle, and is ejected into the ascending aorta to feed the cerebral arteries and upper extremities.

The remainder of the right atrium blood mixes with the unoxygenated superior vena cava

FIGURE 1-8 ▲ Lung volumes and capacities.

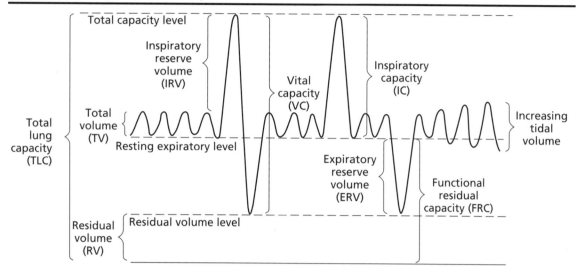

From: Fraser RG, and Paré JA. 1979. *Diagnosis and Diseases of the Chest,* 2nd ed., vol. 4. Philadelphia: WB Saunders. Reprinted by permission.

blood returning from the upper body and enters the right ventricle. This mixed blood is ejected through the pulmonary arteries toward the lungs. The high pulmonary vascular resistance allows only 5–10 percent of the blood to enter the lungs, the majority being shunted across the ductus arteriosus into the thoracic aorta, which services the lower segments of the body (Figure 1-7).

With clamping of the umbilical cord, the placenta, which is a low-resistance organ (contributing to the low systemic vascular resistance found in the fetal state) is unavailable. The net result is an increase in pulmonary blood return to the heart and a decrease in systemic blood return. These changes modify the pressures within the atria. Left atrial pressure increases above the right and leads to functional closure of the foramen ovale. The increase in PaO_2 and decrease in prostaglandin levels facilitate functional closure of the ductus arteriosus. These modifications in blood flow and pressure indicate the change from "in series" to parallel circulation and herald cardiovascular conversion.

Once the first breath is taken and cardiovascular conversion in initiated, the infant must be able to attain sustained rhythmic respirations. This requires the central nervous system to be "turned on" so it can take over the regulation of respiratory activity.

ANATOMY OF RESPIRATION

LUNG VOLUMES

The neonate has a total lung capacity of approximately 63 ml/kg of body weight. As shown in Figure 1-8, this encompasses both the portion of lung volume used in the normal course of breathing and the reserve and dead space volumes. As clinicians, we are primarily concerned with two components of the total lung capacity: tidal volume and functional residual capacity. Table 1-3 outlines the distribution of total lung capacity in the neonatal lung.

Tidal Volume

Tidal volume (the volume of gas inspired with each breath) plays a major role in alveolar minute ventilation and ultimately in the effectiveness of gas exchange. It normally ranges

TABLE 1-3 ▲ Infant Static Lung Volumes (ml/kg)

Total lung capacity (TLC)	63
Inspiratory capacity (IC)	33
Thoracic gas volume (Vtg)	30–36
Functional residual capacity (FRC)	30
Vital capacity (VC)	40
Closing capacity (CC)	35
Tidal volume (V_T)	6
Expiratory reserve volume (ERV)	7
Closing volume (CV)	12
Residual volume (RV)	23
ERV/FRC	0.23
RV/TLC	0.37
FRC/TLC	0.48
V_T/FRC	0.20

From: Smith CA. 1959. *The Physiology of the Newborn Infant,* 4th ed. Springfield, Illinois: Charles C. Thomas, 327. Reprinted by permission.

between 6–8 ml/kg but may be altered by a variety of disease states.

Functional Residual Capacity

Functional residual capacity (the gas remaining in the lungs at the end of expiration) is established during the initial breaths, forming the alveolar reservoir at end expiration, allowing for continuous gas exchange between respiratory efforts and stabilization of PaO_2. FRC normally comprises 30–40 percent of the total capacity of the lung and may change in volume from breath to breath.

Immediately following birth and the initial breath, FRC is low, but it increases rapidly with successive breaths. In preterm infants, FRC will stay low until lung disease resolves. The goal is to keep FRC above the passive resting volume of the lung (reached after a totally relaxed expiration). The neonate's pliable chest wall, which lends itself to a low FRC, makes this difficult.

The role of FRC in the energy expenditure of the respiratory musculature is crucial. It minimizes the work of breathing while optimizing system compliance and maintaining a gas reservoir during expiration.[60]

RESPIRATORY PUMP

The movement of gas in and out of the lungs is based on the functioning of the respiratory pump, which consists of the rib cage and respiratory muscles. The pump must move sufficient oxygen and carbon dioxide into and out of the lungs to replace the oxygen consumed and wash out the carbon dioxide that accumulates in the alveoli. Ventilatory efforts in the neonate depend on the strength and endurance of the diaphragm; when these are insufficient, the neonate requires ventilatory assistance.[60]

Diaphragm

The diaphragm insets on the lower six ribs, the sternum, and the first three lumbar vertebrae. It is innervated bilaterally by the phrenic nerves and exercises its efforts on the lung, the rib cage, and the abdomen. For the diaphragm to work optimally, the intercostal muscles must stabilize the rib cage, and the abdominal muscles should stabilize the abdomen.[61,63] In infants, the coordination of these efforts is almost nonexistent. During REM (rapid eye movement) sleep (the predominant sleep state in the neonate), the intercostal and abdominal muscles are ineffective, contributing to respiratory instability.[75]

The composition of the muscle fibers in the neonate differs from that of the adult. The neonatal diaphragm and intercostal muscles have a lower proportion of fatigue-resistant (Type I) fibers (20 percent, as compared to 60 percent in adults).[60,75,76] Type I fibers increase in number from 24 weeks gestation, when they comprise 10 percent of total fiber content, to reach the adult proportion at eight months postnatal age.[75] Because of this developmental pattern, the neonate is particularly vulnerable to diaphragmatic muscle fatigue—especially when the work of breathing is increased.[60,75] This vulnerability is potentiated with decreasing gestational age.

The infant's diaphragm is attached to a chest wall that is more pliable than that of the adult. This can lead to distortion of the lower portion of the chest wall during contraction, especially if the contraction is forceful. The decreased efficiency of the contraction and reduced tidal volume can make ventilation less effective and require adjustments in respiratory pattern.[60]

Rib Cage and Chest Wall Muscles

The muscles of the rib cage consist of the external intercostal muscles (used during inspiration), the internal intercostal muscles (used during expiration), and the accessory muscles, including the sternocleidomastoid, pectoral, and scalene. The major role of these muscles is stabilization of the chest wall by tonic contraction during diaphragmatic excursion. If they are unable to accomplish this goal, collapse and distortion of the chest wall are likely to occur during inspiratory efforts.

If these muscles are able to provide the stability needed, the contraction of the rib cage inspiratory muscles can contribute to the thoracic volume. During sighing, the increase in tidal volume is due largely to increased chest wall excursion.[77]

Rib Cage Compliance

The infant's chest wall is cartilaginous, soft, and pliable. This design allows for compression during passage through the birth canal without rib fractures and then for further growth and development.[6,78,79] Nelson describes the infant's chest wall as a loose-fitting glove surrounding the neonatal lung.[68] The characteristic high compliance of the neonate's lung dictates that for any given change in volume there is almost no change in pressure.[79] This increased compliance is highest in the preterm infant, but it is significant in the term infant as well.

The clinical implications of this highly compliant chest are related to the ease with which lung collapse is possible in the neonate. The low elastic recoil pressure of the neonatal lung and the high compliance of the thorax result in the majority of tidal breathing being done at near the closing capacity (volume at which lung regions are closed to the main bronchi). This contributes to the possibility of collapse and affects gas distribution.

The mechanical liabilities of a highly compliant chest wall after delivery include a compromised ability to produce large tidal volumes, which require the generation of larger pressures. Consequently, the infant must do more work to move the same amount of tidal volume as an older infant.[79] This is especially true in preterm infants with lung diseases associated with decreased lung compliance. Lung disease increases the respiratory drive in an attempt to generate stronger contractions with high inspiratory pressures that will expand stiff, noncompliant lungs.

The diaphragmatic force and the pliable chest wall lead to chest distortion.[80] Therefore, a portion of the energy and force of the contraction is wasted. Retractions are the clinical signs of these distortions and indicate the degree of rib cage inward collapse during forceful diaphragmatic contraction.[79] This increase in the work of breathing can lead to fatigue and eventually apnea.

Chest wall compliance combined with lung compliance affects the closing volume, closing capacity, expiratory reserve volume, and functional residual capacity. For the neonate, this means a high closing volume and capacity combined with a low expiratory reserve volume and low FRC—and a propensity toward lung collapse.[68]

RESPIRATORY PHYSIOLOGY

CONTROL OF RESPIRATION

The goal of respiration is to meet the organism's oxygen and carbon dioxide metabolic demands by extracting oxygen from the atmosphere and removing carbon dioxide produced by the organism. The respiratory center is responsible for matching the level of ventilation to the metabolic demand. The assessment of metabolic needs and alteration of ventilation are accomplished by the chemoreceptors.

The peripheral chemoreceptors (carotid and aortic bodies) sense oxygen and carbon dioxide tension; the central chemoreceptors (medullary) are sensitive to CO_2 and hydrogen ion concentrations in the extracellular fluid of the brain. When the PaO_2 falls below the acceptable range, the chemoreceptors increase the efferent neural activity to the brain's respiratory center, which brings about an increase in ventilation. At birth, the fetal PaO_2 of 25 mmHg (sufficient for intrauterine growth) increases to 50 mmHg during the first few breaths and then to 70 mmHg during the first hours.[81] This increase in oxygen tension exceeds the fetal demands for oxygen, resulting in a relative "hyperoxia" at birth.

This change in oxygen tension causes the chemoreceptors to become inactive and to remain so for the first few days of life.[82] Thus, fluctuations in oxygen tension levels may not lead to a chemoreceptor response during these early days of life.[60] After this lag time, however, the chemoreceptors reset, becoming oxygen-sensitive and playing a major role in the control of respiration.[83,84]

Sustained hyperventilation efforts during hypoxia cannot be maintained by the neonate. Studies in infants and animals demonstrate that an initial hyperventilatory response is usually followed by a subsequent fall in ventilation and oxygen tensions.[58,85] The reasons for this lack of sustained response are unknown. Davis and Bureau speculate that it may be due to the feeble chemoreceptor output, the central inhibitory effect of hypoxia on ventilation, or changes in pulmonary mechanics.[60]

The neonate's response to carbon dioxide, though more mature than his response to hypoxia, is also limited during the early neonatal period. Neonates can increase ventilation by only three to four times their baseline ventilation in comparison to the 10- to 20-fold increase adults can achieve.[86,87] Along with this, the threshold of carbon dioxide tolerance is higher initially, progressively declining over the first month of life.[86] This, too, may be due to the increased arterial carbon dioxide tension ($PaCO_2$) levels found in the fetal state (45–50 mmHg) and the need to reset chemoreceptors.

Modification of ventilatory patterns is dependent upon inspiratory muscle strength, rib cage rigidity, airway resistance, and lung compliance. The status of these factors and the performance of the respiratory pump are controlled through specific reflex arcs.[60] Chemoreceptors provide information about the metabolic needs of the infant, mechanoreceptors provide information about the status of the respiratory pump, and the respiratory center integrates this information and establishes the ventilatory pattern that most efficiently meets the infant's needs.

Each respiratory cycle during a stable state (such as quiet sleep) is uniform in amplitude, duration, and waveform. Behavioral influences as well as sleep state (REM sleep) alter the regularity of breathing. The information received determines the inspiratory time, the expiratory time, the lung volume at which the breath should occur (FRC), the rate of inspiration, and braking of the expiration.[88] The recruitment and adjustment of the various respiratory muscle groups result in the predetermined lung volume being achieved.[60]

LUNG COMPLIANCE

The pressure gradient necessary to overcome the elastic recoil force in the lung depends on tidal volume and lung compliance. Compliance represents the ease with which tissue, such as lung or chest wall, can be stretched by an external force. It is expressed as the change in volume caused by a change in pressure.[89] This can be demonstrated in a curve that relates lung volume to the change in the alveolar to intrapleural pressure gradient (transpulmonary pressure). The slope of the curve is the compliance. The flatter the curve, the stiffer the lung.[79] (See Figure 2-3.)

Compliance is the opposite of elastic recoil, where tissue seeks to return to the resting position after stretching. Consequently, compliance is largely determined by the amount of elastic recoil that must be overcome before inflation is possible.[90]

Lung compliance in the healthy preterm infant is similar to that in the term infant. Changes in lung compliance are sensed by stretch receptors of the lung. Coupled with the signals from spindle fibers of the respiratory muscles, information is transmitted to the respiratory center to modify the drive necessary to maintain ventilation. Lung disease usually leads to a decrease in lung compliance, which translates to a reduced volume change for a given pressure change.

Lung compliance depends on the tissue elastic characteristics of the parenchyma, connective tissue, and blood vessels as well as the surface tension found in the alveoli and the initial lung volume before inflation. Changes in lung compliance occur with age; however, it takes just as much pressure to produce a normal tidal volume in the newborn as in the adult. The smaller the individual the smaller the volume change for a given pressure change (4 to 6 ml per centimeter of water in infants and 100 to 150 ml in adults).[51]

The most significant determinant of the elastic properties of the lung is the air-liquid interface found in the alveoli. The increase in elastic recoil seen in the presence of an air-liquid interface is caused by the forces of surface tension. When molecules are aligned at the interface they lack opposing molecules on one side (the air side). The intermolecular attractive forces are then unbalanced and the molecules move away from the interface. This movement reduces the surface area to a minimum, reduces the internal surface area of the lung, and augments the elastic recoil of the lung.[51]

Pulmonary surfactant forms an insoluble surface film at the alveolar interface. This phospholipid-protein complex absorbs to the interface to reduce the surface tension and establish lung stability. Surfactant is stretched upon inhalation and compressed upon expiration, the latter allows for the pressure from surface tension to be lowered to physiologically near zero values. The ability to achieve a low surface tension at low lung volumes (end-expiration) tends to stabilize the air spaces and prevent their closure. Without surfactant, the smaller alveoli would tend to empty into the larger ones. This is in accordance with the Laplace relationship which relates the pressure across a surface or collapsing pressure (P) to surface tension (T) and the radius (r) of a curvature ($P = 2T/r$). Consequently, the smaller the radius, the greater the collapsing pressure.

Alveolar collapse occurs in a number of diseases, the most notable being respiratory distress syndrome. In this condition, surfactant deficiency is directly related to developmental immaturity of the lungs and gestational age. Surfactant synthesis also depends on normal pH and pulmonary perfusion. Therefore, any pathology (such as asphyxia, hemorrhagic shock, or pulmonary edema) that interferes with these processes may lead to surfactant deficiency.[2,91,92]

LUNG RESISTANCE

Lung resistance, or reduced airflow caused by friction between molecules, depends on the (1) size and geometric arrangements of the airways, (2) viscous resistance of the lung tissue, and (3) proportion of laminar to turbulent airflow. Resistance varies inversely with lung volume. Therefore, the greater the lung volume, the less resistance, and vice versa. This is because airway diameter increases with the expansion of the parenchyma.

Two types of resistance play a significant role in the adequate ventilation of the neonatal lung:

1. **Viscous resistance** to airflow is created by tissue that is moving against tissue within the lungs themselves or against the chest wall. Secondary to increased tissue density due to organ immaturity and increased fluid in the neonatal lung (delayed resorption, basement membrane leaking, and left-to-right shunting through a patent ductus arteriosus), viscous forces are altered in the neonate with lung pathology. These alterations require increased pressure generation to move air through the airways.

2. **Airway resistance** is generated between individual moving molecules in a gaseous stream or between moving molecules of gas and the walls of the conducting airways.[93] Airway resistance plays the more significant role in impeding airflow, being responsible for as much as 80 percent of total pulmonary resistance. The smallness of the neonate's airways and nasopharynx increases airway resistance inherently, and further pathology can exponentially alter resistance, contributing to ventilatory instability. Unfortunately, the use of endotracheal tubes and ventilatory circuits can also impede the flow of gas and may need to be compensated for in the pressures utilized to deliver adequate support.

In neonates and children less than five years of age, the peripheral airways contribute most to airway resistance. This is secondary to the decreased diameter of airways, especially in the periphery. The distal airway growth in diameter and length lags behind proximal growth dur-

ing the first five years of life. Therefore, a small decrement in airway caliber can lead to a very large increase in peripheral airway resistance.[94] This is seen in the early onset of clinical signs when disease is encountered in the neonate.

Resistance increases with decreasing gestational age and with specific lung diseases that are more prominent in low birth weight infants (such as respiratory distress syndrome and bronchopulmonary dysplasia [BPD]). The increased resistance is sensed by respiratory muscles, which leads to an increase in ventilatory drive. In the infant with BPD, this may lead to an increase in pleural pressure to as much as 20–30 cm H_2O.

Changes in the caliber of the larynx or trachea because of edema and intubation also increase resistance. This effect may be quite pronounced because the resistance is generated in the large airways, where resistance should be lowest.

Airway and chest wall compliance can affect resistive forces in the preterm infant through increased susceptibility to collapse and compression during expiration. Along with this, the reduced functional residual capacity dramatically increases resistance in the preterm infant. Adequate ventilatory support can reduce resistance and stabilize the chest wall, making spontaneous respirations more effective.

TIME CONSTANTS

A time constant—the time needed for a given lung unit to fill to 63 percent of its final capacity—measures the product of lung resistance and compliance. The alveoli with shorter time constants fill faster than those with longer time constants. Nichols and Rogers observe that if resistance and compliance are equal in two adjacent lung units, the time constant will be the same, and there will be no redistribution of gases between the alveoli.[79] If the time constant of one unit is longer but the compliances remain equal, the two alveoli will eventually reach the same

FIGURE 1-9 ▲ **Effect of changes in pleural pressure in the lung.**

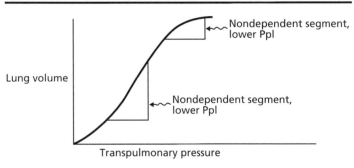

From: Nichols DG, and Rogers MC. 1987. Developmental physiology of the respiratory system. In *Textbook of Pediatric Intensive Care,* vol. 1, Rogers MC, ed. Baltimore: Williams & Wilkins, 88. Reprinted by permission.

volume. The longer the time constant, however, the slower the filling will be because of increased resistance.

The time constant can also be lengthened when compliance is increased but resistance remains the same. In this circumstance, the less compliant alveoli will fill faster than their adjacent, more compliant neighbor. This is due to the decreased volume of the alveoli that are less compliant. Redistribution of gas will occur if inflation is interrupted prematurely because of the increased pressure in the less compliant alveoli as compared to the adjacent lung unit.[79]

This redistribution of gases in the lung is not a major factor in the normal lung, in that the alveoli are relatively stable and do not change much in size because of the effect of surfactant upon the lung.[79]

DISTRIBUTION OF VENTILATION

DEAD SPACE VENTILATION

A variable portion of each breath is not involved in gas exchange and is therefore wasted. This is considered "dead space ventilation." There are two types of dead space: (1) anatomic dead space, that volume of gas within the conducting airways that cannot engage in gas exchange, and (2) alveolar dead space, the volume of inspired gas that reaches the alveoli but does not participate in gas exchange because of inadequate perfusion to that alveoli.

The total (anatomic plus alveolar) dead space is termed "physiologic dead space." Physiologic dead space is usually expressed as a fraction of the tidal volume, approximately 0.3 in infants and adults.[95] Patients experiencing respiratory failure have elevated ratios of dead space to tidal volume, which results in hypoxia and hypercarbia unless counteracted by an increase in the amount of air expired per minute.[79]

PLEURAL PRESSURE

The differences in pleural pressure within the lung play a significant role in determining the distribution of gases. During spontaneous breathing, a greater proportion of gas is distributed to the dependent regions of the lung.[96] It is assumed that the increased negative intrapleural pressure in the bases is the reason for this distribution pattern. Nichols and Rogers note that the smaller alveoli in the dependent lung regions lie on the steeper slope of the transpulmonary pressure to lung volume curve (Figure 1-9), resulting in a greater portion of tidal volume being directed to the dependent alveoli during normal breathing.[79] A greater portion of the pulmonary perfusion goes to the dependent regions as well, thereby matching ventilation and perfusion more closely (Figure 1-10). In addition, this distribution pattern is related to the preferential distribution of gases upon inspiration to non-gravity dependent areas of the lung until just after the FRC is reached. What this means is that at normal FRC the apical alveoli are larger than the basal alveoli, and the largest volume of resting gas is in the upper lung zones. As gas continues to fill the non-dependent lung regions the alveoli in the upper regions will become so

FIGURE 1-10 ▲ Gravity dependence of perfusion.

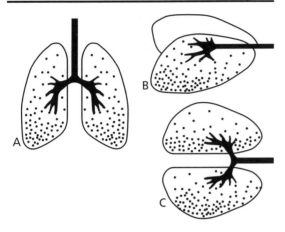

Blood is distributed to the most gravity-dependent areas of the lung.

A = upright; B = supine; C = side-lying

From: Malley WJ. 1990. *Clinical Blood Gases.* Philadelphia: WB Saunders, 65. Reprinted by permission.

full that further inflation is more difficult than expanding the alveoli in the lower lung regions. At this point, which is reached when the inspired gas volume is slightly above the normal FRC, additional gas will preferentially ventilate the bases. Consequently, most of the gas inhaled during normal breathing actually ventilates the bases.

Pleural pressure increases from the apex to the base of the lung, so alveoli become smaller at the base. Smaller alveoli are on the steep portion of the pressure-volume (compliance) curve; thus, a given change in transpulmonary pressure produces a greater increase in volume in the smaller alveoli.

CLOSING CAPACITY

During quiet breathing in the neonate (especially the preterm infant), lung volumes can be reduced below FRC, with dependent regions of the lung being closed to the main bronchi (closing capacity). When the closing capacity exceeds the FRC, the ventilation: perfusion ratio drops, and hypoxia and hypercarbia can be seen. If total atelectasis ("whiteout") exists, then closing capacity exceeds not only FRC but also

tidal volume, and the alveoli in the affected portions of the lung are closed during expiration and inspiration.

The use of end-expiratory pressure in the form of positive end-expiratory pressure or continuous distending pressure is designed to raise FRC above closing capacity.[79] This is used in the neonatal population when chest wall compliance leads to marked distortion and altered lung volumes as well as during disease states associated with alveolar collapse (such as respiratory distress syndrome).

The greater closing capacity seen in children under 6 years of age and in adults over 40 is probably as a result of decreased elastic recoil in the lung.[92,97] Elastic recoil is the property that allows the lung to retract away from the chest wall, creating a subatmospheric pressure in the intrapleural space. The decrease in elastic recoil leads to an increase in subatmospheric pressure in the intrapleural spaces and airway closure in dependent regions.[79]

PERFUSION

Alveolar ventilation is dependent upon the airways and pulmonary vasculature. Pulmonary vascular muscle thickness is a function of gestational age—the preterm infant having smooth muscle that is less well developed. This incomplete development results in a drop in pulmonary vascular resistance much sooner after delivery, predisposing the preterm infant to a faster onset of congestive heart failure and left-to-right shunting.[79] This relatively rapid reduction in pulmonary vascular resistance, combined with the potential for fluid overload, can result in opening of extrapulmonary shunts, leading to hypoxia and further respiratory deterioration.

VASCULAR PRESSURES AND RESISTANCE

There are three categories of intravascular pressure associated with the pulmonary circulation: pulmonary artery pressure, transmural pressure, and perfusion pressure. The interaction and relationships between these pressures affect the flow of blood in the lung and are implicated in the distribution of blood flow.

Pulmonary Artery Pressure

Pulmonary artery pressure measures the systolic, diastolic, and mean arterial pressures in the pulmonary artery in reference to atmospheric pressure at the level of the heart. After birth, pulmonary artery pressure falls as the lungs inflate; however, adult pressures are not achieved until several months have passed.[98] Normal systolic, diastolic, and mean pressures in the adult are 22, 8, and 15, respectively (normal values for the neonate have not been established).[68,79]

Transmural Pressure

Transmural pressure is the difference between the pressures inside and outside the vessel. This is measured differently, depending on the level of the measurement. At upper levels, it is the gradient between pulmonary artery pressure and pleural pressure; at the pulmonary capillaries, it is the difference between pleural pressure and alveolar pressure.[99]

Capillary transmural pressure provides the hydrostatic pressure that tends to force fluid out of the capillaries and into the pulmonary interstitium. This is counterbalanced by oncotic pressure forces. The greater the capillary transmural pressure, the more distended the vessel, the greater the flow.

Perfusion Pressure

Perfusion pressure is the pressure gradient between two points in the circulation (downward flow). This cascade is needed for blood to flow appropriately. In the pulmonary circulation, this is measured as the difference between pulmonary artery pressure and left atrial pressure.

Perfusion pressure divided by pulmonary blood flow provides a calculated value for pulmonary vascular resistance. An increase in

FIGURE 1-11 ▲ Pulmonary perfusion zones.

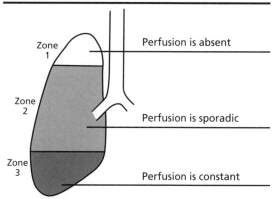

From: Malley WJ. 1990. *Clinical Blood Gases.* Philadelphia: WB Saunders, 65. Reprinted by permission.

flow, as occurs with activity, produces a drop in pulmonary vascular resistance secondary to the recruitment of additional pulmonary capillaries.[100,101]

NORMAL PULMONARY BLOOD FLOW

In the adult, the majority of pulmonary blood flow is distributed to the dependent regions of the lungs because of gravitational forces. In zone 1 (apex of the lung), the alveolar pressure is greater than the pulmonary artery and venous pressures. As a result, the pulmonary vessels collapse, and there is a concomitant loss of gas exchange and wasted ventilation.[102]

In zone 2 (middle of the lung), pulmonary artery pressure exceeds alveolar pressure, and blood flow resumes. The perfusion pressure increases as blood flows downward, which results in a linear increase in blood flow. Slowing of blood occurs when the pulmonary venous and alveolar pressures are equal.[102]

In zone 3 (base of the lung), pulmonary venous and pulmonary artery pressures increase, exceeding alveolar pressure. In the more dependent regions of this zone, the transmural pressure increases (resulting in dilation of the vessels), and blood flow increases.[102] Figure 1-11 illustrates the zonal distribution of perfusion.

FIGURE 1-12 ▲ Components of physiologic shunting and dead space.

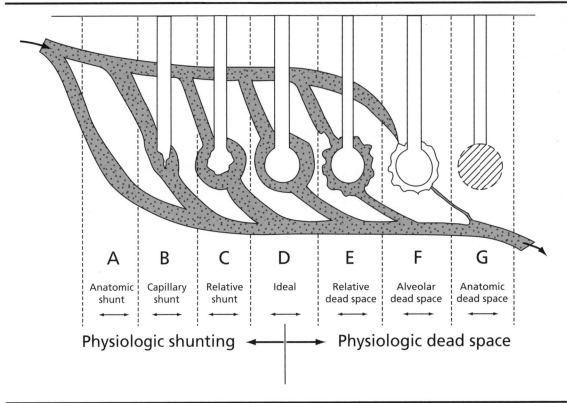

Adapted from: Burke JF. 1983. *Surgical Physiology*. Philadelphia: WB Saunders, 407. Reprinted by permission.

Posture differences between the upright adult and supine-lying infant probably explain pulmonary blood distribution in the infant, but this has not been explicated. The general principles probably still apply, however. Wasted ventilation in the apices resulting from lack of perfusion is presumably much less likely in the supine position, helping to balance some of the limitations of the neonatal lung.

ABNORMAL DISTRIBUTION OF PULMONARY BLOOD FLOW

Numerous factors may influence the distribution of pulmonary blood flow in the lung. One of the most significant for the neonate is hypoxia. Vasoconstriction results from alveolar hypoxia. If generalized, hypoxia may result in an increase in intravascular pulmonary artery pressure, which is more intense in infants than in adults.[92,103]

VENTILATION-PERFUSION MATCHING

Efficient gas exchange in the lungs requires matching pulmonary ventilation ($\dot{V}_A$) and perfusion ($\dot{Q}_C$). Ventilation-perfusion mismatching is the most common reason for hypoxia in the newborn and a frequent result of the neonatal respiratory system liabilities. The interaction between ventilation and perfusion is expressed as a ratio ($\dot{V}_A/\dot{Q}_C$) and reflects the relationship between alveolar ventilation and capillary perfusion for the lung as a whole.

Air space ventilation should be adequate to remove the carbon dioxide delivered to it from the blood, and air space perfusion should be no greater than that which allows oxygenation and complete saturation of the blood in its brief passage through the alveolar capillaries. Ideal efficiency would occur if ventilation were perfectly matched to perfusion, yielding a ratio of 1:1. This ideal relationship is demonstrated in Figure 1-12.

In the healthy adult, capillary blood spends 0.75 seconds in the alveolus, and oxygen-carbon dioxide exchange occurs across the 0.5 micron alveolar-capillary membrane. As the blood leaves the alveolus, the blood gas tensions are identical with those of the alveolar gas. The gas tensions achieved at equilibrium depend on the following factors:[104–107]

1. Ventilation rate
2. Membrane thickness
3. Membrane area
4. Capillary blood flow
5. Venous gas tensions
6. Inspired gas tensions

The ability to achieve equilibrium rapidly depends on (1) the area of exchange being large enough to allow the blood to be spread thinly over the vessel wall and (2) the blood and gas being actively mixed together.[104]

Matching of ventilation to perfusion depends largely on gravity. Both ventilation and perfusion increase with further distance down the lung, perfusion increasing more than ventilation. The right ventricular pressure is inadequate to fully perfuse lung apices. Lung weight leads to a relatively greater negative intrapleural pressure at the apex than at the base. This means, according to Krauss, that "apical alveoli are better expanded and receive a smaller portion of each tidal volume than those at the bases."[105] Along with this, there is reduced perfusion in the apices, creating a high ratio of ventilation to perfusion.[80,107]

A ventilation:perfusion ratio of zero indicates a shunt. In this situation, no ventilation takes place during the passage of blood through the lungs. The pulmonary capillary blood arrives in the left atrium with the same gas tensions it had when it was mixed with venous blood. An example of an intrapulmonary shunt would be the perfusion of an atelectatic area of the lung.

High $\dot{V}_A/\dot{Q}_C$ ratios are the result of increased dead space and occur if the blood is spread in an extremely thin film over a very large surface area or if blood is vigorously mixed with large volumes of air. In these circumstances, equilibrium occurs, but a large amount of ventilation is required.[104] There is wasted ventilation either in anatomical conducting airways and/or poorly perfused alveoli (alveolar dead space). Thus a large amount of ventilation is wasted on a relatively small amount of blood without significantly changing the oxygen content. This inefficient gas exchange will eventually result in carbon dioxide retention.

Alveolar underventilation will result in low $\dot{V}_A/\dot{Q}_C$ ratios. In this situation, ventilation is low in relation to perfusion but not entirely absent. It is also found in persons with disease in which airway obstruction reduces ventilation to alveolar units (such as asthma or cystic fibrosis).

The blood perfusing the underventilated alveoli is not completely oxygenated, and a smaller amount of carbon dioxide is removed. These partial venoarterial shunts contribute this blood to the arterial stream, creating venous admixture, which is reflected in an elevated $PaCO_2$ and decreased PaO_2.

Abnormalities of $\dot{V}_A/\dot{Q}_C$ may be secondary to (1) too much or too little ventilation to an area with normal blood flow, (2) too much or too little blood flow with normal ventilation, or (3) some combination of the two (Figure 1-13). Whatever occurs, the lung's regulatory mechanisms work to achieve and maintain the ideal. In areas where $\dot{V}_A/\dot{Q}_C$ is high and carbon dioxide levels are low, local airway constriction reduces the amount of ventilation going to the area. When the opposite occurs, the airways dilate to increase ventilation to the area and improve carbon dioxide exchange.

FIGURE 1-13 ▲ Blockage of ventilation or perfusion.

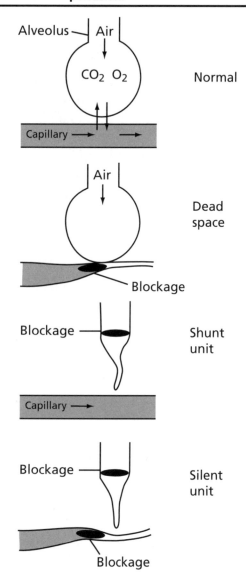

From: Malley WJ. 1990. *Clinical Blood Gases.* Philadelphia: WB Saunders, 77. Reprinted by permission.

Where oxygenation is also affected and low alveolar oxygen concentrations are found, the lung reduces blood flow to the region. These mechanisms are finite, however.

In the newborn, most of the ventilated areas are well perfused, and there is little dead space. But significant amounts of perfusion are wasted on unexpanded air spaces (intrapulmonary shunts). The newborn's lower PaO_2 demonstrates the widened alveolar to arterial oxygen tension gradient, reflecting the increased venous admixture. Although perfusion of unexpanded air spaces may play a significant role in venous admixture, the continued right-to-left shunting through transitional circulatory circuits contributes to the situation. Because of developmental immaturity, the premature infant is at even greater risk of shunting and venous admixture.[108,109]

Shunting and wasted ventilation are normal features of the newborn lung, the latter resulting from the transition from fluid-filled to air-filled lungs, where alveoli are underventilated but normally perfused. These effects begin to dissipate after one or two hours of air breathing. During the first few days of life, the neonatal lung has a greater shunt component and a larger proportion of low $\dot{V}_A/\dot{Q}_C$ areas as compared to the adult lung, although tidal volume, alveolar volume, and dead space volume per breath are similar (when expressed in ml/kg).

SUMMARY

Although the newborn's respiratory system is not fully developed at birth, he does demonstrate capabilities and strategies to achieve sustained respirations. Beyond this, he is capable of achieving gas tension and acid-base homeostasis and of employing compensatory mechanisms to maintain that balance in disease states.

Transition must be seen as an event that takes several days to achieve, with initial responses being aligned with the fetal state. Knowledge of these differences and the progression toward extrauterine stability can guide clinical assessment and therapeutic interventions.

Recognizing that the infant has prepared throughout his gestation for this transition can provide us with an appreciation of the accomplishment. The respiratory muscles have exercised and trained to take over the function of the respiratory pump although fatigue may develop quickly. Intercostal muscles can stabilize the chest wall, so effective ventilation can be achieved.

Difficulties arise when disease or immaturity is encountered. There is little reserve to increase ventilatory efforts. Sustaining increased respiratory activity may also be limited. The ability to recruit accessory muscles, the use of laryngeal braking (grunting), and the recruitment of new alveoli help improve gas exchange and increase the pulmonary surface area.[60]

For those infants greater than 28 weeks gestation, these mechanisms may be employable, though to what degree and efficiency we do not know. Each infant responds uniquely to the process of transition and to pathology. The development of refined clinical skills and further research may give us more clues as to when and how the respiratory system prepares for and achieves its sustained activity.

REFERENCES

1. Reid LM. 1984. Structural development of the lung and pulmonary circulation. In *Respiratory Distress Syndrome,* Ravio K, et al., eds. London: Academic Press, 1–18.

2. Bucher U, and Reid L. 1961. Development of the intrasegmental bronchial tree: The pattern of branching and development of cartilage at various stages of intra-uterine life. *Thorax* 16(3): 207–218.

3. Emery JL. 1970. The postnatal development of the human lung and its implications for lung pathology. *Respiration* 27(supplement): S41–S50.

4. Inselman LS, and Mellins RB. 1981. Growth and development of the lung. *Journal of Pediatrics* 98(1): 1–15.

5. Wessels NK. 1977. *Tissue Interactions and Development.* Menlo Park, California: Benjamin Cummings.

6. Agostoni E. 1959. Volume pressure relationships of the thorax and lung in the newborn. *Journal of Applied Physiology* 14: 909–913.

7. Harned HS. 1978. Respiration and the respiratory system. In *Perinatal Physiology,* Stave U, ed. New York: Plenum, 53–101.

8. Hislop A, and Reid LM. 1977. Formation of the pulmonary vasculature. In *Development of the Lung,* Hodson WA, ed. New York: Marcel Dekker, 37–86.

9. Mendelson CR, et al. 1981. Multihormonal regulation of surfactant synthesis by human fetal lung *in vitro. Journal of Clinical Endocrinology and Metabolism* 53(2): 307–317.

10. Thurlbeck WM. 1975. Postnatal growth and development of the lung. *American Review of Respiratory Disease* 111(6): 803–844.

11. Hallman M. 1984. Development of pulmonary surfactant. In *Respiratory Distress Syndrome,* Ravio K, et al., eds. London: Academic Press, 33–50.

12. Meyrick B, and Reid LM. 1977. Ultrastructure of alveolar lining and its development. In *Development of the Lung,* Hodson WA, ed. New York: Marcel Dekker, 135–214.

13. Bryan AC, and Bryan MH. 1978. Control of respiration in the newborn. *Clinics in Perinatology* 5(2): 269–281.

14. Bleasdale JE, and Johnston JM. 1985. Developmental biochemistry of lung surfactant. In *Pulmonary Development: Transition from Intrauterine to Extrauterine Life,* Nelson GH, ed. New York: Marcel Dekker, 47–73.

15. Farrell PM, and Ulane RE. 1981. The regulation of lung phospholipid metabolisms. In *Physiological and Biochemical Basis for Perinatal Medicine,* Monset-Couchard M, and Minkowski A, eds. New York: S. Karger, 11–31.

16. Milner AD, Saunders RA, and Hopkin IE. 1978. Effects of delivery by cesarean section on lung mechanics and lung volume in the human neonate. *Archives of Disease in Childhood* 53(7): 545–548.

17. Smith BT. 1979. Biochemistry and metabolism of pulmonary surface-active material. In *The Surfactant System and the Neonatal Lung, Mead Johnson Symposium on Perinatal and Developmental Medicine,* no. 14. Evansville, Indiana: Mead Johnson, 12–16.

18. Van Golde LMG. 1976. Metabolism of phospholipids in the lung. *American Review of Respiratory Disease* 114(5): 977–1000.

19. Liggins GC. 1969. Premature delivery of fetal lambs infused with glucocorticoids. *Endocrinology* 45: 515–523.

20. Kresch MJ, and Gross I. 1987. The biochemistry of fetal lung development. *Clinics in Perinatology* 14(3): 481–507.

21. Ballard PL. 1981. Hormonal regulation of the surfactant system. In *Physiological and Biochemical Basis for Perinatal Medicine,* Monset-Couchard M, and Minkowski A, eds. New York: S. Karger, 42–53.

22. Hitchcock KR. 1979. Hormones and the lung. Part I: Thyroid hormones and glucocorticoids in lung development. *Anatomical Record* 194(1): 15–39.

23. Kitterman JA, et al. 1981. Prepartum maturation of the lung in fetal sheep: Relation to cortisol. *Journal of Applied Physiology* 51(2): 384–390.

24. Brehier A, et al. 1977. Corticosteroid induction of phosphatidic acid phosphatase in fetal rabbit lung. *Biochemical and Biophysical Research Communications* 77(3): 883–890.

25. Pope TS, and Rooney SA. 1987. Effects of glucocorticoid and thyroid hormones on regulatory enzymes of fatty acid synthesis and glycogen metabolism in developing fetal rat lung. *Biochimica et Biophysica Acta* 918(2): 141–148.

26. Rooney SA, et al. 1986. Glucocorticoid stimulation of choline-phosphate cytidyltransferase activity in fetal rat lung: Receptor-response relationships. *Biochimica et Biophysica Acta* 888(2): 208–216.

27. Ballard PL, et al. 1980. Transplacental stimulation of lung development in the fetal rabbit by 3,5-dimethyl-3'-isopropyl-L-thyronine. *Journal of Clinical Investigation* 65(6): 1407–1417.

28. Whitsett JA, et al. 1987. Induction of surfactant protein in fetal lung. Effects of cAMP and dexamethasone on SAP-35 RNA and synthesis. *Journal of Biological Chemistry* 262(11): 5256–5261.

29. Fiascone J, et al. 1986. Differential effect of betamethasone on alveolar surfactant and lung tissue of fetal rabbits. *Pediatric Research* 20: 428A.

30. Smith BT. 1979. Lung maturation in the fetal rat: Acceleration by injection of fibroblast-pneumocyte factor. *Science* 204(4397): 1094–1095.

31. Gonzales LW, et al. 1986. Glucocorticoids and thyroid hormones stimulate biochemical and morphological differentiation of human fetal lung in organ culture. *Journal of Clinical Endocrinology and Metabolism* 62(4): 678–691.

32. Gross I, and Wilson CM. 1982. Fetal lung in organ culture. Part IV: Supra-additive hormone interactions. *Journal of Applied Physiology* 52(6): 1420–1425.

33. Ballard PL, et al. 1986. Human pulmonary surfactant apoprotein: Effects of development; culture and hormones on the protein and its mRNA. *Pediatric Research* 20: 422A.

34. Pope TS, and Rooney SA. 1987. Opposing effects of glucocorticoid and thyroid hormones on the fatty acid synthetase activity in culture fetal rat lung. *Federation Proceedings* 46: 2005.

35. Cuestas RA, Lindall A, and Engel RR. 1976. Low thyroid hormones and respiratory distress syndrome of the newborn: Studies on cord blood. *New England Journal of Medicine* 295(6): 297–302.

36. Ballard PL, Hovey ML, and Gonzales LK. 1984. Thyroid hormone stimulation of phosphatidylcholine synthesis in cultured fetal rabbit lung. *Journal of Clinical Investigation* 74(3): 898–905.

37. Rooney SA, et al. 1979. Thyrotropin-releasing hormone increases the amount of surfactant in lung lavage from fetal rabbits. *Pediatric Research* 13: 623–625.

38. Dobbs LG, and Mason RJ. 1979. Pulmonary alveolar type II cells isolated from rats. Release of phosphatidylcholine in response to beta-adrenergic stimulation. *Journal of Clinical Investigation* 63(3): 378–387.

39. Corbet AJ, et al. 1978. Effect of aminophylline and dexamethasone on secretion of pulmonary surfactant in fetal rabbits. *Pediatric Research* 12(7): 797–799.

40. Hayden W, Olson EB, and Zachman RD. 1977. Effect of maternal isoxsuprine on fetal rabbit lung biochemical maturation. *American Journal of Obstetrics and Gynecology* 129(6): 691–694.

41. Walters DV, and Olver RE. 1978. The role of catecholamines in lung liquid absorption at birth. *Pediatric Research* 12(3): 239–242.

42. Smith BT, et al. 1975. Insulin antagonism of cortisol action on lecithin synthesis by cultured fetal lung cells. *Journal of Pediatrics* 87(6): 953–955.

43. Gross I, et al. 1980. The influence of hormones on the biochemical development of fetal rat lung in organ culture. Part II: Insulin. *Pediatric Research* 14(6): 834–838.

44. Gewolb IH, et al. 1982. Delay in pulmonary glycogen degradation in fetuses of streptozotocin diabetic rats. *Pediatric Research* 16(10): 869–873.

45. Sosenko IR, Hartig-Beecken I, and Frantz ID. 1980. Cortisol reversal of functional delay of lung maturation in fetuses of diabetic rabbits. *Journal of Applied Physiology* 49(6): 971–974.

46. Strang LB. 1967. Uptake of liquid from the lungs at the start of breathing. In *Ciba Foundation Symposium: Development of the Lung,* DeReuck AVS, and Porter R, eds. London: JA Churchill, 348–391.

47. Milner AD, and Vyas H. 1982. Lung expansion at birth. *Journal of Pediatrics* 101(6): 879–886.

48. Bland RD. 1992. Formation of fetal lung liquid and its removal near birth. In *Fetal and Neonatal Physiology,* vol I, Polin RA, and Fox WW, eds. Philadelphia: WB Saunders, 782–789.

49. Mescher EJ, et al. 1975. Ontogeny of tracheal fluid, pulmonary surfactant, and plasma corticoids in the fetal lamb. *Journal of Applied Physiology* 39(6): 1017–1021.

50. Strang LB. 1977. Pulmonary circulation at birth. In *Neonatal Respiration, Physiological and Clinical Studies.* Oxford: Blackwell Scientific Publications, 111–137.

51. Burgess WR, and Chernick V. 1982. *Respiratory Therapy in Newborn Infants and Children.* New York: Thieme-Stratton.

52. Alcorn D, et al. 1977. Morphological effects of chronic tracheal ligation and drainage in the fetal lamb lung. *Journal of Anatomy* 123(3): 649–660.

53. Perlman M, Williams J, and Hirsch M. 1976. Neonatal pulmonary hypoplasia after prolonged leakage of amniotic fluid. *Archives of Disease in Childhood* 51(5): 349–353.

54. Weibel ER, and Gil J. 1977. Structure-function relationships at the alveolar level. In *Bioengineering Aspects of the Lung,* West JB, ed. New York: Marcel Dekker, 1–81.

55. Zapletal A, Paul T, and Samanek M. 1976. Pulmonary elasticity in children and adolescents. *Journal of Applied Physiology* 40(6): 953–961.

56. Avery ME, Fletcher BD, and Williams RG. 1981. *The Lung and Its Disorders in the Newborn Infant.* Philadelphia: WB Saunders.

57. Liggins GC, and Kitterman JA. 1981. Development of the fetal lung. In *The Fetus and Independent Life, Ciba Foundation Symposium.* London: Pitman, 308–330.

58. Marchal F. 1987. Neonatal apnea. In *Neonatal Medicine,* Stern L, and Vert P, eds. New York: Masson, 409–427.

59. Chernick V. 1978. Fetal breathing movements and the onset of breathing at birth. *Clinics in Perinatology* 5(2): 257–268.

60. Davis GM, and Bureau MA. 1987. Pulmonary and chest wall mechanics in the control of respiration in the newborn. *Clinics in Perinatology* 14(3): 551–579.

61. Mantell CD. 1976. Breathing movements in the human fetus. *American Journal of Obstetrics and Gynecology* 125(4): 550–553.

62. Avery ME, and Taeusch HW. 1984. *Schaffer's Diseases of the Newborn,* 5th ed. Philadelphia: WB Saunders.

63. Boddy K, Dawes GS, and Robinson J. 1975. Intra-uterine fetal breathing movements. In *Modern Perinatal Medicine,* Gluck L, ed. Chicago: Year Book Medical Publishers, 381–389.

64. Patrick JE, et al. 1978. Human fetal breathing movements and gross fetal body movements at weeks 34 to 35 of gestation. *American Journal of Obstetrics and Gynecology* 130(6): 693–699.

65. Patrick J. 1977. Measurement of human fetal breathing movements. In *Mead Johnson Symposium on Perinatal and Developmental Medicine,* no. 12. Evansville, Indiana: Mead Johnson.

66. Kitterman JA, and Liggins GC. 1980. Fetal breathing movements and inhibitors of prostaglandin synthesis. *Seminars in Perinatology* 4(2): 97–100.

67. Milner AD, Saunders RA, and Hopkin IE. 1978. Effects of delivery by cesarean section on lung mechanics and lung volume in the human neonate. *Archives of Disease in Childhood* 53(7): 545–548.

68. Nelson NM. 1976. Respiration and circulation after birth. In *Physiology of the Newborn Infant,* 4th ed., Smith CA, and Nelson NM, eds. Springfield, Illinois: Charles C. Thomas, 117–262.

69. Karlberg P. 1960. The adaptive changes in the immediate postnatal period, with particular reference to respiration. *Journal of Pediatrics* 56: 585–589.

70. Jaykka S. 1954. A new theory concerning the mechanism of the initiation of respiration in the newborn. *Acta Paediatrica Scandinavica* 43: 399–410.

71. Gruenwald P. 1963. Normal and abnormal expansion of the lungs of newborn infants obtained at autopsy. *Laboratory Investigation* 12: 563–567.

72. Karlberg P, et al. 1962. Respiratory studies in newborn infants. Part II: Pulmonary ventilation and mechanics of breathing in the first minutes of life, including the onset of respiration. *Acta Paediatrica Scandinavica* 51: 121–136.

73. Klaus M, et al. 1962. Alveolar epithelial cell mitochondria as a source of the surface-active lung lining. *Science* 137: 750–751.

74. Haworth SG. 1981. Normal structural and functional adaptation to extrauterine life. *Journal of Pediatrics* 98(6): 915–918.

75. Escobedo MB. 1982. Fetal and neonatal cardiopulmonary physiology. In *Practical Neonatal Respiratory Care,* Schreiner RL, and Kisling JA, eds. New York: Raven Press, 1–18.

76. Keens DH, and Ianuzzo CD. 1979. Development of fatigue-resistant muscle fibers in human ventilatory muscles. *American Review of Respiratory Disease* 119(2 part 2): 139–141.

77. Thach BT, and Taeusch HW. 1976. Sighing in newborn human infants: Role of inflation-augmenting reflex. *Journal of Applied Physiology* 41(4): 502–507.

78. Avery ME, and Cook CD. 1961. Volume pressure relationship of lungs and thorax in fetal, neonatal, and adult goats. *Journal of Applied Physiology* 16: 1034–1038.

79. Nichols DG, and Rogers MC. 1987. Developmental physiology of the respiratory system. In *Textbook of Pediatric Intensive Care,* vol. 1, Rogers MC, ed. Baltimore: Williams & Wilkins, 83–111.

80. Bryan AC, Mansell AL, and Levinson H. 1976. Development of the mechanical properties of the respiratory system. In *Development of the Lung,* Hodson WA, ed. New York: Marcel Dekker, 445–468.

81. Strang LB. 1978. *Neonatal Respiration: Physiological and Clinical Studies.* London: Mosby-Year Book.

82. Blanco CE, Hanson MA, and McCooke HB. 1985. Studies *in utero* of the mechanisms of chemoreceptor resetting. In *The Physiologic Development of the Fetus and the Newborn,* Jones CT, and Nathanielsz PW, eds. London: Academic Press, 639–642.

83. Bureau MA, and begin R. 1982. Postnatal maturation of the respiratory response to O_2 in awake newborn lambs. *Journal of Applied Physiology* 52(2): 428–433.

84. Girard F, Lacaisse A, and Dejours P. 1960. Le stimulus O_2 ventilatoire a la periode neonatale chez l'homme. *Journal de Physiologie* 52: 108–109.

85. Albersheim S, et al. 1976. Effects of CO_2 on immediate ventilatory response to O_2 in preterm infants. *Journal of Applied Physiology* 41(5 part 1): 609–611.

86. Davis GM, and Bureau MA. 1987. Pulmonary and chest wall mechanics in the control of respiration in the newborn. *Clinics in Perinatology* 14(3): 551–579.

87. Guthrie RD, et al. 1981. Development of CO_2 sensitivity: Effects of gestational age, postnatal age, and sleep state. *Journal of Applied Physiology* 50(5): 956–961.

88. Widdicombe JG. 1981. Nervous receptors in the respiratory tract. In *Regulation of Breathing,* part 1, Hornbein TF, ed. New York: Marcel Dekker, 429–472.

89. Algren S, and Lyman LE. 1993. Mechanics of ventilation: Compliance. *Neonatal Network* 12(4): 63–67.

90. Kersten L. 1989. *Comprehensive Respiratory Care: A Decision Making Approach.* Philadelphia: WB Saunders.

91. Henry JN. 1968. The effect of shock on pulmonary alveolar surfactant. Its role in refractory respiratory insufficiency of the critically ill or severely injured patient. *Journal of Trauma* 8(5): 756–773.

92. Said SI, et al. 1965. Pulmonary surface activity in induced pulmonary edema. *Journal of Clinical Investigation* 44: 458–464.

93. Algren S, and Lynman LE. 1993. Mechanics of ventilation: Resistance. *Neonatal Network* 12(6): 83–86.

94. Hogg JC, et al. 1970. Age as a factor in the distribution of lower-airway conductance and in the pathologic anatomy of obstructive lung disease. *New England Journal of Medicine* 282(23): 1283–1287.

95. Polgar G, and Weng TR. 1979. The functional development of the respiratory system from the period of gestation to adulthood. *American Review of Respiratory Disease* 120(3): 625–695.

96. Rehder K, et al. 1979. Ventilation-perfusion relationship in young healthy awake and anesthetized-paralyzed man. *Journal of Applied Physiology* 47(4): 745–753.

97. Mansell A, Bryan C, and Levinson H. 1972. Airway closure in children. *Journal of Applied Physiology* 33(6): 711–714.

98. Dawes GS, et al. 1953. Changes in the lung of the newborn lamb. *Journal of Physiology* 121: 141–147.

99. Boyden EA. 1977. Development and growth of the airways. In *Development of the Lung,* Hodson WA, ed. New York: Marcel Dekker, 3–35.

100. Robotham JL, et al. 1980. A physiologic assessment of segmental bronchial atresia. *American Review of Respiratory Disease* 121(3): 533–540.

101. Macklem PT. 1971. Airway obstruction and collateral ventilation. *Physiological Reviews* 51(2): 368–436.

102. West JB, Dollery CT, and Naimark A. 1964. Distribution of blood flow in isolated lung: Relation to vascular and alveolar pressures. *Journal of Applied Physiology* 19: 713–724.

103. James LS, and Rowe RD. 1957. The pattern of response of pulmonary and systemic arterial pressures in newborn and older infants to short periods of hypoxia. *Journal of Pediatrics* 51: 5–14.

104. Marshall BE, and Marshall C. 1980. Continuity of response to hypoxic pulmonary vasoconstriction. *Journal of Applied Physiology* 49(2): 189–196.

105. Krauss RV. 1979. Ventilation-perfusion relationship in neonates. In *Neonatal Pulmonary Care,* Thibeault DW, and Gregory GA, eds. Menlo Park, California: Addison-Wesley, 54–69.

106. Farhi LE. 1966. Ventilation-perfusion relationship and its role in alveolar gas exchange. In *Recent Advances in Respiratory Physiology,* Caro CG, ed. Baltimore: Williams & Wilkins, 148–197.

107. West JB. 1966. Regional differences in blood flow and ventilation in the lung. In *Recent Advances in Respiratory Physiology,* Caro CG, ed. Baltimore: Williams & Wilkins, 198–254.

108. West JB. 1970. *Ventilation, Blood Flow, and Gas Exchange,* 2nd ed. Oxford: Blackwell Scientific Publications.

109. Koch G, and Wendel H. 1968. Adjustment of arterial blood gases and acid base balance in the normal newborn infant during the first week of life. *Biology of the Neonate* 12(3): 136–161.

NOTES

THE AUTHORS: Ms. Signor is a respiratory nurse clinician at Saint Mary's Hospital, Grand Rapids, Mich. Dr. del Bueno is assistant dean of continuing education at the University of Pennsylvania School of Nursing, Philadelphia.

Produced by Freda Baron Friedman

also a factor. If the ABGs indicate hypoxemia (decreased oxygen in the blood), then hypoxia (decreased oxygen to the tissues) might also be present. Under these conditions, anaerobic metabolism occurs, with lactic acid produced as a by-product. Lactic acid cannot be

continued on page 47

101. Macklem PT. 1971. Airway obstruction and collateral ventilation. *Physiological Reviews* 51(2): 368–436.

102. West JB, Dollery CT, and Naimark A. 1964. Distribution of blood flow in isolated lung: Relation to vascular and alveolar pressures. *Journal of Applied Physiology* 19: 713–724.

103. James LS, and Rowe RD. 1957. The pattern of response of pulmonary and systemic arterial pressures in newborn and older infants to short periods of hypoxia. *Journal of Pediatrics* 51: 5–14.

104. Marshall BE, and Marshall C. 1980. Continuity of response to hypoxic pulmonary vasoconstriction. *Journal of Applied Physiology* 49(2): 189–196.

105. Krauss RV. 1979. Ventilation-perfusion relationship in neonates. In *Neonatal Pulmonary Care,* Thibeault DW, and Gregory GA, eds. Menlo Park, California: Addison-Wesley, 54–69.

106. Farhi LE. 1966. Ventilation-perfusion relationship and its role in alveolar gas exchange. In *Recent Advances in Respiratory Physiology,* Caro CG, ed. Baltimore: Williams & Wilkins, 148–197.

107. West JB. 1966. Regional differences in blood flow and ventilation in the lung. In *Recent Advances in Respiratory Physiology,* Caro CG, ed. Baltimore: Williams & Wilkins, 198–254.

108. West JB. 1970. *Ventilation, Blood Flow, and Gas Exchange,* 2nd ed. Oxford: Blackwell Scientific Publications.

109. Koch G, and Wendel H. 1968. Adjustment of arterial blood gases and acid base balance in the normal newborn infant during the first week of life. *Biology of the Neonate* 12(3): 136–161.

NOTES

63. Boddy K, Dawes GS, and Robinson J. 1975. Intrauterine fetal breathing movements. In *Modern Perinatal Medicine,* Gluck L, ed. Chicago: Year Book Medical Publishers, 381–389.

64. Patrick JE, et al. 1978. Human fetal breathing movements and gross fetal body movements at weeks 34 to 35 of gestation. *American Journal of Obstetrics and Gynecology* 130(6): 693–699.

65. Patrick J. 1977. Measurement of human fetal breathing movements. In *Mead Johnson Symposium on Perinatal and Developmental Medicine,* no. 12. Evansville, Indiana: Mead Johnson.

66. Kitterman JA, and Liggins GC. 1980. Fetal breathing movements and inhibitors of prostaglandin synthesis. *Seminars in Perinatology* 4(2): 97–100.

67. Milner AD, Saunders RA, and Hopkin IE. 1978. Effects of delivery by cesarean section on lung mechanics and lung volume in the human neonate. *Archives of Disease in Childhood* 53(7): 545–548.

68. Nelson NM. 1976. Respiration and circulation after birth. In *Physiology of the Newborn Infant,* 4th ed., Smith CA, and Nelson NM, eds. Springfield, Illinois: Charles C. Thomas, 117–262.

69. Karlberg P. 1960. The adaptive changes in the immediate postnatal period, with particular reference to respiration. *Journal of Pediatrics* 56: 585–589.

70. Jaykka S. 1954. A new theory concerning the mechanism of the initiation of respiration in the newborn. *Acta Paediatrica Scandinavica* 43: 399–410.

71. Gruenwald P. 1963. Normal and abnormal expansion of the lungs of newborn infants obtained at autopsy. *Laboratory Investigation* 12: 563–567.

72. Karlberg P, et al. 1962. Respiratory studies in newborn infants. Part II: Pulmonary ventilation and mechanics of breathing in the first minutes of life, including the onset of respiration. *Acta Paediatrica Scandinavica* 51: 121–136.

73. Klaus M, et al. 1962. Alveolar epithelial cell mitochondria as a source of the surface-active lung lining. *Science* 137: 750–751.

74. Haworth SG. 1981. Normal structural and functional adaptation to extrauterine life. *Journal of Pediatrics* 98(6): 915–918.

75. Escobedo MB. 1982. Fetal and neonatal cardiopulmonary physiology. In *Practical Neonatal Respiratory Care,* Schreiner RL, and Kisling JA, eds. New York: Raven Press, 1–18.

76. Keens DH, and Ianuzzo CD. 1979. Development of fatigue-resistant muscle fibers in human ventilatory muscles. *American Review of Respiratory Disease* 119(2 part 2): 139–141.

77. Thach BT, and Taeusch HW. 1976. Sighing in newborn human infants: Role of inflation- augmenting reflex. *Journal of Applied Physiology* 41(4): 502–507.

78. Avery ME, and Cook CD. 1961. Volume pressure relationship of lungs and thorax in fetal, neonatal, and adult goats. *Journal of Applied Physiology* 16: 1034–1038.

79. Nichols DG, and Rogers MC. 1987. Developmental physiology of the respiratory system. In *Textbook of Pediatric Intensive Care,* vol. 1, Rogers MC, ed. Baltimore: Williams & Wilkins, 83–111.

80. Bryan AC, Mansell AL, and Levinson H. 1976. Development of the mechanical properties of the respiratory system. In *Development of the Lung,* Hodson WA, ed. New York: Marcel Dekker, 445–468.

81. Strang LB. 1978. *Neonatal Respiration: Physiological and Clinical Studies.* London: Mosby-Year Book.

82. Blanco CE, Hanson MA, and McCooke HB. 1985. Studies *in utero* of the mechanisms of chemoreceptor resetting. In *The Physiologic Development of the Fetus and the Newborn,* Jones CT, and Nathanielsz PW, eds. London: Academic Press, 639–642.

83. Bureau MA, and begin R. 1982. Postnatal maturation of the respiratory response to O_2 in awake newborn lambs. *Journal of Applied Physiology* 52(2): 428–433.

84. Girard F, Lacaisse A, and Dejours P. 1960. Le stimulus O_2 ventilatoire a la periode neonatale chez l'homme. *Journal de Physiologie* 52: 108–109.

85. Albersheim S, et al. 1976. Effects of CO_2 on immediate ventilatory response to O_2 in preterm infants. *Journal of Applied Physiology* 41(5 part 1): 609–611.

86. Davis GM, and Bureau MA. 1987. Pulmonary and chest wall mechanics in the control of respiration in the newborn. *Clinics in Perinatology* 14(3): 551–579.

87. Guthrie RD, et al. 1981. Development of CO_2 sensitivity: Effects of gestational age, postnatal age, and sleep state. *Journal of Applied Physiology* 50(5): 956–961.

88. Widdicombe JG. 1981. Nervous receptors in the respiratory tract. In *Regulation of Breathing,* part 1, Hornbein TF, ed. New York: Marcel Dekker, 429–472.

89. Algren S, and Lyman LE. 1993. Mechanics of ventilation: Compliance. *Neonatal Network* 12(4): 63–67.

90. Kersten L. 1989. *Comprehensive Respiratory Care: A Decision Making Approach.* Philadelphia: WB Saunders.

91. Henry JN. 1968. The effect of shock on pulmonary alveolar surfactant. Its role in refractory respiratory insufficiency of the critically ill or severely injured patient. *Journal of Trauma* 8(5): 756–773.

92. Said SI, et al. 1965. Pulmonary surface activity in induced pulmonary edema. *Journal of Clinical Investigation* 44: 458–464.

93. Algren S, and Lynman LE. 1993. Mechanics of ventilation: Resistance. *Neonatal Network* 12(6): 83–86.

94. Hogg JC, et al. 1970. Age as a factor in the distribution of lower-airway conductance and in the pathologic anatomy of obstructive lung disease. *New England Journal of Medicine* 282(23): 1283–1287.

95. Polgar G, and Weng TR. 1979. The functional development of the respiratory system from the period of gestation to adulthood. *American Review of Respiratory Disease* 120(3): 625–695.

96. Rehder K, et al. 1979. Ventilation-perfusion relationship in young healthy awake and anesthetized-paralyzed man. *Journal of Applied Physiology* 47(4): 745–753.

97. Mansell A, Bryan C, and Levinson H. 1972. Airway closure in children. *Journal of Applied Physiology* 33(6): 711–714.

98. Dawes GS, et al. 1953. Changes in the lung of the newborn lamb. *Journal of Physiology* 121: 141–147.

99. Boyden EA. 1977. Development and growth of the airways. In *Development of the Lung,* Hodson WA, ed. New York: Marcel Dekker, 3–35.

100. Robotham JL, et al. 1980. A physiologic assessment of segmental bronchial atresia. *American Review of Respiratory Disease* 121(3): 533–540.

2 Pathophysiology of Acute Respiratory Distress

Susan Orlando, RNC, MS

Considering the complex series of cardio-respiratory changes that occur at birth, it is not surprising that the transition to extrauterine life does not always proceed smoothly. Neonatal respiratory disorders account for the majority of admissions to intensive care units and result in significant morbidity and mortality.

Once the infant shows signs of respiratory distress, prompt diagnosis is essential. Respiratory distress may be related to structural problems, such as poor lung development, or to chest wall or diaphragmatic defects. Biochemical and physical immaturity may exist. Abnormalities in the central nervous system may cause alterations in the respiratory regulatory apparatus. Perfusion abnormalities may impair gas exchange. Aspiration and infection can also occur.

Not all infants with respiratory distress have a respiratory disease (Table 2-1). In some cases, congenital heart disease may be difficult to distinguish from primary lung disease. Labored breathing may result from a metabolic problem. The coexistence of other factors, such as cold stress and polycythemia, may compound respiratory distress. Most neonatal respiratory

problems are treated medically, but surgical intervention may be required for a number of conditions that present with respiratory distress. Institution of appropriate therapy requires an accurate diagnosis. Knowledge of pathophysiology of neonatal pulmonary diseases is essential to ensure comprehensive management. This chapter discusses the pathophysiology of the most common pulmonary disorders that present as acute respiratory distress in the newborn period.

RESPIRATORY DISTRESS SYNDROME (HYALINE MEMBRANE DISEASE)

Respiratory distress syndrome (hyaline membrane disease, RDS) is the major pulmonary problem occurring in the neonate. This syndrome affects approximately 40,000 infants annually in the U.S. Nearly 65 percent of these infants are born at gestational ages of 30 weeks or less.[1] An infant of 37–40 weeks gestational age will rarely develop RDS. The prematurity rate is the major reason RDS remains a major neonatal problem: The frequency of RDS, which primarily affects preterm infants less than 35 weeks of age, increases inversely with gestational age. However, susceptibility to RDS

TABLE 2-1 ▲ Differential Diagnosis of Respiratory Distress in the Newborn Period

Presentation with ± cyanosis, ± grunting, ± retractions, ± tachypnea, ± apnea, ± shock, ± lethargy

Respiratory			Extrapulmonary			
Common	*Less Common*	*Rare*	*Heart*	*Metabolic*	*Brain*	*Blood*
Respiratory distress syndrome (hyaline membrane disease)	Pulmonary hemorrhage	Airway obstruction (upper), e.g., choanal atresia	Congenital heart disease	Metabolic acidosis	Hemorrhage	Acute blood loss
Transient tachypnea	Pneumothorax	Space-occupying lesion, e.g., diaphragmatic hernia, lung cysts, etc.	Patent ductus arteriosus (acquired)	Hypoglycemia	Edema	Hypovolemia
Meconium aspiration	Immature lung syndrome			Hypothermia	Drugs	Twin–twin transfusion
Primary pulmonary hypertension (persistent fetal circulation)		Hypoplasia of the lung		Septicemia	Trauma	Hyperviscosity
Pneumonia, especially Group B Streptococcus						

Modified from: Klaus MH, Fanaroff AV, and Martin RJ. 1993. Respiratory Problems. In *Care of the High-Risk Neonate*, Klaus MH, and Fanaroff AV, eds. Philadelphia: WB Saunders; and Polin RA, Yoder MC, and Burg FO. 1993. *Workbook in Practical Neonatology*, 2nd ed. Philadelphia: WB Saunders, 165. Reprinted by permission.

appears to depend more on the neonate's stage of lung maturity than on precise gestational age. Risk factors known to predispose the neonate to developing RDS are listed in Table 2-2.

Despite significant advances in understanding the pathophysiology of the disease, RDS remains a major cause of neonatal death. RDS is often the most acute problem of the very immature infant. Numerous complications associated with preterm birth can prolong hospitalization and add enormous costs. Most infants with RDS do not die from primary lung disease but from complications directly associated with RDS such as air leak syndrome, intraventricular hemorrhage, pulmonary hemorrhage, or from extreme prematurity.[2] In randomized, clinical trials, maternal antenatal steroid therapy has resulted in reduced neonatal mortality and incidence of RDS in preterm infants. However, only 15 percent of women who deliver preterm infants less than 1,500 gm birth weight are currently treated with corticosteroids antenatally.[3] As the use of antenatal steroid therapy increases, the incidence of RDS is expected to decrease.

Other factors thought to produce a "sparing effect," or to lessen the severity of the disease in the at-risk population include maternal toxemia, heroin addiction, prolonged rupture of the membranes, and chronic intrauterine stress leading to fetal growth retardation. Stress appears to be the mechanism that accelerates lung maturity in the fetus. Chronic fetal stress increases production of endogenous corticosteroids and results in accelerated lung maturity. Similarly, antenatal administration of glucocorticoids accelerates fetal lung maturity in some infants by enhancing surfactant production.

CLINICAL PRESENTATION

Infants with RDS develop typical signs of respiratory distress immediately after birth or within the first six hours. The usual presentation includes a combination of grunting, intercostal retractions, cyanosis, nasal flaring, and tachypnea. In the very small infant, the disease usually manifests itself as respiratory failure at birth. The presence of apnea in the early stage of the disease is an ominous sign: It usually

TABLE 2-2 ▲ Risk Factors for Development of RDS

Prematurity
Male sex
Maternal diabetes
Perinatal asphyxia
Second-born twin
Familial predisposition
Cesarean section without labor

FIGURE 2-1 ▲ **AP view of the chest of an infant with respiratory distress syndrome (hyaline membrane disease).** Note the reticulogranular appearance of the lung fields and the extension of air bronchograms.

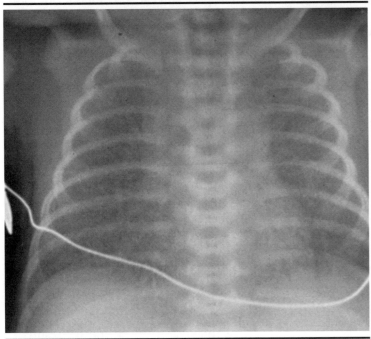

indicates hypoxemia and respiratory failure; it may also reflect thermal instability or sepsis.

The clinical course is variable in terms of severity. There is usually a pattern of increasing oxygen dependence and poor lung function, in which surfactant use exceeds the rate of surfactant production. After 48 to 72 hours of age most infants begin to show signs of recovery. Oxygenation and ventilation improve while retractions and respiratory rates decrease. The timing of clinical improvement coincides with a spontaneous diuresis.

Infants with RDS are predisposed to developing symptomatic patent ductus arteriosus (PDA)—left-to-right shunting through the ductus arteriosus causing compromised cardiovascular or pulmonary function relative to the magnitude of the shunt. The incidence in infants less than 30 weeks gestational age with RDS is 75–80 percent.[4] In infants with the most severe RDS, a large left-to-right shunt

may be present on the first day of life without the characteristic ductal murmur (Chapter 6).

A significant degree of shunting through the patent ductus results in diminished blood flow to the lower aorta and systemic hypoperfusion. Most of the left ventricular output is diverted back to the lungs. The brain, gut, kidneys, and myocardium may not receive adequate perfusion. Tissue mottling, diminished capillary filling, acidemia, and oliguria may result and mimic the clinical picture of septicemia, intracranial hemorrhage, or a metabolic disorder. In a very small infant, pharmacologic measures may fail to close the PDA, resulting in a prolonged recovery phase and ventilator dependency. Surgical intervention becomes necessary for these infants.

RADIOGRAPHIC FINDINGS

The features of RDS on x-ray are characteristic (Figure 2-1). Both lung fields show a fine reticulogranular pattern and marked underaeration, leading to a small lung volume. The most distinguishing finding is peripheral extension and persistence of air bronchograms.[5] Prominent air bronchograms represent aerated bronchioles superimposed on a background of nonaerated alveoli. Granularity is attributed to the presence of distended terminal airways (alveolar ducts and terminal bronchioles) seen against a background of alveolar atelectasis.

Treatment with positive-pressure ventilation commonly results in a coarser appearance of the lung fields. Granularity is replaced by a pattern of small bubbles. This finding reflects overdistention of the terminal airways. Upon expiration, these bubbles can empty and a

FIGURE 2-2 ▲ The pathophysiology of RDS.

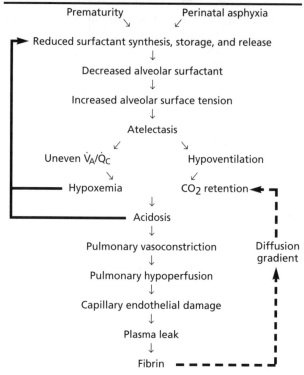

From: Fanaroff AA, and Martin RJ. 1992. *Neonatal-Perinatal Medicine: Diseases of the Fetus and Infant,* 5th ed. St. Louis: Mosby-Year Book, 811. Reprinted by permission.

"whiteout" effect may be seen. This pattern occurs because the alveoli are underaerated and lack residual air (functional residual capacity), which results in empty lungs upon expiration. In the recovery phase, alveolar aeration occurs, and granularity disappears as surfactant production and function improves. The lung fields clear from the periphery inward and from the upper lobes to lower. The lungs become large and radiolucent and frequently appear hyperaerated.[6]

ETIOLOGY AND PATHOPHYSIOLOGY

Normal postnatal pulmonary adaptation requires the presence of adequate amounts of surface-active material to line the air spaces. In the normal lung, surfactant is continually formed, oxidized during breathing, and replenished. Surfactant provides alveolar stability by decreasing the forces of surface tension and pre-

venting alveolar collapse at expiration. This allows more complete gas exchange between the air space and capillary blood. Additional advantages of surfactant include increased lung compliance, decreased work of breathing, decreased opening pressure, and enhanced alveolar fluid clearance. (A more detailed discussion of surfactant can be found in Chapters 1 and 9.)

The development of RDS is thought to begin with surfactant deficiency (Figure 2-2). This deficiency may be due to insufficient quantity, abnormal composition and function, or disruption of surfactant production. A combination of these factors may be present. The phospholipid composition of surfactant changes with gestational age. (Chapter 1 discusses the physiology of surfactant production and function.)

Inability to maintain a residual volume of air in the alveoli on expiration results in extensive atelectasis. The reduced volume at the end of expiration requires the generation of high pressures to re-expand the lung with each breath (Figure 2-3).

Infants with RDS will have ventilation-perfusion relationship abnormalities. Hypoxia results from right-to-left shunting of blood through the foramen ovale, causing significant venous admixture of arterial blood. The ductus arteriosus relaxes in response to hypoxia, allowing left-to-right shunting of blood. In addition, intrapulmonary shunting occurs as blood is directed away from areas of the lung that are ventilated, resulting in hypercarbia. Acidemia, hypercapnia, and hypoxia result in increased pulmonary vasoconstriction.

The presence of large amounts of fetal lung fluid in preterm infants contributes to early alveolar flooding. The development of alveolar pulmonary edema adds to the compromised lung function as protein-rich interstitial fluid fills the alveolar air spaces. When ventilation is initiated, distal lung units tend to remain fluid filled and undistended while more proximal airways dilate to accommodate the ventilatory volume. With expiration, the fluid moves to the proximal airways as the lung collapses. The cyclic movement of fluids results in erosion of the bronchiolar epithelium. Within hours of birth, hyaline membranes are formed from serum proteins such as fibrinogen and albumin, and cell debris is created from bronchiolar and epithelial damage.[1]

TREATMENT

Therapy for infants with RDS is directed at providing support for respiratory and cardiovascular insufficiency. Immediate appropriate therapy can be life saving. Preventing alveolar atelectasis, hypoxia, and hypercarbia are the main goals of therapy. General supportive measures must also be maximized. (See Chapter 3 for a detailed discussion of nursing care.) Maintenance of adequate oxygenation is a nursing care priority.

Oxygen must be carefully administered to provide adequate tissue oxygenation without risk of oxygen toxicity. (See Chapter 6 for a detailed discussion of complications of therapy.) An arterial oxygen tension (PaO_2) between 50 and 70 torr is satisfactory for most infants. A very high inspired oxygen concentration may be required to maintain the arterial oxygen tension within an acceptable range. Frequent or continuous monitoring of arterial blood gases is essential during the acute phase of the disease. Transcutaneous oxygen monitors and pulse oximeters provide a noninvasive means of obtaining immediate information on the infant's oxygenation status.

The decision to initiate ventilator therapy should be made on an individual basis. Variables that must be considered include birth weight, gestational age, postnatal age, results of the chest x-ray, progression of disease, and blood gas values. More immature and smaller

FIGURE 2-3 ▲ Pressure-volume curves of normal newborn lung and RDS lung. In the RDS lung, there is very little increase in lung volume with high inflation pressure. The lung collapses to subnormal volume with expiration.

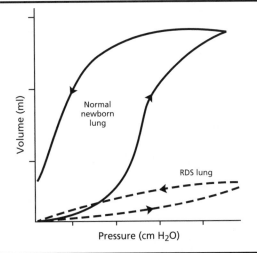

From: Harris TR, and Wood BR. 1996. Physiologic principles. In *Assisted Ventilation of the Newborn*, 3rd ed., Goldsmith JP, and Karotkin EH, eds. Philadelphia: WB Saunders, 32. Reprinted by permission.

infants, who will have a greater incidence of fatigue and apnea, generally require mechanical ventilation even when oxygen requirements are low. Some larger infants may be managed with continuous positive airway pressure (CPAP) and will not require intubation and ventilator therapy.

The goal of ventilator therapy is to provide the most effective gas exchange with the least risk of lung damage. Complications such as barotrauma, air leaks, oxygen toxicity, subglottic stenosis, pulmonary infections, cerebral hemorrhage, and retinopathy of prematurity are known to occur with intubation and ventilation.

New therapeutic modalities used in the prevention and treatment of RDS are undergoing clinical trials. Combination therapy for the mother utilizing tocolytic agents and antenatal steroid therapy has been shown to reduce mortality, morbidity, and RDS in infants weighing less than 1,000 gm.[7] Advances in high-risk obstetrics, such as tocolytic therapy and home monitoring of uterine activity, as well as educational programs for early detection of premature labor, may affect the prematurity rate. Surfactant replacement therapy offers hope in reducing the severity of RDS and, in some cases, eliminating it (Chapter 9).[8] High-frequency ventilation and extracorporeal membrane oxygenation (ECMO) have been tried in cases where conventional ventilator therapy has failed (Chapters 13 and 14).[9,10]

TRANSIENT TACHYPNEA OF THE NEWBORN

Transient tachypnea of the newborn (TTN), also called "wet lung disease" and Type II respiratory distress syndrome, represents one of the most common causes of respiratory distress in the immediate newborn period. Full-term and near-term infants usually present with an increased respiratory rate and mild cyanosis. Frequently, there is a history of maternal sedation resulting in mild depression at birth.[11] Substernal retractions and expiratory grunting may be present in varying degrees of severity. The clinical signs and symptoms of TTN may mimic those seen in the early phase of RDS or Group B streptococcal pneumonia. The diagnosis of TTN is usually made by excluding other, less benign, causes of respiratory distress (see Table 2-1).

The most common presentation is one in which the respiratory rate is normal for the first hour of life and gradually increases during the next 4 to 6 hours. The rate usually peaks between 6 and 36 hours, then gradually returns to normal by 48 to 72 hours. The maximum rate may reach 120 breaths per minute. Mild hypercarbia, hypoxia, and acidosis may be present at 2 to 6 hours.[11]

Blood gases most frequently show a mild respiratory acidosis, which resolves within 8 to 24 hours. Retained lung fluid interferes with alveolar ventilation and results in hypercarbia.

Maldistribution of ventilation and ongoing perfusion of nonventilated areas of the lung cause mild to moderate hypoxemia.

Physical examination may reveal a barrel-shaped chest. Consequently, subcostal retractions may be less prominent. As the respiratory symptoms improve, the chest will resume a more normal size.[12] Retained lung fluid may obstruct the lower airway, resulting in overdistention from a ball-valve effect. Grunting in these infants may be associated with forced expiration due to partial airway obstruction from retained lung fluid rather than being a means of increasing intra-alveolar pressure as lung compliance worsens.[11]

ETIOLOGY AND PATHOPHYSIOLOGY

Delayed postnatal resorption of normal lung fluid is the most likely explanation for the clinical findings in infants with TTN. *In utero,* the potential airways and air spaces are filled with fluid formed by the fetal lung. This fluid is normally cleared from the chest prior to the first breath by the "thoracic squeeze" that occurs during vaginal delivery. The remainder of the fluid is quickly cleared by the pulmonary veins and lymphatics.

Factors that predispose the infant to wet lung disease include prematurity, cesarean section, breech delivery, hypervolemia, and hypoproteinemia. A premature infant undergoes less thoracic compression than a term infant because of his smaller thorax. The normal thoracic squeeze is absent in infants delivered by cesarean section, resulting in an increased volume of interstitial and alveolar fluid and a decreased thoracic gas volume during the first few hours after birth.[13] Premature infants are more hypoproteinemic than term infants. A lower plasma oncotic pressure may result in delayed resorption of lung fluid. Hypervolemia may increase the capillary and lymphatic hydrostatic pressure. Elevated central pressure may result from placental transfusion and delay clearance of lung fluid through the thoracic duct.

An excess of interstitial fluid in the lung causes air trapping. The resulting hyperinflation is one mechanism that can raise pulmonary vascular resistance. When pulmonary vascular resistance is higher than systemic vascular resistance, the fetal pattern of circulation may occur, with shunting through the ductus arteriosus and foramen ovale. Severe hypoxemia results. This manifestation of TTN may be seen more frequently than expected.[14,15]

RADIOGRAPHIC FINDINGS

Because the presenting signs of transient tachypnea are commonly found in other neonatal respiratory diseases, the radiographic pattern becomes the key to diagnosis. The characteristic finding is prominent perihilar streaking and fluid in the interlobar fissures. The prominent perihilar streaking may represent engorgement of the periarterial lymphatics that function in the clearance of alveolar fluid. There may be small collections of liquid, particularly at the costophrenic angles. There is progressive clearing of the lung fluid from the alveoli from peripheral to central and from upper to lower lung fields. Within 48 to 72 hours, the chest x-ray is normal.[6]

Hyperaeration of the lungs is evidenced by flattened hemidiaphragms and an increased anterior-posterior diameter of the chest. One factor differentiating infants with RDS from those with transient tachypnea is lung size. The lungs appear small and granular in infants with RDS; in those with TTN, the lungs are usually large and granular (Figure 2-4).[5]

TREATMENT

Transient tachypnea of the newborn is a self-limited condition requiring supplemental oxygen and supportive care. Continuous positive airway pressure may be used in severe cases (Chapter 11). Pulse oximetry or transcutaneous

FIGURE 2-4 ▲ AP view of the chest in an infant with transient tachypnea of the newborn. There is a typical pattern of streaky perihilar densities representing resorption of fluid through the pulmonary veins and lymphatics. The lungs are overaerated.

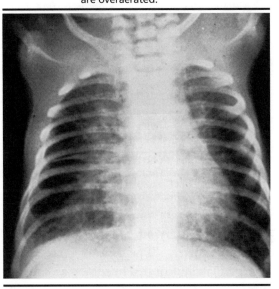

monitoring allows noninvasive assessment of oxygenation. The infant should be maintained in a neutral thermal environment.

Fluid and electrolyte requirements should be met with intravenous fluids during the acute phase of the disease. Oral feedings are contraindicated because of rapid respiratory rates. If pneumonia is suspected initially, antibiotics may be administered prophylactically. When hypoxemia is severe and tachypnea continues, persistent pulmonary hypertension may complicate the infant's clinical condition, and aggressive medical management may be required to break the cycle of hypoxemia (Figure 2-5).

NEONATAL PNEUMONIA

Pneumonia must be considered in every newborn infant with asphyxia or respiratory distress at birth. Pneumonia is the most common neonatal infection, resulting in significant morbidity and mortality. Nearly 20 percent of all stillborn infants autopsied have a congenitally

FIGURE 2-5 ▲ Cycle of hypoxemia in persistent pulmonary hypertension of the newborn.

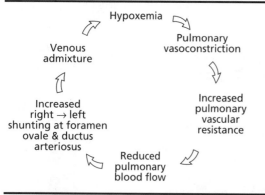

From: Harris TR, and Wood BR. 1996. Physiologic principles. In *Assisted Ventilation of the Newborn,* 3rd ed., Goldsmith JP, and Karotkin EH, eds. Philadelphia: WB Saunders, 53. Reprinted by permission.

acquired pulmonary infection.[16] Mortality rates are approximately 20 percent for infants who have perinatally acquired pneumonias; the rate approaches 50 percent for infants who acquire infection in the postnatal period.[17]

ETIOLOGY AND PATHOPHYSIOLOGY

Neonatal pneumonia may occur as a primary infection or a part of generalized sepsis. It is often difficult to distinguish the two. Infectious agents include bacteria, viruses, protozoa, mycoplasmas, and fungi.

Pneumonia may be acquired *in utero,* during labor or delivery, or postnatally. Examination of the placenta and umbilical cord may provide the first evidence suggesting the presence of congenital pneumonia, which may result from the transplacental passage of organisms such as cytomegalovirus, herpes, varicella, and enterovirus. Listeria, *M. tuberculosis,* and *T. pallidum* are less common agents.

Ascending infection from the maternal genital tract before or during labor is the more common route of contamination. The major predisposing factor is prolonged rupture of fetal membranes, although bacteria can enter the amniotic fluid through intact membranes. Rup-

ture of the membranes for more than 24 hours, excessive obstetrical manipulation, prolonged labor with intact membranes, maternal urinary tract infection, and maternal fever have all been linked to congenital pneumonia. Fetal tachycardia and loss of beat-to-beat variability in the fetal heart rate pattern during labor may reflect the fetal response to infection.

Organisms that normally inhabit the maternal genital tract are responsible for infecting the neonate at risk. Bacterial contamination of the infant always occurs during vaginal delivery. Organisms enter the oropharynx and gastrointestinal tract *in utero* when the fetus swallows contaminated amniotic fluid. Aspiration of contaminated secretions present in the oropharynx may follow a complicated labor and delivery. Chlamydia, herpes simplex, and *Candida albicans* can infect the fetus during passage through the birth canal; however, manifestations of pneumonia may not appear until days after birth. Genital mycoplasmas are gaining increased recognition as a significant cause of perinatal infection.

Ureaplasma urealyticum and *Mycoplasma hominis* may be transmitted vertically from the mother to the developing fetus *in utero* or at delivery. *Ureaplasma urealyticum* has been the agent most commonly linked with histologic chorioamnionitis and is also linked to the development of chronic lung disease in the low birth weight infant.[18,19]

Pneumonia during the postnatal period may also result from nosocomial infection. The neonate may acquire pathogenic organisms by droplets spread from hospital personnel, other infected infants, or parents. Unwashed hands, contaminated blood products, infected human milk, and open skin lesions are common modes of transmitting various pathogens to the susceptible neonate. Viral pneumonia caused by respiratory syncytial virus (RSV) or adenovirus may occur in epidemic proportions in the

BD 3/5/94 0928 hrs. 37 wks
Mom BC + 3/5/94 2200 hrs.
3/18/94 ileocolostomy
(bowel resected)

Benj DeLong   Lisa DePriest

Adm. 2/26/94
28 y.o. oligo ↓ fetal mavemt @ 26 3/7, vag spotting.
G4 P2 Ab1   Corebx, D+C '89

>2 phs/d cigs   Preg
                                          84 ─ ♂→ 5/34
3/1 amnio for culture, chrom, fluid given + dye ─   (34-36 wks?)
     no leak noted → oligo 2° to plac. insuff   91 ─ ♀
                                                  MGM ─ died
Abx started, steroids given, Mg SO4 x 24 hrs   age 28 2°
in L+D x 1 wk → 2nd course steroids.   cervical Ca.
     U/S for persistent vag bleeding ─ c/w
          chr. plac abruption

3/5 ↑ bleeding / breech → classical c/s + BTL done.

⊖ lupus anticoagulant, E coli sepsis 3/5

8/94 → 4/95 @ CHOP → Ped. Center (disch 1/98
     Trach / vent / reop for obst (signif loss of bowel)
     Feeding tube
SCHC   Billmire ─ Nissen/gastrostomy 2/12/96
adm 2/11   xrays ─ organoaxial rotation stomach
disch 2/20   SCHC 11/18/96 BPD, air trapping
                    Non obst passage barium   thru GI tract

7/94 eye f/up ─ vascularized
              retinas

→ SCHC Panitch ─
     Outpt 4/2/97 ─ (7/13/98) ─ Summary 4 yrs 32 lb 38 1/2" gastrostomy no
                        7/21 ─ ill again → steroids   (5-10%)   longer used
  (readm to St Lukes shortly p d/c from Ped. Center ─ O2, steroids)
     several meds for asthma/BPD/   Flovent 2 puffs bid, albuterol, chromolyn 4 x/d
                        RAD   itropropium inhal 3x/d
                              nasal corticosteroids, antihist/decong in allergy season
* MRI Brain 9/19/97 : SCHC   sl. prom vents (mild hydrocephalus)
                    diffuse gen'l ized cerebral atrophy: prom. gsulci + bilat frontal
                         CSF collections

BD 3/5/94 0928 27 1/2 wks
Mom BC ⊕ 3/5/9 2200 hrs E coli
3/18/94 ─ ileocolostomy c
              resection
4/27 ─ closure 1700 gm.
6/8 ─ 93 days old d/c 2659 gm

January 21, 2001

John J. Snyder
McDonald and Snyder, P.C.
Two Penn Center Plaza
Philadelphia PA 19102-1755

      Re: DePriest (De Long) v. Unger, MD., et al
             Your File No. 40-255

Dear Mr. Snyder,

You asked for a copy of my curriculum vitae which I am enclosing with this letter.

My charge for time spent reviewing medical records and in preparing a letter concerning a case is $200/hour. I have spent approximately 6 hours reviewing the case and submit a bill for $1200. My Social Security No. is 127-30-6425.

I wonder about not being an apt expert in this case for a couple of reasons. First, since the infant was admitted both to Children's Hospital and St. Christopher's Hospital at times that I have been on the staffs of these hospitals, will that suggest to the plaintiff and/or jury that I am biased? I believe I am unbiased since there is no complaint against these hospitals and I do not believe anything significant in the long run happened at these hospitals. Secondly, I have become acquainted with Dr. Unger recently via phone contacts regarding a tiny infant he sent to St. Christopher's for surgery during a time that I was the neonatology attending covering the NICU (December 21-27, 2000). Thirdly, Dr. Unger, now the solo neonatologist at St. Luke's, is forming a loose liaison with St. Christopher's for coverage and at least one of my partners has and will continue to cover St. Luke's nursery as a moonlighting neonatologist. I do not plan to cover that nursery as a moonlighter or in any other capacity.

Please let me know if I should continue.

Sincerely,

Jeanette Pleasure MD
Associate Professor of Pediatrics, MCP-Hahnemann Univ. School of Medicine
Neonatologist at St. Christopher's and Hahnemann University Hospital

3/26 Andrew McInincy

BD 3/5/94 0928 hrs. 27wks
Mom BC + 3/5/94 2200 hrs.
3/18/94 ileocolostomy
(bowel resected)
4/27 closure 1700gm.
6/8 93Days d/c 2659gm.

intensive care unit. The most common noso-comial fungal infection is caused by *Candida albicans.* Widespread use of broad-spectrum antibiotics and central lines place the very low birth weight infant at high risk for pulmonary candidiasis.

Immaturity of the lungs and immune sys-tem causes the neonate to be more suscepti-ble to pulmonary infection. An immature ciliary apparatus leads to suboptimal removal of inflammatory debris, mucus, and pathogens. In addition, the neonatal lung has an insuffi-cient number of pulmonary macrophages for intrapulmonary bacterial clearance.[20] That new-born infants have deficiencies in the neutrophil inflammatory system is suggested by several clinical observations: frequency of neutropenia during serious infection, high bacterial attack rate, high mortality rate, and lack of significant pulmonary neutrophil accumulation (observed at postmortem examination in neonates with pneumonia).[21]

Infants who require admission to intensive care units are at higher risk for colonization of the upper respiratory tract with pathogenic organisms than those who are not admitted. Factors predisposing the NICU patient to pneu-monia include liberal use of antibiotics, over-crowding and understaffing, invasive procedures such as endotracheal intubation and suction-ing, contaminated respiratory support equip-ment, and frequent invasion of the protective skin barrier for blood sampling and parenteral fluid administration.[22] The specific organisms that colonize the respiratory tracts of NICU infants are influenced by the choice of anti-biotics routinely used and the resident flora of the nursery.

CLINICAL PRESENTATION

Clinical signs characteristic of neonatal infec-tion are nonspecific. Some infants with pneu-monia demonstrate no pulmonary symptoms.

More often, the presentation will include sub-tle neurologic signs. The key to early diagno-sis is a high index of suspicion. Temperature instability, lethargy, poor peripheral perfusion, apnea, tachycardia, and tachypnea are common early signs. The presence of tachypnea, cyanosis, grunting, retractions, and nasal flaring will focus attention on the pulmonary system. These clini-cal signs indicative of possible pneumonia are also present in other causes of respiratory dis-tress (see Table 2-1).

More specific clinical signs, such as charac-teristic skin lesions, may be found in associa-tion with congenital pneumonia caused by Candida, herpes simplex, or *T. pallidum.* Hep-atosplenomegaly and jaundice suggest a con-genital viral infection. Symptoms of intrapartal infection may be delayed for hours following aspiration of infected amniotic fluid because of the incubation period before the onset of infec-tion. In preterm infants, it is often difficult ini-tially to distinguish between pneumonia and respiratory distress syndrome. Some at-risk infants may have pneumonia in combination with RDS or TTN.

DIAGNOSTIC WORKUP

The chest film is the most reliable examina-tion for detecting pneumonia; however, appro-priate bacterial and viral cultures are needed to identify the specific organism. Rapid viral screening tests allow earlier initiation of appro-priate therapy.

Latex agglutination assay of body fluids detects specific antigens and aids in rapid diag-nosis of early neonatal sepsis and pneumonia. It is recommended, however, that antigen test kits be used only as an adjunct to other diag-nostic tests and not as a substitute for bacteri-al culture.[23] Blood cultures, which are usually positive in infants with congenital pneumonia, should be obtained on all infants with suspected pneumonia.[24]

FIGURE 2-6 ▲ AP view of the chest in an infant with pneumonia. Note the patchy, asymmetric pulmonary infiltrates.

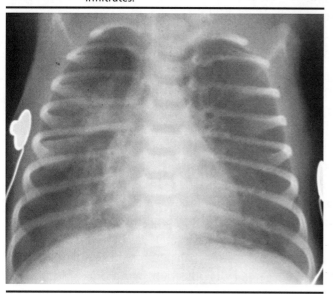

The best indirect indication of congenital infection and pneumonia is the presence of bacteria on a Gram's stain of tracheal aspirates obtained during the first eight hours of life.[25] A culture of tracheal secretions obtained through a newly inserted endotracheal tube or by tracheal aspiration through a catheter under direct laryngoscopy during the first 12 hours of life has proved useful in diagnosing neonatal bacterial pneumonia.[17] Because of rapid colonization, results of tracheal cultures obtained later may be difficult to interpret. The most definitive method of diagnosis is culture and Gram's stain of pleural fluid, but the procedural risks may result in increased morbidity and outweigh any benefits.

The neutrophil count is valuable in identifying infants with congenital pneumonia or septicemia. Neutropenia in the presence of respiratory distress during the first 72 hours of life suggests bacterial disease. Additionally, an increase in the ratio of immature to total neutrophils on the leukocyte differential is frequently observed during neonatal infection.[26]

RADIOGRAPHIC FINDINGS

Chest x-ray examinations are required to support the diagnosis of pneumonia and to distinguish it from other causes of respiratory distress. In some cases, no abnormalities will be found if the studies are performed soon after the onset of symptoms, but radiologic diagnosis should be possible within 24 to 72 hours. Patchy opacifications become more impressive during subsequent days. In some infants, an area of radiopacification is present but may be attributed to atelectasis. Bilateral homogenous consolidation is a common finding when the pneumonia has been acquired *in utero.*

A wide spectrum of findings is commonly seen following aspiration of infected amniotic fluid: Mild cases may be evidenced by patchy, bilateral bronchopneumonic infiltrates; severe cases may show diffuse bilateral alveolar infiltrate in the lungs with moderate hyperaeration.[6] Although it is difficult to distinguish RDS from Group B β–Streptococcus pneumonia radiologically, the presence of pleural effusions suggests pneumonia. Serial chest films are useful in following the course of the disease and assessing the effectiveness of treatment (Figure 2-6).

TREATMENT

Antibiotic therapy should be instituted immediately following appropriate diagnostic studies and before identifying a pathogenic organism. The initial choice of therapy is broad-spectrum parenteral antibiotics. Therapeutic agents such as ampicillin and gentamicin or cefotaxime will provide coverage for the majority of neonatal infections caused by organisms found in the maternal genital flora. Erythromycin is the drug of choice for neonatal infections due to *Ureaplasma urealyticum* as well as *Chlamydia trachomatis.*[27]

Many nosocomial infections are caused by organisms that have developed resistance to commonly used antibiotics. Once the pathogen has been identified and sensitivity patterns obtained, therapy can be altered to provide the most effective agent. A combination of antibiotics may be used for synergistic effect. The length of antibiotic therapy should be guided by the response of the infant and the identity of the pathogen. The average duration of therapy is 10 to 14 days but may be longer in severe cases.

Viral pathogens may respond to a limited number of drugs. Ribavirin therapy may be instituted following the diagnosis of respiratory syncytial virus. When herpes simplex infection is suspected, acyclovir or vidarabine should be used.

In addition to antimicrobial therapy, the neonate with pneumonia requires careful monitoring of oxygenation and acid-base status.

Supplemental oxygen and ventilatory assistance are often necessary. Volume expanders, blood products, and buffers may be needed for the infant with cardiovascular collapse from septic shock. Exchange transfusion, granulocyte transfusion, and administration of intravenous gamma globulin have been utilized in cases of overwhelming sepsis when conventional therapy has failed.[28] Extracorporeal membrane oxygenation has also been used in attempts to improve survival rates in neonates with little chance of survival.[10]

MECONIUM ASPIRATION SYNDROME

The passage of meconium by the fetus *in utero* is estimated to occur in 8 to 29 percent of all deliveries.[29] However, this occurrence is seen primarily in fetuses born at term or postterm or among those who are small for gestational age. During breech deliveries meconium passage is common and is often ignored.

When meconium-stained amniotic fluid is detected, careful and continuous monitoring of fetal well-being is required during labor. The passage of meconium into the amniotic fluid is considered a sign of fetal distress when accompanied by fetal heart rate abnormalities.[30] Increased stillbirth and neonatal mortality rates have been associated with meconium staining. In the United States, approximately 520,000 infants born annually are meconium stained. Five percent of these infants (~26,000) will develop meconium aspiration syndrome. Thirty percent of these infants (~7,800) will require mechanical ventilation. Pneumothoraces will occur in at least 2,900 of these babies. More than 4 percent (~1,000) will die from meconium aspiration syndrome.[31]

ETIOLOGY AND PATHOPHYSIOLOGY

Meconium is first produced during the fifth month of gestation. It is free of bacteria and contains residuals of gastrointestinal secretions.[29] The pathophysiologic stimuli that trigger the fetal passage of meconium are not clearly understood.

The following theories have been proposed to explain the relationship between fetal hypoxia and the passage of meconium *in utero:*[29]
- Fetal gut ischemia resulting from decreased perfusion during the "diving reflex"
- Hyperperistalsis following an episode of intestinal ischemia
- Vagal stimulation elicited by umbilical cord compression, resulting in increased peristalsis and anal sphincter dilation

Meconium passage *in utero* is considered by some to be a normal physiologic function of the term and postterm fetus, indicating fetal maturity.[30] It is rarely observed in fetuses of less than 37 weeks gestation.

Fetal breathing movements occur in the healthy fetus at a rate of 30–70 times per minute. Normally, fluid from the airways moves out into the amniotic fluid with fetal respiratory

FIGURE 2-7 ▲ Pathophysiology of meconium aspiration syndrome.

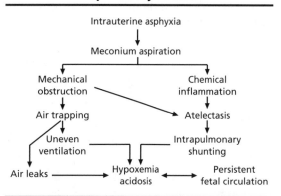

From: Fanaroff AA, and Martin RJ. 1992. *Neonatal-Perinatal Medicine: Diseases of the Fetus and Infant,* 5th ed. St. Louis: Mosby-Year Book, 835. Reprinted by permission.

movements. During an episode of fetal asphyxia, these movements cease and apnea occurs. As the asphyxial episode continues, apnea is replaced by deep gasping. Amniotic fluid containing particulate material may be inhaled into the trachea and large bronchi, and the infant may demonstrate airway obstruction at birth. After the onset of air breathing, meconium migrates rapidly to the distal airways.

The amount of meconium passed into the amniotic fluid will affect the appearance and viscosity of the fluid. As a result, the amniotic fluid may have a light green tinge or have the consistency and appearance of thick pea soup. Yellow or "old" meconium indicates prolonged fetal hypoxia and is an ominous sign.[32]

Mechanical obstruction of the airways with meconium particles results in a ball-valve phenomenon. With complete obstruction of the smaller airways, atelectasis of alveoli distal to the obstruction occurs. Partial airway obstruction results in areas of overexpansion as air passes around the obstruction to inflate the alveoli. As the airway collapses around the obstruction during expiration, residual air becomes trapped distally. Pneumothorax occurs when the overdistended alveoli rupture and air leaks out into the pleural space. Pneumomediastinum results

when extra-alveolar air moves through interstitial tissue to the mediastinum.

The chemical composition of meconium causes local toxic effects. Bile salts, pancreatic enzymes, desquamated intestinal epithelium, and biliverdin in meconium initiate a chemical pneumonitis that further compromises pulmonary function (Figure 2-7).[33]

CLINICAL PRESENTATION

Typically, an infant with meconium aspiration syndrome has a history of fetal distress and meconium-stained amniotic fluid. The classic postmature infant will show signs of weight loss with little subcutaneous fat remaining. The umbilical cord may be thin with minimal Wharton's jelly. The nails, umbilical cord, and skin may be meconium stained. Respiratory distress at birth may be mild, moderate, or severe.

Tracheal occlusion by a meconium plug causes severe gasping respirations, marked retractions, and poor air exchange. The severity of meconium aspiration syndrome is related to the amount of aspirated meconium. In mild cases, hypoxemia is present but easily corrected with minimal oxygen therapy; tachypnea is present but usually resolves within 72 hours. A low partial pressure of carbon dioxide in arterial blood ($PaCO_2$) and normal pH may be seen. Infants with moderate disease will gradually worsen during the first 24 hours.

Severely affected infants have neurologic and respiratory depression at birth resulting from the hypoxic insult precipitating the passage of meconium. They develop respiratory distress with cyanosis, nasal flaring, grunting, retracting, and tachypnea. The chest appears overinflated. Coarse crackles are common. Diminished breath sounds or heart tones may indicate a pulmonary air leak. Arterial blood gases typically show hypoxemia and acidosis. These infants will have combined respiratory and metabolic acidosis secondary to respiratory failure and asphyxia. Because of large intrapulmonary shunts and persistence of fetal circulation patterns, hypoxemia is often profound despite administration of 100 percent oxygen.

RADIOGRAPHIC FINDINGS

The classic radiographic picture of meconium aspiration syndrome includes coarse, patchy, irregular pulmonary infiltrates. Areas of irregular aeration are common, with some appearing atelectatic and others appearing emphysematous. Hyperaeration of the chest with flattening of the diaphragm is frequently seen. Pneumothorax and pneumomediastinum are common.[6] Chemical pneumonitis may be apparent after 48 hours.[5] Massive aspiration is characterized by a "snowstorm" appearance. The extent of clinical and radiographic findings will depend upon the amount of meconium aspirated into the lungs (Figure 2-8).

FIGURE 2-8 ▲ **AP view of the chest in an infant with meconium aspiration syndrome.** There are areas of patchy, asymmetric alveolar consolidation and volume loss in addition to areas of overexpansion due to obstruction (ball-valve effect). The lung fields are hyperexpanded.

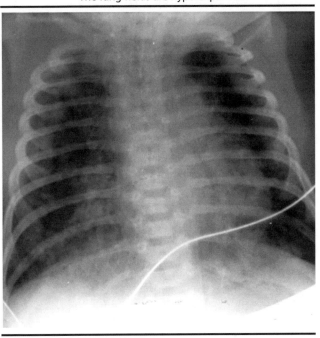

TREATMENT

Prevention is the key to managing the infant at risk for meconium aspiration. Amnioinfusion during labor has been used to correct oligohydramnios and decrease vagal stimulation caused by cord compression.[34] In a prospective randomized study, patients identified with thick meconium who received amnioinfusion had significantly fewer low one-minute Apgar scores, less meconium below the cords, and a significantly lower incidence of operative delivery.[35] Interventions aimed at reducing the incidence of meconium below the cords are important because the incidence of meconium aspiration remains at 2 percent despite the use of aggressive tracheal suctioning protocols.

Several studies have demonstrated decreased mortality and morbidity when meconium is removed from the mouth, pharynx, and trachea before the onset of breathing.[36–38] This requires an obstetrical and pediatric team approach. The obstetrician should begin the resuscitation by suctioning the nose and pharynx with a DeLee catheter or wall suction apparatus immediately after the head is delivered. The infant should then be handed to a designated member of the resuscitation team who is skilled in intubating the trachea under direct laryngoscopy.

If the infant is depressed at birth or the meconium is thick and particulate, direct suctioning of the trachea should be accomplished before the infant makes inspiratory efforts. Universal precautions should be taken. Suctioning should always precede positive-pressure ventilation. Meconium aspirator devices and regulated wall suction should be utilized to effectively clear meconium from the airway. The urgent need for oxygenation and ventilation in these infants should not be ignored.

Some investigators have questioned the need for routine tracheal suctioning at birth of meconium-stained infants who are delivered vaginally and have a one-minute Apgar score of more than 8. In a prospective study, meconium-stained but vigorous infants who made their first inspiratory effort before being handed to the pediatrician did not benefit from immediate tracheal suction.[39] Furthermore, case reports have demonstrated that aggressive airway management during and immediately after birth does not always prevent aspiration of meconium.[40]

NURSERY MANAGEMENT

Supportive respiratory therapy is required for infants who develop meconium aspiration syndrome. The infant should be monitored continuously for tachypnea. Frequent assessment of blood gases is essential. The need for oxygen and assisted ventilation will be dictated by arterial blood gas values. Continuous monitoring of oxygenation by pulse oximetry or transcutaneous oxygen pressure will alert the nurse to early deterioration. Vigorous pulmonary toilet with percussion, vibration, and suctioning should be performed frequently in the first few hours to remove any residual meconium. Chest x-ray films should be obtained to confirm the diagnosis of meconium aspiration and to rule out pulmonary air leaks.

Broad-spectrum antibiotic therapy is indicated when infection is suspected. Appropriate cultures should be obtained before starting therapy. There is no objective evidence to suggest that prophylactic antibiotic therapy improves the outcome in neonates with meconium aspiration syndrome. Prophylactic use of antibiotics is a common practice in infants with this disease because it is difficult to distinguish it on the chest x-ray film from superimposed bacterial pneumonia. The use of steroid therapy to minimize airway inflammation caused by the presence of meconium is controversial.[41]

The infant should be carefully monitored for signs of seizure activity reflecting anoxic cerebral injury. Anticonvulsant therapy may be required. Metabolic derangements such as hypoglycemia and hypocalcemia require appropriate therapy and monitoring. Fluid balance is critical in these infants because cerebral edema and inappropriate secretion of antidiuretic hormone often occur following an asphyxial insult. Fluid restriction may be initiated early in the course of the disease. Careful monitoring of urine output is essential in the postasphyxial stage. Hematuria, oliguria, and anuria may indicate anoxic renal damage.

Ventilatory assistance is indicated when adequate oxygenation cannot be achieved or maintained in a high concentration of oxygen. Respiratory failure commonly occurs in severe cases of meconium aspiration and may necessitate prolonged assisted ventilation. Once the infant requires assisted ventilation, morbidity and mortality increase. Sedatives and neuromuscular blocking agents may be added to the therapeutic regime when the infant's own ventilatory efforts interfere with the effectiveness of mechanical ventilation.

Recovery from meconium aspiration syndrome usually occurs within three to seven days in infants who do not require assisted ventilation. Those requiring assisted ventilation are usually ventilator dependent for three to seven days. Although the infant may be weaned successfully from assisted ventilation, tachypnea may persist for weeks. Pulmonary air leaks, persistent pulmonary hypertension, and pulmonary barotrauma often complicate the course of the disease. Prolonged ventilator therapy predisposes these infants to bronchopulmonary dysplasia with resulting oxygen dependency. More long-term deficits may be seen as sequelae of asphyxia.

The major cause of death in infants with meconium aspiration syndrome is respiratory failure.[42] In some cases, the infant cannot be adequately oxygenated and ventilated with conventional respiratory support. Extracorporeal membrane oxygenation has been used in many of these infants to improve survival.[43]

PERSISTENT PULMONARY HYPERTENSION OF THE NEWBORN

Persistent pulmonary hypertension of the newborn (PPHN) is a clinical syndrome characterized by cyanosis secondary to shunting of unoxygenated blood through the ductus arteriosus and foramen ovale. Gersony, Duc, and Sinclair originally described this condition in infants with no parenchymal lung disease or cardiac lesion who developed central cyanosis shortly after birth; they applied the term "persistence of the fetal circulation" to these infants.[44] A variety of other terms has also been used to describe infants with cyanosis and respiratory disease during the first few days of life who have no structural cardiac lesion, including progressive pulmonary hypertension, persistence of fetal cardiopulmonary circulation, pulmonary vascular obstruction, as well as persistence of fetal circulation and persistent pulmonary hypertension of the newborn.

Because of the variable criteria used to define the syndrome, the true incidence of PPHN is unknown. Although elevated pulmonary vascular resistance is the key pathophysiologic element in the syndrome, there is a wide spectrum of etiologies. Classification according to etiology helps us understand the pathophysiology and manage the condition.

ETIOLOGY AND PATHOPHYSIOLOGY

Pulmonary artery pressure is the product of pulmonary blood flow and pulmonary vascular resistance. The majority of infants with

TABLE 2-3 ▲ Clinical Conditions Associated with Persistent Pulmonary Hypertension of the Newborn

Pathophysiologic	Anatomic
Uteroplacental insufficiency	Diaphragmatic hernia
Perinatal asphyxia	Hypoplastic lungs
Hematologic	**Cardiac**
Polycythemia	Myocardial dysfunction
Hyperviscosity	Congenital heart defects
Metabolic	**Respiratory**
Hypocalcemia	Aspiration syndromes
Hypoglycemia	Infection (GBS*)
Hypothermia	Hyaline membrane disease
	Transient tachypnea of the newborn
Other	
Maternal drugs (aspirin, indomethacin, phenytoin, lithium)	

* Group B β Streptococcus

PPHN will have elevated pulmonary vascular resistance; few will have increased pulmonary blood flow as an important component of PPHN. Pulmonary artery pressure may be equal to or greater than systemic arterial pressure in infants with PPHN. Right ventricular and right atrial pressures rise.

When right atrial pressure exceeds left atrial pressure and pulmonary arterial pressure is greater than systemic pressure, blood flow follows the path of least resistance through the foramen ovale and ductus arteriosus. This right-to-left shunt causes hypoxemia secondary to venous admixture. Hypoxemia increases pulmonary vasoconstriction, and the cycle continues (see Figure 2-5).

Persistent pulmonary hypertension may occur in association with a wide spectrum of neonatal diseases (Table 2-3). Gersony classified the causes of pulmonary hypertension in terms of cardiopulmonary pathophysiology as follows: (1) pulmonary venous hypertension, (2) functional obstruction of the pulmonary vascular bed, (3) pulmonary vascular constriction, (4) decreased pulmonary vascular bed, and (5) increased pulmonary blood flow.[45]

The time period during which pulmonary vasoconstriction occurs may clarify the pathophysiology of PPHN. Etiologies can be categorized into intrauterine, intrapartum, or postpartum periods. The terms primary, or idiopathic, and secondary have also been used to describe PPHN. Regardless of the classification used, it is essential to understand that a combination of etiologies may be responsible for PPHN.

CLINICAL PRESENTATION

Infants presenting with clinical evidence of PPHN are usually more than 32 weeks gestational age and born following complications of pregnancy, labor, and delivery. The syndrome occurs most commonly in term or postterm infants following an intrauterine or intrapartum asphyxial episode. Onset of symptoms is usually immediate in infants with congenital diaphragmatic hernia or severe asphyxia. Others may have a more subtle presentation, but most infants at risk will have clinical manifestations before 24 hours of age. Clinical symptoms may initially be indistinguishable from those of cyanotic congenital heart disease.

There is marked variability in the clinical course. Evidence of respiratory distress may be mild to severe. Signs of heart failure may be present in more adversely affected infants. Central cyanosis may be present despite a high inspired oxygen concentration. Arterial blood gases reveal severe hypoxemia and metabolic acidosis. Arterial PaO_2 values or transcutaneous oxygen values may fluctuate widely when the infant is handled or stressed. The $PaCO_2$ is usually normal but may be mildly elevated. Physical examination reveals varying degrees of respiratory distress and cyanosis.

A single, loud second heart sound or a narrowly split second heart sound with a loud pulmonic component is heard. A long, harsh systolic murmur may be heard at the lower left sternal border. This is due to tricuspid insufficiency. Inspection of the chest reveals a hyperactive precordium with a prominent right ventricular impulse that is visible or easily palpable at the lower left sternal border.

The chest may be barrel shaped following aspiration of meconium or the use of high positive inflating pressures with mechanical ventilation. Retractions are present when pulmonary compliance is decreased. Peripheral perfusion is often poor, and pulses are diminished.

X-RAY FINDINGS

There is no classic x-ray for PPHN because the etiologies are varied. The chest x-ray may show normal or decreased pulmonary vascular markings. When the syndrome is complicated by pulmonary disease such as meconium aspiration, pneumonia, or hyaline membrane disease, the x-ray findings will reflect the primary pulmonary disorder. Cardiomegaly is a frequent finding on the initial chest x-ray and may be present without clinically detectable cardiac dysfunction.[46] The more severely affected infants with PPHN may show signs of heart failure. Pleural effusions, pulmonary venous congestion, and marked cardiomegaly may be seen when there is myocardial dysfunction.

DIAGNOSTIC WORKUP

The diagnosis of PPHN should be suspected in any infant who has hypoxemia that is out of proportion to the severity of lung disease. Parenchymal lung disease is the most common etiology of hypoxemia. However, persistent pulmonary hypertension often complicates the clinical course of infants with primary lung disease.

The most important differential diagnosis to exclude in these infants is cyanotic heart disease. A series of noninvasive bedside tests can be performed using arterial blood gas determinations and ventilation techniques to differentiate between cyanotic heart disease and pulmonary parenchymal disease. These include the hyperoxia test, preductal and postductal arterial blood sampling, and the hyperoxia-hyperventilation test.[47]

The hyperoxia test is used in term infants to differentiate between the fixed right-to-left shunt in congenital heart disease or PPHN and a ventilation-perfusion mismatch as seen in parenchymal lung disease. The infant is placed in 100 percent oxygen concentration for five to ten minutes before an arterial or trans-cutaneous oxygen pressure is determined. If a ventilation-perfusion problem is the cause of the hypoxemia, oxygen will diffuse into the poorly ventilated areas of the lung, and the PaO_2 will usually rise above 100 mmHg. A right-to-left shunt is demonstrated when the PaO_2 remains low in 100 percent oxygen. However, this shunt may be secondary to congenital heart disease or PPHN. Further evaluation is needed to determine if the right-to-left shunt is occurring at the ductal level.

Preductal and postductal arterial sampling is used to demonstrate the presence of a right-to-left shunt through the ductus arteriosus. Preductal samples can be obtained from the right radial or either temporal artery; postductal sites most frequently sampled include the umbilical, femoral, and posterior tibial arteries (Figure 2-9). The left radial artery may represent a mixture of preductal and postductal blood because of the proximity of the left subclavian artery to the ductus arteriosus.

Preductal and postductal samples must be obtained simultaneously from the quiet infant if they are to be considered reliable. In the hypoxemic infant, a PaO_2 difference greater than 15–20 mmHg indicates significant right-to-left shunting at the ductal level. If the test reveals no difference in PaO_2 between preductal and postductal sites, pulmonary hypertension is not ruled out because shunting may be primarily at the atrial level (see Figure 2-9). Additional testing is needed to differentiate between PPHN and cyanotic heart disease.

FIGURE 2-9 ▲ **A.** Preductal and postductal sampling sites. **B.** Right-to-left shunt across the patent ductus arteriosus. **C.** Right-to-left shunt across the foramen ovale.

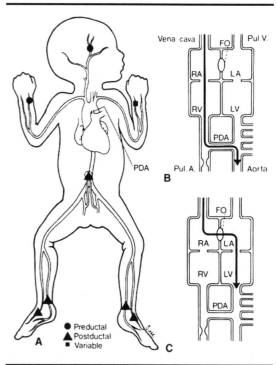

From: Durand DJ, and Phillips BL. 1996. Blood gases: Technical aspects and interpretation. In *Assisted Ventilation of the Newborn*, 3rd ed., Goldsmith JP, and Karotkin EH, eds. Philadelphia: WB Saunders, 267. Reprinted by permission.

The hyperoxia-hyperventilation test is the next step in evaluation. This test is most effectively done with infants who are intubated. Their oxygen requirements are generally high. An anesthesia bag with an in-line pressure manometer is used to hyperventilate the infant using 100 percent oxygen at rates between 100 and 150 per minute. Inflating pressure is determined by adequacy of chest wall movement.

The clinical response to adequate hyperventilation is assessed by observing color change in the infant or visually examining the umbilical artery catheter blood sample, which will change from dark to bright red, and closely monitoring blood gases by transcutaneous monitors or direct blood gas determinations.

Once hyperoxygenation is achieved, it is important to note the carbon dioxide pressure level at which the change occurred. Hyperventilation has been shown to decrease pulmonary artery pressure and alveolar-arterial oxygen difference.[48] The critical carbon dioxide pressure can serve as a useful index for guiding ventilator therapy.[49] The need to use inflating pressures above 35–40 cm H_2O and ventilatory rates above 130 to obtain a critical carbon dioxide pressure of 20 torr or less signifies a poor prognosis.[50]

Echocardiography is used to confirm the presence of a structurally normal heart in infants with PPHN. Additionally, it can be utilized to measure the ratio of the systolic time intervals of the right ventricle: The ratio of the right ventricular pre-ejection period (RPEP) to the right ventricular ejection time (RVET) is elevated in infants with pulmonary hypertension.[51]

Contrast echocardiography can be used to demonstrate shunting through the foramen ovale. When myocardial ischemia is present, the electrocardiogram will show ST-segment depression. Invasive diagnostic tests such as cardiac catheterization and pulmonary artery pressure monitoring are rarely needed to make the diagnosis of PPHN.

TREATMENT

When the fetus has been identified to be at risk for persistent pulmonary hypertension, the first step in prevention is skilled resuscitation and stabilization. Preventing hypoxemia, acidosis, and hypothermia during the immediate newborn period is essential. The time, site, and delivery route of the fetus with a known risk factor such as congenital diaphragmatic hernia may be scheduled in order to minimize intrapartum and postnatal stress.

The aim of therapy for infants with PPHN is to correct hypoxemia by reversing the right-to-left shunt. This is accomplished by decreasing pulmonary artery pressure or elevating the systemic arterial blood pressure. Treatment includes mechanical ventilation, drug therapy, and supportive care.

Mechanical Ventilation

Initially, the fraction of inspired oxygen (FiO_2) should be increased until the PaO_2 is greater than 50 mmHg postductally. In most cases, the infant will require an FiO_2 of 0.70 or more to maintain a PaO_2 of 50 or greater. Mechanical ventilation is most effective when it is begun early in the course of the disease. The goal is to reduce the $PaCO_2$ to a level at which the PaO_2 rises above 100 mmHg. Each infant has a critical level of $PaCO_2$ at which optimum oxygenation occurs because of decreased pulmonary vascular resistance and a decrease in right-to-left shunt.[49]

Ventilator rates of 120–150 breaths per minute may be required to reach the critical level of carbon dioxide. It may be necessary to hand ventilate the infant if the critical carbon dioxide level is not achieved with the use of a mechanical ventilator. The initial peak inflating pressure is determined by the minimal pressure required to move the chest wall while decreasing the $PaCO_2$ to the critical level. The oxygen concentration should be sustained at a level that will result in the infant maintaining a PaO_2 greater than 120 mmHg.

Weaning should be done cautiously while the pulmonary vasculature is reactive because aggressive changes in FiO_2 may result in pulmonary vasospasm and sudden hypoxemia. Inspired oxygen concentration is decreased cautiously, 1 percent at a time. If the PaO_2 remains greater than 120 mmHg, weaning should be continued. High peak inflating pressure should also be decreased 1 cm each time, provided that critical carbon dioxide pressure and adequate oxygenation are maintained.

The transitional phase of PPHN is the point in the disease process when the hypoxemia is no longer due to pulmonary artery hypertension but to chronic parenchymal lung disease.[52] During the transition phase, the $PaCO_2$ may be allowed to rise by decreasing ventilator settings without causing a sudden decline in the PaO_2. This is usually seen after two or three days. Failure to wean from high pressures and rates during the transition phase can result in severe barotrauma.

Mechanical hyperventilation using high rates and high inspiratory pressure to induce hypocarbia is widely used in treating pulmonary hypertension. There are many unanswered questions regarding risks versus benefits of this therapy. Induced hypocarbia and alkalosis shift the oxygen-hemoglobin dissociation curve farther to the left, which reduces oxygen release at the tissue level. Venous blood return to the heart is impeded, and cardiac output is reduced when extremely high inspiratory pressure and ventilatory rates are used. Hypotension and reduced cardiac output cause a further reduction in oxygenation. Induced hypocarbia can diminish cerebral blood flow and increase cerebrospinal fluid lactate levels.[53]

Another approach in ventilatory treatment of PPHN is to minimize barotrauma while maintaining a PaO_2 between 50 and 70 mmHg; $PaCO_2$ is maintained in the 40–60 mmHg range. The appropriate peak inspiratory pressure is determined by clinical assessment of chest excursion. This conservative approach has been used successfully to manage a group of infants with PPHN and severe respiratory failure.[54]

Drug Therapy

A variety of pharmacologic agents has been used in managing PPHN. Sedation may be utilized early in the course of treatment if the infant's spontaneous respiratory effort is out of synchrony with the ventilator. Morphine sulfate is administered to decrease the infant's spontaneous activity and resistance to controlled ventilation. The use of fentanyl as an alternative to morphine for sedation of mechanically ventilated neonates is gaining popularity.[55,56]

Skeletal muscle paralysis may be pharmacologically induced with agents such as pancuronium bromide (Pavulon) when sedation fails to produce a desired improvement in oxygenation and ventilation. Meticulous nursing care and continuous assessment of all bodily functions are required when neuromuscular blocking agents are used.

Vasodilator therapy has been utilized in attempts to reverse the direction of shunting by decreasing pulmonary vascular resistance. To date, no available drug selectively dilates the pulmonary vessels in infants with PPHN. The most widely used drug at present is tolazoline (Priscoline), but serious complications such as hypotension, hemorrhage, and renal dysfunction have been reported following its use. The systemic vasodilator effects of tolazoline often predominate over its pulmonary vascular effects and result in increased right-to-left shunt.[57]

Volume expanders and pressor agents may be required to maintain normal blood pressure. When vascular volume has been restored and hypotension still exists, dopamine may be utilized to increase myocardial contractility and cardiac output. Dobutamine is sometimes used in combination therapy with dopamine (Chapter 5).

Success with pharmacologic therapy for infants with PPHN has been varied and unpredictable (Chapter 10). However, recent studies indicate that some critically ill infants with severe hypoxemia and evidence of pulmonary hypertension respond to inhaled nitric oxide with significant improvement in oxygenation (Chapter 15).[58–61]

Supportive Care

Protocols for minimal stimulation are utilized in many neonatal centers for infants with PPHN. The infant may be secluded in a quiet, darkened room with restricted caregivers and

TABLE 2-4 ▲ Causes of Apnea

Prematurity	**Central Nervous System Disorders**
	Intracranial hemorrhage
Respiratory Disorders	Asphyxia
Respiratory distress syndrome	Seizures
Airway obstruction	Congenital anomalies
Congenital anomalies of the airway	Kernicterus
Atelectasis	
Acidosis	**Hematopoietic Disorders**
Hypoxia	Anemia
	Polycythemia
Cardiovascular Disorders	
Patent ductus arteriosis	**Iatrogenic Factors**
Hypotension	Hypothermia
Congestive heart failure	Hyperthermia
Arrhythmias	Rapid rewarming
	Vigorous suctioning
Infection	Passage of feeding tubes
Pneumonia	Obstruction of airway
Septicemia	
Meningitis	**Drugs**
Viral infections	MATERNAL
	Narcotics
Gastrointestinal Disorders	Anesthesia
Gastroesophageal reflux	Magnesium sulfate
Necrotizing enterocolitis	Cocaine
	NEONATAL
Metabolic Disorders	Narcotics
Hypoglycemia	Prostaglandin E
Hypocalcemia	Anticonvulsants
Hyponatremia	
Hypermagnesemia	
Hypernatremia	
Hyperammonemia	

Adapted from: Beachy PJ, and Deacon J. 1993. *Core Curriculum for Neonatal Intensive Care.* Philadelphia: WB Saunders, 128–129. Reprinted by permission.

visitors. Sedation and skeletal muscle paralysis are used to facilitate ventilation. Sensitivity to noise and handling during the acute stage of the disease is manifested by sudden and prolonged periods of hypoxia. Nursing care should be organized and coordinated to prevent unnecessary disturbances.

Pulse oximetry or transcutaneous oxygen monitors may be utilized simultaneously at preductal and postductal sites. Continuous arterial blood pressure monitoring is imperative. In term infants, the mean arterial pressure should be maintained above 50 mmHg. Maintaining systolic pressures between 60 and 80 mmHg reduces the systemic and pulmonary pressure gradient, resulting in a decreased right-to-left shunt.[50] Vasopressor therapy is usually required.

Fluid balance must be maintained to ensure adequate intravascular volume and blood pressure. Central venous pressure monitoring may aid in determining adequacy of fluid replacement. General nursing care measures to ensure maintenance of skin integrity are essential because these infants may not tolerate frequent position changes.

Despite ventilatory, pharmacologic, and supportive therapies, many infants do not survive. Others have been saved with ECMO therapy.[62] Recent studies suggest inhaled nitric oxide therapy may prevent the need for ECMO in some infants with pulmonary hypertension (Chapter 15). Whatever the treatment, the outcome will vary according to etiology and severity of the disease.

APNEA

Apnea is one of the most common respiratory problems encountered in the high-risk neonate. In the premature infant, the incidence correlates inversely with gestational age and weight. Apnea is observed during the first ten days of life in 25 percent of infants weighing less than 2,500 gm at birth.[63] More than 80 percent of infants weighing less than 1,000 gm will experience episodes of apnea during the neonatal period. The frequency of episodes decreases with increasing postconceptional age, and episodes usually cease by the time the infant reaches a postconceptional age of 40 weeks.

DEFINITIONS

There have been many definitions of apnea in the literature. The lack of consistency has caused confusion when discussing these clinical events. The National Institutes of Health consensus statement on infantile apnea and home monitoring clarifies the terminology:[64]

- *Apnea* is the cessation of respiratory airflow.
- *Pathologic apnea* occurs when the respiratory pause is greater than 20 seconds or of shorter duration and associated with cyanosis, bradycardia, marked pallor, or hypotonia.
- *Periodic breathing* occurs when there are three or more respiratory pauses lasting more than 3 seconds with less than 20 seconds of respiration between pauses. This breathing pattern occurs frequently and is considered normal in the immature infant.
- *Apnea of prematurity* is defined as periodic breathing with pathologic apnea in a premature infant.

More specific definitions of abnormal breathing patterns assist clinicians in distinguishing the clinical significance of these events.

CLASSIFICATION

Apnea is classified by the presence or absence of upper airway obstruction during the episode. In *central apnea*, there is no inspiratory effort. Airflow and chest wall movement cease simultaneously. During an episode of *obstructive apnea*, there is evidence of breathing efforts demonstrated by chest wall movement, but nasal airflow is absent. *Mixed apnea* occurs when there is a lack of breathing effort either preceded or followed by airway obstruction. The infant may appear to have central apnea, but when respiratory effort resumes, there is no airflow. Heart rate and oxygen saturation will continue to fall despite chest movement. Mixed apnea accounts for more than 50 percent of all

apnea in premature infants; obstructive apnea and central apnea account for less than 25 percent each.[65] The distribution of these types of apnea changes over time with advancing postconceptional age. Central apnea predominates in larger premature infants weighing more than 2,000 gm at birth.[66]

ETIOLOGY AND PATHOPHYSIOLOGY

There is a variety of clinical conditions that may predispose an infant to apnea (Table 2-4). Almost any illness affecting the neonate can present with apnea as the initial manifestation. Although the majority of apneic episodes occur in premature infants who have no organic disease, all other etiologies should be excluded before apnea of prematurity is diagnosed.

Prematurity

Premature infants are at increased risk for developing apnea because of immaturity of brainstem function. The incidence and severity of apneic episodes increase with decreasing gestational age. Central respiratory drive improves as dendritic and other synaptic interconnections multiply in the maturing brain.[67] As postconceptional age increases, the number of apnea episodes generally decreases.

Respiratory control is affected by sleep states. Apnea occurs more frequently during active or REM sleep. In the premature infant, up to 80 percent of sleep time may be spent in REM sleep. During this sleep state, there is variability in the respiratory rhythm and paradoxical chest wall movements. The inward movement of the rib cage during abdominal expansion results in a decrease in functional residual capacity and a fall in PaO_2.[68] Diaphragm activity increases as a compensatory mechanism. Muscle fatigue can result from the increased diaphragm activity. As more negative pressure is generated during inspiration, the upper airway may collapse. These mechanisms increase vulnerability to apnea in preterm infants.

Respiratory Disorders

Premature infants less than 33 weeks post-conceptional age have diminished ventilatory and respiratory muscle responses to increased inspired carbon dioxide.[69] The term infant responds to an increase in $PaCO_2$ concentration by increasing minute ventilation. This response is blunted in the preterm infant. Furthermore, the decreased respiratory center output and depressed ventilatory response to hypercarbia are even more pronounced in preterm infants with apnea than in a group matched for gestational age who were without apnea.[70] A central disturbance in the regulation of breathing is the cause of apnea in these infants.

Newborn infants have a unique ventilatory response to hypoxemia. Hypoxemia causes a brief period of increased ventilation followed by respiratory depression. This response is seen during the first two to three weeks after birth.[67] Inability to maintain hyperventilation in response to sustained hypoxia can destabilize respiratory control. Any neonatal disorder that leads to hypoxemia can result in apnea due to decreased oxygen delivery to the respiratory center.

Airway obstruction is a cause of apnea in preterm infants. The muscles involved in generating an inspiratory effort activate in synchrony to maintain a patent oropharynx. The negative pressure produced during inspiration causes the soft tissues of the upper airway to collapse. Opposing force from the genioglossus muscle helps prevent obstruction to airflow. Contraction of the muscle pulls the tongue forward and the hyoid bone toward the mandible. Other muscle groups produce dilating forces in the pharynx. Upper airway obstruction occurs when the negative pharyngeal pressure exceeds the distending pressure exerted by the upper airway muscles. In the preterm infant, neck flexion interferes with neuromuscular regulation of pharyngeal patency and increases the incidence of apnea due to upper airway obstruction.[71]

Pulmonary disorders associated with a decreased functional residual capacity or decreased compliance can be a cause of apnea. Infants recovering from RDS may demonstrate apnea as the lungs improve and attempts are made to wean them from ventilatory support. Muscle fatigue is common in these infants because of the high energy expenditure required to move the diaphragm and achieve an adequate lung volume with stiff lungs and chest wall distortion.[69]

Apnea in the near-term or term infant is always abnormal. An increase in the number of apneic episodes experienced by a preterm infant warrants investigation. Respiratory distress syndrome, infection, central nervous system hemorrhage, and patent ductus arteriosus are the most frequent causes of apnea due to pathologic conditions.

Infection

Infection should always be considered as a cause of apnea, particularly when episodes occur during the first hours of life. Pneumonia may cause apnea due to hypoxemia. Infants with meningitis may have respiratory center depression. Respiratory syncytial virus frequently causes apnea in infants up to 44 weeks postconceptional age.[72] Nosocomial infection should always be considered in hospitalized, low birth weight infants.

Cardiovascular Disorders

Patent ductus arteriosus is a common finding in infants with respiratory distress syndrome. Apnea may be seen in infants with PDA when a decrease in alveolar ventilation occurs from increased pulmonary blood flow and decreased pulmonary compliance. Anemia affects oxygen transport and may predispose the infant to apnea due to decreased oxygen-carrying capacity to the central nervous system or a decreased blood volume and central nervous system perfusion pressure.[73]

Central Nervous System Disorders

Central nervous system abnormalities may cause respiratory center depression. Apnea may be a manifestation of neonatal seizures. Intracranial hemorrhage should be considered a risk factor for apnea in all high-risk infants. Perinatal asphyxia causes hypoxemia and respiratory center depression. More severe cases result in brain injury. Transplacental passage of maternal drugs may result in a depressed neonate at birth. The effects of maternal general anesthesia and narcotic analgesia are usually seen immediately after birth. Apnea due to hypermagnesemia in the neonate is a consequence of maternal treatment. Illicit drug use may also cause neonatal apnea.

Metabolic Disorders

Metabolic abnormalities are known to cause neurologic instability and apnea. Infants depend on alternating excitation and inhibition of muscle fibers to establish rhythmic breathing. Hypoglycemic infants may have an acute depletion of the energy supply of diaphragmatic fibers leading to diaphragmatic fatigue and apnea.[74] Other imbalances such as hypocalcemia and hyponatremia may lead to respiratory arrest. Thermal instability affects respiratory control. Environmental temperatures near the upper limit of the neutral thermal zone have been associated with an increased incidence of apnea.[63] Sudden increases in environmental temperature as well as rapid rewarming of the cold-stressed infant increase the risk of apnea.

EVALUATION

Infants at high risk for apnea should be carefully monitored for early detection of respiratory instability. Continuous monitoring for the first 10 to 14 days of life should be routine for all premature infants who weigh less than 1,800 gm or are less than 34 weeks gestational age. Monitoring should continue until no significant apneic episode has occurred for 5 to 7 days.[75] Heart rate should be monitored in addition to respiratory rate. Obstructed breaths may not trigger a respiration alarm, and heart rate does not always drop during an episode of apnea. Concurrent monitoring using pulse oximetry or transcutaneous monitors allows noninvasive detection of hypoxemic episodes that may lead to apnea.

An attempt to determine the cause of apnea is essential. Perinatal and neonatal risk factors can be determined by careful history. A complete physical and neurologic examination should be performed. The infant's response to environmental temperature should be carefully evaluated. The basic laboratory workup may identify sources of infection, common metabolic problems, and alterations in respiration. Additional tests may be ordered if the initial workup fails to identify a cause of apnea.

MANAGEMENT AND TREATMENT

When specific diseases or underlying conditions have been identified, treatment of the primary disease should be initiated. Acute management of apnea is the same for all etiologies and includes establishment of an airway, assurance of adequate ventilation, and evaluation of vital signs. A bag and mask should be set up at the bedside of every monitored infant. In some cases, immediate respiratory support is required before initiating treatment for the underlying cause. If apnea continues after initial treatment of underlying causes, or if there is not a clear etiology, therapeutic interventions should be directed toward decreasing the number and severity of apneic episodes.

Preventive measures such as a stable thermal environment, avoidance of neck flexion, and maintenance of nasal patency should be carried out for all infants with apnea. Continuous monitoring of heart rate, respiratory rate, and oxygenation is essential. Treatment of apnea includes tactile stimulation, continuous positive airway pressure, and drug therapy. Noninvasive interventions may be effective in reducing apneic episodes and should be used first. Cutaneous stimulation can compensate for the decreased number of afferent signals toward the respiratory center and modify the output of respiratory generators.

CPAP of 4 cm H_2O is effective in reducing obstructive, and therefore, mixed apnea but has no effect on central apnea.[65] Nasal or pharyngeal CPAP provides positive pressure throughout inspiration and expiration; this pressure splints the upper airway and maintains patency. Other beneficial effects of CPAP include stabilization of the chest wall, increased functional residual capacity, and improvement in oxygenation (Chapter 11).

Pharmacologic treatment of apnea includes the use of respiratory stimulants such as theophylline, aminophylline, and caffeine. Methylxanthines appear to decrease the incidence of central, mixed, and obstructive apnea. Several mechanisms may account for the reduction of apneic episodes following methylxanthine administration. Central stimulation of the respiratory center results in increased minute ventilation and ventilatory response to hypercapnia. Methylxanthines have peripheral effects on the neuromuscular junction, increasing skeletal muscle tone and decreasing diaphragm fatigue.[74] Treatment with methylxanthines should follow a strict protocol to minimize complications from side effects. The occurrence of gastric irritation, tachycardia, hyperactivity, electrolyte imbalances, and seizures is directly related to serum levels.

Doxapram has been used to treat apnea in infants unresponsive to methylxanthines. It has been shown to increase minute ventilation and tidal volume without any effect on respiratory timing. The drug has limited use in neonates because continuous intravenous infusion is needed to maintain therapeutic levels. In addition, the preparation available in the U.S. contains benzyl alcohol and is not recommended for use in premature infants.[72] Drug therapy for neonatal apnea is discussed further in Chapter 10.

Mechanical ventilation may be required for some infants who continue to have episodes of apnea despite use of CPAP and pharmacologic therapy. The very low birth weight infant may require six to ten breaths per minute to prevent recurring apnea. Minimal peak inspiratory and end-expiratory pressures with a short inspiratory time should be used.[74] In other infants, full ventilatory support may be required until the primary cause of apnea is identified and treated.

Prognosis for infants with apnea will depend on the etiology. Repeated episodes of hypoxia may result in brain injury. Many infants with apnea have other medical conditions that will affect their developmental outcome. Apnea in the preterm infant usually resolves by a postconceptional age of 40 weeks. A select group of infants may require pharmacologic therapy after discharge. Home monitoring may be indicated for some infants.

SUMMARY

Most infants admitted to neonatal intensive care units have respiratory disorders. Understanding the pathophysiology associated with each disease process is essential to ensure timely and comprehensive management. Knowledge of clinical presentation and etiology in relation to gestational age assists in differential diagnosis. The goal of therapy for neonatal respiratory disorders is the maintenance of adequate oxygenation and ventilation. Advances in antenatal care impact the prematurity rate and lessen the incidence of respiratory disorders related to immaturity. Such advances in technology as artifical surfactant, new modes of ventilation, ECMO, and inhaled nitric oxide have improved outcomes for many infants with severe respiratory disease.

REFERENCES

1. Raj JU. 1988. Hyaline membrane disease. In *Neonatal Cardiopulmonary Distress,* Emmanouilides GC, and Baylen G, eds. Chicago: Year Book Medical Publishers, 54–55.

2. Jobe A. 1988. Respiratory distress syndrome: Pathophysiologic basis for new therapeutic efforts. In *Neonatal Cardiopulmonary Distress,* Emmanouilides GC, and Baylen G, eds. Chicago: Year Book Medical Publishers, 317.

3. National Institutes of Health Consensus Statement. 1994. Effect of corticosteroids for fetal maturation on perinatal outcomes, February 28–March 2, 12(2): 1–24.

4. Cotton RB. 1987. Relationship of PDA to respiratory distress in preterm infants. *Clinics in Perinatology* 14(3): 621–633.

5. Swischuk LE. 1989. *Imaging of the Newborn, Infant, and Young Child,* 3rd ed. Baltimore: Williams & Wilkins, 35, 52, 56.

6. Wesenberg RL. 1973. *The Newborn Chest.* Hagerstown, Philadelphia: Harper & Row, 45–46, 62, 74–83, 119–124.

7. Papageorgiou A, et al. 1989. Reduction of mortality, morbidity, and respiratory distress syndrome in infants weighing less than 1,000 grams by treatment with betamethasone and ritodrine. *Pediatrics* 83(4): 493–497.

8. Shapiro D. 1990. Surfactant replacement therapy. In *Current Therapy in Neonatal-Perinatal Medicine,* part II, Nelson NM, ed. Philadelphia: BC Decker, 477–480.

9. Bancalari E, and Goldberg R. 1987. High-frequency ventilation in the neonate. *Clinics in Perinatology* 14(3): 581–597.

10. Short BL, Miller MK, and Anderson KD. 1987. Extracorporeal membrane oxygenation in the management of respiratory failure in the newborn. *Clinics in Perinatology* 14(3): 737–749.

11. Sundell H, et al. 1971. Studies on infants with Type II respiratory distress syndrome. *Journal of Pediatrics* 78(5): 754–764.

12. Auld P. 1978. Respiratory distress syndromes of the newborn. In *Pulmonary Diseases of the Fetus, Newborn and Child,* Scarpelli EM, ed. Philadelphia: Lea & Febiger, 502–503.

13. Milner AD, Saunders RA, and Hopkin IE. 1978. Effect of delivery by cesarean section on lung mechanics and lung volume in the human neonate. *Archives of Disease in Childhood* 53(14): 545–548.

14. Bucciarelli RL, et al. 1976. Persistence of fetal cardiopulmonary circulation: One manifestation of TTN. *Pediatrics* 58(2): 192–197.

15. Bonita BW. 1987. Transient pulmonary vascular lability: A form of mild pulmonary hypertension of the newborn not requiring mechanical ventilation. *Journal of Perinatology* 8(1): 19–23.

16. Merritt TA. 1984. Respiratory distress. In *Assessment of the Newborn: A Guide for the Practitioner,* Ziai M, Clark T, and Merritt TA, eds. Boston: Little, Brown, 168.

17. Dennehy PH. 1987. Respiratory infections in the newborn. *Clinics in Perinatology* 14(3): 667–682.

18. Cassell GH, et al. 1988. Association of *Ureaplasma urealyticum* infection of the lower respiratory tract with chronic lung disease and death in very-low-birth-weight infants. *Lancet* 2(8605): 240–245.

19. Sanchez PJ, and Regan JA. 1988. *Ureaplasma urealyticum* colonization and chronic lung disease in low birth weight infants. *Pediatric Infectious Disease Journal* 7(8): 542–546.

20. Reid L. 1977. Influence of the pattern of structural growth of lung on susceptibility to specific infectious diseases in infants and children. *Pediatric Research* 11(3 part 2): 210–215.

21. Christensen RD, Thibeault DW, and Hall RT. 1986. Neonatal bacterial and fungal pneumonia. In *Neonatal Pulmonary Care,* 2nd ed., Thibeault DW, and Gregory GA, eds. Norwalk, Connecticut: Appleton & Lange, 580.

22. Lott JW. 1994. *Neonatal Infection: Assessment, Diagnosis, and Management.* Petaluma, California: NICU INK, 37, 151–158.

23. Department of Health & Human Services. 1997. FDA safety alert: Risks of devices for direct detection of group B streptococcal antigen. Rockville, Maryland: Food and Drug Administration. March 24.

24. Sherman MP, Chance KH, and Goetzman BW. 1984. Gram's stain of tracheal secretions predict neonatal bacteremia. *American Journal of Diseases of Children* 138(9): 848–850.

25. Sherman MP, et al. 1980. Tracheal aspiration and its clinical correlates in the diagnosis of congenital pneumonia. *Pediatrics* 65(2): 258–263.

26. Manroe BL, et al. 1979. The neonatal blood count in health and disease. Part I: Reference values for neutrophilic cells. *Journal of Pediatrics* 95(1): 89–98.

27. McCracken G, and Freiji B. 1990. Clinical pharmacology of antimicrobial agents. In *Infectious Diseases of the Fetus and Newborn Infant,* 3rd ed., Remington J, and Klein JO, eds. Philadelphia: WB Saunders, 1020–1078.

28. Wasserman RL. 1983. Unconventional therapies for neonatal sepsis. *Pediatric Infectious Disease Journal* 2(6): 421–423.

29. Bacsik RD. 1977. Meconium aspiration syndrome. *Pediatric Clinics of North America* 24(3): 463–479.

30. Fenton AN, and Steer CM. 1962. Fetal distress. *American Journal of Obstetrics and Gynecology* 83: 352–362.

31. Wisell TE, and Bent RC. 1993. Meconium staining and the meconium aspiration syndrome. *Pediatric Clinics of North America* 40(5): 955–981.

32. Desmond MM, et al. 1957. Meconium staining of the amniotic fluid: A marker of fetal hypoxia. *Obstetrics and Gynecology* 9: 91–103.

33. Tyler DC, Murphy J, and Cheney FW. 1978. Mechanical and chemical damage to lung tissue caused by meconium aspiration. *Pediatrics* 62(4): 454–459.

34. Miyazaki FS, and Nevarez F. 1985. Saline amnioinfusion for relief of repetitive variable decelerations: A prospective randomized study. *American Journal of Obstetrics and Gynecology* 153(3): 301–306.

35. Wenstrom KD, and Parsons MT. 1989. The prevention of meconium aspiration in labor using amnioinfusion. *Obstetrics and Gynecology* 73(4): 647–650.

36. Carson BS, et al. 1976. Combined obstetric and pediatric approach to prevent meconium aspiration syndrome. *American Journal of Obstetrics and Gynecology* 126(6): 712–715.

37. Ting P, and Brady JP. 1974. Tracheal suction in meconium aspiration. *American Journal of Obstetrics and Gynecology* 122(6): 767–771.

38. Gregory GA, et al. 1974. Meconium aspiration in infants—a prospective study. *Journal of Pediatrics* 85(6): 848–852.

39. Linder N, et al. 1988. Need for endotracheal intubation and suction in meconium-stained neonates. *Journal of Pediatrics* 112(4): 613–615.

40. Davis RO, et al. 1985. Fatal meconium aspiration syndrome occurring despite airway management considered appropriate. *American Journal of Obstetrics and Gynecology* 151(6): 731–736.

41. Brady JP, and Goldman SL. 1986. Management of meconium aspiration syndrome. In *Neonatal Pulmonary Care,* 2nd ed., Thibeault D, and Gregory G, eds. Norwalk, Connecticut. Appleton & Lange, 497.

42. Vidyasagar D, et al. 1975. Assisted ventilation in infants with meconium aspiration syndrome. *Pediatrics* 56(2): 208–213.

43. Heiss KF, and Bartlett RH. 1989. Extracorporeal membrane oxygenation: An experimental protocol becomes a clinical service. *Advances in Pediatrics* 36: 117–136.

44. Gersony WM, Duc GV, and Sinclair JC. 1969. "PFC" syndrome (persistence of the fetal circulation). *Circulation* 40(supplement 3): S87.

45. Gersony WM. 1984. Neonatal pulmonary hypertension: Pathophysiology, classification, and etiology. *Clinics in Perinatology* 11(3): 517–524.

46. Henry GW. 1984. Noninvasive assessment of cardiac function and pulmonary hypertension in persistent pulmonary hypertension of the newborn. *Clinics in Perinatology* 11(3): 627–640.

47. Fox WW, and Duara S. 1983. Persistent pulmonary hypertension of the neonate: Diagnosis and management. *Journal of Pediatrics* 103(4): 505–514.

48. Peckham GJ, and Fox WW. 1978. Physiologic factors affecting pulmonary pressure in infants with persistent pulmonary hypertension. *Journal of Pediatrics* 93(6): 1005–1010.

49. Fox WW. 1981. Arterial blood gas evaluation and mechanical ventilation in the management of persistent pulmonary hypertension of the neonate. 83rd Ross Conference on Pediatric Research: Cardiovascular Sequelae of Asphyxia in the Newborn, 102.

50. Duara S, and Fox WW. 1986. Persistent pulmonary hypertension of the neonate. In *Neonatal Pulmonary Care,* 2nd ed., Thibeault DW, and Gregory G, eds. Norwalk, Connecticut: Appleton & Lange, 479.

51. Riggs T, et al. 1977. Neonatal circulatory changes: An echocardiographic study. *Pediatrics* 59(3): 338–344.

52. Sosulski R, and Fox WW. 1982. Hyperventilation therapy for persistent pulmonary hypertension of the neonate and occurrence of a transition phase. *Pediatric Research* I6: 309A.

53. Plum F, and Posner J. 1967. Blood and cerebrospinal fluid lactate during hyperventilation. *American Journal of Physiology* 212(4): 864–870.

54. Wung J, et al. 1985. Management of infants with severe respiratory failure and persistence of the fetal circulation, without hyperventilation. *Pediatrics* 76(4): 488–494.

55. Bell SG, and Ellis LS. 1987. Use of fentanyl for sedation of mechanically ventilated infants. *Neonatal Network* 6(2): 27–31.

56. Maguire D, and Maloney P. 1988. A comparison of fentanyl and morphine use in neonates. *Neonatal Network* 7(1): 27–32.

57. Roberts RT. 1984. *Drug Therapy in Infants.* Philadelphia: WB Saunders, 191–192.

58. Kinsella JP, and Abman SH. 1993. Inhalational nitric oxide therapy for persistent pulmonary hypertension of the newborn. *Pediatrics* 91(5): 997–998.

59. Finer NN, et al. 1994. Inhaled nitric oxide in infants referred for extracorporeal membrane oxygenation: Dose response. *Journal of Pediatrics* 124(2): 302–308.

60. Kinsella JP, et al. 1992. Low dose inhalational nitric oxide in persistent pulmonary hypertension of the newborn. *Lancet* 340: 819–820.

61. Roberts JD, et al. 1992. Inhaled nitric oxide in persistent pulmonary hypertension of the newborn. *Lancet* 340: 318–319.

62. O'Rourke P, et al. 1989. Extracorporeal membrane oxygenation and conventional medical therapy in neonates with persistent pulmonary hypertension of the newborn: A prospective randomized study. *Pediatrics* 84(6): 957–963.

63. Daily WJ, et al. 1969. Apnea in premature infants: Monitoring, incidence, heart rate changes, and an effect of environmental temperature. *Pediatrics* 43(4): 510–518.

64. National Institutes of Health. Consensus Statement. 1987. Consensus Developmental Conference on Infantile Apnea and Home Monitoring, September 29–October 1, 1986. *Pediatrics* 79(2): 292–299.

65. Miller MJ, Carlo WA, and Martin RJ. 1985. Continuous positive airway pressure selectively reduces obstructive apnea in preterm infants. *Journal of Pediatrics* 106(1): 91–94.

66. Lee D, et al. 1987. A developmental study on types and frequency distribution of short apneas (3 to 15 seconds) in term and preterm infants. *Pediatric Research* 22(3): 344–349.

67. Martin RJ, Miller MJ, and Carlo WA. 1986. Pathogenesis of apnea in preterm infants. *Journal of Pediatrics* 109(5): 733–740.

68. Miller MJ, and Martin RJ. 1992. Apnea of prematurity. *Clinics in Perinatology* 19(4): 789–808.

69. Rigatto H. 1982. Apnea. *Pediatric Clinics of North America* 29(5): 1105–1116.

70. Gerhardt T, and Bancalari E. 1984. Apnea of prematurity. Part I: Lung function and regulation of breathing. *Pediatrics* 74(1): 58–62.

71. Thatch BT, and Stark AR. 1979. Spontaneous neck flexion and airway obstruction during apneic spells in preterm infants. *Journal of Pediatrics* 94(2): 275–281.

72. Dransfield DA. 1993. Breathing disorders in the newborn infant. In *Workbook in Practical Neonatology,* 2nd ed., Polin RA, Yoder MC, and Burg FD, eds. Philadelphia: WB Saunders, 207–225.

73. Kattwinkel J. 1977. Neonatal apnea: Pathogenesis and therapy. *Journal of Pediatrics* 90(3): 342–347.

74. Marchal F, Bairam A, and Vert P. 1987. Neonatal apnea and apneic syndromes. *Clinics in Perinatology* 14(3): 509–524.

75. Martin RJ, Fanaroff AA, and Klaus MH. 1993. Respiratory problems. In *Care of the High-Risk Neonate,* 4th ed., Klaus MH, and Fanaroff AA, eds. Philadelphia: WB Saunders, 228–259.

3 Nursing Assessment and Care for the Neonate in Acute Respiratory Distress

Kathleen Koszarek, RNC, MSN

Nursing care of the critically ill newborn is a vital component contributing to a positive outcome for the neonate experiencing acute respiratory distress. The caretaker at the bedside integrates knowledge and skills of many aspects of care, including developmental physiology, pathophysiology, and the psychosocial needs of the patient and family. No other health care professional spends as many hours at the patient's bedside. This intense, lengthy contact allows the nurse to become totally familiar with the infant's status and promotes an awareness of the subtle cues that warn of a change in the infant's clinical condition. The impact of nursing care on neonatal morbidity and mortality should never be underestimated, and each nursing unit must be aware of its standards of care and the performance of its individual members.

This chapter discusses components of respiratory care for the neonate, from delivery to admission and routine care measures. Special attention is given to clinical assessment, basic nursing care measures, and parental support issues.

RESUSCITATION

Responsibility for the neonate precedes his admission into the NICU. Preparations for

resuscitation and an orderly admission must be instituted prior to the birth. Essential to this preparation is an awareness of the maternal-fetal factors that place the neonate at risk. Absolute prediction of infant status at delivery is not possible, but a thorough knowledge of the perinatal history allows the clinician to identify risk factors for the neonate and to begin anticipatory measures. Pulmonary immaturity must be anticipated with preterm delivery; asphyxia is seen more often in term infants with congenital anomalies or those experiencing fetal distress. Table 3-1 lists high-risk antepartum and intrapartum conditions that are associated with respiratory depression or distress in the neonate at delivery.

Any institution that provides perinatal health services must have an adequately staffed and equipped resuscitation room. This means having trained personnel available from the moment of delivery to receive the infant for whom acute respiratory distress is anticipated. Any perinatal center delivering intrapartum care must have an individual capable of providing emergency care for the infant. A formal education program, such as the Neonatal Resuscitation Program (NRP) through the American

Academy of Pediatrics and the American Heart Association, will help to ensure that personnel are adequately trained.[1] When resuscitative measures are required, an orderly approach will optimize results (Figure 3-1).

Resuscitative measures are based on the clinical presentation of the infant as well as anticipation of problems. The Apgar score has become a standard for initial clinical assessment throughout the country (Table 3-2). Despite this instrument's simplicity, improper and biased scoring occurs, and an effort must be made by the observer to use the scale as objectively as possible.[2]

Along with the appropriate resuscitation equipment, each delivery area needs to have resuscitation information available for quick reference. This information includes resuscitative drug doses, appropriate endotracheal tube size for weight, depth of insertion for umbilical lines, and emergency phone numbers needed to mobilize a resuscitation team.

Nursing responsibilities during resuscitation include the following:

- Monitor heart rate; recheck heart rate every one to two minutes while aggressive resuscitation is under way; place the infant on a cardiac monitor and pulse oximeter if available.
- Assist with correct airway positioning of the infant and suction airway as needed; deliver oxygen and bag and mask manual ventilation as required.
- Place an orogastric tube and leave open to gravity drainage if mask ventilation continues longer than two minutes; occasionally aspirate tube to ensure patency and relieve gastric distention.
- Initiate and continue chest compressions as per protocol.
- Draw up and administer resuscitation medications as ordered by the physician; verify that dose and route of administration are correct.

TABLE 3-1 ▲ Risk Factors for Neonatal Respiratory Depression

Antepartum Factors
Age >35 years
Maternal diabetes
Pregnancy-induced hypertension
Chronic hypertension
Anemia or isoimmunization
Previous fetal or neonatal death
Bleeding in the second or third trimester
Maternal infection
Hydramnios
Oligohydramnios
Premature rupture of membranes
Postterm gestation
Multiple gestation
Size-dates discrepancy
Drug therapy such as:
    Lithium carbonate
    Magnesium
    Adrenergic-blocking drugs
Maternal substance abuse
Fetal malformation
Diminished fetal activity
No prenatal care

Intrapartum Factors
Emergency cesarean section
Breech or other abnormal presentation
Premature labor
Prolonged rupture of membranes more than 24 hours before delivery
Precipitous labor
Prolonged labor (more than 24 hours)
Prolonged second stage of labor (more than two hours)
Nonreassuring fetal heart rate patterns
Use of general anesthesia
Uterine tetany
Narcotics administered to mother within four hours of delivery
Meconium-stained amniotic fluid
Prolapsed cord
Abruptio placenta
Placenta previa

From: Bloom RS, and Cropley C. 1994. *Textbook of Neonatal Resuscitation*. Dallas: American Heart Association, 1-18. Reprinted by permission.

- Assist with procedures such as endotracheal intubation, umbilical line placement, or chest tube placement.

FIGURE 3-1 ▲ Overview of resuscitation in the delivery room.

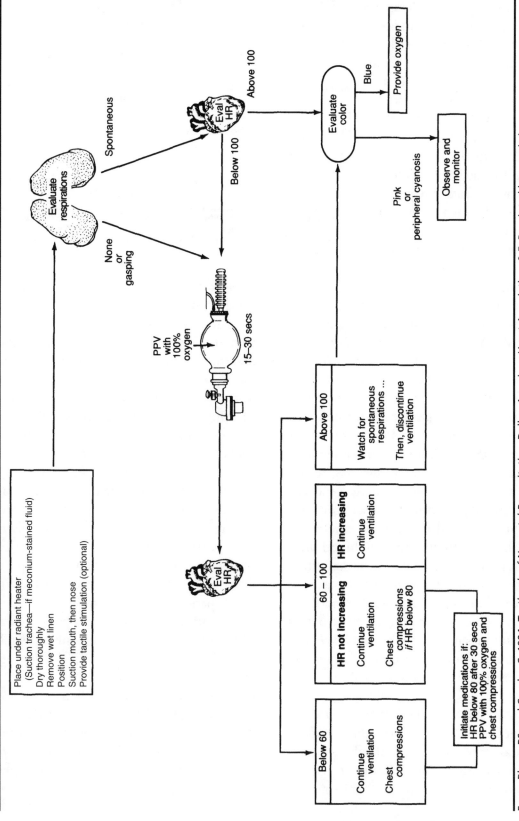

Place under radiant heater
(Suction trachea—if meconium-stained fluid)
Dry thoroughly
Remove wet linen
Position
Suction mouth, then nose
Provide tactile stimulation (optional)

Evaluate respirations

Spontaneous

None or gasping

PPV with 100% oxygen

15–30 secs

Eval HR

Above 100

Below 100

Eval HR

Above 100

Watch for spontaneous respirations ...
Then, discontinue ventilation

60 – 100

HR not increasing
Continue ventilation
Chest compressions *if HR below 80*

HR increasing
Continue ventilation

Below 60
Continue ventilation
Chest compressions

Initiate medications if:
HR below 80 after 30 secs
PPV with 100% oxygen and chest compressions

Evaluate color

Blue

Provide oxygen

Pink or peripheral cyanosis

Observe and monitor

From: Bloom RS, and Cropley C. 1994. *Textbook of Neonatal Resuscitation.* Dallas: American Heart Association, 0-5. Reprinted by permission.

- Monitor the infant's temperature; continue to dry the infant as needed; remove wet linen from the infant; use servomechanism and calibrate radiant warmer controls; use skin probe to continually assess infant temperature.
- Check blood glucose via reagent strip, notify physician; start IV and IV fluids if required.

Obviously, one person cannot handle all of these tasks simultaneously, but the nurse must be aware of the overall care needed by the infant in acute distress.

Further examination of the infant should be done in the delivery room or resuscitation area to identify any abnormalities that require immediate treatment. A brief examination routine can provide valuable information regarding the infant's status (Table 3-3).

Anticipation of problems extends to the nursery as well. A well-prepared nursery environment includes a heat source for temperature stabilization, cardiorespiratory and oxygen saturation monitoring equipment, oxygen and suction availability, manual resuscitator with appropriately sized face masks, emergency drugs, intubation supplies, and blood pressure monitoring equipment. Constant attention to the patient's respiratory status is maintained during the admission procedure. Medical and nursing procedures carried out on any infant in acute distress should be coordinated and modified to minimize stress that could lead to further compromise.

ADMISSION AND TRANSITION

Immediate assessment procedures include auscultation of cardiac and breath sounds as well as vital signs, including heart rate, respiratory rate, blood pressure, and temperature.

TABLE 3-2 ▲ Apgar Scoring Criteria

	Score		
Sign	0	1	2
Heart rate	Absent	Slow (<100 beats/minute)	>100 beats/minute
Respirations	Absent	Weak cry, hypoventilation	Good, strong cry
Muscle tone	Limp	Some flexion	Active motion
Reflex irritability (response to brisk slap on soles of feet)	No response	Grimace	Cough or sneeze
Color	Blue or pale	Body pink, extremities blue	Completely pink

From: Freeman RK, and Poland RL. 1992. *Guidelines for Perinatal Care,* 3rd ed. Elk Grove Village, Illinois: American Academy of Pediatrics, American College of Obstetricians and Gynecologists, 85. Reprinted by permission.

Blood glucose and hematocrit should be measured by the time the infant is one hour of age. Weight may be estimated if the infant is too compromised to tolerate the stressful weighing procedure. If the infant is weighed, the utmost care must be taken to ensure adequate ventilation and oxygenation during the process. Monitoring equipment (cardiorespiratory, temperature, and oxygen saturation) needs to be applied as quickly as is feasible.

Common sense can be used to determine which procedures can be delayed. Although measurements and gestational age assessment are vital pieces of information, they should not be obtained to the detriment of the patient. Table 3-4 provides a list of admitting procedures to be done within a reasonable time frame, patient status permitting.

The first six hours of life are a period of transition for the newborn. Some infants exhibit acute distress at delivery; others develop signs and symptoms of ineffective adaptation to extrauterine life over the first hours. Not every infant who exhibits difficulty during transition will require extraordinary supportive measures, but careful assessment and monitoring will ensure that supportive measures are in place when needed to prevent further infant

TABLE 3-3 ▲ Delivery Room Inspection of Infant

General: Inspect for asymmetry of growth, presence of major birth defects or birth marks, checking trunk front and back as well as extremities and spine. Note head shape, fontanels, and suture lines. Check genitalia for normalcy.

Neurologic: Note posture, activity, responsiveness.

Respiratory: Auscultate breath sounds, assessing air entry and equality. Inspect movement of the thorax and rate of respirations.

Cardiac: Note underlying skin color and assess perfusion. Auscultate cardiac sounds, noting rate, rhythm, and presence or absence of murmur. Note point of maximal impulse (PMI). Palpate brachial and femoral pulses.

Abdomen: Palpate for presence of kidneys and to rule out abdominal masses.

TABLE 3-4 ▲ Admission Procedures

- Weigh infant; measure head circumference and length.
- Obtain vital signs: temperature, heart rate, respiratory rate, blood pressure; measure serum glucose and hematocrit.
- Apply and calibrate monitoring equipment, including setting alarm limits.
- Implement priority orders, including medications and diagnostic studies.
- Obtain perinatal history, perform physical examination and gestational age assessment.

compromise. An awareness of "expected" behavior and clinical presentation can assist the nurse in identifying those infants who are not successfully adapting to extrauterine life.

Normal recovery from the birth process has been outlined by Desmond and coworkers, who describe a characteristic series of changes in vital signs and physical behavior during the first hours of life (Figure 3-2). A normal transition period can be divided into two major periods of reactivity:[3]

1. The first 60 minutes of life has been identified as a period of reactivity characterized by an alert infant, with eyes open, intense activity, and increased muscle tone. This initial period is followed by an unresponsive interval occurring between one and four hours of age and lasting two to four hours.

2. The infant then moves into a second period of reactivity and exhibits variable levels of

FIGURE 3-2 ▲ Newborn adaptations following birth.

Cardiovascular system Heart rate	Rapid Decreasing Regular Irregular Loud and forceful	Visible apical impulse		Labile			
Cord pulsation	Present Absent	Present		Cord oozing			
Color	Transient cyanosis/acrocyanosis	Flushing with cry		Swift changes in color			
Respiratory system	Rapid, shallow Rales and ronchi Flaring alae, grunting, or retraction	Clear "Barrelling" of chest		Variable rate, related to activity			
Mucus	Thin, clear small bubbles				Thick, yellowish		
Temperature	Falling		Low	Rising			
Neurologic system Activity Reactivity Tonus Posture	Eyes open First reactivity period Increased tonus Upper extremities flexed, lower extended	Intense alerting behavior Relatively unresponsive	First sleep Second reactivity period Relaxed in sleep	Variable Variable	(Gagging, swallowing)		
Bowel function Peristalsis Stools	Bowel sounds Abdomen Bowel sounds absent filling present Present at with air delivery	Visible peristalsis	Variable Meconium passage				
Age	Birth 15 Min	1 Hr 2 Hr	3 Hr 4 Hr	5 Hr 6 Hr			

From: Desmond MM, et al. 1963. The clinical behavior of the newly born. Part I: The term baby. *Journal of Pediatrics* 62(3): 311. Reprinted by permission.

responsiveness and a tendency toward increased muscle tone.

The immature infant will exhibit a prolonged period of unresponsiveness following the first period, with the second period of reactivity beginning at a later time. Drugs given to the mother prior to delivery also alter the time sequence, and infants requiring resuscitation exhibit a general neurologic decline, evidenced by hypotonia and decreased response to stimuli, following the first reactivity period.[3,4]

THERMOREGULATION

Excessive cooling or heating is detrimental to the neonate. Heat balance in the newborn is a result of internal heat production and heat supplied by external sources measured against heat loss.

A neonate has three basic methods of heat production, although they are not all fully developed or totally efficient:

1. Shivering. Shivering will produce heat through muscle activity; but the immature nervous system limits this reaction in the term infant, and it is not available to the preterm infant.

2. Voluntary muscle activity. The infant may generate heat by crying or moving, and heat loss is reduced by changing position to limit the exposed skin surface. This response is again limited in preterm or compromised infants, especially those who are sedated or physically restrained. A term newborn may become restless and increase muscular activity in response to cold stress, but a premature infant is likely to show little response or become hypotonic.

3. Metabolic heat production. The main method of heat production is chemical (non-shivering) thermogenesis. This requires an increase in the metabolic rate and increased oxygen consumption. Stimulation of thermal receptors in the skin, especially those located in the trigeminal region of the face, will result

in an increase in the metabolic rate. The central regulating mechanism for temperature control is situated in the hypothalamus. This control center can be impaired by various drugs and by conditions such as intracranial hemorrhage, gross cerebral malformation, trauma, and severe birth asphyxia.[5]

Brown adipose tissue (BAT), which is stored prenatally in the mediastinum, interscapular, paraspinal, and perirenal areas, is used initially as the fuel source. In response to cold stress, norepinephrine and thyroxine are released, resulting in metabolism of the BAT. Brown fat is rapidly metabolized for heat production. Metabolism of this tissue results in the breakdown of triglycerides into glycerol and free fatty acids. Because oxygen is required for the combustion of fatty acids to produce heat, hypoxia may adversely affect the process. Under conditions of stress, epinephrine is also released, activating the utilization of glycogen stores. Glycolysis may be inhibited, however, in the presence of lipolysis, which occurs during the utilization of brown fat.

Heat production abilities can be quickly exhausted in the term infant, and brown fat, once metabolized, is not replaced. Central nervous system damage, sedation, shock, hypoxia, and certain drugs will reduce the metabolic response to cold.[6] Premature infants have limited ability to increase their metabolic rate, have minimal brown fat and glycogen stores, and may have impaired oxygenation secondary to lung disease—all of which put them at increased risk for hypothermia.

HEAT LOSS

Thermoregulation is further complicated by the neonate's susceptibility to heat loss. The body surface is large when compared to total body mass, thereby accelerating heat loss. Heat reaches the body surfaces by direct conduction through body tissue or via the circulation. In the preterm infant, the insulation layer of

TABLE 3-5 ▲ Standard of Care for Thermoregulation[53-59]

Medical Diagnostic Category: Newborns and Other Neonates with Conditions Originating in the Perinatal Period
Medical Diagnosis: All
Nursing Diagnosis: Ineffective Thermoregulation Related to Developmental Immaturity

Related Factors/ Defining Characteristics	Expected Outcome	Nursing Interventions
Abnormal body temperature (normal axillary [ax] temperature of 36.3–37°C) Hypothermia: • Respiratory: increased oxygen needs, apnea, grunting, nasal flaring, tachypnea • Bradycardia • Hypoglycemia • Metabolic acidosis • Pallor, mottling, acrocyanosis • Lethargy, agitation • Feeding intolerance • Poor weight gain Hyperthermia: • Hypoxia • Metabolic acidosis • Peripheral vasodilation, flushing • Hypotension • Tachycardia • Tachypnea • Dehydration, elevated BUN • Poor weight gain • Seizures	Infant will be free of the signs or symptoms of altered thermoregulation as evidenced by ax temperature of 36.3–37°C Vital signs within normal limits for patient Oxygen saturations >85% Blood gases within indicated parameters No evidence of respiratory distress Serum electrolyte and fluid balance within normal limits Acceptable peripheral perfusion with urine output >2 ml/kg/hour Absence of lethargy or agitation Normal feeding pattern Growth within normal parameters as evidenced by growth chart	Maintain in stable thermal environment. Place in radiant warmer or double-walled incubator; set initial skin probe at 36.5°C for incubator and 37°C under warmer. Utilize equipment alarms and servocontrol skin probes; monitor skin probe values. Consult neutral thermal environment chart to estimate initial ambient temperature for incubator. Assess and document: • Temperature every 15–30 minutes until stable, then every 2–4 hours as indicated • Signs of alteration in thermoregulation, as per **Defining Characteristics** • Skin temperature, ambient temperature, and heater output; relate findings to axillary temperatures • Temperature of oxyhood or ventilator circuit if in use Monitor lab values for evidence of instability: elevated BUN, acidosis, hypo- or hyperglycemia. Weigh or bathe infant only if temperature is stable. To avoid hyperthermia: • Keep infant away from direct sunlight • Utilize skin probe to monitor temperature if phototherapy or heat light in use • Use blankets between heating pad and infant to avoid burns • Avoid overheating soaks or bath water • Avoid excess clothing • Check security of servocontrol probe To decrease **evaporative** heat loss: • Keep neonate dry; change wet linen promptly • Bathe under radiant warmer and in a draft-free environment • Cover with heat shield; or if in radiant warmer and intubated, cover with plastic film wrap blanket • Increase incubator humidity if needed for ELBW infants To decrease **convective** heat loss: • Use radiant overhead warmer for procedures • Use porthole sleeves on incubator • Use plastic film wrap stretched over side guards of radiant warmers, especially for the VLBW infant; keep side guards up • Transport infant in enclosed, warmed incubator • Keep infant away from air drafts To decrease **conductive** heat loss: • Prewarm linen and equipment that infant will be placed on • Utilize a warming mattress as needed; set at desired body temperature To decrease **radiant** heat loss: • Keep infant away from outside windows (or cold walls) • Use heat shield in incubator or line incubator with aluminum foil • Keep nursery environmental temperature at at least 75°F • Dress medically stable infants who are in incubators with hats, gowns, and booties Begin weaning to room environment by bundling and discontinuing skin servocontrol.

subcutaneous fat is thin, and the skin density is decreased, thereby allowing greater heat and evaporative water loss.[7,8]

Vasoconstriction of peripheral vessels will keep internal heat, generated by normal metabolic processes, from being lost to the external environment. However, this mechanism is compromised during periods of vasodilation associated with phases of shock and in the presence of certain autonomic drugs (i.e., Tolazoline), that produce vasodilation. Preterm infants have limited subcutaneous tissue to serve as a insulation layer, an extremely thin epidermal skin layer, and impaired ability to limit skin blood flow.

Heat is lost through four mechanisms:

- *Conduction* refers to heat transfer through solids, liquids, or gases; it is dependent on physical contact between surfaces of different temperatures. In the infant, heat from the body core is transferred to the body surface and then from the body surface to objects in contact with the skin.

- *Convection* refers to heat transfer via gas involving a mixing of cooler and warmer air, facilitated by air movement. Air molecules adjacent to the infant's skin are heated by the skin, and these heated molecules expand and diffuse away from the skin. Heat loss is accelerated by air currents.

- *Evaporation* refers to the heat taken from a surface that is required to change a given amount of liquid into a gas. Heat loss is similar to convection, but gas molecules transport water rather than kinetic energy. Heat loss is accelerated by low environmental humidity.

- *Radiation* refers to transmission of heat by electromagnetic waves from the surface of one mass to another; it requires no direct contact. Heat is transferred to cooler objects,

FIGURE 3-3 ▲ Physiologic consequences of cold stress.

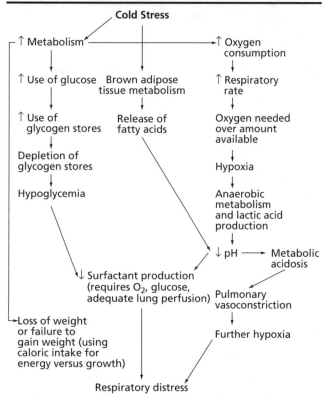

From: Blackburn ST, and Loper DL. 1992. Thermoregulation. In *Maternal, Fetal, and Neonatal Physiology: A Clinical Perspective.* Philadelphia: WB Saunders, 692. Reprinted by permission.

with the rate of transfer dependent on temperature gradient, distance, and surface area.

Practical application of these principles can be made to many aspects of nursing care and incorporated into a standard of care for thermoregulation (Table 3-5).

Ideally, infants will be maintained in environmental temperatures and conditions that permit maintenance of normal core temperature when oxygen consumption and metabolic rate at rest are minimal. This has been called the infant's neutral thermal environment, the components of which are environmental air temperature, radiant surfaces, ambient air flow, and relative humidity. Although environmental air temperature is usually easily monitored and maintained, factors such as temperature of radiant surfaces, air flow, and humidity are more difficult to assess and control. Because thermal

FIGURE 3-4 ▲ Neonatal morbidity by birth weight and age.

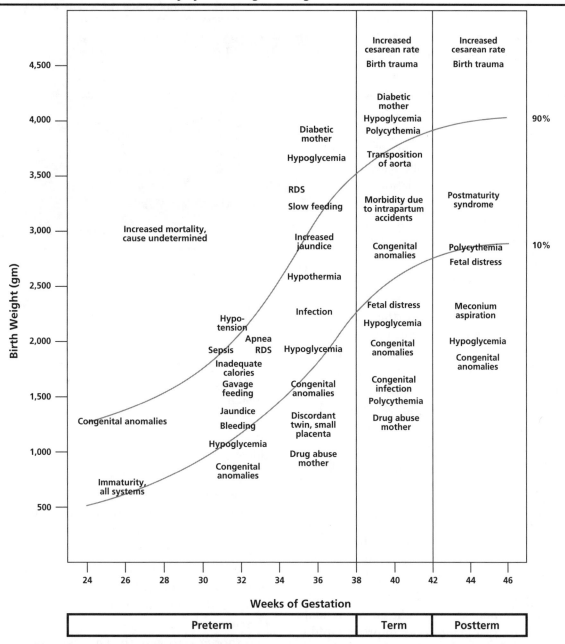

From: Lubchenco LO. 1976. *The High Risk Infant.* Philadelphia: WB Saunders, 122. Reprinted by permission.

needs vary with weight and gestational age, the proper neutral thermal environment for individual infants should be estimated from available graphs and then adjusted accordingly, with the goal of maintaining infant temperature between 36.3°C and 37°C.

THERMAL INSTABILITY

Thermal instability—whether hypothermia or hyperthermia—places the infant at risk for further complications, and diligent nursing care may markedly decrease the incidence of these complications. The cold-stressed infant, if capable, will increase his metabolic rate to produce heat, thereby increasing consumption of calories. Poor weight gain and hypoglycemia are consequences of this caloric consumption. The increased metabolic rate requires oxygen as fuel, and increased oxygen consumption may produce tissue hypoxia and a resultant metabolic acidosis. Secondary effects of cold stress include metabolic acidosis as a consequence of vasoconstriction and fat metabolism. Pulmonary vasoconstriction can occur, leading to further hypoxia, acidosis, and increasing severity of respiratory distress (Figure 3-3).

Although hypothermia is more common, hyperthermia may also occur very readily in the neonate. Hyperthermia is usually iatrogenic in etiology but may also be an indication of sepsis, dehydration, or neurologic compromise. Blood flow to the skin is increased during hyperthermia in an attempt by the overheated neonate to release heat. This can result in hypotension and increased insensible water loss leading to dehydration. Hyperthermia causes increased oxygen consumption and places the infant at risk for apnea and seizures.

Although term newborns have functioning sweat glands to assist with heat dissipation, infants less than 32 weeks gestation have virtually no ability to sweat. Infants between 32 and 37 weeks have limited ability, usually confined to the head and face. The functional ability of the sweat glands does improve rapidly with chronological age and matures rapidly during the first four weeks after birth.[5]

ASSESSMENT OF GESTATIONAL AGE

The American Academy of Pediatrics recommended in 1967 that newborns be classified by birth weight, gestational age, and intrauterine growth to identify existing or potential

FIGURE 3-5 ▲ **Three babies, same gestational age (32 weeks), weighing 600, 1,400, and 2,750 gm, respectively, from left to right.**

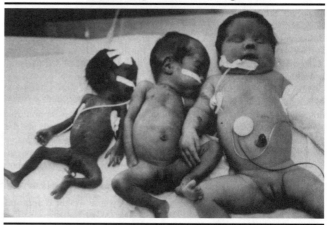

From Korones S. 1986. *High-Risk Newborn Infants,* 4th ed. St. Louis: Mosby-Year Book, 118. Reprinted by permission.

problems (Figure 3-4). Weight alone is an inadequate predictor of gestational age (Figure 3-5), and it is well recognized today that infants have unique problems or risk factors associated with gestational age, birth weight, or appropriateness of growth.

Clinical assessment tools have been developed to assist the clinician in estimating gestational age. In 1970, Dubowitz, Dubowitz, and Goldberg published an assessment tool incorporating both neurologic and physical criteria. Neurologic criteria are usually less biased than physical criteria by intrauterine growth retardation (IUGR) and birth weight, though they may be affected by central nervous system insult or trauma. Use of physical criteria alone may result in an overestimation of maturity in the presence of IUGR.[9]

A shorter version of the Dubowitz tool was developed by Ballard and coworkers, eliminating the more stressful maneuvers of the neuromuscular examination.[10,11] The most current revision of the Ballard Maturational Score may be used on newborns as young as 20 weeks gestation (Figure 3-6).

Numerous other versions of gestational age assessment tools are available, but the criteria

FIGURE 3-6 ▲ Ballard maturational score.

Neuromuscular Maturity

Neuromuscular Maturity Sign	Score							Record Score Here
	−1	0	1	2	3	4	5	
Posture								
Square Window (Wrist)	>90°	90°	60°	45°	30°	0°		
Arm Recoil		180°	140°–180°	110°–140°	90°–110°	<90°		
Popliteal Angle	180°	160°	140°	120°	100°	90°	<90°	
Scarf Sign								
Heel to Ear								
						Total Neuromuscular Maturity Score		

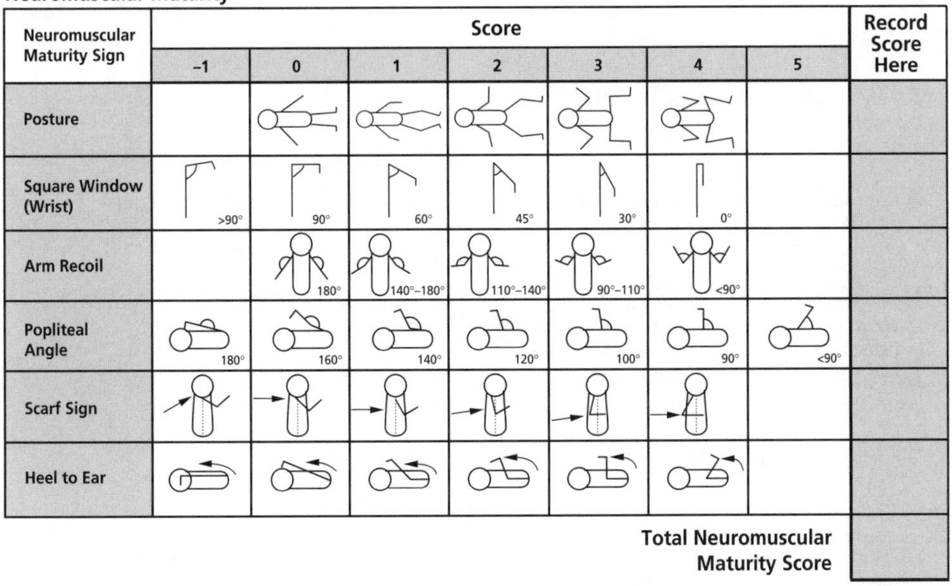

Maturity Rating

Score	Weeks
−10	20
−5	22
0	24
5	26
10	28
15	30
20	32
25	34
30	36
35	38
40	40
45	42
50	44

Physical Maturity

Physical Maturity Sign	Score							Record Score Here
	−1	0	1	2	3	4	5	
Skin	sticky friable transparent	gelatinous red translucent	smooth pink visible veins	superficial peeling and/or rash, few veins	cracking pale areas rare veins	parchment deep cracking no vessels	leathery cracked wrinkled	
Lanugo	none	sparse	abundant	thinning	bald areas	mostly bald		
Plantar Surface	heel-toe 40–50 mm:-1 <40 mm:-2	>50 mm no crease	faint red marks	anterior transverse crease only	creases anterior 2/3	creases over entire sole		
Breast	imperceptible	barely perceptible	flat areola no bud	stippled areola 1–2 mm bud	raised areola 3–4 mm bud	full areola 5–10 mm bud		
Eye/Ear	lids fused loosely: -1 tightly: -2	lids open pinna flat stays folded	sl. curved pinna; soft; slow recoil	well-curved pinna; soft but ready recoil	formed and firm; instant recoil	thick cartilage ear stiff		
Genitals (Male)	scrotum flat, smooth	scrotum empty faint rugae	testes in upper canal rare rugae	testes descending few rugae	testes down good rugae	testes pendulous deep rugae		
Genitals (Female)	clitoris prominent and labia flat	prominent clitoris and small labia minora	prominent clitoris and enlarging minora	majora and minora equally prominent	majora large minora small	majora cover clitoris and minora		
						Total Physical Maturity Score		

From: Ballard JL, et al. 1991. New Ballard score, expanded to include extremely premature infants. *Journal of Pediatrics* 119(3): 418. Reprinted by permission.

FIGURE 3-7 ▲ Finnstrom's gestational age assessment criteria.

Criteria	Score				Total
	1	**2**	**3**	**4**	
Breast size, transverse diameter	Less than 5 mm	5 to 10 mm	More than 10 mm		
Nipple formation by inspection	Barely visible, no areola	Nipple well defined, areola not raised	Nipple well defined, edge of areola raised above the skin		
Skin opacity by inspection of abdomen	Numerous veins, tributaries and venules seen clearly	Veins and tributaries seen	Few large vessels seen	Few large vessels indistinct or no vessels seen	
Scalp hair by inspection	Fine, woolly or fuzzy; strands indistinct	Coarse and silky; each hair appears as a single strand			
Ear cartilage by palpation	No cartilage in antitragus	Cartilage in antitragus	Cartilage in antihelix	Cartilage formation complete in helix	
Fingernails by inspection and palpation	Nails do not reach fingertips	Nails reach fingertips	Nails reach or pass fingertips, edge distinct and relatively firm		
Plantar skin creases by inspection of broad creases	No skin creases present	Anterior transverse creases only	Occasional creases in anterior two-thirds	Whole sole covered with creases	

Gestational age (physical exam)_____   **Total Score_____**

Appropriateness of growth SGA/AGA/LGA

Adapted from: Finnstrom O. 1977. Studies on maturity in newborn infants. Part IX: Further observations on the use of external characteristics in estimating gestational age. *Acta Paediatrica Scandinavica* 66(5): 601–604. Reprinted by permission.

defined by Finnstrom (Figures 3-7 and 3-7A) may be the most useful for assessing critically ill infants who cannot tolerate the manipulation required for neuromuscular assessment.[12,13]

Gestational age assessment should be performed as soon as feasible because early, accurate identification of infants at risk is essential. The results of even a properly done gestational age examination can vary approximately two weeks (plus or minus) from actual gestation. Despite this limitation, it remains a valuable tool. This assessment is usually not as urgent when the mother has received early and continuous prenatal care. Ultrasound dating, especially when it is done during the first or second trimester, provides very accurate dating.

OVERALL CLINICAL ASSESSMENT

Particular attention should be paid to the infant's clinical presentation. Presenting clinical

FIGURE 3-7A ▲ Transforming maturity score to gestational age (days).

Maturity Score (7 criteria)	Gestational Age in Days
7	191
8	198
9	204
10	211
11	217
12	224
13	230
14	237
15	243
16	250
17	256
18	263
19	269
20	276
21	282
22	289
23	295

From: Finnstrom O. 1977. Studies on maturity in newborn infants. Part IX: Further observations on the use of external characteristics in estimating gestational age. *Acta Paediatrica Scandinavica* 66(5): 602. Reprinted by permission.

signs may indicate the etiology of the respiratory distress, and sequential monitoring traces the progression of the respiratory disease. An orderly approach to physical examination provides a consistent, complete assessment.

Assessment interventions must be tempered by an appreciation of the infant's tolerance for such stressful procedures. Any critically ill infant should be monitored with transcutaneous PaO_2 or pulse oximetry to assist in assessing tolerance. Some clinicians prefer to group their caregiving tasks; others space them, assuming that the stress is decreased. The superiority of either method is unclear, but it is certain that the infant should be allowed to recover from any procedure, as evidenced by normalization of transcutaneous oxygen value ($TcPO_2$), pulse oximetry saturation (SpO_2), or heart rate and color, before further stressful procedures are implemented. Evaluation of the infant's tolerance following care measures should guide the caregiver's subsequent approach to interventions with that individual infant.

TABLE 3-6 ▲ **History and Physical**

History	
Maternal:	
Age, gravida, para (term and preterm delivery), abortions, living children	
Blood type, antibody screening (including syphillis and hepatitis B), GBS (vaginal culture), chlamydia	
Complications of pregnancy, recent infections	
Labor and Delivery:	
Labor spontaneous or induced; complications of labor, fetal monitoring	
Rupture of membranes: hours prior to delivery, character of fluid	
Medications given	
Fetal presentation, delivery—vaginal or cesarean section (indication); use of forceps	
Apgar at 1, 5, 10 minutes (if indicated); specify lost points	
Resuscitation measures required	
Family:	
Mother/father: married, single, cohabitating, apart, father in contact	
Environment: living arrangements, telephone	

Physical Examination	
Vital signs:	Temperature (axillary)
	Pulse
	Respirations
	BP (central or peripheral, four limbs)
	Blood glucose
	Hematocrit
General:	Resting posture, activity, gross abnormality or overt distress, color
Skin:	Condition, texture, lanugo, vernix; note meconium staining, jaundice, hemangioma, nevi, rash, excoriation, petechiae, bruises
Head:	General shape; note molding, caput, cephalhematoma, craniotabes; sutures, fontanels (anterior and posterior); hair texture, abnormal hair whorls
Eyes:	Size or shape of eyes, clarity of lenses, reactivity of pupils; note hemorrhage, edema, discharge
Nose:	Shape, patency; note drainage, flaring of nasal alae
Ears:	Cartilaginous development, position of ear lobe, shape of auricle
Mouth:	Palate, tongue (size), lips and mucous membranes (color)
Neck:	Trachea position, movement, note masses
Chest:	Clavicles, symmetry; diameter of breast buds; note retractions, abnormal rate or respiratory pattern
Lungs:	Breath sounds, equality, character; note grunt, crackles, rhonchi, wheezes, stridor
Cardiovascular system:	Point of maximal impulse, heart rhythm and rate; murmur (quality, radiation, location of intensity); peripheral pulses—femoral, brachial, radial (equality); peripheral perfusion
Abdomen:	Shape, muscle tone, number of umbilical vessels, size of liver; note any masses palpated
Genitourinary System:	Female: note discharge, abnormalities in voiding Male: Urethral meatus patency and position; testicular descent and scrotal development (rugae); note hernia or hydrocele, abnormalities in voiding
Anus:	Patency, stools
Extremities:	Symmetry, range of motion; number, shape, length of digits; length of nails; palmar creases
Spine:	Alignment; note sacral dimple, scoliosis, myelomeningocele
Neurologic System:	Tone, responsiveness, cry (character, intensity, frequency); behavior (alertness, irritability); reflexes (suck, grasp, Moro); note tremors, paralysis (facial, brachial, lower extremities)

TABLE 3-7 ▲ Silverman-Andersen Retraction Score

Stage 0	Stage 1	Stage 2
Upper chest and abdomen rise synchronously	Lag or minimal sinking of upper chest as abdomen rises	"See-saw" sinking of upper chest with rising abdomen
No intercostal sinking on inspiration	Just visible sinking of intercostal spaces on inspiration	Marked sinking of intercostal spaces on inspiration
No xiphoid retraction	Just visible xiphoid retraction	Marked xiphoid retractions
No nasal flaring	Nasal flaring minimal	Marked nasal flaring
No expiratory grunt	Expiratory grunt heard with stethoscope only	Expiratory grunt heard with naked ear

Modified from: Silverman WA, and Andersen DH. 1956. A controlled clinical trial of effects of water mist on obstructive respiratory signs, death rate, and necropsy findings among premature infants. *Pediatrics* 17(1): 1–10. Reprinted by permission.

Initial assessment procedures in the nursery are essential to establish a baseline of information. Because this is often the patient's first complete physical examination, each nursing unit needs an established format for this procedure (Table 3-6). The useful nursing admission note will be exact, including name, age, sex, admitting diagnosis, mode of admission, pertinent findings from the examinations, and any significant perinatal history. All of the data will be used to prepare a nursing plan of care for the neonate.

CLINICAL ASSESSMENT OF RESPIRATORY STATUS

Clinical assessment of the infant's respiratory status begins with basic observation. Color is judged, looking at generalized color as well as that of the oral mucous membranes. Cyanosis is a blue discoloration of the skin, nail beds, and mucous membranes resulting from hemoglobin that is unsaturated or not carrying a maximum amount of oxygen. Fetal hemoglobin, which makes up the majority of the newborn's hemoglobin, is easily saturated with oxygen but does not release oxygen as readily as adult hemoglobin does. High saturations are thus associated with lower PaO_2 levels. In the newborn infant, clinical cyanosis does not occur until severe hypoxia is present.

The presence of oral or nasal secretions is noted. Chest movement is evaluated, includ-ing depth of respirations, symmetry, and synchrony. The rate of respiration is counted for a full minute. Tachypnea is the most frequent indicator of respiratory disease, although an infant in severe respiratory failure may exhibit slow, gasping respiration or experience episodes of apnea.

Because the infant's cartilage is soft, airway resistance or lung disease may produce visible retractions. Retractions can be intercostal (between the ribs) or subcostal (immediately below the rib cage). Sternal as well as suprasternal and subxiphoid retractions may be present. Severe lung or airway resistance can also produce "see-saw" respirations, characterized by a collapsing chest and a rising abdomen on inspiration. Nasal flaring may also be identified during inspiration. Flaring is the result of widening of the nasal alae in an attempt to decrease upper airway resistance.

Auscultation is performed to determine air movement and the quality of breath sounds. Grunting, a sound produced when air is exhaled against a partially closed glottis, may be audible without the aid of a stethoscope. This maneuver delays expiration and increases gas exchange by increasing end-expiratory pressure and lung volume.

Auscultation of the chest should progress in an orderly manner, with the examiner comparing and contrasting each side of the chest for equality of breath sounds. Because sound is easily transmitted through the small chest of the newborn, the clinician has to be able to identify subtle differences, assessing and documenting the presence of crackles (coarse or fine), wheezes, grunting, or other extraneous sounds.

A scale (Silverman-Andersen) has been developed to provide an objective means of assessing the progression or improvement of respiratory distress (Table 3-7). This scale is especially useful in assisting the novice during a complete evaluation. As experience is gained in caring for the critically ill neonate, the nurse will be able to recognize patterns of clinical signs and symptoms associated with specific disease states. For example, a round barrel chest is seen with volume trapping (obstructive) disorders such as transient tachypnea of the newborn and meconium aspiration syndrome; retractions and hypoexpansion are present with restrictive (atelectatic) disease such as respiratory distress syndrome (hyaline membrane disease). (Chapter 2 discusses pathophysiology and clinical presentation more specifically.)

Although nursing care will depend on the infant's clinical diagnosis, each unit is responsible for developing a standard of care for the infant experiencing respiratory distress. Table 3-8 provides an example of a standard of nursing care that can be generalized to this patient group. Utilization of such standards of care provides a knowledge base for the nursing and medical staff as well as documentation of minimum care requirements. The individual patient's care plan is based on those established standards for that patient's diagnosis, but this information need not be rewritten on the care plan itself. Instead, the patient's care plan can be used for communicating information unique to that individual patient that falls outside the established standards of care.

INTERPRETATION OF BLOOD GASES

An adjunct to clinical assessment of respiratory disease is chemical assessment via blood gases. The medical plan of care for the patient includes the frequency of blood gas determinations, and it is the responsibility of every nurse to be cognizant of each blood gas sample drawn on her patients. The nurse also needs to be aware of the status of the patient prior to obtaining the sample to assist in the interpretation of the blood gases obtained.

Assessment of any abnormalities identified and institution of treatment is often the responsibility of the staff nurse or respiratory therapist, working within the parameters established by the physician. Although the etiology of abnormalities can be complex and multifactorial, the nurse must have a basic knowledge of acid-base disorders in order to interpret blood gases. Chapter 8 discusses blood gas interpretation and oxygen saturation in the neonate.

RADIOLOGY OF THE NEONATAL CHEST

Radiographic examination is a medical standard of care for the neonate with respiratory distress. The frequency of such examinations is at the discretion of the physician, but in an emergency the nurse is often the first health care worker available to view the film. On transport it is usually the responsibility of the primary transport nurse to interpret available films.

The nurse's responsibility begins with the x-ray examination itself and includes an awareness of appropriate technique. Proper technique includes using the collimator light to identify the x-ray field and then tightly coning down the field size to provide a better quality film as well as reducing radiation scatter. A properly positioned cassette with appropriate coning will expose only those structures that are to be evaluated. Nursing responsibility includes placing a small lead shield over the infant's reproductive organs to further limit radiation exposure and assuring that such objects as shields, which touch the infant, are cleaned properly if used for other patients.

TABLE 3-8 ▲ Standard of Care for Infant with Respiratory Distress[60-62]

Medical Diagnostic Category: Newborns and other neonates with conditions originating in the perinatal period

Medical Diagnosis: Respiratory distress syndrome, transient tachypnea of the newborn, meconium aspiration syndrome, pneumonia, congenital diaphragmatic hernia, persistent pulmonary hypertension of the newborn

Collaborative Problem	Expected Outcome	Nursing Interventions
Respiratory insufficiency	Normal blood gases maintained	Administer ventilation and monitor parameters. Administer muscle relaxants and sedation as ordered. Administer exogenous surfactant as ordered. Maintain normothermia.
Fluid and electrolyte balance/nutrition	Normal fluid and electrolyte balance maintained	Administer parenteral and enteral fluids as ordered. Monitor glucose, electrolyte, and hematocrit values. Weigh and measure growth parameters as required.
Infection	Infection treated appropriately	Administer antibiotics as ordered. Monitor culture reports and complete blood cell count (CBC) results.

Nursing Diagnosis: Impaired gas exchange

Related Factors/ Defining Characteristics	Expected Outcome	Nursing Interventions
Respiratory distress: Grunting, flaring, retractions, apnea, tachypnea Abnormal breath sounds: Crackles, rhonchi, wheezes, stridor, decreased, absent, unequal Cyanosis, pallor Tachycardia, bradycardia Abnormal blood gases, transcutaneous CO_2/O_2, or oxygen saturation	Infant will maintain adequate gas exchange during acute phase as evidenced by: Blood gases within stated parameters Adequate and appropriate breath sounds Lack of cyanosis Oxygen saturation $\geq 88\%$ Vital signs within normal parameters	Assess blood gases: Assess ventilation ($PaCO_2/PaO_2$) and acid-base balance ($pH/HCO_3/PaCO_2$). Follow serially to detect deterioration: acidosis, hypoxia, hypercapnea. Notify MD if deterioration. Assess and document every two hours: Breath sounds. Vital signs. Ventilatory/oxygen parameters and alarm limits; oxygen saturation. Signs of impaired gas exchange secondary to extubation, pulmonary air leak, ventilator malfunction. Assess response to muscle relaxants, note: Duration of effect. Change in cardiovascular or pulmonary status. Need for continuation of paralysis. Minimize handling to prevent hypoxia, use readings from pulse oximeter to modify care. Explain treatment rationale to infant's family.

Nursing Diagnosis: Ineffective airway clearance

Related Factors/ Defining Characteristics	Expected Outcome	Nursing Interventions
Presence of endotracheal tube, nasal prongs, nasal pharyngeal tube Excessive amounts of mucus Atelectasis on chest film Abnormal breath sounds Cyanosis Hypercapnia	Clear airway will be maintained as evidenced by: Clear and equal breath sounds Lack of respiratory difficulty Normal blood gases	Ensure that chest physiotherapy treatments and administration of aerosol medications are done on schedule. Follow two-person suctioning procedure for endotracheal tube; individualize to prevent hypoxia. Suction nares PRN when utilizing nasal prongs or nasal pharyngeal tube. Reposition infant every two hours as tolerated. Place small roll under neck to promote maintainance of airway. Report absent or unequal breath sounds, tenacious secretions, or clinical deterioration.

The NICU staff nurse should have the basic knowledge necessary to recognize acute or dramatic changes in the infant's x-ray film and to convey this information to the physician if he or she is not immediately available to view the films. The best way for nurses to develop this skill is through consistent exposure to the diagnostic interpretation of such films. Attending radiographic rounds, if the unit has them, is an excellent way to gain such exposure.

Interpretation of the x-ray film requires a systematic approach, beginning with evaluation of the quality of the film. Exposure, seen as density and contrast, is noted. Overpenetration results in a dark film, with the infant's lungs appearing hyperlucent or overaerated. Underpenetration produces a "white" film, giving the false impression of atelectasis or hypoexpansion.

Density and contrast can be evaluated by looking at the appearance of the stomach, which is usually partially filled with air, providing a baseline for comparison. The technician documents on each film the settings used when obtaining that film. Use of consistent settings, with appropriate modification of the technique, is the best means of obtaining quality films.

Film interpretation continues with a survey of the infant's positioning. Rotation, if any, should be identified. On a nonrotated film, the ribs appear of equal length on either side of the vertebral column, and the clavicles appear symmetric. A rotated film will skew the appearance of the lung fields and prevent the evaluation of a mediastinal shift. One side may falsely appear atelectatic, and the heart may obscure the left lung field.

If the area to be exposed is not perpendicular to the beam from the x-ray tube, an oblique view will be obtained. Such a film would slant all structures and misrepresent positioning of indwelling tubes and lines. With proper angulation the clavicles will be at a 90 degree angle to the vertebral column. Errors can be avoided by proper positioning of the infant, who should be held flat and prevented from rolling to one side or the other. If the infant is to be held during the procedure, the staff member must wear a lead apron, and the staff member's hand must be coned out of the field.

Motion during the film could make assessment of the lung fields inaccurate. Evidence of motion is best detected by the blurring of normally distinct structures such as electrocardiograph lead wires.

Next the film should be evaluated for extraneous objects that may prevent interpretation or lead to a false conclusion. Radiopaque objects will appear clearly on the film and are thus easily identified. If possible, these objects should be removed from the field prior to the x-ray study to prevent an obstruction of body structures. Electrocardiograph leads, temperature probes, and transcutaneous sensors will block viewing of structures and should be moved, if feasible. For an anterior-posterior chest film, it is best to place electrocardiograph leads in the axillary line and to place skin sensors on the shoulder or abdomen.

Nonradiopaque objects will not appear clearly on the film but will leave shadows that may be difficult to differentiate from pathologic findings in the chest. Warming mattresses produce a waffle-like appearance that prevents any realistic interpretation of the film. Bunched linen or plastic tubings lying under or over the infant will produce extraneous lines. Incubator tops often have a small hole used for the insertion of tubings into the incubator. If an x-ray film is shot through this Plexiglas top, a small, circular bleb may appear on the film. Skin folds may be falsely interpreted as a pneumothorax. These are best identified on the film by following the skin fold line outside the thoracic cavity.

After the film has been assessed for technical difficulties, a clinical examination can be started. Air or gas is radiolucent and leaves a dark gray or black image. Tissue and water have increased density and are therefore more radiopaque with a lighter image. Bone and metal, with the highest density, will leave a light gray or white image.

FIGURE 3-8 ▲ Sketch showing the method for determining the cardiac-to-thoracic ratio.

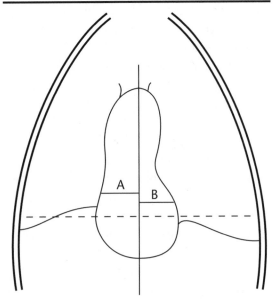

The sum of the horizontal projections from the vertical line (lines marked A and B) is the transverse diameter of the heart. The dotted line is the greatest internal diameter of the chest. The ratio between the transverse cardiac diameter and the internal diameter of the chest is the cardiac-to-thoracic ratio.

Adapted from: Crummy AB. 1987. The cardiovascular system. In *Paul and Juhl's Essentials of Radiologic Imaging*, Juhl J, and Crummy A, eds. Philadelphia: JB Lippincott, 974–976. Reprinted by permission.

Examine the film systematically:

1. **Evaluate heart size, position, and shape**. Cardiac borders should be clear and distinct. The cardiac silhouette of the newborn is large, especially in the first 24 hours of life. Cardiac size is estimated by determining the cardiothoracic ratio. The longest horizontal diameter of the heart is divided by the greatest internal diameter of the chest (Figure 3-8). The heart will normally measure half the distance of the thorax, with a cardiothoracic ratio of 0.5, although the ratio in normal newborns may be slightly larger. This measurement, used to determine cardiomegaly, is further limited in the neonate because a large thymic shadow or areas of atelectasis will create a generous cardiac sil-

houette that may exceed this ratio. An expiratory film will do likewise.[14]

Cardiomegaly is seen in infants with volume overload, and an extremely small silhouette will be seen in infants who are hypovolemic or dehydrated or who have high intrathoracic pressure that is causing decreased venous return. Initially the apex of the heart is elevated secondary to right ventricular hypertrophy associated with fetal circulation. Because the left ventricle predominates in extrauterine life, the cardiac apex will descend caudally. The configuration is affected by the size of the thymus, but abnormal shapes still can be seen with various congenital heart diseases. A globular shape is seen with hypoplastic left heart or coarctation of the aorta, an egg shape is seen with transposition of the great vessels, and a boot shape is seen with tetralogy of Fallot.

2. **Evaluate the mediastinum.** The space between the lungs contains esophagus, trachea, thymus, heart, and major vessels. Displacement of the mediastinum is associated with free air in the pleural space.

3. **Survey the lung fields.** Pulmonary expansion can be determined by locating the level of the diaphragm. The right diaphragm is normally slightly higher than the left because of the liver. During inspiration, the dome of the right hemidiaphragm will usually move to the level of the eighth rib or below. The diaphragm will be higher if the lungs are severely hypoventilated or if the film was taken during the expiratory phase. Overinflated lungs appear hyperlucent, with their normally domed diaphragms flattened.

4. **Determine the aeration of the lungs.** Are they clear (dark) or opaque (white)? Is there evidence of granularity, seen as coarseness or a "ground glass" appearance? Are there areas of streaking, haziness, or consolidation? Lung tissue should extend fully to the pleura.

TABLE 3-9 ▲ Disorders Indicated by Abnormal X-Ray Patterns

Granular: hyaline membrane disease, TTN, neonatal pneumonitis (especially Group B Streptococcus)

Bubbly: hyaline membrane disease with overdistended terminal airways (associated with mechanical ventilation), pulmonary interstitial emphysema, bronchopulmonary dysplasia, Wilson-Mikity syndrome

Opaque: absent or greatly reduced FRC, pulmonary hemorrhage, bilateral chylothorax or hydrothorax

Vascular Congestion: TTN, congenital heart disease >12 hours of age, myocardial dysfunction with congestive heart failure

Infiltrate: pulmonary infections (viral and bacterial), meconium aspiration, amniotic fluid aspiration, segmental atelectasis, pulmonary hemorrhage, vascular congestion secondary to cardiac disease, TTN, early Wilson-Mikity syndrome

Hazy: underaeration, pulmonary edema, healing phase of hyaline membrane disease, bilateral diaphragmatic paralysis

Overaerated, Clear: hyperventilation, congenital heart disease with decreased pulmonary vascularity, central obstructing lesions (vascular ring or mediastinal mass)

Unequal Aeration: mucus plugging or improper placement of endotracheal tube, unilateral pulmonary hypoplasia, congenital lobar emphysema

Hyperlucent: pulmonary air leak

Adapted from: Swischuk LE. 1986. Radiology of pulmonary insufficiency. In *Neonatal Pulmonary Care*, Thibeault D, and Gregory G, eds. Norwalk, Connecticut: Appleton & Lange, 235–279.

Hyperlucency (extremely clear) areas over the entire lung or at its margins may indicate a pneumothorax (free air in the thoracic cavity surrounding the lung). A decubitus film (obtained by placing the unaffected side down and taking the film as an anteroposterior penetration) will more clearly define a pneumothorax because the free air will rise to the upmost area. Free air in the mediastinal area, called a pneumomediastinum, will outline the thymus, producing a sail or butterfly appearance. A pneumopericardium (free air around the heart) will be seen as a complete halo encircling the heart.

5. **Assess pulmonary vascularity**. Vascular markings branch in a treelike fashion from the hilum, decreasing in size as they extend through the lung fields. The margins should be sharp. Hazy, indistinct margins suggest early pulmonary interstitial edema. Decreased pulmonary vascularity suggests persistent pulmonary hypertension of the newborn with a right-to-left shunt, or congenital heart disease with obstructed pulmonary blood flow.

Table 3-9 lists the classical radiographic findings associated with the major neonatal respiratory pathologies. Because many of the abnormalities have similar radiographic findings, a knowledge of the patient's history and clinical presentation is essential. A basic competence in x-ray film interpretation and familiarity with associated respiratory pathophysiology will be of invaluable assistance to the nurse in providing the appropriate patient care—including the ability to knowledgeably communicate patient status to the physician.

ROUTINE CARE

After the admission of the infant, a routine should be established regarding the frequency of assessment. Table 3-10 provides an example of routine nursing orders for the critically ill patient. Premature infants often tolerate handling poorly, so the relative importance of all interventions has to be weighed against their potential disturbance of the patient.

Monitoring vital signs does not necessarily mean that the baby must be disturbed. Heart rate, blood pressure, and skin temperature values can usually be obtained from monitoring equipment. At least once each shift, verify the monitored vital signs by counting pulse and respirations for one minute, and correlate direct blood pressure readings with an indirect (cuff pressure) reading method.

The nurse is responsible for verifying the proper functioning of all monitoring equipment, setting appropriate alarm limits for the patient, and analyzing the information gathered for significant changes. The nurse reviews

TABLE 3-10 ▲ Nursing Care Guidelines for Critically Ill Infants

Vital Signs

1. Temperature (axillary), pulse, and respirations:
   - every 1 hour or more frequently on critically unstable infants
   - every 2–3 hours on all mechanically ventilated, CPAP, or oxyhood patients
   - every 3–4 hours on stable infants not in supplemental oxygen
2. Record blood pressure every 1 hour on all infants with arterial lines (lines must be recalibrated every 12 hours and should be correlated with an indirect, peripheral BP measurement)
3. Take peripheral BP (documenting extremity used):
   - every 4 hours on all acute care infants without arterial lines
   - every 12 hours on all infants
4. Record oxygen saturation:
   - every 1 hour or more frequently on unstable infants

Laboratory tests

1. Hematocrit (label as central or peripheral):
   - On admission and every 8 hours on all unstable infants
   - Daily on stable NICU patients; extending to twice weekly when out of supplemental oxygen
2. Blood glucose:
   - On admission and every 1–2 hours until stable (60–150 mg %)
   - every 8 hours on NPO patients
   - every 12 hours while patient on IV fluids
3. Urine specific gravity, pH, glucose, protein (reagent strip):
   - every 12 hours on all patients receiving parenteral fluids

Intake and Output

1. Compute every 8–12 hours
2. Calculate urine output (ml/kg/hour) every 4–8 hours if urine output low or excessively high
3. Record all fluid intake, including medications, flush solution used, and blood products
4. Record all output, including urine, blood, stool, gastric output, and drainage

and interprets changes in vital signs, evaluates temperature fluctuations and thermal environment, calculates urine output (ml/kg/hour), and compares fluid intake with output. Normal parameters for vital signs are as follows:

- Temperature (axillary): 36.3°–37°C
- Heart rate:
  80–160 beats/minute (term infant)
  120–160 beats/minute (preterm infant)

- Respiratory rate: 30–60 breaths/minute
- Blood pressure (term infant):
  Systolic 50–70 mmHg, increasing by four days of age to 60–90 mmHg
  Diastolic 25–45 mmHg, with a slight rise by four days of age

A rule of thumb for premature infants is to use their gestational age as a guideline for minimal mean blood pressure in the first few days of life. For example, a 26-week infant should have a mean BP of at least 26 torr and a 34-week infant should have a mean BP of at least 34 torr (Figure 3-9).

The nurse also reviews hematocrit and serum glucose values, urine checks (specific gravity, glucose, protein, pH), stool checks (occult blood, reducing substance), acid-base status, recent laboratory studies, and outstanding laboratory test results. Each NICU should have available to the nursing staff a listing of normal laboratory values specific for its hospital's laboratory. These values, properly interpreted, along with sound nursing judgment of overall status, can provide an accurate picture of the neonate's clinical condition.

ADMINISTRATION OF MEDICATION

A major nursing responsibility is the prompt and accurate administration of medication. Dosages of drugs given to the neonate are based on body weight, and each nurse must be capable of calculating such doses. Because doses and volumes are relatively small, extreme care is needed in the preparation and administration of medications. Complicating this are the patient's possible fluid restriction and dependence on a continuous infusion of glucose. Drugs infused over several minutes or hours should be mixed with glucose solutions when compatible to provide optimal calories.

The literature is rich with information on drug doses, routes, and intervals but often lacks the necessary information on minimum dilution volumes, administration rates, and drug

FIGURE 3-9 ▲ Systolic, diastolic, mean, and pulse pressures for newborns (based on birth weight) during the first 12 hours of life.

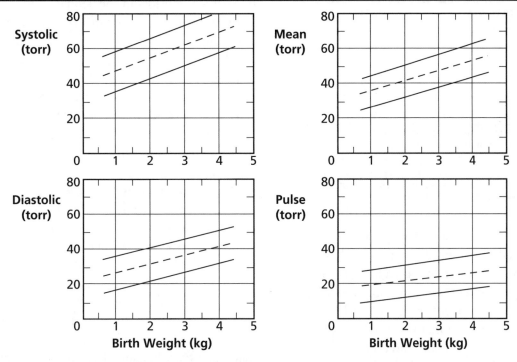

Linear regressions (broken lines) and 95% confidence limits (solid lines) of systolic (top left) and diastolic (bottom left) aortic blood pressures and mean pressure (top right) and pulse pressure (bottom right) on birth weight in healthy newborn infants during the first 12 hours after birth.

Adapted from: Versmold HT, et al. 1981. Aortic blood pressure during the first 12 hours of life in infants 610 to 4,220 grams. *Pediatrics* 67(5): 611. Reprinted by permission.

compatibilities. Table 3-11 is a protocol sheet listing the information that should be available to the nurse for every drug administered in the NICU.

FLUID REQUIREMENTS

Infants in respiratory distress are usually managed initially with intravenous fluids. Umbilical catheters and percutaneously inserted intravenous catheters are used. Central venous lines may be utilized if prolonged parenteral fluids are required. Nursing personnel are responsible for ongoing assessment of these fluids, to assure both accuracy of infusion rates and patency of the line. Intravenous infiltrates or catheter accidents result in major iatrogenic complications.

Fluid requirements vary with gestational and chronological age. Table 3-12 illustrates how fluid requirements are calculated for the term infant. Fluid is required to replace water retained for growth and water lost in urine,

TABLE 3-11 ▲ Protocol of Essential Drug Information

Name: Generic name with trade names (indexed by both names)

Indication/Action: Class, indication/action of drug

Dose/Route/Interval: Dose (listed by single dose, not by total daily dose), route, and interval of administration

Preparation: Type of fluid for reconstitution and for dilution; preferred fluids listed first (see drug label for reconstitution instructions)

Administration Rate: Desired rate of administration

Other Pertinent Information: Drug levels, side effects, antidotes, incompatibilities, etc.

TABLE 3-12 ▲ Estimated Fluid Requirement for Term Infants

To Replace Loss by	ml/kg
Insensible water loss	15–20
Urine	60–90
Stool*	10
Growth*	10–15
Water of oxidation	−15
Total	80–120

*On day 1 of life, these values should be zero, rising to the stated numbers by day 3.

From: Wassner SJ. 1990. Fluid therapy. In *Current Therapy in Neonatal-Perinatal Medicine,* part II, Nelson N, ed. Toronto: BC Decker, 153. Reprinted by permission of Mosby-Year Book.

stool, and other body drainage such as gastro-intestinal or wound drainage as well as fluid lost from the respiratory tract and via the skin (insensible water loss). Insensible water loss is especially significant in the infant because it increases proportionally as birth weight and gestational age decrease, and 80 ml fluid/kg or more may be lost through the skin each day in an infant less than 30 weeks gestation.[15] Table 3-13 lists factors that can increase or decrease insensible water loss in the neonate.

During the first week of life, physiologic extracellular dehydration normally causes a 5–20 percent weight loss. A higher fraction of weight loss is experienced by smaller, more preterm infants because of their proportionately larger extracellular water (59 percent of body weight at 24 weeks gestation compared to 44 percent at term) and greater tissue catabolism.[16]

Fluid requirements increase with postnatal age and the introduction of enteral feedings. Fecal water losses are greater and urine output increases in response to the increased renal solute load when feedings begin. Oxidation of metabolic fuels (carbohydrates, fats, and protein) results in a gain in fluid as some water is generated by cells as a by-product of cell metabolism, but this is offset by the deposit of water in tissue associated with growth. Clinical assessment of hydration includes evaluation of vital signs, skin turgor,

TABLE 3-13 ▲ Factors Affecting Insensible Water Loss in Newborn Infants

Factor	Effect on Insensible Water Loss
Level of maturity	Inversely proportional to birth weight and gestational age
Respiratory distress (hyperpnea)	Respiratory insensible water loss increases with rising minute ventilation if dry air is being breathed
Environmental temperature above neutral thermal zone	Increased in proportion to increment in temperature
Elevated body temperature	Increased by as much as 300%
Skin breakdown or injury	Increased by uncertain magnitude
Congenital skin defects (gastroschisis, omphalocele, neural tube defects)	Increased by uncertain magnitude until defect is surgically corrected
Radiant warmer	Increased by about 50%
Phototherapy	Increased by about 50%
Motor activity and crying	Increased by up to 70%
High ambient or inspired humidity	Reduced by 30% when ambient vapor pressure is increased by 200%
Plastic heat shield	Reduced by 10–30%
Plastic blanket	Reduced by 30–70%
Semipermeable membrane	Reduced by 50%
Topical agents	Reduced by 50%

From: Bell EF, and Oh W. 1994. Fluid and electrolyte management. In *Neonatology: Pathophysiology and Management of the Newborn,* Avery G, Fletcher MA, and MacDonald MM, eds. Philadelphia: JB Lippincott, 315. Reprinted by permission.

TABLE 3-14 ▲ Neonatal Enteral Feedings[21,23,63,64]

Route	Advantages	Disadvantages
Gastric (bolus)	Utilizes stomach capacity and digestive capabilities Potential for greater absorption More physiologic than continuous Tube easier to place and less likely to perforate GI tract	Potential compromise in neonates with severe respiratory distress, delayed gastric emptying, esophageal chalasia, or during the use of nasal CPAP Bradycardia with tube placement
Gastric (continuous)	Minimizes volume given at any one time, may be better tolerated by VLBW infants or infants with bowel disease, or severe cardiopulmonary disease	Higher risk of bacterial contamination of formula or breast milk Decreased fat content of breast milk
Transpyloric (continuous)	Useful in infants with delayed gastric emptying or gastroesophageal reflux and aspiration Used in infants on respiratory support, such as nasal CPAP	As per continuous gastric feedings Risk of bowel perforation Increased radiation exposure because of more frequent x-ray exams for placement May experience decreased absorption of potassium and fat

mucous membranes, anterior fontanel, body weight, and urine output.

NUTRITIONAL REQUIREMENTS

The neonate has high nutrition requirements to support growth, and the ill neonate's needs are even greater. Enteral feedings are the ideal method of providing caloric needs in a balanced diet. Unfortunately, the critically ill neonate may not be a candidate for enteral feedings for several days or weeks.

Parenteral nutrition is begun with glucose infusions, usually 5 or 10 percent dextrose in water, depending on the infant's tolerance of the glucose load. The glucose intake is increased during the first week of life, with a usual goal of 11–12 mg/kg/minute of glucose. A minimum of 50–60 kcal/kg/day is needed for maintenance, and additional calories are required for growth. Glucose intolerance, as evidenced by a blood glucose level greater than 150 mg/dl and/or glucosuria, can be precipitated by stress, thermal instability, sepsis, acidosis, or respiratory failure.

Protein, provided as parenteral amino acids, can be started by one or two days of age, if the infant is receiving at least maintenance calories as carbohydrate (glucose). The infant is started on 0.5–1 gm/kg/day of protein, which is

gradually increased over a week's time to 2–3 gm/kg/day as long as renal and liver functions are adequate. Electrolytes, vitamins, minerals, and trace elements must also be provided as part of the parenteral solution.

Fat, given as an intravenous fat emulsion, can also be started by one to two days of age. The infant is given 0.5–1 gm/kg/day of fat, which is usually increased 0.5 gm/kg/day to a maximum of 3 gm/kg/day, although preterm infants may not be able to tolerate the higher amounts. Serum turbidity is a poor predictor of hyperlipidemia; therefore blood levels must be monitored. Serum triglyceride levels higher than 150 mg/dl or total cholesterol greater than 200 mg/dl usually require a decrease in fat administration. Lipids provide an excellent source of calories in minimal fluid volumes as they are calorie dense compared to carbohydrates and protein. Up to 50 percent of the neonate's calories can be given as fat.[17]

Enteral feedings should be started as soon as feasible. They remain the best source of nutrition for the neonate—especially for the low birth weight infant who is particularly vulnerable to malnutrition. Even infants requiring mechanical ventilation should be considered candidates for early enteral feedings (Table 3-14). Determination of the formula, volume, and route of feeding is based on the infant's gestational age, weight, and clinical status. The time when suck, swallow, and respirations are coordinated varies, but generally infants can begin successful nippling by 32–34 weeks gestation if they are alert and vigorous without respiratory distress. For breastfeeding infants, "practice" sessions can be initiated when the infant is medically stable.

A previously ill neonate or a preterm infant usually must be started on gavage feedings in small volumes that are gradually increased over several days time. Each nursery should have personnel capable of properly placing a gavage tube and correctly administering the feeding to the neonate.[18] Infants who use pacifiers during feedings have been found to nipple feed earlier, gain weight better, and be discharged home earlier.[19,20]

The infant's clinical status is assessed with each feeding, or every two to four hours if feedings are continuous. Abdominal distention, regurgitation, absence of bowel sounds, bile-stained aspirates, and large feeding residuals are indications of feeding intolerance.

Formula for term infants contains 20 calories per ounce. This is considered the caloric content of breast milk as well, although the actual caloric content can vary greatly. Utilization of breast milk requires special care measures by the mother and the nursery staff to prevent excessive bacterial contamination. Use of breast milk in continuous feedings is associated with high bacterial growth and loss of fat content.[21,22]

Steady growth can normally be achieved when the infant is receiving 110–120 kcal/kg/day. If the infant cannot tolerate the high fluid volumes necessary to achieve this goal, a modified formula of increased caloric density (24 kcal/oz) can be utilized.[23] Also available are formulas and breast milk supplements that provide the additional calories, vitamins, and minerals required by the premature infant.

SKIN CARE

Skin integrity relates directly to neonatal well-being, and skin care has been recognized as a vital nursing care function. Skin maturity and integrity greatly affect thermoregulation, insensible water loss, and susceptibility to infection.

The skin is composed of the epidermis and the dermis. The outer layer of the epidermis, known as the stratum corneum (horny layer), is itself composed of several layers of flattened and dehydrated cells. It is tough, fairly impermeable, and constitutes a barrier against bacteria while decreasing water and heat loss. The dermo-epidermal junction is a specialized attachment between the epidermis and the papillary or outer layer of the dermis. The dermis lies beneath the epidermis and is formed of connective tissue containing lymphatics, nerves and nerve endings, blood vessels, sebaceous and sweat glands, and elastic fibers. Underlying this is subcutaneous tissue, first appearing around 14 weeks gestation but not significant in quantity until near term.

When an infant is born prematurely, the stratum corneum is underdeveloped, and the dermo-epidermal junction is weak, which results in a markedly increased permeability of the skin—especially in infants less than 32 weeks gestation and two weeks chronological age. Premature infants also display functional immaturity of sweat glands, altered vasomotor tone, and a deficit in the shivering reflex. Consequently, they are at increased risk for temperature instability, high insensible water loss, and skin injury.[24,25]

Normally the stratum corneum is a diffusion barrier, aided by skin surface lipids (sebum). The premature infant's skin is highly susceptible to percutaneous absorption of substances because of an underdeveloped

TABLE 3-15 ▲ Standard of Care for Neonatal Skin[26,60,65,66]

Medical Diagnostic Category: Newborns and other neonates with conditions originating in the perinatal period
Medical Diagnosis: All
Nursing Diagnosis: Skin integrity, impaired: high risk

Related Factors/ Defining Characteristics	Expected Outcome	Nursing Interventions
Developmental factors: Less than two weeks postnatal age; premature	Skin integrity maintained	Assess skin and document integrity, color, perfusion, turgor, temperature, and edema each shift and PRN.
	Trauma to skin minimized	Notify physician of significant findings requiring medical intervention.
Altered tissue perfusion	Skin moist or slightly dry, flaky	Minimize use of adhesives; avoid benzoin preparations; use alcohol sparingly.
Altered nutritional status		Utilize pectin barriers and hydrogel-backed or water-based gel adhesive electrodes; change as indicated by infant's skin integrity.
Altered skin turgor		Remove adhesives from infants with patience and water-soaked cotton balls.
External factors:		Utilize pressure gauze dressings for stasis of bleeding.
Excretions and secretions		Allow transparent dressings to peel off naturally.
Physical immobility		
Humidity (excessive or decreased)		Avoid hot packs or heat-retaining plastic.
Iatrogenic		Avoid use of emollients and agents with preservatives and dyes.
• *Mechanical* factors: epidermal stripping from removal of adhesives; restraints; pressure points		Using sterile water, remove povidone-iodine on skin after procedures and before dressing wounds.
		Rotate sites for temperature probes every 24 hours.
		Prevent pressure points by turning infant every 2 hours and PRN and utilizing eggcrate foam or water mattress.
• *Chemical* burns: external burns from topical agents such as alcohol or povidone-iodine; internal burns from intravenous infiltrates		Avoid causing pressure points or constriction of blood flow (with dressings, tubing, probes, or clothes).
		Bathe the acutely ill infant only in diaper area or where skin is soiled, as tolerated; bathe convalescent infants with soap only once or twice per week.
		Utilize less alkaline soaps such as Lowila, Aveeno, Basis, Neutrogena, Purpost, Oilatum.
• *Thermal* burns from heating units or transcutaneous probes		Treat excessively dry skin with a nonperfumed emollient, such as Eucerin creme or Aquaphor ointment.
		Treat IV infiltrates with hyaluronidase or phentalamine (if dopamine infiltrate); elevate and immobilize area of infiltrate; do not use moist heat on IV infiltrates.

stratum corneum and a thin layer of keratinocytes. Factors influencing absorption are temperature, hydration, perfusion, surface lipids, chronological and gestational age, condition of the skin, and the chemical and vehicle used.

An acidic skin pH develops during the first four days after delivery, providing an acid mantle that has a bactericidal quality. Bathing alters the status of the skin, so care must be exercised to promote the acid mantle that provides protection.[26]

The skin care needs of the sick infant include preventing physical injury (stripping the epidermis, thermal burns, pressure necrosis), preventing chemical injury (chemical infiltrates, chemical burns), minimizing insensible water loss, minimizing risk of infection, and avoiding excessive transdermal absorption of topical agents. Table 3-15 provides a standard of care, listing nursing interventions designed to protect the integrity of the neonate's skin.

TABLE 3-16 ▲ **Standard of Care for Developmental Growth**[33,60,67,68]

Medical Diagnostic Category: Newborns and other neonates with conditions originating in the perinatal period
Medical Diagnosis: All
Nursing Diagnosis: Alteration of growth and development related to overstimulation in the environment

Related Factors/ Defining Characteristics	Expected Outcome	Nursing Interventions
Prematurity Neonatal disease Overstimulation in the environment Inability to meet own basic needs Impaired physical growth	Infant will maintain equilibrium of physiologic status.	Recognize and minimize signs of overstimulation: • *Mild stress response:* gaze aversion, yawning, hiccups, grimacing, tongue thrusting, slack jaw, bowel movements, sneezing, and coughing • *Moderate stress response:* flushing, mottling, sighing, regurgitation, finger splaying, extension of arms and legs, jitteriness, jerky movements, limpness • *Severe stress response:* hypoxia, pallor, cyanosis, tachypnea, apnea, tachycardia, bradycardia, arrhythmia
Abnormal tone	Infant will rest in flexed position, free from hyperextended positioning; infant will tolerate handling and stimulation with minimal stress responses.	Promote flexed position: Support with blanket rolls or swaddle with blanket. Place in a prone position with arms and knees flexed, or on side with hands in midline, as often as possible. Avoid sudden position changes; contain limbs during and after position changes. Avoid hyperextended positioning: Avoid large neck rolls. Do not lift feet when in prone position; rather lift hips for diaper change. Avoid supine, "spread eagle" positioning.
	Infant will maintain restful sleep states for weight gain.	Decrease/minimize overstimulation and stress response: Shade eyes and cover ears with soft gauze or blanket when in open warmer. Coordinate care to minimize unnecessary handling. Talk in a soft voice, then lightly touch before handling. Provide a calm, quiet environment in unit. Provide pacifier, stroking, and/or touch to comfort at least BID and PRN during painful procedures. Shade incubator, close portholes gently. Do not awaken for routine vital signs. Keep dressed if condition warrants. Schedule periods to turn lights down in nursery to support circadian rhythms.
	Parents will participate in infant's care.	Provide consistent caregivers. Teach/demonstrate to parents how to recognize early signs of stress and provide social interaction based on infant's readiness and response.

DEVELOPMENTAL CARE

Research during the last decade has begun to look aggressively at the developmental needs of the NICU patient. There is improved survival, but many infants continue to be at risk for poor neurodevelopmental outcomes. Researchers are assessing the caregiving environment and its impact on the growth and development of the fragile infant. Studies have documented that the NICU can be overstimulating and the complexity of the setting exceeds the ability of infants to cope or adapt, especially those born preterm.[27–31]

Adaptation is defined as a process by which bodily functions and behavioral responses are modified to promote an equilibrium between self and environment. According to Als and associates, adaptation in the infant is a function of neurophysiologic development and requires integrated functioning between the infant's physiologic and behavioral systems.[32] Lack of adaptability can be attributed to a disruption in the infant's attempts to cope with environmental events such as light, noise, pain, and touch. As a result of this disruption, imbalances in autonomic, motor, and state subsystem functioning may occur. The preterm infant is especially vulnerable because he has not attained integrated functioning between the physiologic and behavioral systems. If he is developmentally able, the infant will attempt to utilize self-regulatory mechanisms to maintain balance and cope with disruptions. Again, these self-regulatory mechanisms, such as sucking and hand-to-mouth maneuvers, are absent or limited in the preterm infant.

Concern exists that these imbalances, if not corrected, may result in late neurobehavioral sequelae and subsequent developmental delays.[27] Because there is potential association between infant organization and developmental outcomes, all nursing care and the caregiving environment should support optimal infant development.[29]

Nurses can support the infant's developmental agenda by allowing and supporting stabilization of physiologic and behavioral functioning, which may ultimately improve developmental outcome. Table 3-16 is an example of a developmental care plan. The National Association of Neonatal Nurses has published *Infant and Family-Centered Developmental Care Guidelines,* which contains more extensive information on this topic.[33]

There is wide variation in NICU environments and care practices. Because of the growing concern regarding intensive care facilities and their impact on the medical and developmental state of sick infants, a federally funded project, known as The Physical and Developmental Environment of the High-Risk Infant, is presently under way, reviewing current and past research dealing with specific NICU issues and relating these to potential impact on the outcome of the high-risk infant.

One of the goals of this project is to identify beneficial and potentially detrimental care practices and NICU physical environment factors.

Multiple study groups are looking at areas such as light, sound, touch, position, sleep, physical environment, developmental promotion and intervention, family issues, and staff issues. A comprehensive knowledge base is being developed as a basis for appropriate recommendations for care practices and formulation of research questions. This information will be disseminated through publications and regional conferences, and the reader is advised to be alert for this ongoing work.

CARE OF PARENTS

An essential component of care for the neonate is care for the parents. It begins with a respect for their rights as parents and an understanding that they are individuals in a crisis situation. A crisis develops when an individual's coping skills cannot deal with a problem or threat. It is important to remember that it is the parents and not the health care team members who define the magnitude or significance of the crisis. Reaction to the crisis causes a temporary disruption of the normal psychological equilibrium, resulting in tension and discomfort. Feelings of guilt, anxiety, fear, shame, and helplessness may occur. As a result of this affective upset, the cognitive process may be impaired, resulting in confusion and disorganized behavior.[34,35]

Because parents usually anticipate a normal birth and a healthy infant, a crisis situation develops when these do not occur. Parents, specifically the mother, prepare during the pregnancy for the perfect child. Even the premature infant may be perceived by the parents as defective. The birth of a premature or critically ill infant may also be viewed as failure by the woman to produce a normal or complete child. The guilt feelings arising from such perceptions often discourage or prohibit a closeness between the parent and the child as well as between the parents themselves. Guilt, coupled with a life-threatening situation, interferes with the parents' ability to understand and deal with the problem.[36]

The following techniques may assist the nurse when communicating bad news or diagnostic information to the parents:[37]

1. Maintain eye contact; use touch and space appropriately.
2. Use the client's name.
3. Begin with a tone-setting statement.
4. Give a brief description of the problem in layman's terms.
5. Follow with the correct medical term(s), verbal and written.
6. End with a continuity statement, explaining what will happen next.

Parents of a premature infant have not had time to psychologically prepare for the birth of their child. The last weeks of a pregnancy are spent physically and mentally preparing for the birth of an infant. With a preterm delivery, the parent's state of unpreparedness combined with what may be viewed as a life-threatening situation to both the mother and the infant all lead to an extremely high level of stress. The birth experience and the delivered infant are not what the parents had wanted or expected. Perceptual distortions are often out of proportion to the severity of the situation. Parents are hampered by both physical and mental barriers in their attempt to become acquainted with and form emotional ties to their child. Going home without the baby also reinforces their feelings of disappointment and failure.[38]

According to the findings of Kaplan and Mason, parents of premature infants have four developmental tasks following the birth of their child: (1) expressing grief, in anticipation of the loss of the infant, (2) acknowledging maternal failure to produce a term or healthy infant,

(3) resuming the process of relating to the infant when the infant begins to recover, and (4) understanding the special needs of their infant.[39] To provide appropriate support, the nurse needs to recognize the stage at which the individual parent is functioning.

Throughout the infant's hospitalization, parents' needs should be identified along with those of their infant. The perceptive nurse will identify the family's strengths and capitalize on them to assist them though a difficult time. The family's weaknesses, which are sometimes easy to see and other times hidden, will eventually impact the parents' ability to deal with their infant's problems.

The initial phase of crisis is usually marked by a period of physical, functional, and emotional disorganization. Parents feel they cannot take on the parental role because they do not have a child to care for. The hospital staff assumes the care of their child, and the feelings of inadequacy and disorganization intensify. Parents may mimic the physician or nurses in an attempt to define their role as parent. When they cannot perform at the same level, further feelings of inadequacy develop.

Denial may be used as a coping mechanism in order to control the disorganization precipitated by the crisis. Withdrawal may be a form of denial as well as a part of the anticipatory grief for the potential loss of their child. Anger and resentment are also seen during this phase. The anger may be directed at themselves or displaced to others, including family, friends, or health care workers.[40]

Caplan has described three coping patterns used by mothers in dealing successfully with this type of crisis situation: (1) The mother masters the situation by cognitive understanding of the cause and consequence of the prematurity. (2) The mother copes emotionally, verbalizing her feelings and sharing them with others. (3) The mother actively seeks help from others.[41] The nurse can attempt to identify the successful coping strategies employed by the parents and assist them in their attempt to deal with the situation.

Once the parents move through their phase of grief and work through their sense of failure, they can begin a phase of emotional adaptation and enter a more positive relationship with their child. They begin to focus on their infant as an individual and resume the task of interacting with the infant that began during the pregnancy.

The parents are getting acquainted with their child during their early days together. The acquaintance process has been described as consisting of three main components. Participants in the process (1) acquire information about each other, (2) assess one another's attitudes, and (3) then continue to collect data to change or reinforce existing impressions and to develop further impressions about each other.[42]

Applying this information to parent-infant interaction, it can be seen that the parents gather information about their infant and assess the infant's attitude toward them. The well, term infant can communicate in various ways, focusing on the human face and listening attentively to the human voice. The child will latch to the mother by grasping, sucking, or rooting, and the mother interprets these behaviors as methods of seeking contact. Parents identify signals such as crying, smiling, babbling, and arm gestures as personal communications from the infant.[43]

Infant cues play a major part in the acquaintance process. Research has shown that for many mothers the first positive maternal feelings toward their infants are associated with the baby's responses to them.[44] The mother uses the infant's behavior to judge or assess the infant's attitude toward her. Fathers also attempt to assess their infant's attitudes early in the acquaintance process by interpreting infant behaviors. Success in gaining information and in assessing infant attitudes may influence the development of a positive parent-infant relationship.[45]

Unfortunately, the premature or critically ill newborn does not respond in the typical manner. During the acute phase of illness, these infants may be hypotonic or motionless. As they recover, they may be irritable, inconsolable, or easily exhausted. Parents may perceive the premature infant's immature reflexes as abnormal.[46] Such behaviors, as well as those exhibited by a neurologically abnormal infant, can hinder parent-infant interaction, and parents need to find ways to come to terms with the infant's abilities and inabilities. Skin-to-skin (kangaroo) care has been implemented in many nurseries to support positive parent-child interaction. During kangaroo care, the diaper-clad infant is placed directly on the mother's or father's chest, under their clothing. Infants may be held for several hours, and medically stable infants are allowed to nurse at the breast as desired.[47,48] In a study by Affonso and colleagues, mothers reported an increased sense of mastery and enhanced self-esteem following several weeks of holding their babies in the skin-to-skin kangaroo position.[49] However, mothers also needed periods of respite. Nurses must be sensitive to the parents' emotional status, allowing them to decline kangaroo care without guilt. Table 3-17 provides a care plan dealing with general principles that health care team members can utilize to assist the NICU parent through this crisis situation.

As parents of critically ill and premature infants emotionally adapt and attach to their infant, they should be encouraged to assume caretaking responsibilities that take into consideration the individuality of each parent, infant, and situation. Mastering caretaking skills reinforces their roles as parents and diminishes feelings of inadequacy. Reluctance to assume

TABLE 3-17 ▲ Standard of Care for Optimizing Parental Coping

Medical Diagnostic Category: Newborns and other neonates with conditions originating in the perinatal period
Medical Diagnosis: All
Nursing Diagnosis: Ineffective individual coping

Related Factors/ Defining Characteristics	Expected Outcome	Nursing Interventions
Inability to meet own basic needs	Parent(s) get appropriate meals and rest.	Assist individual in recognizing own health care needs. Collaborate with social services in finding alternate housing, such as boarding home or hotel, or assistance with meals when appropriate. Encourage parents' utilization of their family support system.
Inability to express fears and concerns	Parent(s) will verbalize feelings about infant's illness and hospitalization.	Provide supportive climate in which parent(s) may feel comfortable sharing their concerns. Allow parent(s) to fully express their feelings; do not minimize or repudiate their stated concerns.
Failure to understand rationale for prescribed treatment regimen	Parent(s) will verbalize an understanding of infant's condition, treatment, and progress, after initial shock and/or denial.	Interpret hospital environment and events for parent(s). Offer brief explanation of infant's condition and treatment. Refer pertinent questions to physician. Reinforce or clarify explanations.
Inappropriate anger toward staff	Parent(s) will collaborate with health care team members regarding decisions about infant.	Recognize parent's ethnic/cultural background and identify customs or attitudes that will affect interaction with health care personnel. Utilize primary nursing to provide a consistent caretaker who can develop a trusting relationship with parent(s). Allow ventilation of anger with a nondefensive response from staff. Offer additional support avenues such as social workers, pastoral care, or parent support group. Arrange multidisciplinary family conferences for difficult or complex patient or family.

Nursing Diagnosis: High risk for altered parenting

Related Factors/ Defining Characteristics	Expected Outcome	Nursing Interventions
Unwillingness to participate in infant care

Inappropriate visual, tactile, or auditory stimulation of infant

Lack of parental attachment behavior

Frequent identification of negative characteristics of infant | Parent(s) will demonstrate positive attachment behaviors toward infant.

Parent(s) will participate in infant's care. | Provide an open visiting policy. Involve parent(s) in decisions about infant's care, offering choices whenever possible. Encourage participation in basic care; be aware that parents can easily be intimidated by the expertise of the hospital staff. Identify and avoid attachment behavior by hospital staff that supersedes the parent's role. Provide privacy at the bedside. When medically appropriate, provide periods of skin-to-skin contact between parent(s) and infant (kangaroo care). Identify special characteristics of infant to assist parent(s) in seeing infant as a unique individual. Encourage the bringing of clothes, small toys, or small religious articles. Encourage picture taking. If parent(s) cannot visit, maintain contact by arranging times to call parent(s) to provide updates and send weekly information letters (Figure 3-10). Develop discharge plan early in hospitalization, encouraging parental input. |

(continued on page 87)

this role may indicate that the parents are still grieving the anticipated loss of their child, and forcing them to assume responsibilities prematurely may reinforce feelings of disorganization.

TABLE 3-17 ▲ Standard of Care for Optimizing Parental Coping (continued)

Medical Diagnostic Category: Newborns and other neonates with conditions originating in the perinatal period
Medical Diagnosis: All
Nursing Diagnosis: Knowledge deficit (high-risk infant)

Related Factors/ Defining Characteristics	Expected Outcome	Nursing Interventions
Verbalization of inadequate information or of inadequate recall of information Parent(s) requesting information Parent(s) relate incorrect information to other family members or to the health care team	Parent(s) will be able to verbalize their understanding of infant's present condition, planned treatment, and likely progress.	Prepare parent(s) for first contact with infant when possible. Provide tours of the NICU to parent(s) identified by the obstetrician as high risk for delivering a preterm or ill infant. Explain what equipment is being used and why. Encourage parent(s) to ask questions frequently. Coordinate information and explanations within the health care team so that information given to the parent(s) is consistent. Carefully plan timing and content of information to avoid information overload. Periodically reclarify with parent(s) understanding of infant's status. Provide significant information to both parent(s) to avoid confusion. Provide written literature when appropriate.

Adapted from: McFarland GK, and McFarlane EA. 1993. *Nursing Diagnosis and Intervention: Planning for Patient Care*, 2nd ed. St. Louis: Mosby-Year Book.

As parents move through this phase, they start to recognize the special needs of their child. How is this infant like other "normal" infants, and how does he differ? As parents recognize the uniqueness of their infant and develop an understanding of that child's needs, they are accepting and integrating him into their family. These tasks may be only partially completed at the time of the infant's discharge but eventually must be accomplished to foster a positive relationship.

DISCHARGE PLANNING

Throughout hospitalization the goal remains focused on successful discharge of the infant. This, itself, can be a crisis event for parents. Depending on his or her stage of adjustment, each family member may be at a different level of readiness to learn, and parental readiness must be achieved before successful learning can take place. As parents work through the emotional upheaval of the infant's hospitalization, the nurse continually assesses their status and introduces health information and caregiving skills that they are capable of handling.

Effective discharge planning ensures continuity of care while decreasing delays. Appropri-

ate discharge will decrease the risk of nosocomial infection to the infant, reduce costs for both fam-

FIGURE 3-10 ▲ Example of weekly update note sent home to parents.

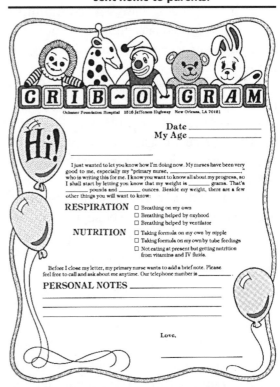

From: Ochsner Foundation Hospital. *Primary Nursing Care Manual.* Reprinted by permission.

TABLE 3-18 ▲ Guidelines for Effective Parent Teaching

1. Use "everyday" terms.
2. Utilize two or more modes of communication.
3. Recognize parent's limitations.
4. Make comparisons.
5. Repeat information.
6. Progress from simple to difficult.
7. Summarize information.
8. Check for understanding.
9. Encourage questions.
10. Allow expression of feeling.

Adapted from: Sumrall BC: Personal communication.

ily and hospital, provide earlier assimilation of the infant into the family unit, and hopefully provide an atmosphere more conducive to infant stimulation and development.[50,51]

If discharge planning is done ineffectively or if excessively early discharge is advocated because of financial constraints or other rationale, the infant is at higher risk for illness and rehospitalization. If the discharge teaching is incomplete, if community resources are inadequate, if the family or home situation is unacceptable, then discharge is inappropriate.

Successful discharge planning and discharge teaching will achieve maximum parental confidence and competence while maintaining the health of the infant. The stress of transition to the home will be decreased, and the family unit will be successfully re-established.

To achieve these goals, the entire process of discharge planning needs to be approached systematically. The process begins as a part of the initial assessment at the time of admission to the NICU and continues as further information becomes available. Ongoing patient and family assessment is required throughout the hospitalization to promote effectiveness and efficiency.

The planning process should be organized through a single individual with input from the entire health care team. A discharge coordi-nator provides the expertise necessary to link the family and patient to community services. The multidisciplinary team usually includes the primary nurse, neonatologist, nurse practitioner or resident, social worker, and discharge planner. Other health care services, such as respiratory therapy, occupational therapy, physical therapy, dietary, along with the necessary community services, participate as required.

To be ready for discharge, the high-risk infant should meet the following criteria:[52]

- The infant is physiologically stable, able to maintain temperature in an open crib wearing appropriate clothing.
- The infant is nippling or nursing all feedings. If an alternate feeding method is required, the parents or other care providers are able to perform the procedure appropriately.
- The infant is gaining weight steadily.
- The infant is free of apnea or receiving appropriate treatment and provisions have been made for home monitoring.
- Parental competence (in the ability to gavage feed or administer medication, for example) is confirmed.
- The home situation is appropriate.

Discharge teaching is part of the implementation of discharge planning. The effective nurse will use every teaching opportunity to its fullest. To help the family move forward, the nurse will recognize and deal professionally with obstacles to learning, such as insecurity, anger, frustration, or guilt. Other common obstacles to learning may involve parents' intellectual capabilities or their willingness to make the required time commitment. Table 3-18 lists some general guidelines for effective parent teaching.

Because inconsistency in information given to parents can be extremely stressful, standardized discharge teaching protocols will promote continuity of care among those providing direct patient care. Written teaching materials given to the family in advance of rooming-in are helpful if they have the educational ability to read and understand the information. Rooming-in with the infant provides a less intense environment than the NICU for the parents and allows extensive caretaking opportunities.

Evaluation of the discharge process is ongoing. A discharge checklist will document progress and ensure completion of the teaching or planning requirements. Follow-up visits and phone calls complete the evaluation process.

Key points for discharge planning include the following:[51]

1. Begin at the time of admission to the NICU.
2. Utilize a multidisciplinary team approach.
3. Confirm patient and family readiness for discharge.
4. Clarify family involvement; develop an informal but written contract for the complex, technology-dependent neonate.
5. Coordinate through one individual, such as a primary nurse, social worker, or discharge planner.
6. Utilize a written, individualized discharge teaching plan.
7. Encourage rooming-in.
8. Arrange appropriate follow-up: pediatric care, specialty services (such as surgery, neurology, ophthalmology), early intervention programs, newborn follow-up, medical equipment supply, community support agencies, home health nursing, respite care services.
9. Follow up with a telephone call two to three days after discharge.

SUMMARY

Nursing care of the infant in acute respiratory distress is all encompassing. Responsibilities begin with direct patient care and extend to the family of the infant. Although the focus of patient care activities will be directed by the patient's diagnosis, the nurse provides total assessment and care. Each intervention with the neonate has a purpose and will impact the patient's status. The effective nurse looks at each aspect of the neonate's care with the awareness that nursing activities are creating the environment in which the infant lives. The neonate's well-being is truly in the hands of his nurse.

REFERENCES

1. Committee on Perinatal Health. 1993. *Toward Improving the Outcome of Pregnancy: The 90s and Beyond.* White Plains, New York: March of Dimes Birth Defects Foundation.
2. Clark DA, and Hakanson DO. 1988. The inaccuracy of Apgar scoring. *Clinics in Perinatology* 8(3): 203–205.
3. Desmond MM, Rudolph AJ, and Phitakshphraiwan P. 1966. The transitional care nursery: A mechanism for preventative medicine in the newborn. *Pediatric Clinics of North America* 13(3): 651–667.
4. Brazelton TB. 1961. Psychophysiologic reactions in the neonate. *Journal of Pediatrics* 58(4): 513–518.
5. Hey E. 1994. Thermoregulation. In *Neonatology: Pathophysiology and Management of the Newborn,* 4th ed., Avery GB, Fletcher MA, and MacDonald MG, eds. Philadelphia: JB Lippincott, 357–365.
6. Perlstein P. 1992. Physical environment. In *Neonatal-Perinatal Medicine: Diseases of the Fetus and Infant,* 5th ed., Fanaroff AA, and Martin RJ, eds. St. Louis: Mosby-Year Book, 401–419.
7. LeBlanc MH. 1992. Neonatal heat transfer. In *Fetal and Neonatal Physiology,* Polin RA, and Fox WW, eds. Philadelphia: WB Saunders, 483–488.
8. Topper WH, and Stewart TP. 1984. Thermal support for the very-low-birth-weight infant: Role of supplemental conductive heat. *Journal of Pediatrics* 105(5): 810–814.
9. Dubowitz L, Dubowitz V, and Goldberg C. 1970. Clinical assessment of gestational age in the newborn infant. *Journal of Pediatrics* 77(1): 1–10.
10. Ballard JL, Novak KK, and Driver M. 1979. A simplified score for assessment of fetal maturation of newly born infants. *Journal of Pediatrics* 95(5): 769–774.
11. Ballard JL, et al. 1991. New Ballard score, expanded to include extremely premature infants. *Journal of Pediatrics* 119(3): 417–423.
12. Finnstrom O. 1977. Studies on maturity in newborn infants. Part IX: Further observations on the use of external characteristics in estimating gestational age. *Acta Paediatrica Scandinavica* 66(5): 601–604.
13. Constantine NA, et al. 1987. Use of physical and neurologic observations in assessment of gestational age in low birth weight infants. *Journal of Pediatrics* 110(6): 921–928.
14. Park MK. 1988. *Pediatric Cardiology for Practitioners,* 2nd ed. Chicago: Year Book Medical Publishers, 54.
15. Cartlidge P, and Rutter N. 1992. Skin barrier function. In *Fetal and Neonatal Physiology,* Polin RA, and Fox WW, eds. Philadelphia: WB Saunders, 569–585.

16. Bell EF, and Oh W. 1994. Fluid and electrolyte management. In *Neonatology: Pathophysiology and Management of the Newborn,* 4th ed., Avery GB, Fletcher MA, and MacDonald MG, eds. Philadelphia: JB Lippincott, 312–329.

17. D'Harlingue AE, and Byrne WJ. 1991. Nutrition in the newborn. In *Diseases of the Newborn,* 6th ed., Taeusch HW, Ballard RA, and Avery ME, eds. Philadelphia: WB Saunders, 709–727.

18. Weibley TT, et al. 1987. Gavage tube insertion in the premature infant. *American Journal of Maternal Child Nursing* 12(1): 24–27.

19. Bernbaum JC, et al. 1983. Nonnutritive sucking during gavage feeding enhances growth and maturation in premature infants. *Pediatrics* 71(1): 41–45.

20. Goldson E. 1986. Nonnutritive sucking in the sick infant. *Journal of Perinatology* 8(1): 30–34.

21. Greer F, McCormick A, and Locker J. 1984. Changes in fat concentration of human milk during delivery by intermittent bolus and continuous mechanical pump infusion. *Journal of Pediatrics* 105(5): 745–749.

22. Lemons P, et al. 1983. Bacterial growth in human milk during continuous feeding. *American Journal of Perinatology* 1(1): 76–80.

23. American Academy of Pediatrics Committee on Nutrition. 1985. Nutritional needs of low birth weight infants. *Pediatrics* 75(5): 976–986.

24. Rutter N. 1988. The immature skin. *British Medical Bulletin* 44(4): 957–970.

25. Solomon LM, and Esterly NB. 1973. *Neonatal Dermatology.* Philadelphia: WB Saunders, 1–22.

26. Rutter N. 1987. Percutaneous drug absorption in the newborn: Hazards and uses. *Clinical Pediatrics* 14(4): 911–930.

27. Graven S, et al. 1992. The high-risk infant environment. Part I: The role of the neonatal intensive care unit in the outcome of high-risk infants. *Journal of Pediatrics* 12(2) 164–172.

28. DePaul D, and Chambers SE. 1995. Environmental noise in the neonatal intensive care unit: Implications for nursing practice. *Journal of Perinatal and Neonatal Nursing* 8(4): 71–76.

29. Als H, et al. 1986. Individualized behavioral and environmental care for the very low birth weight preterm infant at high risk for bronchopulmonary dysplasia: Neonatal intensive care unit and developmental outcome. *Pediatrics* 78(6): 1123–1132.

30. Gottfried AW, Hodgman JE, and Brown KW. 1984. How intensive is newborn intensive care? An environmental analysis. *Pediatrics* 74(2): 292–294.

31. Wolke D. 1987. Environmental neonatology. *Archives of Disease in Childhood* 62(10): 987–988.

32. Als H, et al. 1982. Toward a research instrument for the Assessment of Preterm Infant's Behavior (APIB). In *Theory and Research in Behavioral Pediatrics,* Fitzgerald HE, Lester BM, and Yogman MW, eds. New York: Plenum, 35–63.

33. National Association of Neonatal Nurses. 1994. *Infant and Family-Centered Developmental Care Guidelines.* Petaluma, California: NANN.

34. Aguilera DC, and Messick JM. 1978. *Crisis Intervention: Theory and Methodology.* St. Louis: Mosby-Year Book, 62–79.

35. Lam C. 1982. Crisis intervention in respiratory distress. *Journal of the California Perinatal Association* 2(2): 104–107.

36. Klaus JH, and Kennell MH. 1982. *Parent-Infant Bonding,* 2nd ed. St. Louis: Mosby-Year Book, 151–161.

37. Sumrall BC. 1990. Personal communication.

38. Mercer R. 1990. *Parents at Risk.* New York: Springer, 154–166.

39. Kaplan D, and Mason E. 1960. Maternal reactions to premature birth viewed as an acute emotional disorder. *American Journal of Orthopsychiatry* 30: 359–552.

40. Sammons W, and Lewis J. 1985. *Premature Babies—A Different Beginning.* St. Louis: Mosby-Year Book, 42–45.

41. Caplan G. 1960. Patterns of parental response to the crisis of premature birth. *Psychiatry* 23: 365–367.

42. Newcomb T. 1961. *The Acquaintance Process.* New York: Holt, Rinehart and Winston, 4–23.

43. Brazelton TB, Koslowski B, and Main M. 1974. The origins of reciprocity: The early mother-infant interaction. In *The Effect of the Infant on Its Caregiver,* Lewis M, and Rosenblum L, eds. New York: Wiley, 49–76.

44. Robson K, and Moss H. 1970. Patterns and determinants of maternal attachment. *Journal of Pediatrics* 77(6): 976–985.

45. Gay JT. 1981. A conceptual framework of bonding. *Journal of Obstetric, Gynecologic, and Neonatal Nursing* 10(6): 440–444.

46. Johnson SH, and Grubbs J. 1975. The premature infant's reflex behaviors: Effects on the maternal-child relationship. *Journal of Obstetric, Gynecologic, and Neonatal Nursing* 4(3): 15–20.

47. Anderson GE. 1991. Current knowledge about skin-to-skin (kangaroo) care for preterm infants. *Journal of Perinatology* 11(3): 216–226.

48. Ludington-Hoe SM, et al. 1994. Kangaroo care: Research results, and practice implications and guidelines. *Neonatal Network* 13(1): 19–27.

49. Affonso D, et al. 1993. Reconciliation and healing for mothers through skin-to-skin contact provided in an American tertiary level intensive care nursery. *Neonatal Network* 12(3): 25–32.

50. Brooten D, et al. 1986. A randomized clinical trial of early hospital discharge and home follow-up of very-low-birth-weight infants. *New England Journal of Medicine* 315(15): 934–939.

51. Zotkiewicz TT. 1996. Home at last. In *Newborn Intensive Care: What Every Parent Needs To Know,* Zaichkin J, ed. Petaluma, California: NICU INK, 305–341.

52. American Academy of Pediatrics. Committee on Fetus and Newborn and the ACOG Committee on Obstetrics: Maternal and Fetal Medicine. 1992. Postpartum and follow-up care. In *Guidelines for Perinatal Care,* 3rd ed., Freeman RK, and Poland RL, eds. Elk Grove Village, Illinois: American Academy of Pediatrics, American College of Obstetricians and Gynecologists, 108–115.

53. Baumgart S, et al. 1981. Effect of heat shielding on convective and evaporative heat losses and on radiant heat transfer in the premature infant. *Journal of Pediatrics* 99(6): 948–956.

54. Blackburn ST, and Loper DL. 1992. Thermoregulation. In *Maternal, Fetal, and Neonatal Physiology: A Clinical Perspective.* Philadelphia: WB Saunders, 677–697.

55. Glatzl-Hawlik MA, and Bell EF. 1992. Environmental temperature control. In *Fetal and Neonatal Physiology,* Polin RA, and Fox WW, eds. Philadelphia: WB Saunders, 483–488.

56. Greer PS. 1988. Head coverings for newborns under radiant warmers. *Journal of Obstetric, Gynecologic, and Neonatal Nursing* 17(4): 265–271.

57. Kaplan M, and Eidelman AI. 1984. Improved prognosis in severely hypothermic newborn infants treated by rapid rewarming. *Journal of Pediatrics* 105(3): 470–474.

58. Malin SW, and Baumgart S. 1987. Optimal thermal management for low birth weight infants nursed under high-powered radiant warmers. *Pediatrics* 79(1): 47–54.

59. Sinclair JC. 1992. Management of the thermal environment. In *Effective Care of the Newborn Infant,* Sinclair JC, and Bracken MB, eds. New York: Oxford University Press, 40–58.

60. McFarland GK, and McFarlane EA. 1993. *Nursing Diagnosis and Intervention: Planning for Patient Care,* 2nd ed. St. Louis: Mosby-Year Book.

61. Nugent J. 1983. Acute respiratory care of the newborn. *Journal of Obstetric, Gynecologic, and Neonatal Nursing* 12(3 supplement): 31–44.

62. Sconyers S, Ogden B, and Goldberg H. 1987. The effect of body position on the respiratory rate of infants with tachypnea. *Journal of Perinatology* 7(2): 118–121.

63. Parker P, Stroup S, and Greene H. 1981. A controlled comparison of continuous versus intermittent feeding in the treatment of infants with intestinal disease. *Journal of Pediatrics* 99(3): 68–71.

64. Pereira GR, and Lemons JA. 1981. Controlled study of transpyloric and intermittent gavage feeding in the small preterm infant. *Pediatrics* 67(1): 68–71.

65. Lund C, et al. 1986. Evaluation of a pectin-based barrier under tape to protect neonatal skin. *Journal of Obstetric, Gynecologic, and Neonatal Nursing* 15(1): 39–44.

66. NAACOG. 1992. Neonatal skin care. *OGN Nursing Practice Resource,* January, 1–9.

67. Als H. 1984. *Guidelines for the Practical Implementation of Individualized Care and Intervention in the NICU.* Boston: Children's Hospital.

68. Gardner S, et al. 1993. The neonate and the environment: Impact on development. In *Handbook of Neonatal Intensive Care,* 3rd ed., Merenstein GB, and Gardner SL, eds. St. Louis: Mosby-Year Book, 564–608.

NOTES

NOTES

4 Historical and Present Application of Positive Pressure Ventilation

V. L. Cassani III, RNC, MSN, MSNA, NNP, CRNA

As we enter the era of surfactant replacement therapy, extracorporeal membrane oxygenation (ECMO), high-frequency ventilation, and nitric oxide administration—all designed to enhance survival and decrease morbidity in babies afflicted with respiratory failure—it is important to reflect on the progress made in the past 30 years in the application of positive pressure ventilation. As has often been stated, those who are not aware of history are doomed to repeat it. Having a clear grasp of the development of mechanical ventilation to treat the newborn will foster rational application of the technique by practitioners. Clinicians also need to understand the pioneering changes made in the social milieu by our predecessors, for these changes have enabled neonatal intensive care to flourish.

This chapter not only discusses the historical development of newborn mechanical ventilation, but also provides the reader with a clear understanding of some of the underlying physiologic principles of positive pressure ventilation. The effects of applying newly acquired scientific knowledge to the clinical arena are highlighted.

HISTORICAL PERSPECTIVE

The first recorded report of death secondary to respiratory failure in a newborn occurred during the reign of H Wang T, emperor of China (2698–2599 BC). Incidents of a resuscitation of a newborn are also mentioned in Eber's Papyrus (1552 BC) and the Bible (2 Kings 4: 34–35).[1–4]

Birth asphyxia and respiratory failure of newborns continued to attract the attention of medical scholars throughout the ages. Hippocrates (400 BC) published the technique of endotracheal intubation, but this technique did not become a standard of care until the mid-twentieth century.[4] Robert Boyle (AD 1670) reported the results of resuscitation of asphyxiated kittens, and Chaussier (1806) described endotracheal intubation of asphyxiated infants.[1,2]

In the late 1880s, Alexander Graham Bell designed and built a body-enclosing ventilator for newborn resuscitation; a similar device was described in the *Boston Medical and Surgical Journal* by O. W. Doe in 1889. Respiratory failure of the newborn remained an apparently unsolvable problem until a serendipitous cascade of events was set in motion by several key findings during the 1950s and 1960s. The result was the advent of neonatal intensive care.[5-7]

The knowledge of physiologic principles necessary to adequately ventilate newborns had developed slowly. Laplace first described the phenomenon of surface tension in 1806 in a treatise on the movement of the planets and stars.[8] This phenomenon was widely studied by physicists and chemists over the succeeding century, but physiologists did not apply this information until the 1920s.[5]

In 1929, von Neergaard demonstrated the principle of alveolar surface tension at an air-liquid interface. He included this information in his discussion of lung elasticity and mechanics.[9]

Twenty-five years later, Macklin applied this information to infer the presence of surface-active material in alveoli.[10] Subsequent work by basic researchers whose work was supported by the Medical Research Laboratories of the U.S. Army Chemical Center and the British Chemical Defense Experimental Establishment helped to unravel the mystery of surfactants.[5]

In 1956, Pattle demonstrated the presence of stable foam in the trachea of rabbits with lung edema. He observed that these foams were stable and unaffected by antifoams. Pattle attributed the stability to an insoluble mucus surface layer that formed the original lining of the alveoli. He further reasoned that if the alveolar surface tension were that of an ordinary liquid, the imbalance of Starling's forces between the capillaries and the alveoli would exert enough pressure to fill the alveoli with capillary transudate. Therefore, the mucus protein layer must mitigate the surface tension.[11]

A year later, Cook, Sutherland, and Segal demonstrated markedly decreased pulmonary compliance in newborns with respiratory distress.[12] In 1957, Clements first described the changing surface tension of lung extracts at varying surface areas. The surface tension decreased as the surface film was compressed, thus confirming Macklin's supposition.[13]

Avery and Mead took this elegant observation of Clements and in 1959 applied it to their patients dying of hyaline membrane disease (HMD).[14] They found that the surface tension of lung extracts of infants who died of HMD was significantly higher than that of infants who died from other causes. This suggested to Avery and Mead that HMD resulted not from the presence of hyaline membranes (the supposed etiology) but from a lack of surface-active material and an increased surface tension during expiration, which led to atelectasis.[14]

Thus, respiratory distress syndrome (RDS)—a morbid condition that had had 13 different labels—finally had a proposed etiology: *absence* of surface-active material. These researchers provided the rationale for continuous positive airway pressure (CPAP) in 1959. It remained for several other pieces of the puzzle to come together before this became an accepted form of treatment in the l970s.

THE WEDDING OF BASIC SCIENCE AND CLINICAL PRACTICE

These findings of Clements, Pattle, Avery, Mead, and others prompted a renewed focus on RDS research in an attempt to characterize surfactant, determine where it came from, and utilize these findings to improve the outcome of infants suffering from RDS.[5,12] At the International Congress of Pediatrics in 1959, several concerns regarding survival were voiced, including avoiding birth asphyxia and providing adequate metabolic support. Another concept discussed at the congress was important to future development and application of mechanical ventilation: the idea that grunting must come from the glottis. It had previously been assumed that grunting resulted from bronchial or bronchiolar obstruction and that the infant's condition would therefore improve with clearing of the obstruction.[3,6]

During the 1960s, Clements, Pattle, Thomas, Klaus, Gluck, Hallman, and others continued basic research to characterize the components of surfactants.[5,15] Slowly, the different biochemical pieces of surfactants were elucidated, and, coincidentally, the behavior of surfactants *in vitro* was described.[15,16]

As the story of surfactant composition and behavior was unfolding, the site of surfactant production was being identified. In 1962, Buckingham and Avery reported that the appearance of surfactant coincided with the appearance of lamellar bodies in the Type II alveolar cells.[17] Klaus and coworkers concluded that the surface-active lining of the lung develops during the process of lamellar transformation of the mitochondria in the alveolar epithelial cell.[18] When direct and indirect evidence was assembled by these basic researchers, the site of surfactant production and release was clearly identified as Type II alveolar cells.[19–21]

How was all of this basic science benefiting the infants afflicted with RDS? Once the properties, components, and time of appearance of surfactants were known, patients at risk for developing RDS could be identified, and a plan for treatment could be developed.

During the 1950s and early l960s, newborn care was quite different from what it is today. Delivery room care was provided by obstetricians and labor and delivery nurses. In-hospital well-baby care was provided by pediatricians, but it was not reimbursed by insurance companies. Intensive care units did not exist, and there was no economic incentive for hospitals to develop neonatal intensive care units because insurers did not provide reimbursement for any in-hospital newborn care.[7]

Laboratory support was rudimentary. Direct measurement of arterial oxygen tension (PaO_2)

via a Clarke electrode was not available.[22,23] Incubators did not have access ports to maintain a warm environment while care was performed. Blood pressure monitoring for newborns was unavailable. Total parenteral nutrition did not exist. Drug pharmacokinetics in the newborn was a rudimentary science. As with other things, necessity was the mother of invention.[22,23]

All of this was changed rapidly during the 1960s by an escalating series of events and discoveries. Gluck and coworkers initiated the first NICU in 1960.[24] In 1964, Stahlman described an NICU with a machine containing a Clarke electrode for measuring PaO_2 directly in the unit.[25] Health care providers successfully passed legislation requiring insurance reimbursement for newborn care.[23] Severinghaus contributed an arterial blood gas machine to measure pH, partial pressure of carbon dioxide in arterial blood ($PaCO_2$), and PaO_2 on microsamples of blood.[6,22] Gluck and coworkers evolved a means of predicting RDS with amniocentesis.[24]

A means of obtaining blood samples through umbilical vessel catheterization was described.[26] Incubators with the ability to provide constant thermoneutral environments were added to the armamentarium.[27,28] Methods to directly measure blood pressure and heart rate in infants were developed. Thus, the wedding of basic research with clinical practice resulted in the rapid development of neonatal intensive care. However, there were many lessons to be learned along the way.

The first description of the use of patient-controlled ventilation for newborns was made by Donald and Lord in 1953.[29] Use of mechanical ventilation was reserved for treating moribund infants with intractable respiratory insufficiency because there was limited success (less than 10 percent lived) and the procedure was technically difficult.[30–34] Stahlman, Young, and Payne described the use of positive pressure ventilation in treating infants with RDS in 1962.[34]

Despite the renewed interest in applying positive pressure ventilation to treat these infants, the method was adopted slowly. Experimental data in animals and adults showed that the increased intra-alveolar pressure obtained was transmitted to the thorax and impeded venous return and cardiac output.[35] It remained for the clinicians to develop and evaluate methods of applying positive pressure ventilation to infants with decreased pulmonary compliance and to apply a scientific, physiologically based solution to the problem.

THE BEGINNINGS OF NEONATAL VENTILATOR SUPPORT

In 1962, several centers began providing ventilation to newborns with respiratory insufficiency.[23] The success was varied, with one center reporting a 60 percent survival rate while others had limited success.[23,30,36] The variability was understandable; each unit was adapting adult ventilators and designing its own equipment. In addition, the patients selected for treatment were moribund by the time therapy was started, and the staff providing care were venturing into uncharted waters.[22,23]

Standards of care were developed as the care was being provided.[22,23] The ability to rapidly evaluate and adjust therapy was lacking because a microtechnique measurement of PaO_2, $PaCO_2$, pH, bicarbonate, and base excess did not yet exist.[22,23] Many lessons remained to be learned.

Reports of these early attempts at ventilation stimulated further debate about the efficacy of this treatment.[35–37] In the milieu of health care in the 1960s, the use of mechanical ventilation was *not* an accepted method of treatment for infants with RDS despite the early success of Donald and Lord and the promising results of Thomas and coworkers.[29,30]

The primary debate centered around the teleologic arguments and inferences made concerning the physiologic effects of mechanical ventilation, which some authors argued contributed to the progressive acidosis of the infants who died.[35,38,39] The basic error in logic was assuming that positive pressure ventilation impeded the cardiac return and output of the patient.[35,36,38,39] Many years and meticulous studies were needed to refute the assumption that lung compliance and resistance in the infant with RDS were the same as that in the normal adult where interstitial and intra-alveolar pulmonary edema, peribronchiolar and perivascular hemorrhage, and terminal airway and alveolar collapse were not issues.[5,6,22]

In addition, development of the adjuncts to therapy and a physiologically based method of ventilation required accumulation of scientific knowledge acquired from basic and clinical research.[5–7] Not only did this information need to be obtained; it also needed to be shared among clinicians.[5] This was a significant problem because the condition we now call respiratory distress syndrome was still not labeled consistently. This inhibited interchange of information among clinicians; literature searches needed to cross-reference 13 different labels to obtain all the current information on the problem.

THE SEEDS OF FUTURE THERAPY

Coincident with the initial reports of attempts at ventilation by Smith, Daily and Papodopulus during the 1970s, the stage was being set to develop the information and support necessary to move forward.[5–7,31] In 1963, Tooley, Clements, Klaus, and colleagues conducted a clinical trial of *surfactant replacement therapy* in Kandang Kerbau Hospital in Singapore.[40] Although the therapy did initially improve the physiologic states of the infants, it did not improve their long-term outcomes. The investigators attributed the poor outcomes to an inadequate mechanism for delivering the surfactant, lack of adequate monitoring, and inability to measure blood gases and provide thermoneutrality.[6,40] This experiment was an attempt to marry the clinical acumen of Tooley and Klaus with the scientific data that many investigators had acquired regarding surface-active materials.

Application of the lessons learned in Singapore led to development of clinical research facilities that rapidly overcame the initial limitations. The subsequent development of instruments to measure blood gases and blood pressure and to provide temperature regulation resulted in improved outcomes.[5-7] Still, the solution to the problem of providing adequate mechanical ventilation remained elusive.

All mechanical ventilators used were either modifications of adult mechanical ventilators or home-built adaptations of adult ventilators. Treatment included using a neuromuscular blocking agent to relax the infant and providing nutrition via gastrostomy tube.[30] The development of an infant ventilator awaited the serendipitous alignment of resources and personnel.

In 1968, an anesthesiologist was assigned full-time to the nursery at the University of California-San Francisco (UCSF), but not as an anesthesiologist.[5,6,22] George Gregory had no responsibilities other than ventilator research and providing care to the moribund patients in the nursery. He had developed an interest in RDS as a medical student in 1961. As a resident, he had worked extensively with the pediatric staff during the development of intensive care for newborns. Following his fellowship, Gregory was assigned to the intensive care nursery by the Anesthesia Department chairperson.

Along with Tooley, Phibbs, Kitterman, and members of the nursing staff, such as Lilly Yoshida, he labored to develop better methods of care. One of their concerns was to treat neonates with RDS using the knowledge developed by von Neergaard, Macklin, Pattle, Mead, Avery, Clements, and others. After noting the information published by Harrison, Hesse, and Klein,[37] that grunting improved the metabolic status of infants with RDS, Gregory and colleagues reasoned that applying continuous positive airway pressure would *improve* their metabolic and ventilatory status by maintaining lung volume and not impairing cardiac output.[22,37,41]

Previous work had shown that compromised infants were relatively hypovolemic and hypoproteinemic, so the infants at UCSF had these problems corrected by meticulous volume replacement.[6] In addition, Gregory's team showed that only 20 percent of the airway pressure applied to the infants with RDS was transmitted to intrathoracic structures.[42]

The staff continued to experiment with intermittent positive pressure ventilation (IPPV), but without consistent success. Ventilating patients with the Bird Mark VIII with a J-circuit or a Bournes LS1000, the group attained a survival rate of only 20 percent. There were several reasons for these poor outcomes. At respiratory rates of 20 or less, these ventilators did not provide a continuous flow of fresh gas to patients or maintain continuous positive pressure. Ventilation at more rapid rates (60/minute or greater) maintained both continuous positive pressure and an almost continuous provision of fresh gas.[43] But new problems emerged: The infants were unable to be weaned from rapid rates without compromise.

In 1968, Gregory and colleagues decided to try an alternative therapy—CPAP—for any infant with RDS who was breathing spontaneously. This therapy delivers a continuous flow of fresh, humidified gas with a selected fraction of inspired oxygen (FiO_2) while maintaining a continuous distending pressure on the infant's lungs. Of the 20 patients treated, 16 survived.[31] Preliminary results were reported at the meeting of the Society for Pediatric Research in 1970, and final results were reported in 1971.[31]

This success was marked, especially considering the 70 percent survival rate of infants weighing less than 1.5 kg. The four infants who died had complications of patent ductus arteriosus (PDA).[6,31] Later progress was a direct result of this change in therapy.

A cadre of nurses with special skills and abilities in the recently developed intensive care nursery provided CPAP and other therapy. These staff nurses, who learned along with the pediatricians, could monitor heart rate and blood pressure, manage thermoregulation, manipulate complex electronic equipment, and safely manage umbilical arterial and venous catheters while anticipating problems and identifying patients developing these problems.

When Gregory reported the preliminary data and mode of therapy at the Society for Pediatric Research in 1970, he piqued the interest of many of his colleagues in the audience. Included in this group were Robert Kirby, an Air Force anesthesiologist, and Robert de Lemos, an Air Force pediatrician.

Kirby and de Lemos applied the information presented by Gregory and his colleagues as well as that from Thomas and associates and other researchers to the problem of providing adequate mechanical ventilation.[30,31] The adaptation of adult mechanical ventilators to the neonatal population had been singularly unsuccessful. Various centers had modified Bennett PR-2, Bird Mark VIII, MA-1, or Bournes LS1000 ventilators. These ventilators provided a continual flow of gas only during mandatory mechanical breaths, not during spontaneous breathing.

Kirby and de Lemos reasoned that the benefits of Gregory's CPAP system should be incorporated into mechanical ventilation. Kirby designed a pneumatically driven, time-cycled, pressure-limited ventilator that delivered a continual flow of gas, CPAP, and intermittent mandatory ventilation (IMV) to the patient being ventilated. IMV became a mainstay of neonatal mechanical ventilation in the 1970s and early 1980s.

Thus, the treatment of RDS had progressed from attempting to maintain the baby's lung volume by attaching a towel clip around the xiphoid process and suspending it from the incubator roof with a rubber band[43] to application of the knowledge of physiologic principles of surface-active materials by maintaining CPAP.[42] Gregory and his colleagues had brought to fruition the knowledge accumulated by von Neergaard, Gruenwald, Macklin, Radford, Clements, Avery, Mead, and Tooley. However, the benefit of this new therapy proved to be a double-edged sword: the ability to support premature infants versus the inherent risk of complications such as pneumothorax and BPD. To wield this sword effectively would require accumulation of clinical data in controlled trials.

POSITIVE PRESSURE VENTILATION: IMPROVING OUTCOME THROUGH TECHNOLOGICAL DEVELOPMENT

For mechanical ventilation of the newborn, 1970 and 1971 were watershed years. Kirby and de Lemos described IMV; Daily, Smith, and colleagues published their series "Mechanical Ventilation of the Newborn Infant: III, IV, V," in *Anesthesiology*; and Gregory and colleagues reported their data on CPAP.[31–33,44] Whether the therapy was warranted, however, continued to be a subject of debate. It remained for clinical researchers to develop the principles of mechanical ventilation and its applications.

Gregory and associates' application of CPAP resulted in markedly improved survival, but some infants continued to require ventilatory support, which was provided with modified adult ventilators.[31–33] Because of their inherent limitations, these ventilators were not always able to correct the abnormalities of atelectasis, reduced functional residual capacity (FRC), ventilation/perfusion ($\dot{V}_A/\dot{Q}_C$) abnormalities, and right-to-left intrapulmonary shunting.

There were many problems to overcome. The small tidal volumes (V_T) required by infants (25 ml or less) were difficult to regulate accurately in modified adult ventilators designed to deliver greater than 1,000 ml. In addition, there was an effort to mimic the ventilatory pattern of infants with RDS by designing infant ventilators capable of patient-triggered frequencies of 100 breaths per minute or more. These capabilities were not possible, given the technical limitations of the equipment. Carbon dioxide retention was markedly increased when ventilator failure resulted in uncoordinated attempts at spontaneous ventilation without machine cycling and gas flow to the patient.[44]

These limitations were overcome when IMV was introduced. Intermittent mandatory ventilation provided a continuous flow of gas in excess of the infant's minute ventilation for spontaneous breathing as well as a means of delivering mandatory breaths by occluding the gas outflow tract, resulting in inflation of the infant's lungs. Thus, there was a means of providing the level of support infants required by varying from totally manual to completely spontaneous breathing. Intermittent mandatory ventilation enabled clinicians to select ventilatory patterns for specific purposes with minimal physiologic consequences such as hypercarbia.[44]

THE SEARCH FOR A COMMON LANGUAGE

As NICUs began to proliferate and mechanical ventilation evolved, a common language for discussing therapy became necessary. Many authors coined new phrases while describing therapy, and confusion started to creep into scientific discussions. A precise language was necessary to ensure accurate exchange of information among clinicians.

There was and continues to be confusion about the differences among controlled and assisted ventilation, IPPV, IMV, time-cycled ventilators, positive end-expiratory pressure (PEEP), and CPAP. An understanding of these differences is essential for rational application of therapy.

Intermittent positive pressure ventilation, a therapy developed to treat adults, provides intermittent gas flow under pressure through the ventilator circuit. Therefore, spontaneous breathing between mechanical breaths results in rebreathing of previously exhaled gases.[44]

Controlled ventilation, which allows the clinician to determine the ventilatory pattern, results when the rate of respiration is determined by the rate of the ventilator without patient-initiated breaths. Neuromuscular blocking agents are administered to block voluntary respiratory effort, or deliberate hyperventilation is employed to achieve controlled ventilation.[45]

Assisted ventilation, which clinicians attempted to utilize without success in the neonatal population, is mechanical ventilation that the patient triggers with each inspiratory attempt, establishing the ventilator rate and pattern. This technique requires a sophisticated triggering device that detects airflow through the circuit as the patient inspires in order to initiate the mechanical breath.[45] As previously noted, assisted ventilation led to significant morbidity secondary to asynchronous breathing and the resultant hypercarbia.[44]

Synchronized intermittent mandatory ventilation (SIMV) has more recently been used successfully to ventilate babies with RDS.[46] The reported success with this therapy is a direct result of refinements in the triggering device that decreases response times. The result has been that the ventilator triggers the mechanical breath with the patient's inspiration.

Intermittent mandatory ventilation, the conceptual breakthrough of Kirby and de Lemos, provides a continuous flow of gas through the ventilator circuit even when the ventilator is not delivering a mechanical breath.[47,48] This is a departure from IPPV, which provides gas flow only during mechanical ventilation. Positive pressure breaths are thus delivered on a predetermined schedule while the patient continues to breathe voluntarily and receive fresh, humidified gas at a predetermined airway pressure with a selected FiO_2. This allows the infant to breathe efficiently, independent of the mandatory ventilations, and it prevents development of biochemical disruptions such as respiratory acidosis as long as the infant does not breathe asynchronously.

Time-cycled ventilators end the inspiratory phase of the mechanical breath after a preset time has passed. This cycling occurs regardless of the volume of gas delivered or pressure buildup within the ventilator circuit.[47]

Pressure-limited ventilators end the inspiratory phase when a preset pressure is reached within the ventilator circuit. The inspiratory phase ends regardless of the volume of gas delivered during the inspiration.[47,48]

Volume-limited ventilators end the inspiratory phase when a preset volume of gas is delivered. This volume is delivered regardless of the pressure that is reached within the ventilator circuit.[47,48] Not all of the volume of gas is delivered to the patient; some volume is lost in the dead space and compliance of the circuit.

Continuous positive airway pressure, also called continuous distending airway pressure (CDAP), continuous distending pressure (CDP), and several other names, maintains lung volume in patients with high alveolar surface tension by applying airway pressure sufficient to overcome the tendency for alveolar closure. There are several methods of providing CPAP, including use of an endotracheal tube, head-enclosing box, face mask, and nasal prongs. These devices may be attached to a ventilator circuit or anesthesia bag with underwater pressure relief valve.[48] All ventilation is supplied by the patient's own breaths.[48]

Positive end-expiratory pressure maintains positive airway pressure during expiration and between mandatory breaths of the ventilator. It is not synonymous with CPAP. During CPAP, pressure remains constant throughout the patient's voluntary respirations; PEEP is the residual airway pressure maintained at the end of a positive pressure ventilation.[47,48]

Peak inspiratory pressure (PIP) is the maximal inspiratory pressure generated with each mechanical breath of the ventilator. Pressure is selected and preset on the ventilator. The mechanical breath will not be delivered at a higher pressure than the preset PIP.[47,48]

Neonatal IMV ventilators incorporate both time and pressure limits to determine the amount of gas delivered during the inspiratory phase of the mechanical breath. The inspiratory time limits the amount of time the positive pressure breath is delivered. The PIP limits the maximal airway pressure generated during the mechanical breath.

Clearly, neonatal positive pressure ventilation has evolved rapidly during the past 34 years and has become more technically complex. This brief discussion of some of the concepts should serve as a guide for clearer understanding of the principles; it is not intended to supplant the extensive treatises available on design and function of mechanical ventilators.[47,48]

Readers are encouraged to become familiar with the specific mode of operation of the mechanical ventilators employed in their units. Particular attention should be paid to the safe operation and monitoring of the ventilator used. Clinicians should be acutely aware of a product's limitations.

FIGURE 4-1 ▲ Physiologic lung volumes.

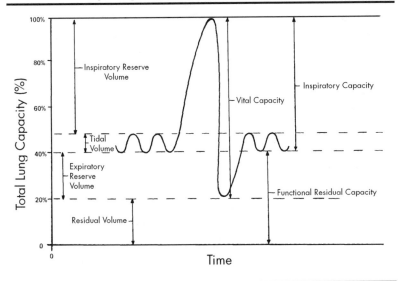

PULMONARY PHYSIOLOGY: A REVIEW

In order to have an understanding of the basic principles of ventilation, it is important to understand some concepts of pulmonary physiology. After the review of physiology, the science and art of marrying physics and physiology will be discussed.

Practitioners are often intimidated by the myriad of terms used in discussing mechanical ventilation and pulmonary physiology. Dead space (D), dynamic and static compliance (C), resistance (R), FRC, V_T, ventilation of the alveoli per unit time ($\dot{V}_A$), perfusion per unit time in the alveolar capillary ($\dot{Q}_C$), elastic recoil, surface tension, mean airway pressure ($\overline{Paw}$), transpulmonary pressure, air trapping, FiO_2, partial pressure of oxygen in alveolar gas (P_AO_2), PaO_2, $\dot{V}_A/\dot{Q}_C$, arterial blood gases (ABGs), and many other terms can be blended to form an incomprehensible foreign language to the novice. It is one of the rites of passage in the NICU to master this new lexicon. To smooth the way, the following discussion focuses on the practical aspects of pulmonary physiology as they apply to patients in the NICU. A word of

caution: All these concepts interrelate in a *dynamic* system that requires a broad understanding.

Ventilation ($\dot{V}_A$) is the bulk flow of gas per unit time into and out of the alveoli to effect oxygen uptake and carbon dioxide (CO_2) elimination. Most practitioners refer to CO_2 elimination as ventilation and reserve the term "oxygenation" for discussing oxygen (O_2) uptake. These two concepts are intertwined to the extent that an increase in **alveolar minute ventilation** ($\dot{V}_A$)—the volume of gas moved into the alveoli per unit time—will increase oxygen content and carbon dioxide elimination within certain limits.[48–51]

Alveolar ventilation ($\dot{V}_A$) is *not* equal to the volume of gas inspired with each breath (the **tidal volume [V_T]**) multiplied by the number of breaths per minute (f). Instead, it is the V_T minus the **respiratory dead space** (V_D) (the volume of the anatomic passages between the external environment and the alveoli that do not function in gas exchange) times the number of inspirations per minute:[48–51]

$$\dot{V}_A = V_T - V_D \times f$$

In addition to the volumes previously defined, there is another physiologic volume that is important to understand: **functional residual capacity (FRC)**. This refers to the point at which the elastic recoil of the lungs and chest wall balance out. It is the lung volume that remains at the end of expiration. This is the volume that allows continual O_2 uptake and CO_2 elimination even when there are no active inspirations. FRC is difficult to establish and maintain in patients with RDS because the surface tension in the alveoli of these babies is four times greater than in normal subjects; therefore, atelectasis with resultant hypoxemia and hypercarbia supervenes. Functional residual capacity and other physiologic lung volumes are illustrated in Figure 4-1.[48–51]

Surface tension results from the intermolecular attraction of structures at a surface. When air and liquid interface, as in the alveoli, the intermolecular attraction among liquid molecules exceeds the forces of attraction between air and liquid molecules. These forces work to minimize the area of interface between air and liquid, and this accounts for the lung's retractive forces, which are calculated according to the Laplace relationship in which pressure (P) is equal to two times the surface tension (ST) divided by the radius (r) of the alveolus.[8,49,50]

$$P = 2ST/r$$

According to this relationship, the surface tension must increase as the alveolar radius decreases. Lung surfactants act at low lung volume and small alveolar radii to minimize these forces of attraction and stabilize the alveolus before it collapses.

Reducing surface tension at the end of expiration helps to maintain FRC by preventing atelectasis. The goal of maintaining oxygenation and ventilation is achieved when atelectasis is prevented and the elastic recoil of the lung is balanced.[47–51]

The lung naturally returns to the smallest resting volume because of its property of **elastic recoil** and the surface tension at the air-liquid interface. This tendency of stretched objects to return to their resting state results in a balance of chest wall (both soft tissue and bony rib cage tissue) and lung elastic recoil, which, in the absence of pathology, returns the lung to FRC at end expiration.[48–51] Figure 4-2 illustrates this concept.

FIGURE 4-2 ▲ Elastic recoil of the lung and chest wall.

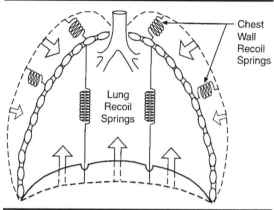

From: Harris TR, and Wood BR. 1996. Physiologic principles. In *Assisted Ventilation of the Neonate,* Goldsmith J, and Karotkin E, eds. Philadelphia: WB Saunders, 32. Reprinted by permission.

The ability to distend the chest wall and increase the volume of the thorax depends on the **compliance** of the system. The relationship of unit change in volume per unit increase in intrathoracic pressure expresses the compliance and thus is a measure of the ability to increase the lung volume with minimal work.[48–51]

Compliance is expressed both in static and dynamic terms. **Static compliance** is measured by holding volume constant, at different levels of inflation, and measuring the pressure within the system needed to maintain the volume. **Dynamic compliance** is measured at the top of inspiration and the bottom of expiration.[49–51] In the absence of pathology, the compliance of the lung is marked. A change in volume is achieved with a minimum change in pressure. Distensibility is quite apparent, as demonstrated in Figure 4-3.

Lung compliance (C$_L$) is equal to change in volume (ΔV) divided by change in pressure (ΔP):

$$C_L = \Delta V/\Delta P$$

Pathophysiology of the lung directly affects compliance and thus requires the clinician to adjust the ventilatory therapy employed.[50,51]

Lung disease decreases compliance markedly, and the pressure required to achieve increases in tidal volume rises. An example of pathophysiology that changes C_L is the RDS compliance curve in Figure 4-3. This is a snapshot of a dynamic system that is constantly changing. Therefore, the astute clinician will be alert for any improvement or deterioration in lung disease that will dictate a change in compliance and thus require an adjustment in ventilation. Unrecognized changes in C_L can drastically alter the FRC of the patient. If compliance improves and the airway pressure remains the same, overdistention of the lung can occur. Conversely, as the disease state worsens and compliance deteriorates, atelectasis occurs if airway pressure remains the same. These concepts are represented in Figure 4-4.

Compliance changes are not restricted to infants with RDS. They occur in all diseases of the newborn lung, including pneumonia, Group B β-hemolytic streptococcal sepsis, meconium aspiration syndrome, fluid overload, and PDA.

As the curve in Figure 4-4 shows, lung compliance is greatest (the largest change in volume occurs with the least change in pressure) when normal FRC is maintained. This information can be applied clinically by evaluating chest wall excursion, and hence lung expansion, with each ventilator cycle. As C_L improves, the chest wall excursion increases. When this happens, ventilatory support can be decreased to avoid overdistention and its concomitant deleterious effects.[49–59] These effects include decreased cardiac output and surfactant production.[14,50,51]

FIGURE 4-3 ▲ Pressure-volume curves of normal and diseased newborn lungs.

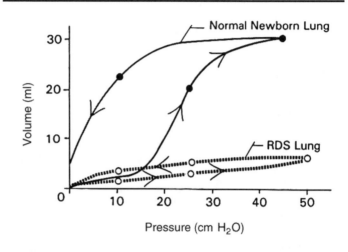

Adapted from: Harris TR, and Wood BR. 1996. Physiologic principles. In *Assisted Ventilation of the Neonate,* Goldsmith J, and Karotkin E, eds. Philadelphia: WB Saunders, 32. Reprinted by permission.

Reduced cardiac output results from increased intrathoracic pressure causing splinting, which impedes venous return to the right atrium.[52] Surfactant production and release are influenced by the mechanical distention of the lungs, and researchers have inferred that lung overdistention diminishes production and release.[56]

FIGURE 4-4 ▲ Compliance curves at various FRCs.

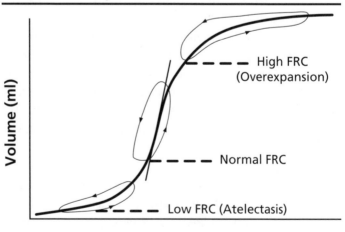

Adapted from: Harris TR, and Wood BR. 1996. Physiologic principles. In *Assisted Ventilation of the Neonate,* Goldsmith J, and Karotkin E, eds. Philadelphia: WB Saunders, 32. Reprinted by permission.

TABLE 4-1 ▲ Pathophysiologic Mechanisms Affecting Ventilation and Perfusion

$\dot{V}_A$	$\dot{Q}_C$
Hypoventilation	Pulmonary hypoperfusion or
Apnea	Pulmonary hyperperfusion due to:
Lung restriction from: Extrinsic factors such as mass effects Intrinsic factors due to space-occupying changes/lesions within the lung	Left-to-right shunting Venous admixture Right-to-left shunting from: Intrapulmonary shunting when ventilation to a segment of lung is zero but perfusion persists
Atelectasis	
Lung volume reduction	
Airway obstruction due to: Aspiration Infection Bronchospasm Gas trapping	Extrapulmonary or intracardiac shunting (shunting at the atrial or ductal level)
Alveolar overdistention	

As lung compliance changes over time, so does resistance. **Resistance** results from friction, such as the viscous resistance of the lungs, as well as resistance to the gas flow in airways and the ventilator circuit.[48,55,57] Airway resistance is directly proportional to the length of any tube through which the gas is flowing and inversely proportional to the fourth power of the radius of the tube, if the flow is laminar. If flow is turbulent, then the resistance increases by the gas flow rate's square. In addition, resistance depends primarily upon the cross-sectional area of the smallest diameter tube in the system.[48,57] Therefore, as the radius decreases and the length of the tube the gas must flow through increases, the pressure required to drive the gas may rise by a factor of 16 just to overcome the resistance of the system and move gas through the tubing and airways.

Anatomic structures and ventilatory appliances that increase resistance include nasal passages, glottis, trachea, bronchi, and endotracheal tubes. Application of CPAP has been reported to both increase[58] and decrease[59] airway resistance. Some data indicate that endotracheal tubes increase the resistance of the system, but

increasing FRC decreases resistance.[59] As can readily be appreciated, resistance depends on a number of interrelated and dynamic variables, including airway diameter, endotracheal tube diameter, and gas flow rates. Clinicians must be alert to changes in resistance that result from secretion accumulation in the airway that can increase the work of breathing.

Resistance and compliance interrelate to determine the **time constant** of the lung: a measure of how quickly pressure generated in the proximal airway results in a 63 percent pressure change in the alveoli. The time constant is a calculated value obtained by multiplying the resistance by the compliance:

$$\textit{time constant (seconds)} = \textit{resistance (cm } H_2O/\textit{liter/second)} \times \textit{compliance (liter/cm } H_2O)$$

When either the resistance or compliance changes, the time constant changes as well. Thus, an increase in resistance results in a prolonged time constant and a need to adjust ventilation therapy.[50,60]

Perfusion is the flow of blood through the lung capillaries per unit time. This is usually expressed in liters per minute.[50]

The ventilation-to-perfusion ($\dot{V}_A/\dot{Q}_C$) ratio expresses the relationship between alveolar ventilation and the blood flow to the lung's capillaries. If the alveolus is ventilated but not perfused, the ratio will approach infinity and PaO_2 will be diminished. Conversely, if the alveolus is not ventilated but is perfused, an intrapulmonary right-to-left shunt will supervene.[50]

Matching of ventilation and perfusion at the alveolar level is the goal of ventilation therapy. Through meticulous adjustment of therapy, the consequences of atelectasis and right-to-left shunting may be avoided; and FiO_2, which affects P_AO_2, can be diminished while PaO_2 is maintained.[49–51]

TABLE 4-2 ▲ Clinical Conditions Affecting Ventilation and Perfusion

Conditions Leading to Decreased $\dot{V}_A$	Conditions Leading to Decreased $\dot{Q}_C$
Hypoventilation from:	**Pulmonary Hypoperfusion Caused by:**
Extreme prematurity	Persistent pulmonary hypertension of the newborn (PPHN) (resulting from increased pulmonary vascular resistance secondary to hypoxemia and acidosis)[50,83]
Abnormalities of the muscles of respiration (including phrenic nerve palsy, spinal cord injury, myasthenia gravis, and Werdnig-Hoffmann syndrome)	
Drug intoxication	**Pulmonary Hyperperfusion from:**
Birth asphyxia	Patent ductus arteriosis (PDA)
Tetanus neonatorum	or
	Ventricular septal defect (VSD)
Apnea from:	(Both PDA and VSD can lead to pulmonary edema, which results in hypoxemia and increased pulmonary vascular resistance and eventually leads to pulmonary hypoperfusion)
Seizures	
Ondine's curse	
Hypoxic-ischemic encephalopathy	Venous admixture (results in hypoxemia and acidosis, which increase pulmonary vascular resistance)
Intracranial hemorrhage	
Apnea of prematurity	
Extrinsic Lung Restriction from:	
Congenital diaphragmatic hernia	
Tumor	
Chylothorax	
Pneumothorax	
Intrinsic Lung Restriction from:	

Congenital malformations such as:
  Lobar emphysema
  Cystic adenomatoid malformation
  Lymphangiectasis	

Pulmonary interstitial emphysema	
Bronchopulmonary dysplasia	
Pulmonary edema	
Pulmonary hemorrhage	
Wilson-Mikity syndrome	
Airway Obstruction from:	
Laryngomalacia	
Choanal atresia	
Pierre-Robin syndrome	
Macroglossia	
Micrognathia	
Nasopharyngeal tumor	
Subglottic stenosis	
Aspiration pneumonia	
Malpositioned endotracheal tube	

Numerous pathophysiologic mechanisms affect both $\dot{V}_A$ and $\dot{Q}_C$ (Table 4-1), and these mechanisms are triggered by a variety of conditions (Table 4-2).

No matter what the pathophysiology causing the alteration in ventilation or perfusion, the ultimate result is the same vicious cycle.

The final common pathway is seen in Figure 4-5. The infant is at risk for slipping into this final common pathway if clinicians do not recognize the prodromal signs of decreased alveolar ventilation or decreased perfusion:

- Increased $PaCO_2$
- Decreased pH

FIGURE 4-5 ▲ Final common pathway of both hypoventilation and hypoperfusion.

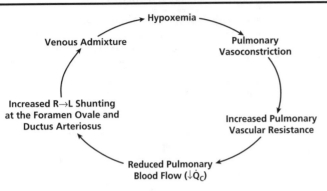

- Decreased PaO_2
- Ductal shunt
- Hypotension
- Hyperinflation
- Decreased C_L
- Decreased cardiac output (CO)

Clinicians direct their intervention at improving $\dot{V}_A$ and $\dot{Q}_C$ to maintain $PaCO_2$, PaO_2, and pH within normal limits, thus minimizing capillary fluid leaks. Preventing capillary fluid leaks helps improve lung compliance and reduces the infant's ventilatory requirements.

When compliance changes, the transpulmonary pressure necessary to increase lung volume also changes. **Transpulmonary pressure** is the difference in pressure between the alveolus and the intrapleural space. When compliance decreases, the transpulmonary pressure necessary to increase lung volume must increase. In other words, the pressure gradient generated across the lung must increase to compensate for the lung's stiffness. However, as intra-alveolar pressure is increased with CPAP, the lung may become overdistended and air trapping may occur within it.[49–51]

Air trapping, which can cause significant increases in $PaCO_2$, results

from alveolar overdistention, which can lead to proximal airway collapse prior to complete emptying of the tidal volume. Because the V_T is not completely exhaled, the carbon dioxide released in the alveolus is not exhausted; instead, it remains available for reuptake into the capillary blood flowing by the alveolus. Judicious use of CPAP and/or mechanical ventilation can improve this physiologic aberration, but inappropriate use results in further complications.[50,51]

MEAN AIRWAY PRESSURE: WHERE THE MONEY IS

The patient's clinical status is improved by establishing and maintaining FRC. This is done by adjusting the PEEP or other ventilator parameters to alter the **mean airway pressure** (P$\overline{aw}$) within the ventilator circuit. All the components of ventilation previously discussed— V_T, f, gas flow, PIP, PEEP, and inspiratory time—interrelate to determine P$\overline{aw}$. As with any dynamic, fluid system, any adjustment in one parameter influences the others.[49–51]

FIGURE 4-6 ▲ The positive pressure ventilator cycle.

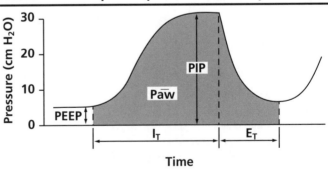

PIP—peak inspiratory pressure
PEEP—positive end-expiratory pressure
I$_T$—inspiratory time
E$_T$—expiratory time
P$\overline{aw}$—mean airway pressure (the total area under curve—shaded)

Adapted from: Coulter D. 1981. *Neonatal Transport Manual*. Salt Lake City: University of Utah; and Cassani VL III. 1985. *Neonatal Transport Manual*. Reno, Nevada: Washoe Medical Center. Reprinted by permission.

Mean airway pressure is the algebraic sum of the PIP, PEEP, inspiratory time (I_T), flow rate of the gas through the ventilator circuit, and rate of mechanical ventilation. It is the average pressure transmitted to the airways over a series of ventilator cycles. Mean airway pressure is the area under the pressure-time curve of the ventilator cycle, as illustrated in Figure 4-6 and expressed algebraically as follows:

$$P\overline{aw} = \frac{(f)\ (I_T)\ (PIP) + [60 - (f)\ (I_T)]\ (PEEP)}{60}$$

There are numerous ways of altering the components of $P\overline{aw}$. If the rate of mechanical ventilation is held constant, $P\overline{aw}$ may be increased by increasing inspiratory flow rate, PIP, or PEEP or by reversing the inspiratory-to-expiratory (I:E) ratio.[62,63] This is a powerful tool for managing patients with respiratory failure.

Mean airway pressure has a pivotal role in maintaining FRC and $\dot{V}_A$ during mechanical ventilation. Clinical researchers have evaluated the effects of altering frequency, PIP, PEEP, and pressure waveform on oxygenation of infants with RDS.[58–72] Reynolds as well as Smith and colleagues have shown that increasing f and PIP within certain limits improves oxygenation.[62,63,64,66,67] Changes in inspiratory flow rate, and hence the pressure waveform of the ventilator, also alter oxygenation.[66] Fox and associates demonstrated that increased PEEP improved oxygenation of infants with RDS.[68] Reversing the I:E ratio has also improved oxygen content in some patients.[64,65,70,71]

When evaluated on an individual basis, these data appear to be conflicting. However, the underlying principle that weaves through all these studies is that altering mean airway pressure changes oxygenation and ventilation in newborns with RDS. Each of the para-

FIGURE 4-7 ▲ Ventilator changes that increase mean airway pressure.

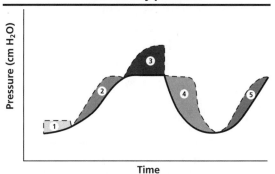

1. Positive end-expiratory pressure higher
2. Inspiratory flow rate increased
3. Peak inspiratory pressure higher
4. Inspiratory time longer
5. Increased ventilator rate

Adapted from: Coulter D. 1981. *Neonatal Transport Manual*. Salt Lake City: University of Utah; and Cassani VL III. 1985. *Neonatal Transport Manual*. Reno, Nevada: Washoe Medical Center. Reprinted by permission.

meters evaluated by these researchers—PIP, PEEP, I:E ratio, f, and gas flow—directly affects $P\overline{aw}$. In the dynamic system of an infant with RDS and a continuous flow ventilator, changes in any one of these components may result in a significant change in mean airway pressure.

Boros and coworkers, in an elegantly designed study, independently varied I:E ratio, PEEP, and inspiratory flow rate during IMV. Oxygenation improved during severe RDS as mean airway pressure increased when any of the three variables was manipulated. These investigators argued that mean airway pressure has a central role in maintaining FRC and that manipulation of the ventilator variable is important only in terms of its direct effect on mean airway pressure.[69]

Diagrammatically, this idea is simple. As shown in Figure 4-7, changes in (1) inspiratory flow rate, (2) PIP, (3) I:E ratio, (4) ventilator rate, and (5) PEEP change the shape of the pressure waveform. However, the mean airway pressure, which is the area under the curve of the pressure waveform, may be the *same* when one of these parameters is decreased while another is increased.

Before this underlying principle was recognized, great debates raged among clinicians about what parameters are important to manipulate when providing IMV and weaning mechanical ventilation. When discussing IMV, clinicians at one center would advocate rapid rate ventilation with low PIPs; others would employ lower ventilatory frequencies with higher PIPs. As the understanding of the physics and physiology became clearer, it was apparent that both methods of ventilation were successful because they both maintained FRC by increasing P$\overline{aw}$ to the point necessary to overcome the resistive forces of the atelectatic lung.

These are not the only manipulations that can affect mean airway pressure. Changing the diameter of the endotracheal tube or ventilator circuit tubing will also change mean airway pressure.[72] The ventilator and patient are a dynamic system that changes from moment to moment. As the infant's lung disease lessens, compliance improves, the time constant of the lung lengthens, and the upstroke of the inspiratory cycle will rise rapidly. The PIP will be reached more rapidly, and the ventilator will deliver more tidal volume with each breath.[72,73] This is synonymous with a change to a more "square wave" ventilatory pattern and results in increased minute ventilation.[57,72] Thus, an increase in mean airway pressure will occur as compliance improves. This may be beneficial, up to a point. Mirro and coworkers demonstrated that increased mean airway pressure in normal lungs decreases cardiac output in a linear relationship and increased mean airway pressure in diseased lungs reduces heart, kidney, and intestinal blood flow despite arterial blood pressure remaining the same.[74] Thus, application of mechanical ventilation requires continual adjustments in therapy.

PATIENT APPLICATION: MORE ART THAN SCIENCE

In the early 1970s, after Gregory and coworkers rekindled interest in applying positive pressure in treating RDS and Daily, Smith, and colleagues demonstrated that mechanical ventilation, judiciously applied, improved the outcome of infants with RDS, an avalanche of articles and books appeared on the subject.[31–33,39,44,45,63,67–82] The discussions ranged from proper techniques for modifying adult ventilators for neonatal application to the introduction of IMV.[33,39,44,52,64,66,79]

As sophistication in utilizing mechanical ventilation developed, three basic mechanical ventilator variants evolved: (1) negative pressure ventilators, derivatives of the "iron lung" utilized for poliomyelitis victims, (2) positive pressure, volume-cycled ventilators, and (3) positive pressure ventilators that are time cycled and pressure limited.[24,76,82] More recently, SIMV ventilators that use microprocessors and triggering devices with rapid response times have become available. A detailed review of ventilator design, controls, and fact sheets is available in the literature.[46–48]

Inherent limitations in both the negative pressure and volume-cycled ventilators have decreased their use.[47] Since the mid-1970s, the ventilators produced for use in neonates have been pressure limited and time cycled. Therefore, this discussion focuses on use of pressure-limited, time-cycled ventilators for treatment of neonatal respiratory failure.

Mechanical ventilation is employed to accomplish effective gas exchange.[60,82] However, the optimal application of mechanical ventilation remains a controversial topic more than four decades after Donald and Lord first described the use of the technique in newborns.[29] One problem is that clinicians have become victims of their own initial success.

When first introduced, mechanical ventilators were employed for treating infants weighing more than 1,500 gm. As clinicians became more adept, survivors weighing less than 1,000 gm became the rule rather than the exception.[80] Today, infants weighing less than 500 gm survive.[79] Therefore, the patient population receiving mechanical ventilation became larger and more diverse physiologically.

Organized, blinded, randomized, controlled studies of mechanical ventilation in newborns have been difficult to establish because of this diversity and the ethical dilemma of using control groups. As the initial successes were reported and led to widespread use of mechanical ventilation, the crush of events has pushed the application of technology forward. Scientific inquiries have, unfortunately, not been performed to evaluate all of the arguments of some very expert clinicians.

The use of IMV in the NICU is directed at correcting two fundamental problems of respiratory failure in the newborn: atelectasis and obstructive disease processes. Chapter 5 describes in detail the application of IMV and SIMV for treatment of these problems.

SUMMARY

Mechanical ventilation of newborns has developed rapidly since 1964. The technique is recognized as the standard of care for treating respiratory failure in the newborn. It requires meticulous application of basic physiologic principles and careful titration of therapy to maintain adequate gas exchange. Early reports of success have resulted in widespread use of the technique without blinded, controlled trials to demonstrate efficacy of a particular technique. Clinicians have applied mechanical ventilation to treat atelectatic and obstructive diseases of the newborn respiratory system.

DEDICATION

This chapter is dedicated to Jennifer Marie Day and all the other babies who proved the efficacy of IMV.

REFERENCES

1. Strang LB, ed. 1977. *Neonatal Respiration: Physiology and Clinical Studies.* Philadelphia: JB Lippincott.
2. Milner AD, and Martin RJ. 1985. *Neonatal and Pediatric Respiratory Medicine.* Philadelphia: JB Lippincott.
3. Stern L, ed. 1984. *Hyaline Membrane Disease: Pathogenesis and Pathophysiology.* New York: Grune & Stratton.
4. Kirby RR, and Greybar GB. 1980. Intermittent mandatory ventilation. *International Anesthesiology Clinics* 18(2).
5. Comroe JH. 1977. *Retrospectroscope: Insights into Medical Discovery.* Menlo Park, California: Von Gehr.
6. Gregory GA. October 7, 1987. Personal communication.
7. Sunshine P. October 7, 1987. Personal communication.
8. Laplace PS. *Traite' de Me'canique Ce'leste,* 5 vols. Paris: Crapelet, Courcier, 1798–1827.
9. von Neergaard K. 1929. *Neve auffassungen uber einen grundbegriff der atemmechanik. Die retraktionskraft der lunge, abhangig von der oberflachenspunnung in den alveoleh.* English translation by Comroe JH Jr, ed. 1976. In *Pulmonary and Respiratory Physiology: Benchmark Papers in Human Physiology,* part I. Stroudsberg, Pennsylvania: Dowden, Hutchinson and Ross, 214–234.
10. Macklin CC. 1954. The pulmonary alveolar mucoid film and the pneumocytes. *Lancet* 1: 1099–1104.
11. Pattle RE. 1956. A test of silicone anti-foam treatment of lung oedema in rabbits. *Journal of Pathology and Bacteriology* 72: 203.
12. Cook C, Sutherland J, and Segal S. 1957. Studies of respiratory physiology in the newborn infant. Part III: Measurements of mechanics of respiration. *Journal of Clinical Investigation* 36: 440.
13. Clements JA. 1957. Surface tension of lung extracts. *Proceedings of the Society for Experimental Biology and Medicine* 95: 170.
14. Avery ME, and Mead J. 1959. Surface properties in relation to atelectasis and hyaline membrane disease. *American Journal of Diseases of Children* 17: 517.
15. Klaus MH, Clements JA, and Havel RJ. 1961. Composition of surface-active material isolated from beef lung. *Proceedings of the National Academy of Sciences of the United States of America* 47: 1858.
16. Thannhauser SJ, Benotti J, and Boncoddo NF. 1946. Isolation and properties of hydrolecithin (dipalmityl lecithin) from lungs, its occurrence in the sphingomyelin fraction of animal tissues. *Journal of Biological Chemistry* 166: 669.
17. Buckingham S, and Avery ME. 1962. Time of appearance of lung surfactant in the foetal mouse. *Nature* 193: 688.
18. Klaus MH, et al. 1962. Alveolar epithelial cell mitochondria as a source of the surface-active lung lining. *Science* 137: 750.
19. Gil J, and Reiss OK. 1973. Isolation and characterization of lamellar bodies and tubular myelin from rat lung homogenates. *Journal of Cellular Biology* 58(1): 152–171.

20. Williams MC, and Mason RJ. 1977. Development of the Type II cell in the fetal rat lung. *American Review of Respiratory Disease* 115(6 part 2): 37–47.

21. Campiche MA, et al. 1963. An electron microscope study of the fetal development of human lung. *Pediatrics* 32: 976.

22. Gregory GA. October 10, 1987. Personal communication.

23. Sunshine P. October 10, 1987. Personal communication.

24. Gluck L. February 22, 1988. Personal communication.

25. Stahlman M. 1964. Treatment of cardiovascular disorders of the newborn. *Pediatric Clinics of North America* 11(2): 363.

26. Kitterman JA, Phibbs RH, and Tooley WH. 1970. Catheterization of umbilical vessels in newborn infants. *Pediatric Clinics of North America* 17(4): 895–912.

27. Hey E, and Mount L. 1966. Temperature control in incubators. *Lancet* 2(456): 202–203.

28. Hey E, and O'Connell B. 1970. Oxygen consumption and heat balance in the cot-nursed baby. *Archives of Disease in Childhood* 45(241): 335–343.

29. Donald I, and Lord J. 1953. Augmented respiration studies in atelectasis neonatorum. *Lancet* 1: 9.

30. Thomas DV, et al. 1965. Prolonged respirator use in pulmonary insufficiency of the newborn. *Journal of the American Medical Association* 193(3): 183.

31. Gregory GA, et al. 1971. Treatment of the idiopathic respiratory distress syndrome with continuous positive airway pressure. *New England Journal of Medicine* 284(24): 1333–1340.

32. Daily WJR, et al. 1971. Mechanical ventilation of newborn infants. Part III: Historical comments and development of a scoring system for selection of infants. *Anesthesiology* 34(2): 119–126.

33. Smith PC, and Daily WJR. 1971. Mechanical ventilation of newborn infants. Part IV: Technique of controlled intermittent positive-pressure ventilation. *Anesthesiology* 34(2): 127–131.

34. Stahlman MT, Young WC, and Payne G. 1962. Studies of ventilatory aids in hyaline membrane disease. *American Journal of Diseases of Children* 104: 526.

35. Cournand A, et al. 1948. Physiological studies of the effects of intermittent positive pressure breathing on cardiac output in man. *American Journal of Physiology* 152: 162.

36. Swyer PR. 1965. An assessment of artificial respiration in the newborn. In *Problems of Neonatal Intensive Care Units, Report of the 59th Ross Conference on Pediatric Research.* Columbus, Ohio: Ross Laboratories.

37. Harrison VC, Hesse H de V, and Klein M. 1968. The significance of grunting in hyaline membrane disease. *Pediatrics* 41(3): 549–559.

38. Kirby RR. 1981. Mechanical ventilation of the newborn, pitfalls and practice. *Perinatology-Neonatology* July/August: 47–51.

39. deLemos RA, and Kirby RR. 1980. Early development: Intermittent mandatory ventilation in neonatal respiratory support. *International Anesthesia Clinics* 18(2): 39–51.

40. Tooley WH. 1977. Hyaline membrane disease: Telling it like it was. *American Review of Respiratory Disease* 115(6 part 2): 19–28.

41. Hesse H de V, et al. 1970. Intermittent positive pressure ventilation in hyaline membrane disease. *Journal of Pediatrics* 76(2): 183–193.

42. Gregory GA, et al. 1977. The time course changes in lung function after a change in CPAP. *Clinical Research* 25: 193A.

43. Love J, and Tillery N. 1953. New treatment of atelectasis of the newborn. *American Journal of Diseases of Children* 86: 423.

44. Daily WJR, Sunshine P, and Smith PC. 1971. Mechanical ventilation of newborn infants. Part V: Five years experience. *Anesthesiology* 34(2): 132–138.

45. Kirby RR, et al. 1971. Continuous flow ventilation as an alternative to assisted or controlled ventilation in infants. *Anesthesia and Analgesia* 51(6): 871–875.

46. Visveshwara N, et al. 1991. Patient-triggered synchronized assisted ventilation of newborns. Report of a preliminary study and three years' experience. *Journal of Perinatology* 11(4): 347–354.

47. Yoder BA, et al. 1986. Design of mechanical ventilators. In *Neonatal Pulmonary Care,* Thibeault DW, and Gregory GA, eds. Menlo Park, California: Addison-Wesley, 281–307.

48. Kirby RR, Smith RA, and Desautels DA, eds. 1985. *Mechanical Ventilation.* New York: Churchill Livingstone.

49. Carlo WA, and Martin RJ. 1986. Principles of neonatal assisted ventilation. *Pediatric Clinics of North America* 33(1): 221–237.

50. Mines AH. 1981. *Respiratory Physiology.* New York: Raven Press.

51. Harris TR, and Wood BR. 1996. Physiologic principles. In *Assisted Ventilation of the Neonate,* Goldsmith JP, and Karotkin EH, eds. Philadelphia: WB Saunders, 21–68.

52. Suter PM, Fairley B, and Isenberg MD. 1975. Optimum end-expiratory airway pressure in patients with acute pulmonary failure. *New England Journal of Medicine* 292(6): 284–289.

53. Kumar A, et al. 1970. Continuous positive pressure ventilation in acute respiratory failure. *New England Journal of Medicine* 283(26): 1430–1436.

54. Richards CC, and Backman L. 1961. Lung and chest wall compliance of apneic paralyzed infants. *Journal of Clinical Investigation* 40(1): 73.

55. Polgar G. 1967. Opposing forces to breathing in newborn infants. *Biology of the Neonate* 11(1): 1–22.

56. Truog WE. 1984. Surface active material: Influence of lung distension and mechanical ventilation on secretion. *Seminars in Perinatology* 8(4): 300–307.

57. Polgar G, and String ST. 1966. The viscous resistance of the lung tissues in newborn infants. *Journal of Pediatrics* 69(5): 787–792.

58. Briscal WA, and Dubois AB. 1958. The relationship between airway resistance, airway conductance and lung volume in subjects of different age and body size. *Journal of Clinical Investigation* 37: 1279.

59. Saunders RA, Milner AD, and Hopkins IE. 1976. The effects of continuous positive airway pressure on lung mechanics and lung volume in the neonate. *Biology of the Neonate* 29(3–4): 178–186.

60. Stark AR, and Frantz ID. 1986. Respiratory distress syndrome. *Pediatric Clinics of North America* 33(3): 533–544.

61. Fox WW, and Duara S. 1983. Persistent pulmonary hypertension in the neonate: Diagnosis and management. *Journal of Pediatrics* 103(4): 505–514.

62. Reynolds EOR. 1974. Pressure waveform and ventilator settings for mechanical ventilation in severe hyaline membrane disease. *International Anesthesiology Clinics* 12(4): 259–280.

63. Reynolds EO. 1971. Effects of alterations in mechanical ventilator settings on pulmonary gas exchange in hyaline membrane disease. *Archives of Disease in Childhood* 46(246): 152–159.

64. Herman S, and Reynolds EOR. 1973. Methods for improving oxygenation in infants mechanically ventilated for severe hyaline membrane disease. *Archives of Disease in Childhood* 48(8): 612–617.

65. Owen-Thomas JB, Ulan OA, and Swyer PR. 1968. The effect of varying inspiratory gas flow rate on arterial oxygenation during IPPV in the respiratory distress syndrome. *British Journal of Anaesthesia* 40(7): 493–502.

66. Smith PC, Schach E, and Daily WJR. 1972. Mechanical ventilation of newborn infants. Part II: Effects of independent variation of rate and pressure on arterial oxygenation. *Anesthesiology* 37(5): 498–502.

67. Smith PC, et al. 1969. Mechanical ventilation of newborn infants. Part I: The effect of rate and pressure on arterial oxygenation of infants with respiratory distress syndrome. *Pediatric Research* 3(3): 244–254.

68. Fox WW, et al. 1977. The PaO_2 response to changes in PEEP in RDS. *Critical Care Medicine* 5(5): 226–229.

69. Boros SJ, et al. 1977. The effect of independent variations in inspiratory-expiratory ratio and end expiratory pressure during mechanical ventilation in hyaline membrane disease: The significance of mean airway pressure. *Journal of Pediatrics* 91(5): 794–798.

70. Spahr A, et al. 1980. Hyaline membrane disease: A controlled study of inspiratory to expiratory ratio in its management by ventilator. *American Journal of Diseases of Children* 134(4): 373–376.

71. Eriksson I, et al. 1977. The influence of ventilatory pattern on ventilation, circulation and oxygen transport during continuous positive-pressure ventilation: An experimental study. *Acta Anaesthesiologica Scandinavica (Supplement)* 64: 149–163.

72. LeSouef PN, England SJ, and Bryan AC. 1984. Total resistance of the respiratory system in preterm infants with and without an endotracheal tube. *Journal of Pediatrics* 104(1): 108–111.

73. Cunningham MD, and Desai NS. 1986. Methods of assessment and findings regarding pulmonary function in infants less than 1,000 grams. *Clinics in Perinatology* 13(2): 299–313.

74. Mirro R, et al. 1987. Relationship between mean airway pressure, cardiac output, and organ blood flow with normal and decreased respiratory compliance. *Journal of Pediatrics* 111(1): 101–106.

75. Belton H, et al. 1974. Ventilatory support of the newborn infant with respiratory distress syndrome and respiratory failure. *International Anesthesiology Clinics* 12(4): 81–110.

76. Mannino F, et al. 1976. Early mechanical ventilation in RDS with a prolonged inspiration. *Pediatric Research* 10(1): 464A.

77. Hakanson DO. 1996. Positive pressure ventilation: Volume cycled ventilators. In *Assisted Ventilation of the Neonate*, Goldsmith JP, and Karotkin EH, eds. Philadelphia: WB Saunders, 187–197.

78. Fox WW, and Spitzer AR. 1996. Positive pressure ventilation: Pressure and time cycled ventilators. In *Assisted Ventilation of the Neonate*, Goldsmith JP, and Karotkin EH, eds. Philadelphia: WB Saunders, 167–186.

79. Bhat R, and Zikos-Labropoulou E. 1986. Resuscitation and respiratory management of infants weighing less than 1,000 grams. *Clinics in Perinatology* l3(2): 285–297.

80. Krauss AN. 1980. Assisted ventilation: A critical review. *Clinics in Perinatology* 7(1): 61–74.

81. Reynolds EOR. 1979. Ventilator therapy: Principles of management of pulmonary insufficiency in the neonate. In *Neonatal Pulmonary Care*, Thibeault DW, and Gregory G, eds. Menlo Park, California: Addison-Wesley, 217–236.

82. Mannino F, and Merritt TA. 1986. The management of respiratory distress syndrome. In *Neonatal Pulmonary Care*, Thibeault DW, and Gregory G, eds. Menlo Park, California: Addison-Wesley, 427–460.

83. Turner GR, and Levin DL. 1984. Prostaglandin synthesis inhibition in persistent pulmonary hypertension of the newborn. *Clinics in Perinatology* 11(3): 581.

NOTES

NOTES

5 Application of Mechanical Ventilation

V. L. Cassani III, RNC, MSN, MSNA, NNP, CRNA
Debbie Fraser Askin, RNC, MN

There have been many changes in ventilatory management of sick newborns since 1991. Surfactant replacement therapy for respiratory distress syndrome (RDS), helium-oxygen ventilation for treatment of pulmonary interstitial emphysema, high-frequency ventilation (oscillatory, jet, and flow interrupter), synchronized intermittent mandatory ventilation (SIMV), liquid ventilation with perfluorochemicals for respiratory failure, and nitric oxide therapy have all been aggressively researched. The results of the initial trials in each of these areas have changed the way clinicians view and manage ventilation of the newborn, much as Gregory's landmark study regarding the benefits of continuous positive airway pressure (CPAP) for treatment of respiratory distress syndrome changed respiratory management of the newborn in the early 1970s.[1]

This new technology has directly affected how newborns with varying types of lung disease are managed. Although these new therapies have a place in the world of neonatology, not all will be used for the majority of sick newborns. Rational application of the basic underlying physiologic principles of intermittent mandatory ventilation (IMV) remains the mainstay of therapy for babies with respiratory failure. This chapter reviews the components of conventional mechanical ventilation, explains how the fundamentals of IMV described in Chapter 4 can be applied to selected patients in the NICU, describes how surfactant replacement therapy affects the management of IMV, outlines the various adjuncts to mechanical ventilation, and describes the application of SIMV.

CRITERIA FOR MECHANICAL VENTILATION

During the 1970s, after Gregory and associates' evaluation of continuous positive airway pressure,[1] Reynolds' studies seemed to indicate that prolonged inspiratory time and lower peak inspiratory pressure (PIP) would improve oxygenation and decrease the likelihood of sequelae.[2-4] Mannino and colleagues showed improved survival with fewer sequelae in infants treated with early mechanical ventilation without prior application of CPAP, when compared to infants receiving conventional management of RDS, which at that time consisted of hood oxygen and CPAP.[5] The criteria for initiating mechanical ventilation changed. The use of

CPAP as an initial treatment for RDS and meconium aspiration syndrome gave way to use of IMV for initial therapy in many centers.[6,7]

This practice has been modified in some centers. Presently, some clinicians still initially manage respiratory distress of varying etiologies with nasal CPAP (Chapter 11) and reserve intubation and ventilation for more clinically distressed patients.

The following are commonly accepted criteria for intubation and ventilation:

1. Respiratory acidosis with pH <7.25
2. Severe hypoxemia (PaO_2 <50 mmHg despite FiO_2 [fraction of inspired oxygen] >0.8)
3. Apnea complicating the clinical course of RDS

These criteria must be evaluated in light of each individual clinical situation. A term infant with respiratory distress secondary to a pneumothorax may benefit from hood oxygen rather than from IMV. An extremely premature infant who was not exposed to steroids *in utero* may benefit from immediate intubation and ventilation followed by surfactant administration. In addition, term infants with congenital diaphragmatic hernia benefit from immediate intubation and ventilation to prevent development of persistent pulmonary hypertension of the newborn (PPHN): hypercarbia, acidosis, and hypoxemia.

COMPONENTS OF CONVENTIONAL MECHANICAL VENTILATION

Effective mechanical ventilation depends on adequate oxygenation and removal of carbon dioxide. In the case of conventional mechanical ventilation, this can be achieved through

TABLE 5-1 ▲ Ventilator Manipulations to Improve Ventilation and Decrease PaCO$_2$

Parameter	Advantage	Disadvantage
↑ Rate	Easy to titrate Minimizes barotrauma	Maintains same dead space/tidal volume May lead to inadvertent PEEP
↑ PIP	Better bulk flow (improved dead space/tidal volume)	More barotrauma Shifts to stiffer compliance curve
↓ PEEP	Widens compression pressure Decreases dead space Decreases expiratory load Shifts to steeper compliance curve	Decreases P$\overline{aw}$ Decreases oxygenation Stops splinting obstructed/closed airways
↑ Flow	Permits shorter T$_I$, longer T$_E$	More barotrauma
↑ T$_E$	Allows longer expiration for passive expiration in face of prolonged time constant	Shortens T$_I$ Decreases P$\overline{aw}$ Decreases oxygenation

Modified from: Richardson D. 1991. Mechanical ventilation. In *Manual of Neonatal Care*, 3rd ed., Cloherty JP, and Stark AR, eds. Boston: Little, Brown, 204. Reprinted by permission.

manipulation of six components: (1) ventilator rate, (2) PIP, (3) positive end-expiratory pressure (PEEP), (4) inspiratory-to-expiratory (I:E) ratio, (5) flow of gases through the ventilator, and (6) FiO_2. Manipulation of these variables determines the shape or waveform of the mechanical breath and the mean airway pressure (P$\overline{aw}$).

VENTILATOR SETTINGS

The following general principles apply to ventilator settings:

- Alveolar and arterial carbon dioxide levels depend on minute ventilation and are most directly affected by ventilator rate, PIP, PEEP, and I:E ratio (Table 5-1). Acceptable levels of $PaCO_2$ depend on the infant's gestational age and disease process.
- Oxygenation is most directly affected by FiO_2, PIP, PEEP, and I:E ratio (Table 5-2).
- Mean airway pressure is determined by PIP, rate, flow, I:E ratio, and PEEP (Figure 5-1).
- The impact of various ventilator settings will depend on the infant's compliance and resistance.

The initial settings chosen for neonatal ventilation should be based on the infant's

TABLE 5-2 ▲ Ventilator Manipulations to Improve Oxygenation

Parameter	Advantage	Disadvantage
↑ FiO_2	Minimizes barotrauma Easily administered	Fails to affect V̇/Q matching Direct toxicity, expecially >0.60
↑ PIP	Critical opening pressure Improves V̇/Q	Barotrauma: air leak, BPD
↑ PEEP	Maintains FRC/prevents collapse Splints obstructed airways Regularizes respiration	Shifts to stiffer compliance curve Obstructs venous return Increases expiratory work and CO_2 Increases dead space
↑ T_I	Increases P̄aw without increasing PIP "Critical opening time"	Necessitates slower rates, higher PIP Lower minute ventilation for given PIP-PEEP combination
↑ Flow	Square wave—maximizes P̄aw	Greater shear force, more barotrauma Greater resistance at greater flows
↑ Rate	Increases P̄aw while using lower PIP	Inadvertent PEEP with high rates or long time constants

Note: All manipulations (except FiO_2) result in higher mean airway pressure.

From: Richardson D. 1991. Mechanical ventilation. In *Manual of Neonatal Care,* 3rd ed., Cloherty JP, and Stark AR, eds. Boston: Little, Brown, 202. Reprinted by permission.

compliance and resistance, disease process, and gestational age and size.

PIP

As the name implies, peak inspiratory pressure refers to the maximum level of pressure

FIGURE 5-1 ▲ The positive pressure ventilator cycle.

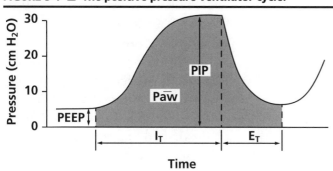

PIP—peak inspiratory pressure
PEEP—positive end-expiratory pressure
I_T—inspiratory time
E_T—expiratory time
P̄aw—mean airway pressure (the total area under curve—shaded)

Adapted from: Coulter D. 1981. *Neonatal Transport Manual.* Salt Lake City: University of Utah; and Cassani VL III. 1985. *Neonatal Transport Manual.* Reno, Nevada: Washoe Medical Center. Reprinted by permission.

generated during inspiration. With a pressure-limited ventilator, PIP is attained and held at the preset limit until the inspiratory time is complete and exhalation is triggered. PIP is depicted in Figure 5-1.

Increasing the PIP has the effect of increasing tidal volume and mean airway pressure, therefore improving both ventilation and oxygenation.[8] High PIPs will expand those alveoli with high opening pressures but contribute to barotrauma and may impede venous return.[9] To avoid adverse effects, the lowest pressure necessary to adequately move the chest should be chosen.

PEEP

Positive end-expiratory pressure represents a constant pressure applied to the airway between inspirations (illustrated in Figure 5-1). The infant with normal lungs maintains a physiologic level of PEEP—approximately +2 cm H_2O—by closing the glottis.[10] Inadvertent PEEP develops when expiratory time is too short for the alveoli to empty adequately. Inadvertent PEEP may be of particular concern with certain types of ventilator modes such as high-frequency ventilation.

Infants with RDS benefit from the application of PEEP because it acts to increase functional residual capacity (FRC), stabilize alveoli, and prevent collapse. The level of PEEP used will affect tidal volume and minute ventilation because transmural airway pressure (Δp) is determined by PIP minus PEEP.[11] Adequate levels of PEEP

FIGURE 5-2 ▲ Comparison of ventilator waveforms: A, sine wave (relative); B, square wave (relative).

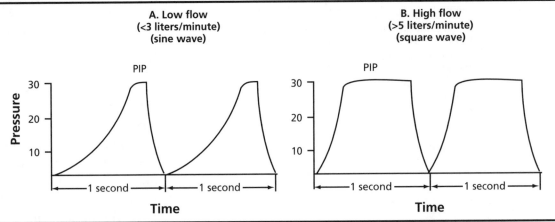

From: Spitzer AR, and Fox WW. 1996. Positive-pressure ventilation: Pressure-limited and time-cycled ventilators. In *Assisted Ventilation of the Neonate,* 3rd ed., Goldsmith JP, and Karotkin EH, eds. Philadelphia: WB Saunders, 169. Reprinted by permission.

improve the relationship between ventilation and perfusion in the lung.[8,11]

Elevated levels of PEEP may impede venous return, decrease cardiac output and lung compliance, and contribute to air leak.[11,12] PEEP can also increase pulmonary vascular resistance by compressing the pulmonary vascular bed.

Ventilator Rate

Minute ventilation and hence carbon dioxide levels are largely determined by ventilator rate. Physiologic rates of 40–60 breaths per minute are commonly chosen as initial ventilator settings, but hyperventilation or slower rates are advocated in some clinical situations. Higher ventilator rates necessitate a shorter expiratory time and may contribute to inadvertent PEEP and air trapping. Lower rates are used in weaning the infant from conventional mechanical ventilation, but when low rates are used early in the course of lung disease, a higher PIP may be required to ensure adequate ventilation.

I:E Ratio

This ratio can be determined by setting either inspiratory or expiratory time or by directly setting the ratio (depending on the type of ventilator used). With a ventilator rate of 60, a 1:1 ratio is commonly used, indicating that the time for inspiration equals the time for expiration in the respiratory cycle. Another option is to choose an inspiratory time of 0.35–0.45 seconds, but this will depend on the desired ventilator rate.[10]

Other options include (1) inverse ratios in which the inspiratory time is longer than the expiratory time (used in some clinical situations to improve oxygenation) and (2) prolonged expiratory times (used in weaning and in some obstructive lung problems). Changing the I:E ratio primarily affects mean airway pressure and therefore oxygenation.[8]

Flow Through the Ventilator Circuit

Flow is measured in liters per minute and refers to the flow of gas through the patient circuit.[12] A flow rate of at least twice the infant's minute ventilation ensures that the ventilator can reach the desired pressure.[9] Flow rates of 4–8 liters/minute are common.

The amount of flow will determine the shape of the ventilator breath by determining how quickly the desired PIP is reached. A sine wave has a slow, smooth progression from the level of PEEP to the level of PIP. It resembles a normal breath and results in a lower mean airway pressure. A square wave results when high flows are used to move the ventilator rapidly from the resting or expiratory pressure level to the peak inspiratory pressure. A longer time is spent at the PIP, which may assist in opening atelectatic areas but may also result in increased barotrauma (Figure 5-2 illustrates sine and square waves).[9]

Fraction of Inspired Oxygen

Ranging from concentrations of 21 to 100 percent, oxygen can be administered to maintain adequate levels of arterial oxygenation. Increasing the FiO_2 is the most direct way to improve oxygenation. Oxygen toxicity, associated with retinopathy of prematurity and bronchopulmonary dysplasia (BPD), is of particular concern in the premature infant.[13–17] Desired PaO_2 levels should be individually determined for each infant according to gestational age and disease process. Once an FiO_2 of 0.6 is reached, other alternatives for improving oxygenation such as increased PEEP or P$\overline{aw}$ are usually considered.[12]

Mean Airway Pressure

This is a major determinant of oxygenation. As illustrated in Figure 5-1, mean airway pressure refers to the average pressure applied to the lungs during a respiratory cycle and can be calculated by dividing the area under the pressure curve by the length of the cycle.[8]

Although it is not directly determined by the ventilator operator, mean airway pressure can be altered by manipulating several variables such as PIP, I:E ratio, PEEP, flow, and ventilator rate. To increase mean airway pressure and attain the greatest improvement in oxygenation, PEEP may be increased within certain limits.[13] See Figure 4-7 for an illustration of the effects of these variables on mean airway pressure. The side effects of high levels of mean airway pressure are similar to those of PEEP.

BASIC MANAGEMENT USING IMV

Coincident with the initial reports of improved outcome, students of mechanical ventilation appreciated the need for tailoring therapy to treat the two primary problems faced in NICUs: atelectasis and obstructive diseases in neonates with respiratory failure.[6,7,14] Respiratory failure, as defined here, is limited to impaired pulmonary gas exchange. Physiologic alterations in gas exchange from primary lung disease result in hypercarbia and acidosis. Patients require mechanical ventilation to correct these problems and prevent further compromise.

ATELECTASIS

Decreased FRC and diminished gas exchange are the result of the atelectatic processes seen with congenital pneumonia, RDS, and Group B β-hemolytic streptococcal sepsis.[6,7,15] Currently, there are two basic approaches to managing respiratory failure caused by atelectasis in neonates:

1. **Slow-rate IMV.** Initially, adherents of slow-rate IMV recommended that inspiratory time be up to one second or longer and that PIP be as high as 35 cm H_2O in infants weighing >1,500 gm.[6,7,14,15] These parameters are adjusted as follows: PEEP is applied to assist with "recruitment" of atelectatic alveoli; FiO_2 is adjusted to maintain a PaO_2 of 50–70 mmHg or oxygen saturation of 88–92 percent; rate is 20–30 breaths per minute, and flow through the ventilator circuit 8–12 liters per minute. As hypoxemia and acidosis are corrected, the FiO_2 is gradually reduced until it is <0.6. At that point, inspiratory time is lengthened while IMV rate and PIP are decreased as tolerated to maintain PaO_2 at 50–70 mmHg. These manipulations result in a decrease in mean airway pressure as the lung disease improves. Hyperinflation and increased dead space are avoided as FRC is maintained. This ensures adequate gas exchange and avoids right-to-left intrapulmonary shunts and impaired cardiac output.[6,7,16]

This mode of therapy is not without sequelae. Protein leaks in perialveolar epithelium have been demonstrated following use of high PIPs.[17] Pulmonary interstitial emphysema (PIE), pneumothorax, and bronchopulmonary dysplasia (BPD) have been reported in up to 35 percent of patients receiving this form of IMV.[14–24]

2. **Rapid-rate IMV**. Based on observations of the risks of the slow-rate method, as well as on the findings of Stewart, Finer, and Peters that increases in PEEP more consistently increase PaO_2 and mean airway pressure, Bland and Sedin and others have become proponents of rapid-rate, low-inflation-pressure, intermittent mandatory ventilation.[19,25] Advocates of high-frequency IMV utilize ventilatory rates of 60–120 breaths per minute, PIPs of less than 35 cm H_2O, PEEPs of 4–9 cm H_2O, and inspiratory times of 0.15–0.25 seconds. Following stabilization of gas exchange and improvement of lung disease, the FiO_2, PIP, and PEEP are reduced as tolerated. Rate is kept constant.[19]

This method of ventilation is based on the assumption that the results of previous work by Reynolds and Herman, which demonstrated that improved gas exchange resulted from prolonging inspiratory time, would not hold true if PEEP were employed.[2–4] In addition, Heicher, Kasting, and Harrod showed a decreased incidence of pulmonary air leaks when rapid-rate, low-PIP, low–tidal volume ventilation was employed to treat RDS.[20] Drummond and coworkers have shown this approach to be effective therapy for infants with PPHN.[21]

Bland and Sedin have reported excellent respiratory gas exchange utilizing low peak inflation pressure with rapid ventilation rates.[19] However, this method of ventilation makes the infant particularly susceptible to progressive air trapping, which can lead to increases in dead space volume (V_D) and resultant hypercarbia.[22] As the air trapping increases FRC, thoracic hyperinflation may lead to pneumothorax or thoracic splinting and decreased cardiac output. To avoid air trapping, reduce PIP and PEEP when compliance improves.[22]

There have been modifications of both methods of ventilation since the original descriptions. Because the time constant of the lung is quite short in infants with RDS, the inspiratory time to full lung inflation is also very short. Therefore, I have observed that proponents of low-rate IMV have recently recommended shorter inspiratory times. Recommendations vary from 0.4 to 1 second. Proponents of rapid-rate IMV vary rates between 100 and 120 breaths per minute and inspiratory times between 0.1 and 0.3 seconds.[26–30] These modifications have resulted not only from further clinical experience with these techniques but also from a better understanding of the physiology resulting from direct bedside measurement of pulmonary mechanics.[31,32]

Both methods of ventilation have their own unique risks and benefits. Both methods manipulate mean airway pressure to maintain adequate gas exchange and reduce hypoxemia and acidosis during respiratory failure secondary to atelectasis. PEEP is employed for alveolar "recruitment" and stabilization to maintain FRC, and minute ventilation is maintained through use of PIP, inspiratory time, and ventilator rate. The minute ventilation is similar in both methods of ventilation, but it is achieved in a different manner by varying PIP, inspiratory time, and rate.

EFFECTS OF SURFACTANT THERAPY

Surfactant replacement and prenatal steroid therapies have significantly changed the clinical course of RDS and its ventilatory management. Rescue and prophylactic studies of surfactant therapy demonstrated that dynamic and static compliance and respiratory system compliance increase dramatically following surfactant administration in patients with surfactant deficiency.[32–34] However, compliance and FRC do not improve in patients with sepsis or other causes of respiratory distress.[35,36] In addition, meconium and aspirated blood have been shown to inactivate surfactant in animal models.[36]

Unfortunately, since the advent of exogenous surfactant replacement therapy, there have been no large studies of methods of ventilation. This discussion is based on data available in the reports of surfactant replacement trials.

To avoid alveolar overdistention, clinicians must carefully and frequently evaluate recipients of surfactant therapy for any changes in compliance or FRC and rapidly adjust PIP and/or PEEP accordingly. Making such adjustments on the basis of compliance changes and blood gases will help avoid not only alveolar overdistention but also air trapping, air leak syndrome, and pulmonary interstitial emphysema (PIE). To prevent such risks, here are a few guidelines for monitoring the ventilated infant following surfactant therapy.

- Monitor the patient's compliance changes and blood gases as frequently as every 30 minutes during the early course of surfactant therapy.
- Evaluate compliance changes using static and dynamic compliance measures (if available) performed at the bedside (see Chapter 12 for a detailed discussion of pulmonary function tests).
- Monitor compliance by carefully observing chest excursion. Reduce PIP if chest excursion becomes marked following surfactant administration.
- Reduce PEEP on the basis of increased carbon dioxide levels, decreased pulse pressure, increased heart rate, and decreased blood pressure after obtaining a chest x-ray to con-

firm hyperinflation. Monitor blood pressure waveform at least every hour.

Excellent clinical response following surfactant administration requires rapid weaning to minimal ventilator settings in order to prevent air leak and other risks. Initial ventilator settings for infants with severe lung disease are commonly reduced within 12–24 hours following surfactant administration as follows:

	Initial Settings	After Surfactant
PIP	25–30	10–12
PEEP	4–6	3–5
Ventilator Rate	60–120	5
FiO_2	0.8–1.0	0.21

Rapid improvement may occur within one hour after surfactant administration. It is incumbent upon practitioners, therefore, to rapidly wean the infant from ventilation following clinical improvement. In an attempt to minimize blood draws for arterial blood gases, some centers utilize transcutaneous CO_2, transcutaneous O_2 measurements, and pulse oximetry as guides to rapidly wean the infant from IMV. At a minimum, blood gases should be evaluated hourly for the first four to six hours following surfactant administration.

Low birth weight infants may be successfully extubated to nasal CPAP after being weaned to the minimal ventilator settings listed above. A random survey of clinicians shows that a significant number of them administer a loading dose of aminophylline to these small babies in preparation for extubation. Some clinical data demonstrate that this practice is efficacious,[37,38] but a 1993 study questions it.[38] Successful extubation at one to four days of age has been reported.[37,38] Small babies have a variable response to nasal CPAP (Chapter 11 discusses this mode of therapy).

OBSTRUCTIVE DISEASES

Obstructive airway problems are encountered in retained fetal lung fluid, congenital lobar emphysema, adenomatoid malformation, BPD, meconium aspiration syndrome (MAS), and PIE. They are characterized by severe alveolar ventilation-to-pulmonary capillary perfusion mismatch from uneven distribution of alveolar ventilation. Alveolar ventilation is disrupted by space-occupying lesions or particulate matter in the terminal bronchioles adjacent to the alveolar structure in the form of meconium plugs, amniotic fluid, or distended air dissections in the peribronchiolar parenchyma. Although alveolar inflation usually occurs with each ventilator cycle, complete deflation to FRC does not.

Expiration is impeded by the obstruction, and air trapping results in alveolar overdistention and increased FRC. The air trapping is caused either by the partial airway obstruction, airway collapse when closing volume is reached before FRC, or an exhalation time that is insufficient to allow complete emptying of the alveoli.[11,22,39] The risk of alveolar rupture and pneumothorax, as well as reduced cardiac output, increases with air trapping. Therefore, ventilator therapy is designed to achieve adequate gas exchange while minimizing air trapping.[6,7,39] Because, overall, the time constant of the lung is prolonged in infants with obstructive airway disease, despite normal compliance, clinicians advocate using a prolonged inspiratory time of 0.4–1 second and a ventilator rate of 30–60 breaths per minute. This relatively slow frequency will allow for maximal exhalation of gas from the alveolus before the next positive pressure breath.[11,14] Thus, air trapping is minimized.

In infants with obstructive lung disease, some lung units are not obstructed and have normal resistance and time constants. The alveolar pressures in these areas will equilibrate more rapidly with the mean airway pressure and be preferentially ventilated with each positive pressure breath. Therefore, tidal volume and minute ventilation within these lung units will increase and assist in maintaining gas exchange while minimizing air trapping.[6,7,14] To minimize overdistention and pneumothorax in these normal lung units, PIP should be increased only to the point of achieving chest excursion.

To prevent alveolar overdistention and rupture, some clinicians advocate minimal or no application of PEEP;[7,40] others have employed PEEP without a significant increase in air leaks.[23] In all likelihood, application of PEEP maintains the patency of the obstructed airways and facilitates emptying of the alveoli.[24]

WEANING FROM IMV

Many authors have offered prescriptions for weaning patients from IMV.[6,8,9,11,19,20,22,28] Some advocate reducing FiO_2 to less than 0.6 before reducing PIP, PEEP, or rate.[8] Others advocate decreasing PIP as tolerated to achieve a low inflating pressure as rapidly as possible once gas exchange is established.[19,25] Still others recommend holding rate constant while weaning PIP and PEEP as tolerated.[20] These recommendations have undergone modifications since the advent of better pulmonary function data and the introduction of exogenous surfactant.

Probably the best tactic is to clinically evaluate the infant, decrease any parameter he can tolerate, and re-evaluate after the change has been made. The key factor to evaluate is how the patient's chest wall moves with each ventilatory breath. For example, a low birth weight infant with RDS who initially required a PIP of 30 cm H_2O to achieve chest excursion receives exogenous surfactant and now has extremely generous chest excursion on a PIP of 30 cm H_2O. This baby may tolerate a decrease in PIP to 20 cm H_2O.

In addition, transcutaneous CO_2 and O_2, and pulse oximetry measurements can be used as guides to rapidly wean the infant from IMV while monitoring trends in gas exchange. *Caution:* These measurements provide trending information only, not a hard and fast data point like blood gases. They should be used accordingly.

Applying this basic principle—clinical evaluation; reducing FiO_2, PIP, PEEP, and ventilator rate as tolerated; and re-evaluating the patient after the change—is not a new tactic. However, this process has become more important, and should be carried out more frequently, with the use of surfactant replacement therapy. It is important to remember that any change in PIP, PEEP, or ventilator rate will result in a change in mean airway pressure and thus alter oxygenation and ventilation. Tables 5-1 and 5-2 give overall guidelines for improving both oxygenation and ventilation. The converse maneuver can be used to wean the infant from IMV as clinical improvement occurs.

SYNCHRONIZED INTERMITTENT MECHANICAL VENTILATION

During conventional mechanical ventilation, asynchrony between spontaneous and mechanical breaths often occurs. The result is an infant who "fights the ventilator." When the infant attempts to exhale as the ventilator begins an inspiration, the resulting increase in pressure in the lung contributes to barotrauma and may increase the incidence of air leaks, bronchopulmonary dysplasia, and intraventricular hemorrhage.[41–44] Ventilation that occurs in conjunction with the infant's own inspiratory efforts would, in theory, prevent the problem of asynchrony and allow the use of lower peak inspiratory pressures because of the infant's contribution to transpulmonary pressure.[45]

PATIENT-TRIGGERED VENTILATION

Patient-triggered ventilation (PTV) refers to a system in which ventilator inflation occurs only during the infant's inspiratory phase and does not continue as the infant exhales. Such a system requires a sensor capable of detect-

ing an inspiratory effort and a response time short enough to ensure phase matching.[46] Ideally, the delay time should not exceed 10 percent of the total inflation time.[45]

Early attempts to provide PTV for the neonatal population were hampered by shortcomings in pressure sensitivity and ventilator response times. In 1986, technical advances resulted in the introduction of neonatal PTV.[47]

Most patient-triggered ventilators offer two modes of ventilation:

1. **Assist-control mode** (also referred to as synchronized intermittent positive pressure ventilation) provides mechanical assistance with every spontaneous breath and results in a variable ventilator rate. Most devices providing assist-control ventilation have a refractory window after each breath. To allow adequate time for expiration, another assisted breath cannot be triggered until that time has passed. The length of this refractory period may be fixed or variable, depending on the type of ventilator used. This window also limits the total number of assisted breaths per minute that can be given. For example, with a mandatory expiration time of 0.2 second, a respiratory rate exceeding 100 or 110 breaths per minute would result in assistance for alternate breaths because the infant is taking a breath every 0.6 second.[48] During apneic episodes, ventilator breaths are delivered at a preset control rate.

2. **SIMV mode** uses a selected number of spontaneous breaths to trigger the ventilator, resulting in a predetermined rate of assisted breaths. If the infant becomes apneic, ventilator breaths are delivered at the SIMV rate.[49]

During PTV, the PIP, PEEP, and FiO_2 are determined by the clinician and are usually maintained at the levels used in IMV prior to the switch to PTV. The inspiratory time is shortened to prevent the Hering-Breuer reflex from slowing the infant's spontaneous respiratory rate.[45] The Hering-Breuer inflation and deflation reflexes are activated by stretching or compression of the lungs to prevent overdistention or extreme deflation of the alveoli.

Starting with an inspiratory time of 0.3–0.4 second and decreasing it in small steps until synchrony is observed is one suggested approach to switching an infant to PTV.[50] An inspiratory time of less than 0.2 second is not usually used because it does not allow sufficient volume for adequate ventilation to enter the lung.[45]

The most important component of PTV is the triggering device. This device must be capable of detecting a maximum number of the infant's inspiratory efforts with as short a delay as possible between the onset of those efforts and the commencement of positive pressure.[45] By 1993, the FDA had granted approval for five PTV systems.[51] The four most widely used devices can be categorized according to the type of trigger device employed to detect the infant's inspiratory efforts.

The Star Sync (Infrasonic, Inc., San Diego, California) utilizes a pressure capsule placed on the subxiphisternal area. Because infants are primarily abdominal breathers, inspiration causes abdominal movement that compresses the pressure capsule and triggers the ventilator.[49] Careful placement of the capsule is essential to proper functioning of this device. In addition, shallow respirations or obstructive apnea may interfere with its accuracy.

Impedance pneumography obtained from the cardiorespiratory monitor is the basis for the triggering device designed by Visveshwara and Freeman.[48] The SAVI (Sechrist Industries, Anaheim, California) uses a respiratory waveform obtained from a standard cardiorespiratory monitor to trigger the exhalation solenoid of a conventional neonatal respirator. Changes in the gain setting on the monitor allow variation in the trigger points. A mandatory 0.2-second expiration time is built into the system. Correct placement of the monitoring leads is also essential to accurate triggering in this system. It is suggested that leads be placed along the axillary lines. Adjustment may be needed when the infant is repositioned.[48]

Changes in airflow in the endotracheal tube form the basis for ventilator triggering in the Draeger Babylog 8000 (Draeger, Inc., Luebeck, Germany) and the Bear Cub enhancement module (Bear Medical Systems, Riverside, California).

The Babylog uses a hot-wire anemometer flow sensor contained in an endotracheal tube adapter. One wire is partially shielded, which allows the system to determine the direction of airflow in the endotracheal tube. Sensitivity can be adjusted to trigger the ventilator at various volumes above the threshold of 5 ml/second.[49] The Babylog has a variable refractory period designed to prevent autocycling and air trapping.

The Bear Cub enhancement module also uses a hot-wire anemometer to detect airflow changes. That information is fed to an NVM-1 tidal volume monitor (Bear Medical Systems) that triggers the Bear Cub ventilator. Variable trigger thresholds can also be set with the Bear system.

Weaning From PTV

Strategies for weaning the infant from patient-triggered ventilation depend on the mode of ventilation being used and the infant's gestational age and disease condition. Weaning the infant from SIMV ventilation is achieved in the same manner as with conventional intermittent mandatory ventilation. Experience suggests that weaning may occur more rapidly in the infant on SIMV than IMV.

For infants on assist-control mode ventilation, weaning is carried out by first reducing the PIP. It is important to remember that reducing the backup rate is not effective in weaning the infant from assist-control ventilation because each breath the infant initiates is assisted by the ventilator. Because each breath is assisted to a preset PIP, reducing that pressure will reduce the amount of support the infant is receiving. As the infant's disease process resolves and weaning progresses, the inspiratory time can be adjusted to maintain synchrony between the infant and the ventilator.

Once the assist-control PIP has been reduced to minimal levels (depending on the infant's size and disease condition), the infant can be switched to low settings (rate and PIP) on SIMV and further weaned in the usual manner.

Research

Studies of neonatal PTV have generally demonstrated the safety and efficacy of this type of ventilation in infants greater than 28 weeks gestation. Results in extremely low birth weight infants have been mixed and appear to depend on the type of ventilator system used. General findings in support of patient-triggered ventilation include decreased variability of cerebral blood flow, more consistent airflow patterns, and improved oxygenation.[51–53]

Since patient-triggered ventilation was first introduced, a number of studies have examined its effects in neonates. Early studies focused on the SLE 250 ventilator, a modified adult ventilator that used an abdominal capsule (Graseby capsule) to sense the onset of respirations. Results indicated that this ventilator successfully improved gas exchange and reduced the incidence of pneumothoraces compared to historical controls.[47,54]

Greenough and Pool evaluated this ventilator in a group of 14 neonates ranging in gestational age from 24 to 40 weeks. They found that oxygenation improved in all but one patient and that the greatest improvement occurred in infants in the recovery phase of RDS.[55]

Another early trigger device used an airway pressure monitor connected with noncompliant tubing to a ventilator. Hird and Greenough found the pressure monitor to be superior to the Graseby capsule in detecting infant respiratory efforts but still unacceptable in terms of the length of the trigger delay.[56]

Hird and Greenough also evaluated the Draeger Babylog 8000 and found that oxygenation was improved on patient-triggered ventilation for the group of patients who were more than 28 weeks gestation. $PaCO_2$ was decreased in both patients younger and older than 28 weeks gestational age.[56]

De Boer and colleagues reported on a trial employing an updated version of the SLE ventilator (Model 2000) consisting of a valveless jet ventilator that uses an airway pressure sensor with adjustable trigger sensitivity. This study found that PTV was successful in even the most premature infants.[46] These findings were contrary to those of other researchers and were attributed to the combination of a valveless ventilator design with a very short delay time and a sensitive trigger.[45,50]

Bernstein and associates conducted an extensive comparison among the Star Sync, Bear enhancement module, and Draeger Babylog both in the laboratory and in a group of ten infants with acute respiratory failure. The Star Sync and the Bear were found to trigger successfully 100 percent of the time on assist control and had 1–3 percent rates of asynchrony on SIMV. The Babylog had a success rate of 70 (± 12) percent on assist control and an asynchrony rate of 29 (± 30) percent on SIMV. Reliability problems in the Babylog were attributed to its variable refractory rate.[49]

Visveshwara and Freeman designed the SAVI system and conducted a preliminary study comparing 21 infants receiving PTV with 19 control infants matched for weight, sex, Apgar scores, patent ductus arteriosus, and oxygen index. Infants in the PTV group were found to have a shorter duration of ventilation and oxygen therapy and a trend toward a decreased rate of intraventricular hemorrhage and its progression. Three more years of clinical use encompassing 110 infants confirmed these results.[48]

A study comparing the SAVI and Babylog ventilators in ten premature neonates found that the Babylog was less prone to false triggering and had a shorter response time than the SAVI impedance system. This research team also demonstrated that PTV results in more stable pleural pressures and fewer blood pressure fluctuations in the preterm population.[57]

A multicenter study randomized 306 infants with lung disease to either IMV or SIMV delivered by the Star Sync ventilator. Results demonstrated that for infants with a birth weight of less than 1 kg, the need for supplemental oxygen at 35 weeks postconceptional age was 46 percent in the SIMV group versus 77 percent in the IMV group. For larger infants in this study, SIMV resulted in more rapid improvement with lower FiO$_2$ and a lower requirement for sedation than for smaller infants.[58]

Predicting Success

Gestational age appears to be an important factor in the success of patient-triggered ventilation, particularly for those devices with less sensitive triggers. Factors useful in predicting the failure of PTV include failure of oxygenation to improve within the first hour, failure to achieve synchronicity, and a slow triggering rate relative to the infant's spontaneous respiratory rate.[45,50]

VOLUME VENTILATION

Volume-controlled ventilation has been used extensively in the adult and pediatric populations, but it has only recently enjoyed increased use in neonatal care. Renewed interest in volume ventilation came about because advances in microprocessor technology resolved earlier problems with circuit design flaws, limited rate

capabilities, and incompatibility with IMV and CPAP.

Time-cycled, pressure-limited ventilators complete the inspiratory cycle at a preset time, providing a tidal volume that is determined by a combination of inspiratory time, pressure limit, and patient compliance and resistance. One of the limitations of this type of ventilation is that the continuous flow for the inspiratory phase of ventilation cannot be set independently of the flow available during exhalation. The result may be inadequate tidal volumes in the presence of severe lung disease or an infant who struggles against the ventilator.

Another disadvantage can be seen in the infant with changing pulmonary compliance. As compliance increases or decreases, overdistention or hypoinflation may result from the delivery of a time-cycled, pressure-limited breath.

Volume-controlled ventilators end the inspiratory phase after delivering a preset volume at whatever pressure is needed to achieve the desired volume. Inspiratory time depends on the tidal volume, and inspiratory pressure is determined by tidal volume, airway resistance, and patient compliance.[59]

A disadvantage of volume ventilation is that an unknown amount of the preset volume will be lost in the ventilator circuit and around the uncuffed endotracheal tube. Also, the volume ventilator delivers the same tidal volume with each breath, which may limit the recruitment of atelectatic areas of the lung because higher opening pressures are required for re-expansion.[9]

Volume-controlled ventilation is available in assist-control mode, in which *every* ventilator breath is delivered to a preset volume, and in SIMV, in which a *specific number of breaths* per minute is delivered at the preset volume. Using SIMV, patient-triggered breaths can be given with or without pressure support—mechanical assistance to overcome resistance within the ventilator circuit.[60]

Some ventilators such as the VIP Bird (Bird Products Corporation, Palm Springs, California) offer both volume ventilation and time-cycled, pressure-limited IMV. The Bird also offers synchronized flow triggering of mandatory breaths. The Siemens Servo Ventilator 300 (Siemens Medical Systems, Inc., Danvers, Massachusetts) delivers both pressure-regulated volume control and volume support.

RESEARCH

Although there have been no studies comparing volume ventilation to pressure ventilation, there are several reports on the use of volume ventilation for the neonatal population. Bandy, Nicks, and Donn describe results of trials involving six newborn infants with severe respiratory failure, five of whom were ECMO candidates and one of whom was placed on ECMO. All were switched from time-cycled, pressure-limited ventilation to volume ventilation with a delivered tidal volume of 10–12 ml/kg. All six infants demonstrated dramatic improvements in oxygenation with no increase in mean airway pressure. Analysis of pulmonary mechanics in this group of infants showed that the breath-to-breath variation in tidal volume and minute ventilation during time-cycled, pressure-limited ventilating disappeared during volume ventilation while PIP, consistent during time-cycled, pressure-limited ventilation, varied from breath to breath during volume ventilation.[59]

NURSING IMPLICATIONS

According to Hakanson, "The single most important factor in successful ventilation of the newborn is familiarity with the equipment and its operation.[61] Regardless of the type of ventilator in use, those involved in providing care for the infant need a basic understanding of the mechanics of the ventilator. In particular, attention should be given to those factors that enhance or interfere with the sensitivity of the

triggering device in the PTV and the tidal volume monitor in volume ventilation. Each time the infant is repositioned, suctioned, or disconnected from the ventilator, the infant-ventilator relationship should be checked.

In PTV, careful observation is needed to assess the infant's ability to trigger the ventilator and to determine the effectiveness of PTV for that particular patient. In volume ventilation, the same degree of careful observation is needed to assess the adequacy of the tidal volume actually being delivered to the lungs.

COMPLICATIONS OF MECHANICAL VENTILATION

Unfortunately, patients in the NICU rarely fit exclusively into one of the two categories: atelectasis or obstructive diseases. Respiratory failure and lung disease are dynamic processes that evolve over time.[16,62] The patient's interaction with the ventilator usually results in clinical improvement, but not without a cost.

Since the beginnings of mechanical ventilation in the NICU, extending into the era of surfactant replacement therapy, researchers and clinicians have recognized that RDS is not just a problem of surfactant deficiency. The experience in Singapore in 1963 brought that fact out.[63] Rather, it represents the culmination of a multifactorial process in which barotrauma, oxygen toxicity, and surfactant deficiency result in pulmonary tissue and vascular injury. This pulmonary injury sequence occurs along a continuum starting from small epithelial leaks and alveolar edema, leading to airway stretch and distortion, and progressing to cellular membrane disruption with release of vasoactive substrates and collection of edema and hyaline membranes in alveoli.

When high PIPs are used in experimental models, separation of endothelium from epithelium and basement membrane in the distal airways occurs within five minutes of initiating mechanical ventilation.[16] The progressive protein leak and edema can deactivate surfactant, which leads to more atelectasis and results in a need for increased PIPs and greater airway distortion.[36] The greater the disruption of the intercellular tight junctions which form a barrier between pulmonary interstitium and alveolar air spaces, the more pronounced the disruption of the lung epithelium. The higher airway pressures result in exacerbation of the spiral of protein leak, surfactant deactivation, and atelectasis. The end result is a heterogenous lung disease with components of both atelectasis and obstructive airway disease, which is exacerbated by mediator release, causing more edema and hyaline membrane formation.

The heterogenous lung disease results in differential aeration of bronchial pathways that have the lowest flow resistance.[14] Thus, the more compliant areas of the lung become overdistended while the less compliant portions of the lung require significant opening pressure and collapse between breaths. The overdistended lung units may develop peribronchiolar air leaks, which progress to pulmonary interstitial emphysema. Increased pressure in the less compliant areas can cause distention and rupture at the alveolar terminal bronchiole junction, resulting in PIE. Developing PIE places the infant at risk for air leak from pneumothorax caused by further dissection of the peribronchiolar and perialveolar air leaks.[16]

The goal of treating this complex progressive disease process is to minimize iatrogenic problems while maintaining adequate gas exchange. This goal is accomplished by titrating IMV to maintain gas exchange at the lowest mean airway pressure and FiO_2 possible. The clinician must closely observe chest excursion, transcutaneous CO_2 and O_2, and pulse oximetry values as well as monitor arterial blood gas values. The success of this titration will, in part, determine whether an infant progresses on to develop oxygen dependence and BPD.

Data reported in 1993 by Hallman and colleagues support the contention that initial clinical response to surfactant can be a predictor of outcome. In addition, these investigators demonstrated that patients with initial crystalloid fluid loads of less than 100 ml/kg/day and colloid fluid loads of less than 15 ml/kg/day had better clinical responses to exogenous surfactant.[64] Anticipating and prospectively managing fluid, electrolyte, nutrition, cardiovascular, renal, gastrointestinal, neurologic, and hematologic problems will help to minimize their effects on the infant's outcome.

Underlying reactive airway disease may also complicate the clinical course of infants with BPD.[65] This underlying problem can manifest itself with "tight" breath sounds and wheezes following manipulation of the infant's airway. For example, an infant for whom nasal CPAP has failed because of repeated bouts of severe apnea can require significant IMV or SIMV settings and albuterol nebulizer treatments to break his bronchospasm following placement of an ETT to treat his apnea. Some infants can require PIPs of 30 cm H_2O to move their chests after intubation, despite being on nasal CPAP of 4 cm H_2O.

Unfortunately, a significant number of infants with obstructive airway problems develop a superimposed problem: persistent pulmonary hypertension of the newborn. This problem appears to respond to very aggressive ventilator therapy, including hyperventilation, to correct the hypoxemia and acidosis.[24,62] Some centers have reported successful outcomes for these infants without utilizing hyperventilation.[24] However, all have utilized some form of vasoactive therapy to achieve adequate pulmonary and systemic perfusion.[21,23,24,62,64–72]

Hyperventilation is employed to maintain pH >7.5 and $PaCO_2$ <25 mmHg.[21,62] This therapy is associated with a decrease in pulmonary artery pressure and right-to-left shunting through the patent ductus arteriosus.[23,62,73] More recently, high-frequency ventilation has been utilized to treat infants with PPHN and air leak syndrome. In addition, Kinsella and colleagues as well as Roberts and associates have successfully utilized inhaled nitric oxide (NO) to treat infants with PPHN by selectively dilating the pulmonary vasculature.[74-77] There are also recent reports of combining high-frequency ventilation and NO to treat PPHN.[74,75]

ADJUNCTS TO MECHANICAL VENTILATION

Vasodilators, cardiotonic agents, sedatives, and/or neuromuscular blocking agents are sometimes employed as adjuncts to mechanical ventilation. Application of any of these modalities with ventilated newborns must be weighed against the risks inherent in the therapy. Careful review of the data available on these agents should guide clinicians in their application of the planned intervention. Arguments for employing any of these therapies have not always been supported by clinical data.[41,42,68,70,78-92]

VASODILATORS AND CARDIOTONIC AGENTS

Cardiotonic therapy is utilized to decrease pulmonary vascular resistance (PVR) and/or maintain mean arterial blood pressure. Intravenous vasodilators utilized to decrease PVR include tolazoline, nitroprusside, and prostaglandins. Each has been shown to be beneficial in *some* patients.[21,66-68,70,72,73,78,80] However, clinical response is quite variable and requires the practitioner to have an in-depth knowledge of these agents and to closely, carefully observe the infant prior to and during the therapy. Nitric oxide is an inhaled gas that, when properly administered, selectively decreases PVR without causing systemic effects.[74-77]

Vasodilators and cardiotonic agents are usually employed in the management of critically ill infants with multiple system disease. These infants are able to maintain physiologic function only within a narrow range because, superimposed on their illness are all of the limitations of physiologic function in newborns. Developmentally, all infants' cardiovascular systems are structurally and functionally different from those of adults and older children. Their myocardiums are less organized and relatively unable to demonstrate the classic Frank-Starling response to a volume load.[68] Hence, all infants maintain cardiac output through alterations in heart rate. Sympathetic innervation is incomplete, and target organs have an increased sensitivity to catecholamines. Because resting cardiac output is already maximized and endogenous stores of catecholamines are developmentally subnormal, these infants may very rapidly display signs of cardiac failure.[78,83]

It is incumbent upon all who provide care to these infants to carefully and meticulously monitor heart rate, systemic blood pressure, oxygen content, $PaCO_2$, and urinary output, as well as crystalloid and colloid fluid loads. Vasodilators and cardiotonic drugs alter preload, afterload, the size of the vascular space, renal blood flow, and peripheral vascular resistance in an already compromised infant. Meticulous care is necessary to recognize and prevent complications of these drugs before the patient slips into the spiral of hypoxemia and acidosis, and further cardiac failure. Which cardiotonic agent to use is a question that cannot be clearly answered with the data currently available. Clinical experiences with these drugs and careful review of the literature available are indicated before undertaking such therapy.

Tolazoline Hydrochloride (Priscoline)

An α-adrenergic blocking agent, tolazoline has been utilized as an adjunctive therapy in infants with PPHN to achieve pulmonary vasodilation and decrease pulmonary vascular resistance. Data from two reports published in the 1950s and 1960s seemed to demonstrate improvement in oxygenation of neonates with PPHN. However, re-evaluation of these data does not support the commonly held belief that tolazoline is a pulmonary vessel vasodilator.[93]

Both Drummond and colleagues and Stevenson and associates have described the pharmacologic effects of tolazoline in the neonatal population with PPHN.[21,70] These data indicate that administration of 1–2 mg/kg of tolazoline hydrochloride over ten minutes and an infusion of 1–2 mg/kg/hour resulted in an increase in PaO_2 of more than 20 mmHg on the first arterial blood gas after initiating therapy in 10 of 15 infants with RDS, 13 of 15 infants with meconium aspiration syndrome, and 4 of 9 infants with other pulmonary diseases. The tolazoline also decreased pulmonary artery pressure below systemic arterial pressure in 2 of 5 patients. Apgar scores, diagnoses, or pretolazoline arterial blood gas values did not predict response to tolazoline.[21,70]

The overall survival of these infants did not correlate with response to tolazoline infusion, although survivors did have a greater increase in PaO_2 than nonsurvivors. This effect may be achieved at the expense of having the patient display the following side effects:

- Hypotension
- Hypertension
- Edema
- Oliguria
- Hematuria
- Gastrointestinal bleeding
- Pulmonary hemorrhage
- Seizures

Because tolazoline is excreted unchanged in the urine, its half-life depends on urinary output and varies from 3.3 to 33 hours.[70] The wise clinician will avoid starting an infusion on an oliguric patient. In order to temporize the side effects of hypotension and decreased cardiac output, a cardiotonic infusion and colloid volume support may be necessary.

Sodium Nitroprusside

A direct-acting vasodilator, sodium nitroprusside achieves its effect through action on vascular smooth muscle. Reduction of preload and afterload contributes to improvement of cardiac output, left ventricular function, tissue perfusion, and urinary output. These effects are achieved after blood volume expansion and initiation of a cardiotonic drip to ameliorate systemic hypotension. Benitz and associates report a therapeutic effect in low birth weight infants with RDS and a survival rate in infants with PPHN similar to that reported by Drummond for tolazoline infusion.[21,66] Benitz and associates recommend starting the infusion at 0.25 µg/kg/minute and advancing the rate to a maximum of 6 µg/kg/minute until a therapeutic effect is achieved.[66] Adverse effects are as follows:

- Hypotension
- Tachycardia
- Cyanide poisoning
- Abolition of intrapulmonary autoregulation
- Metabolic acidosis
- Tachyphylaxis
- Thyroid suppression

The half-life of nitroprusside is considerably shorter than that of tolazoline. Thus, it is recommended as the first-line choice when treating PPHN because the drug will clear from the patient's system within minutes.[78,83]

Nitric Oxide

A vasodilator with an extremely short half-life when delivered by inhalation into the lung parenchyma, nitric oxide is reported to selectively reduce pulmonary vascular resistance in patients with PPHN and to mediate reduction of pulmonary vascular resistance immediately after the transition period.[74–77,84–86] NO's mechanism of action involves direct synthesis of cyclic guanosine monophosphate; the result has the same effect as endothelium-derived relaxing factor. This effect is identical to the vasodilatory effect of nitroprusside and nitroglycerin, both of which achieve their actions through formation of nitric oxide, but without the toxic systemic side effects of hypotension. Nitric oxide is an extremely toxic molecule if it is allowed to combine with oxygen to form nitrogen dioxide and NO_3 (peroxynitrate). Dose and response must be carefully monitored to prevent toxic side effects.[74–77,84–86]

Prostaglandins

Prostaglandins are metabolites of arachidonic acid. They decrease pulmonary artery pressure and increase pulmonary blood flow (PBF) in experimental animals. PGI_2, PGE_1, and PGE_2 are nonspecific vasodilators. PGD_2 acts specifically on pulmonary smooth muscle in fetal and newborn animals. However, this specificity was not replicated in human neonates who received infusions of 0.1–10 μg/kg/minute. In these human studies, a nonspecific vasodilation occurred.[69]

The deleterious effects of hypotension are ameliorated by providing cardiotonic pressure support and colloid volume expansion. Infants being infused with PGI_2, PGD_2, PGE_1, or PGE_2 should be observed for pyrexia, apnea, and diarrhea, as well as hypotension. All prostaglandins are rapidly metabolized and their effects clear minutes after the drug infusion is discountinued.[69,83]

Shock and myocardial dysfunction result in decreased cardiac output and all its coincident problems, such as acidosis, hypoxemia, hypoglycemia, and hypovolemia. Sympathomimetic amines such as dopamine, dobutamine, and isoproterenol are employed to improve cardiac output.

Dopamine

An intermediate metabolic precursor of epinephrine, dopamine has a dose-dependent effect on heart rate and contractility. This is achieved through α_1, β_1, β_2, and dopamine receptor stimulation to achieve dopaminergic effects at doses ranging from 2 to 20 μg/kg/minute. Lower doses result in increased renal blood flow and decreased peripheral vascular resistance. Doses of 5–10 μg/kg/minute provide a positive inotropic effect, increase contractility of the heart muscle, and stimulate β_1 receptors. Increasing the dosage beyond 10 μg/kg/minute results in dose-related rises in systemic vascular resistance through α_1 stimulus.

Side effects of dopamine include tachycardia, arrhythmia, hypertension, and gangrenous skin sloughs from IV infiltration. The half-life of dopamine is two minutes, so the cardiac side effects may quickly be corrected by discontinuing the infusion.[21,68,78,83] Sloughs may be prevented with instillation of hyaluronidase or phentolamine at the infiltration site.

Some clinicians mistakenly believe that dopamine achieves its effect by increasing peripheral and central vasoconstriction. Data available from animal and human studies indicate the dopamine has an inotropic effect and causes *central vasodilation* at doses less than 4 μg/kg/minute.[68] Therefore, it is essential to ensure adequate intravascular volume prior to initiating therapy.

Dobutamine

A synthetic β agonist, dobutamine increases myocardial contractility with a minimal effect on heart rate through stimulation of β_1 receptors. It has no effect on renal blood flow and increases peripheral vascular resistance only minimally. It is administered as a continuous infusion at rates of 0.5–20 µg/kg/minute and has a half-life similar to dopamine.[87]

Side effects of dobutamine include arrhythmias and intrapulmonary shunting. There are reports of combining dopamine and dobutamine therapy to achieve an enhanced effect. In combination, low-dose dopamine many increase renal and mesenteric blood flow while dobutamine maintains systemic arterial pressure with a minimal increase in peripheral vascular resistance.[68,78,83]

Isoproterenol

A synthetic catecholamine, isoproterenol stimulates both β_1 and β_2 receptors to increase myocardial activity while decreasing peripheral vascular resistance through vasodilation. Thus, left ventricular afterload reduction may be achieved while heart rate and cardiac output increase and renal blood flow remains unchanged or decreases. Isoproterenol's use is limited by its marked chronotropic effect with the accompanying increase in myocardial oxygen consumption. In addition, the vasodilation may result in decreased central venous pressure (CVP) and hypotension.[68,83]

The patient on isoproterenol must be closely monitored for tachycardia and hypotension, the two most common side effects. Atrial and ventricular arrhythmias have also been reported. All these effects are more marked with this drug than with dobutamine or dopamine.[68,78]

Isoproterenol is administered intravenously at a dosage varying between 0.05 and 0.5 µg/kg/minute. It clears rapidly after discontinuation of the drip and has a half-life similar to the other catecholamines reviewed.[67,68,78]

SEDATION/NEUROMUSCULAR BLOCKADE

Sedation and/or muscle relaxation through neuromuscular blockade remains a controversial topic in neonatal intensive care.[26,27,42,67,79–92]

Sedation

Proponents of sedation with fentanyl or morphine contend that these agents have a minimal cardiovascular effect, prompt onset of action, and minimal side effects while keeping the infant from "fighting the ventilator." Teleologically, they argue that this results in an improved $\dot{V}_A/\dot{Q}_C$ (alveolar ventilation to pulmonary capillary perfusion) ratio and avoids the risks associated with neuromuscular blockers.

Advocates of morphine sedation believe that its longer half-life—four to six hours—achieves sedation without frequent dosing. Proponents of fentanyl sedation point to its minimal cardiovascular effects and lack of histamine response as reasons for its use. Intravenous sedation has not been shown to be efficacious in any recent studies of ventilation. However, continuous infusion of fentanyl at rates of 1–10 µg/kg/hour has been shown to blunt the stress response in neonates and to decrease blood pressure fluctuation in sick newborns.[88–90,92] Additionally, continuous infusion of fentanyl minimizes patient response to external stimuli and appears to keep infants "in synch" with the ventilator.

Neuromuscular Blockade

Proponents of neuromuscular blockade with pancuronium bromide argue that its use plays a role in improving oxygenation while preventing the infant from fighting against the ventilator, hence reducing barotrauma and intracranial hemorrhage.[26,27,29,41,92] Runkle and Bancalari have demonstrated improved oxygenation for infants with meconium aspiration syndrome and PPHN, but not for infants with RDS who received this therapy.[80] Reductions of barotrauma and air leak have been reported.[42] However, Pollitzer and coworkers, in a randomized, controlled trial, demonstrated no difference in the incidence of air leaks between the paralyzed and control groups.[79]

Similarly, there have been reports advocating use of pancuronium to reduce the incidence of intracranial hemorrhage (ICH), as well as reports indicating an increased risk of ICH with pancuronium use.[67,82] Currently, no objective data reliably predict which, if any, infants benefit from pancuronium administration. Traditionally, this therapy has been administered as a therapeutic trial to severely hypoxemic infants and continued if PaO_2 improves.

Pancuronium bromide, a long-acting, competitive neuromuscular blocking agent, prevents transmission of impulses by competing with acetylcholine at the neuromuscular junction. It has an onset of 2–4 minutes and a prolonged half-life of 60–90 minutes, which is increased in infants with acidosis, hypokalemia or decreased renal function, and those receiving aminoglycosides. Dosage varies from 0.06 to 0.1 mg/kg administered as an IV push.[67,82,92] Because pancuronium has a vagolytic effect, tachycardia is an almost universal side effect.

Vecuronium, a steroid analog of pancuronium, has a rapid onset of action (2.5–3 minutes) and a duration of action of 30 minutes. Like pancuronium, it is eliminated by deacetylation in the liver. Its elimination half-life is 68–97 minutes.[83,92]

Atracurium besylate, a bisquaternary isoquinolinium, is primarily degraded by Hoffman elimination and ester hydrolysis in the plasma. Its elimination half-life is 20 minutes. Because its degradation is independent of hepatic or renal function, it can be utilized in infants with oliguria and/or hepatic dysfunction.[81,83,92]

Both atracurium and vecuronium have minimal cardiovascular effects and do not cause a reflex tachycardia because they are not vagolytics. In addition, their short half-lives and rapid onsets of action make them ideal choices for an initial trial of neuromuscular blockade, which can be rapidly reversed if the clinical effect is deleterious.

Side effects of neuromuscular blockade include $\dot{V}_A/\dot{Q}_C$ mismatch, tachycardia, hypotension following vascular pooling, soft tissue edema from capillary leaks, contractures, and pressure sores.[41,81,92] Neuromuscular blockade of infants with RDS results in acute cardiopulmonary effects and a variable response in oxygenation. The most potentially catastrophic hazard is covert extubation. Careful observation and monitoring of oxygenation and changes in heart rate and a meticulous general physical examination are warranted. Because neuromuscular blockade obscures the clinical signs of seizures, some centers advocate loading these infants with phenobarbital and maintaining therapeutic levels of this drug until the infant is weaned from the paralytic agent.

The rapid response of some infants to surfactant replacement therapy has made many clinicians reluctant to employ sedation and/or paralysis because many of these babies rapidly wean to minimal ventilator settings. Another reason for the debate regarding use of intravenous sedation in ventilated neonates is the recent success of utilizing SIMV to ventilate low birth weight infants with RDS.

SUMMARY

Mechanical ventilation of newborns is a well-accepted technique for treating respiratory failure in the newborn. It requires meticulous application of basic physiologic principles and careful titration of therapy to maintain adequate gas exchange. Early reports of success have resulted in widespread use of mechanical ventilation without blinded, controlled trials to demonstrate efficacy of a particular technique.

Clinicians have applied various ventilation techniques to treat atelectatic and obstructive diseases of the newborn respiratory system. Adjuncts to therapy include vasodilators, cardiotonic agents, and neuromuscular blocking agents. Sequelae include pulmonary interstitial emphysema, air leaks, and bronchopulmonary dysplasia.

Patient-triggered ventilation and volume ventilation are two modalities that offer significant benefits for certain groups of neonatal patients. As technology improves and further research is done, these techniques will be further refined to meet the diverse needs of the sick neonate.

REFERENCES

1. Gregory GA, et al. 1971. Treatment of the idiopathic respiratory distress syndrome with continuous positive airway pressure. *New England Journal of Medicine* 284(24): 1333–1340.

2. Reynolds EOR. 1974. Pressure waveform and ventilator settings for mechanical ventilation in severe hyaline membrane disease. *International Anesthesiology Clinics* 12(4): 259–280.

3. Reynolds EOR. 1971. Effects of alterations in mechanical ventilator settings on pulmonary gas exchange in hyaline membrane disease. *Archives of Disease in Childhood* 46(246): 152–159.

4. Herman S, and Reynolds EOR. 1973. Methods for improving oxygenation in infants mechanically ventilated for severe hyaline membrane disease. *Archives of Disease in Childhood* 48(8): 612–617.

5. Mannino F, et al. 1976. Early mechanical ventilation in RDS with a prolonged inspiration. *Pediatric Research* 10(1): 464A.

6. Stark AR, and Frantz ID. 1986. Respiratory distress syndrome. *Pediatric Clinics of North America* 33(3): 533–544.

7. Rhodes PG, et al. 1983. Minimizing pneumothorax and bronchopulmonary dysplasia in ventilated infants with hyaline membrane disease. *Journal of Pediatrics* 103(4): 634–637.

8. Carlo WA, and Martin RJ. 1986. Principles of neonatal assisted ventilation. *Pediatric Clinics of North America* 33(1): 221–237.

9. Fox WW, Spitzer AR, and Shutack JG. 1988. Positive pressure ventilation: Pressure- and time-cycled ventilators. In *Assisted Ventilation of the Neonate,* Goldsmith J, and Karotkin EH, eds. Philadelphia: WB Saunders, 146–170.

10. Gomella TL, and Cunningham MD. 1992. *Neonatology: Management, Procedures, On-Call Problems, Diseases, Drugs,* 2nd ed. Norwalk, Connecticut: Appleton & Lange, 44.

11. Harris TR, and Wood BR. 1996. Physiologic principles. In *Assisted Ventilation of the Neonate,* 3rd ed., Goldsmith J, and Karotkin EH, eds. Philadelphia: WB Saunders, 21–68.

12. Pilbeam SP. 1992. *Mechanical Ventilation: Physiology and Clinical Applications.* St. Louis: Mosby-Year Book.

13. Richardson D, and Stark A. 1992. Blood gas monitoring. In *Manual of Neonatal Care,* Cloherty JP, and Stark AR, eds. Boston: Little, Brown, 209–214.

14. Watts JL, Ariagno RL, and Brady JP. 1977. Chronic pulmonary disease in neonates after artificial ventilation: Distribution of ventilation and pulmonary interstitial emphysema. *Pediatrics* 60(3): 273–281.

15. Thibeault DW, et al. 1973. Pulmonary interstitial emphysema, pneumomediastinum, and pneumothorax: Occurrence in the newborn infant. *American Journal of Diseases of Children* 126(5): 611–614.

16. Ackerman MB, et al. 1984. Pulmonary interstitial emphysema in the premature baboon with hyaline membrane disease. *Critical Care Medicine* 12(6): 512–516.

17. Egan EA, Olver RE, and Strang LB. 1975. Changes in non-electrolyte permeability of alveoli and absorption of lung liquid at the start of breathing in the lamb. *Journal of Physiology* (London) 244(1): 161–179.

18. Northway WH, Rosan RC, and Porter DY. Pulmonary disease following respirator therapy of hyaline-membrane disease: Bronchopulmonary dysplasia. *New England Journal of Medicine* 276(7): 357–368.

19. Bland RD, and Sedin EG. 1983. High frequency mechanical ventilation in the treatment of neonatal respiratory distress. *International Anesthesiology Clinics* 21(3): 125–147.

20. Heicher DA, Kasting DS, and Harrod JR. 1981. Perspective clinical comparison of two methods for mechanical ventilation of neonates: Rapid rate and short inspiratory time versus slow rate and long inspiratory time. *Journal of Pediatrics* 98(6): 957–961.

21. Drummond WH, et al. 1981. The independent effects of hyperventilation, tolazoline, and dopamine on infants with persistent pulmonary hypertension. *Journal of Pediatrics* 98(4): 603–611.

22. Perez-Fontan JJ, et al. 1986. Dynamics of expiration and gas trapping in rabbits during mechanical ventilation at rapid rates. *Critical Care Medicine* 14(1): 39–47.

23. Fox WW, et al. 1975. The therapeutic application of end-expiratory pressure in the meconium aspiration syndrome. *Pediatrics* 56(2): 214–217.

24. Wung JT, et al. 1985. Management of infants with severe respiratory failure and persistence of the fetal circulation, without hyperventilation. *Pediatrics* 76(4): 488–494.

25. Stewart AR, Finer NN, and Peters KL. 1981. Effects of alterations of inspiratory and expiratory pressures and inspiratory/expiratory ratios on mean airway pressure, blood gases, and intracranial pressure. *Pediatrics* 67(4): 474–481.

26. Kano S, et al. 1993. Fast versus slow ventilation for neonates. *American Review of Respiratory Disease* 148(3): 578–584.

27. HIFO Study Group. 1993. Randomized study of high-frequency oscillatory ventilation in infants with severe respiratory distress syndrome. *Journal of Pediatrics* 122(4): 609–619.

28. Clark RH, et al. 1992. Prospective randomized comparison of high-frequency oscillatory and conventional ventilation in respiratory distress syndrome. *Pediatrics* 89(1): 5–12.

29. Kitterman JA, 1993. Transient severe respiratory distress mimicking pulmonary hypoplasia in preterm infants. *Journal of Pediatrics* 123(6): 969–974.

30. OCTAVE Study Group. 1991. Multicenter randomized controlled trial of high against low frequency positive pressure ventilation. *Archives of Disease in Childhood* 66(7): 770–775.

31. Cunningham MD. 1986. Methods of assessment and findings regarding pulmonary function in infants less than 1,000 gm. *Clinics in Perinatology* 13(2): 299–313.

32. Stenson BJ, et al. 1993. Static respiratory compliance in the newborn. Part III: Early changes after exogenous surfactant treatment. *Archives of Disease in Childhood* 70(1): F19–F24.

33. Rider ED, et al. 1993. Treatment responses to surfactants containing natural surfactant proteins in preterm rabbits. *American Review of Respiratory Disease* 147(3): 669–676.

34. Abbasi S, et al. 1991. Pulmonary mechanics in preterm neonates with respiratory failure treated with high-frequency oscillatory ventilation compared with conventional mechanical ventilation. *Pediatrics* 87(4): 487–493.

35. Martin RJ. 1993. Role of surfactant therapy in preventing neonatal lung injury. In *Surfactant Replacement Therapy: A Clinical Symposium.* Columbus, Ohio: Ross Laboratories.

36. Pramanik AK, Holtzman RB, and Merritt TA. 1993. Surfactant replacement therapy for pulmonary diseases. *Pediatric Clinics of North America* 40(5): 913–936.

37. Durand DJ, et al. 1987. Theophylline treatment in the extubation of infants weighing less than 1,250 grams: A controlled trial. *Pediatrics* 80(5): 684–688.

38. Barrington KJ, and Finer NN. 1993. A randomized, controlled trial of aminophylline in ventilatory weaning of premature infants. *Critical Care Medicine* 21(6): 846–850.

39. Mines AH. 1981. *Respiratory Physiology.* New York: Raven Press.

40. Greenough A, Chan V, and Hird MF. 1992. Positive end expiratory pressure in acute and chronic respiratory distress. *Archives of Disease in Childhood* 67(3): 320–323.

41. Greenough A, Morley CJ, and Davis JA. 1983. Interaction of spontaneous respiration with artificial ventilation in preterm babies. *Journal of Pediatrics* 103(5): 769–773.

42. Greenough A, et al. 1984. Pancuronium prevents pneumothoraces in ventilated premature babies who actively expire against positive pressure inflation. *Lancet* 1(8367): 1–3.

43. Rennie JM, South M, and Morley CJ. 1987. Cerebral blood flow velocity variability in infants receiving assisted ventilation. *Archives of Disease in Childhood* 62(12): 1247–1251.

44. Perlman LM, et al. 1985. Reduction in intraventricular hemorrhage by elimination of fluctuating cerebral blood-flow velocity in preterm infants with respiratory distress syndrome. *New England Journal of Medicine* 312(21): 1353–1357.

45. Greenough A, and Milner AD. 1992. Respiratory support using patient triggered ventilation in the neonatal period. *Archives of Disease in Childhood* 67(1): 69–71.

46. de Boer RC, et al. 1993. Long term trigger ventilation in neonatal respiratory distress syndrome. *Archives of Disease in Childhood* 68(3): 308–311.

47. Mehta A, et al. 1986. Patient-triggered ventilation in the newborn. *Lancet* 2(8497): 17–19.

48. Visveshwara N, et al. 1991. Patient-triggered synchronized assisted ventilation of newborns. Report of a preliminary study and three years' experience. *Journal of Perinatology* 11(4): 347–354.

49. Bernstein G, et al. 1993. Response time and reliability of three neonatal patient-triggered ventilators. *American Review of Respiratory Disease* 148(2): 358–364.

50. Mitchell A, Greenough A, and Hird M. 1989. Limitations of patient triggered ventilation in neonates. *Archives of Disease in Childhood* 64(7): 924–929.

51. Bernstein G, Heldt GP, and Mannino FL. 1993. Letter to the editor. *Critical Care Medicine* 21(12): 1984–1985.

52. Govindaswami B, et al. 1993. Reduction in cerebral blood flow velocity variability in infants >1,500 g during synchronized ventilation (SIMV). *Pediatric Research* 33(4 part 2): 1258A.

53. Cleary JP, et al. 1993. Improved oxygenation during synchronized vs. intermittent mandatory ventilation in VLBW infants with respiratory distress: A randomized cross-over design. *Pediatric Research* 33(4 part 2): 1226A.

54. Clifford RD, Whincup G, and Thomas R. 1988. Patient-triggered ventilation prevents pneumothorax in premature babies. *Lancet* 1(8584): 529–530.

55. Greenough A, and Pool J. 1988. Neonatal patient triggered ventilation. *Archives of Disease in Childhood* 63(4): 394–397.

56. Hird MF, and Greenough A. 1991. Patient triggered ventilation using a flow triggered system. (Published erratum, 1992, 67[1]: 71.) *Archives of Disease in Childhood* 66(10): 1140–1142.

57. Hummler H, et al. 1994. Influence of patient triggered ventilation (PTV) on ventilation and blood pressure fluctuations in neonates. *Pediatric Research* 35(4 part 2): 2011A.

58. Bernstein G, et al. 1994. Prospective randomized multicenter trial comparing synchronized and conventional intermittent mandatory ventilation (SIMV vs IMV) in neonates. *Pediatric Research* 35(4 part 2): 1281A.

59. Bandy KP, Nicks JJ, and Donn SM. 1993. Volume controlled ventilation for severe neonatal respiratory failure. *Neonatal Intensive Care* 5(3): 70, 72–73.

60. Goldsmith JP. 1993. Ventilatory management casebook. *Journal of Perinatology* 13(1): 72–75.

61. Hakanson DO. 1988. Volume ventilators. In *Assisted Ventilation of the Neonate,* Goldsmith JP, and Karotkin EH, eds. Philadelphia: WB Saunders, 171–189.

62. Fox WW, and Duara S. 1983. Persistent pulmonary hypertension in the neonate: Diagnosis and management. *Journal of Pediatrics* 103(4): 505–514.

63. Tooley WH. 1977. Hyaline membrane disease: Telling it like it was. *American Review of Respiratory Diseases* 115(6): 19–28.

64. Hallman M, et al. 1993. Association between neonatal care practices and efficacy of exogenous human surfactant: Results of a bicenter randomized trial. *Pediatrics* 91(3): 552–560.

65. Rush MG, and Hazinski TA. 1992. Current therapy of bronchopulmonary dysplasia. *Clinics in Perinatology* 19(3): 563–590.

66. Benitz WE, et al. 1985. Use of sodium nitroprusside in neonates: Efficacy and safety. *Journal of Pediatrics* 106(1): 102–110.

67. Goetzman BW. 1981. Pharmacologic adjuncts. In *Assisted Ventilation of the Neonate,* Goldsmith JP, and Karotkin EH, eds. Philadelphia: WB Saunders, 227–283.

68. Driscoll DJ. 1987. Use of inotropic and chronotropic agents in neonates. *Clinics in Perinatology* 14(4): 931–949.

69. Soifer SJ, and Heymann MA. 1984. Future research directions in persistent pulmonary hypertension of the newborn. *Clinics in Perinatology* 11(3): 745–755.

70. Stevenson DK, et al. 1979. Refractory hypoxemia associated with neonatal pulmonary disease: The use and limitations of tolazoline. *Journal of Pediatrics* 95(4): 595–599.

71. Bacsik RD. 1977. Meconium aspiration syndrome. *Pediatric Clinics of North America* 24(3): 463–479.

72. Drummond WH. 1984. Use of cardiotonic therapy in the management of infants with PPHN. *Clinics in Perinatology* 11(3): 715–728.

73. Turner GR, and Levin DL. 1984. Prostaglandin synthesis inhibition in persistent pulmonary hypertension of the newborn. *Clinics in Perinatology* 11(3): 581–589.

74. Roberts JD, and Shaul PW. 1993. Advances in the treatment of persistent pulmonary hypertension of the newborn. *Pediatric Clinics of North America* 40(5): 983–1004.

75. Roberts JD, et al. 1992. Inhaled nitric oxide in persistent pulmonary hypertension of the newborn. *Lancet* 340(8823): 818–819.

76. Kinsella JP, et al. 1993. Clinical responses to prolonged treatment of persistent pulmonary hypertension of the newborn with low doses of inhaled nitric oxide. *Journal of Pediatrics* 123(1): 103–108.

77. Kinsella JP, et al. 1993. Selective and sustained pulmonary vasodilation with inhalational nitric oxide therapy in a child with idiopathic pulmonary hypertension. *Journal of Pediatrics* 122(5 part 1): 803–806.

78. Yeh TF, ed. 1985. *Drug Therapy in the Neonate and Small Infant.* Chicago: Year Book Medical Publishers.

79. Pollitzer MJ, et al. 1981. Pancuronium during mechanical ventilation speeds recovery of lungs of infants with hyaline membrane disease. *Lancet* 1(8216): 346–348.

80. Runkle B, and Bancalari E. 1984. Acute cardiopulmonary effects of pancuronium bromide in mechanically ventilated newborn infants. *Journal of Pediatrics* 104(4): 614–617.

81. Shaw JE, et al. 1993. Randomized trial of routine versus selective paralysis during ventilation for neonatal respiratory distress syndrome. *Archives of Disease in Childhood* 69(5): 479–482.

82. Costarino AT, and Polin RA. 1987. Neuromuscular relaxants in the neonate. *Clinics in Perinatology* 14(4): 965–989.

83. Wood M, and Wood AJ. 1990. *Drugs and Anesthesia: Pharmacology for Anesthesiologists.* Baltimore: Williams & Wilkins.

84. Geggel RL. 1993. Inhalational nitric oxide: A selective pulmonary vasodilator for treatment of persistent pulmonary hypertension of the newborn. *Journal of Pediatrics* 123(1): 76–79.

85. Finer NN, et al. 1994. Inhaled nitric oxide in infants referred for extracorporeal membrane oxygenation: Dose response. *Journal of Pediatrics* 124(2): 302–308.

86. Kinsella JP, and Abman SH. 1993. Inhalational nitric oxide therapy for persistent pulmonary hypertension of the newborn. *Pediatrics* 91(5): 997–998.

87. Martinez AM, Padbury JF, and Thio S. 1992. Dobutamine pharmacokinetics and cardiovascular responses in critically ill neonates. *Pediatrics* 89(1): 47–51.

88. Goldstein RF, and Brazy JE. 1991. Narcotic sedation stabilizes arterial blood pressure fluctuations in sick premature infants. *Journal of Perinatology* 11(4): 365–371.

89. Arnold JH, et al. 1991. Changes in the pharmacodynamic response to fentanyl in neonates during continuous infusion. *Journal of Pediatrics* 119(4): 639–643.

90. Coulter DM. 1992. Use of fentanyl in neonates. *Journal of Pediatrics* 120(4, part 1): 659–660.

91. Kauffman RE. 1991. Fentanyl, fads, and folly: Who will adopt the therapeutic orphans? *Journal of Pediatrics* 119(4): 558–559.

92. Levene M, and Quinn MW. 1992. Use of sedatives and muscle relaxants in newborn babies receiving mechanical ventilation. *Archives of Disease in Childhood* 67(7): 870–873.

93. Ward RM. 1984. Pharmacology of tolazoline. *Clinics in Perinatology* 11(3): 703–713.

NOTES

6 Complications of Positive Pressure Ventilation

Roxanne Geidel Oellrich, RNC, MSN

Mechanical ventilation has been extremely beneficial in saving the lives of many premature and ill neonates, but it is not without risks. Barotrauma, oxygen toxicity, and the mechanism of positive pressure have harmful effects on many neonatal organs, including the lungs, heart, kidneys, eyes, and brain. Of special importance to all neonatal nurses is the risk for infection and airway trauma resulting from the placement and use of the endotracheal tube. This chapter reviews some of the most common complications of mechanical ventilation: air leak syndromes, airway injury, bronchopulmonary dysplasia (BPD), and pulmonary hemorrhage. Patent ductus arteriosus (PDA) and retinopathy of prematurity (ROP) are also complications frequently associated with conditions requiring mechanical ventilation.

AIR LEAK SYNDROMES

A review of the anatomy and physiology of the thorax and lungs will help the nurse understand why neonates are at especially high risk for developing air leak syndromes. The chest wall or thoracic cage consists of 12 thoracic vertebrae, 12 pairs of ribs, sternum and diaphragm, and intercostal muscles. The cone-shaped tho-racic skeleton is quite flexible because of the presence of cartilage. The major respiratory muscle, the diaphragm, stretches across the bottom of the thorax, separating the thorax from the abdomen. Within the thorax are three subdivisions: the two lungs and the mediastinum. The mediastinum contains the thymus gland, the great vessels, the thoracic duct and small lymph nodes, the heart, a branch of the phrenic nerve, and parts of the trachea and esophagus.

The lungs and the thoracic cavity are lined by a double-layer membrane or pleura: The parietal pleura lines the chest wall, diaphragm, and mediastinum; the visceral pleura covers each lung. These membranes lie in continuous contact with each other and form a potential space, called the pleural space, which contains a thin layer of serous fluid for lubrication and cohesion.

The elastic tissues of the lung and chest wall pull in opposite directions, creating a negative or subatmospheric pressure in the pleural space. These pressures are approximately −2.5 to −10 cm H_2O from base to apex during respiration.[1] Respiratory difficulty develops when air or fluid enters the pleural space, interfering with the

TABLE 6-1 ▲ Sites of Air Leak Syndromes

Site of Extraneous Air	Syndrome
Pulmonary interstitium (perivascular sheaths)	Interstitial emphysema
Alveoli trabeculae-visceral pleura	Pseudocysts
Pleural space	Pneumothorax
Mediastinum	Pneumomediastinum
Pericardial space	Pneumopericardium
Perivascular sheaths (peripheral vessels)	Perivascular emphysema
Vascular lumina (blood)	Air embolus
Subcutaneous tissue	Subcutaneous emphysema
Retroperitoneal connective tissue	Retroperitoneal emphysema
Peritoneal space	Pneumoperitoneum
Intestinal wall	Pneumatosis intestinalis
Scrotum	Pneumoscrotum

From: Korones SB. 1996. *Assisted Ventilation of the Neonate*, 3rd ed. Goldsmith JP, and Karotkin EM, eds. Philadelphia: WB Saunders, 339. Reprinted by permission.

negative pressure and causing a partial or total collapse of the lung.

Neonatal air leaks occur when there are high transpulmonary pressure swings, uneven alveolar ventilation, and air trapping resulting in alveolar overdistention and rupture. Uneven ventilation occurs not only in neonates with immature lungs, but also in those with meconium, blood, or amniotic fluid aspiration or hypoplastic lungs. The air ruptures at the alveolar bases and tracks along the perivascular sheaths of the pulmonary blood vessels or peribronchial tissues to the roots of the lung. Air may then rupture into the pleura, mediastinum, pericardium, or extrathoracic areas (Table 6-1).

Air leaks occur in 1–2 percent of all newborns, but neonates on mechanical ventilation or continuous positive airway pressure (CPAP) are at much higher risk.[2] The incidence of air leaks in the NICU population is quite variable, approximately 2–8 percent, but is much higher among low birth weight infants.[3] Yu and associates report that among 230 infants who weighed 500–999 gm, 35 percent had pulmonary interstitial emphysema (PIE), 20 percent had pneumothorax, 3 percent had pneumomediastinum, and 2 percent had pneumopericardium.[4]

Risk factors for air leak syndromes include respiratory distress syndrome (RDS), meconium aspiration syndrome, hypoplastic lungs, congenital malformation, prematurity, endotracheal tube malposition, and overzealous resuscitation and suctioning.[5] Neonates on mechanical ventilation are especially at risk for air leaks because of alveolar overdistention and air trapping.

Mechanical ventilator factors that may increase the incidence of air leaks include positive end-expiratory pressure (PEEP),

FIGURE 6-1 ▲ Pulmonary interstitial emphysema.

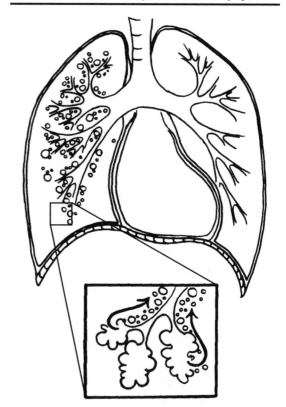

Interstitial emphysema

Modified from: Korones S. 1986. Diseases of the lungs. In *High Risk Newborn Infants*, 4th ed. St. Louis: Mosby-Year Book, 252. Reprinted by permission.

prolonged inspiratory time, high peak pressure, and breathing out of phase with the ventilator. An early study showed a 34 percent incidence of air leaks in infants receiving 3–8 cm H_2O PEEP versus a 21 percent incidence without PEEP.[6] One study reported a 50 percent incidence of air leaks when the inspiratory-to-expiratory (I:E) ratio was 1:1 or higher.[7] In addition, prolonged inspiratory time can cause the infant to breathe against the ventilator, which can cause larger pressure and volume swings and lead to the rupture of alveoli. Studies have reported a higher incidence of air leaks with high peak inspiratory pressures (PIP) and mean airway pressures (P$\overline{aw}$) greater than 12 cm H_2O.[8,9]

PULMONARY
INTERSTITIAL EMPHYSEMA

PIE is a frequent complication in premature neonates with RDS who require mechanical ventilation. Neonates with meconium aspiration may also develop PIE, but premature infants are more prone to develop this condition because of their increased pulmonary connective tissue, which traps extra-alveolar air.[10] Barotrauma from mechanical ventilation causes rupture of small airways and alveoli, which results in air in the interstitial spaces along the peribronchovascular, pleural, and interlobar passages.[11] This free air compromises lung ventilation and pulmonary vascular circulation because it compresses alveoli and blood vessels (Figure 6-1). As a result, there is decreased lung compliance and increased pulmonary vascular resistance.

There are two forms of PIE: a localized variety and a diffuse variety. The localized, unilateral form may involve one or more lobes and may be accompanied by mediastinal shift. Diffuse PIE occurs more often in premature infants on mechanical ventilation because of barotrauma. Morbidity and mortality are highest in low birth weight and gestational age infants

FIGURE 6-2 ▲ Pulmonary interstitial emphysema.

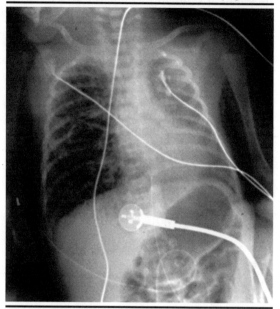

who develop PIE in the first 24 hours of life.[12] Premature infants with PIE are at great risk for developing BPD.

Clinically, the neonate often exhibits a deterioration in respiratory and cardiac status. Additional ventilatory support is often necessary and can lead to a vicious cycle of increasing pressure causing more PIE.

The diagnosis of PIE is made radiographically. The classic picture is a "salt and pepper" pattern in which radiolucent air pockets are visible against the dark background of lung parenchyma. Overinflation may be noted on the affected side (Figure 6-2).

Treatment

Several medical regimens—from conservative to surgical interventions—have been recommended for infants with PIE. Unilateral PIE can be managed by placing the neonate with the affected side down and giving chest physiotherapy.[13] If this is unsuccessful, selective mainstem bronchus intubation and bronchial occlusion are recommended. The bronchus of the unaffected side is intubated for preferential ventilation while the affected lung reabsorbs interstitial air and becomes atelectatic. Improvement is generally seen in 3 to 72 hours.[14,15] Complications of this treatment include difficulty in left-side intubation, bronchial mucosal damage, infection, excessive secretion, hyperinflation of the intubated lung, and further air trapping.[14]

High-frequency ventilation—including high-frequency positive pressure, jet, and oscillating ventilation—has been used effectively to treat diffuse PIE. High-frequency jet ventilation has been shown to be more effective than rapid rate conventional ventilation in treating PIE.[16] High-frequency ventilation allows for adequate minute ventilation while using lower airway pressures, which may reduce the amount of air leaking into the interstitial space.

Other forms of treatment include negative-pressure ventilation and extracorporeal membrane oxygenation (ECMO). Surgical intervention, including pleurotomy, pneumonotomy, pneumonectomy, and lobectomy, has been utilized when the neonate does not respond to medical management.

Nursing Care

Bronchopulmonary dysplasia is a frequent sequela in neonates surviving PIE. Nursing care of the neonate with PIE begins with close monitoring of all intubated and mechanically ventilated neonates. Initially, the nurse will note increasing oxygen and pressure requirements based upon falling oxygen saturations and poor blood gas readings.

Ventilatory management is crucial in preventing the development of further PIE. The endotracheal tube should be maintained in proper position, above the level of the carina. Although the goal is to decrease $\overline{Paw}$, thereby preventing further air leaks, neonates with lung disease often require higher levels of PIP and PEEP. Barotrauma can be reduced by shortening inspiratory time. The nurse should close-

ly monitor oxygen saturations and blood gas levels so that ventilator changes can be made promptly. If the treatment of PIE necessitates the use of high-frequency ventilation, the nurse must be familiar with the equipment and maintain a high level of vigilance.

When treating PIE conservatively, the nurse should position the neonate on the affected side and give physiotherapy as necessary. Oxygen saturations and tolerance of the procedure should be evaluated. Follow-up x-ray examinations will determine if more aggressive therapy is needed.

Neonates who are treated with selective mainstem bronchus intubation should be continuously monitored. Chest physiotherapy and suctioning are vital to prevent plugging of the endotracheal tube and further development of PIE.

PNEUMOMEDIASTINUM

Pneumomediastinum results if the free air from PIE dissects along the perivascular and peribronchial tissue to the level of the hilum of the lung. At the hilum, air may accumulate in the mediastinum, causing a pneumomediastinum. If the pressure increases, it can dissect into the neck, producing subcutaneous emphysema, or into the thoracic cavity, causing a pneumothorax.

Clinical signs associated with pneumomediastinum include respiratory distress. The sternum may be thrust forward; muffled or distant heart sounds and a crunching noise may be heard over the pericardium. Blood gas readings and oxygen saturations indicate hypoxia and hypercarbia as a result of the pressure of free air on the lung and blood vessels.

The diagnosis of pneumomediastinum is made radiographically. The classic finding is the "sail sign": a windblown spinnaker sail appearance of the thymus (Figure 6-3). In addition, the air is usually confined anterior to the

FIGURE 6-3 ▲ Pneumomediastinum.

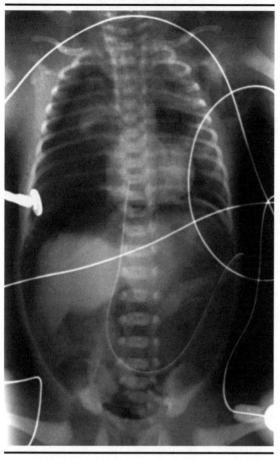

FIGURE 6-4 ▲ Tension pneumothorax.

Air fills the pleural space causing a shift of the trachea, heart, and mediastinum to the opposite side.

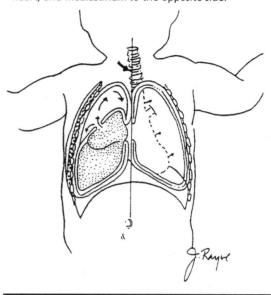

From: Oellrich RG. 1991. *Understanding Chest Drainage in the Neonate.* Fall River, Massachusetts: Pfizer Hospital Products Group, 8. Reprinted by permission.

heart, so on x-ray the heart appears to be in the right hemithorax (dextrocardia).

Medical management for pneumomediastinum involves conservative treatment. As with PIE, the goal is to maintain intrathoracic pressures as low as possible during mechanical ventilation. One treatment used for term neonates is delivering 100 percent oxygen for 6 to 12 hours as a nitrogen washout method.[3] Because of differences in partial pressures of nitrogen and oxygen gases, the air in the pneumomediastinum may be absorbed more quickly. This treatment is not recommended for premature neonates because of their risk of retinopathy of prematurity.

As with any mechanically ventilated neonate, the nurse must monitor closely for respiratory deterioration. Pneumomediastinum often progresses to a pneumothorax.

PNEUMOTHORAX

Spontaneous pneumothorax is known to occur in term and postterm infants. Healthy neonates can generate up to 40–80 cm H_2O with their first breath, which may cause a pneumothorax.

As described earlier, interference with the aeration of the alveoli causes transpulmonary pressure to remain high and results in rupture of the alveoli. The free air develops into PIE and then travels along to the mediastinum, causing a pneumomediastinum. If there is enough air, it moves into the pleura, resulting in a pneumothorax. Pneumothorax may also be caused by air rupturing from subpleural blebs without the development of a pneumomediastinum.[11] Tension pneumothorax can be a severe complication of mechanical ventilation, with free air quickly accumulating in the pleural cavity causing the lung to collapse, shifting the mediastinum, and severely impeding venous return and cardiac output (Figure 6-4).

Infants with RDS are at risk for air leaks because of their stiff, noncompliant lungs. Prior to the use of surfactant, one study reported the incidence of pneumothorax to be 12 percent among infants with RDS not on mechanical ventilation, 11 percent in infants on CPAP, and 26 percent among those on mechanical ventilation.[17] More recent reports indicate that the incidence of pneumothorax among infants treated with surfactant has been reduced.[18,19] Neonates with meconium aspiration are at risk for air leaks because they often require mechanical ventilation, and ball-valve airway obstruction leads to further air trapping. One study reports that 12 percent of neonates with meconium aspiration develop pneumothorax.[20]

Premature neonates having a pneumothorax are at high risk for developing a cerebral hemorrhage because of a combination of intrathoracic pressure fluctuations in association with relative overperfusion of the periventricular circulation, lack of cerebral autoregulation, and inherent weakness of the periventricular capillary beds. Often these neonates on mechanical ventilation for respiratory distress syndrome require high ventilatory pressures, which can increase intrathoracic pressure, thereby reducing venous return. This can increase cerebral blood pressure, causing fragile capillaries to rupture. At the time of a pneumothorax, systemic hemodynamic changes cause a marked increase in cerebral blood flow velocity and increased capillary pressure, which can lead to an intraventricular hemorrhage.[21,22] In some situations there is a loss of cerebral autoregulation. Systemic hypotension caused by the increased intrathoracic pressure can result in cerebral hypotension. As a consequence of altered cerebral perfusion, ischemia and IVH have been reported.[23]

TABLE 6-2 ▲ Signs and Symptoms of Pneumothorax/Air Leaks

Respiratory distress (tachypnea, nasal flaring, grunting, retractions, cyanosis)

Diminished breath sounds on affected side

Decreased arterial blood pressure (initial increase)

Decreased heart rate (initial increase)

Increased diastolic blood pressure

Increased central venous pressure

Decreased pH

Decreased PO_2

Decreased transcutaneous PO_2

Distended abdomen

Palpable liver and spleen

Chest asymmetry

Irritability

Diminished, shifted, or muffled cardiac sounds and point of maximal impulse

Decrease in height of QRS complex on monitor

Poor peripheral perfusion

Cardiopulmonary arrest

Adapted from: Hagedorn M, Gardner S, and Abman S. 1993. Respiratory diseases. In *Handbook of Neonatal Intensive Care*, 3rd ed., Merenstein GB, and Gardner SL, eds. St. Louis: Mosby-Year Book, 335; and Oellrich RG. 1985. Pneumothorax, chest tubes, and the neonate. *MCN: American Journal of Maternal Child Nursing* 10(1): 30. Reprinted by permission.

Premature neonates on mechanical ventilation who have developed one pneumothorax should be monitored for bilateral pneumothoraces. Neonates at highest risk for bilateral pneumothoraces have pulmonary interstitial emphysema at the time of the initial pneumothorax.[24] Any infant who develops a spontaneous pneumothorax should be evaluated for renal anomalies because of a noted correlation between renal anomalies and pulmonary hypoplasia.[25]

Signs and Symptoms

Clinical signs and symptoms of pneumothorax in the neonate are often subtle (Table 6-2). Unusual irritability or restlessness can be an early sign. The most common sign is respiratory distress indicated by grunting, retractions, tachypnea, and cyanosis. In addition, there is a decrease in the pH, PaO_2, and oxygen

FIGURE 6-5 ▲ Pneumothorax.

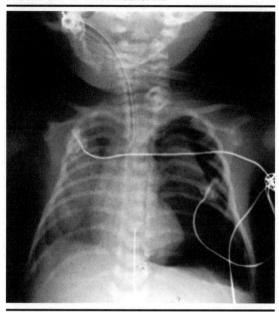

saturations. Diagnosis, however, cannot be made by these signs alone because they also often accompany other causes of respiratory deterioration.

Diminished breath sounds may be heard on the affected side, but this may be difficult to determine because of the small size of the chest and easily transmitted breath sounds in the neonate. It may be difficult to auscultate diminished breath sounds in the neonate with RDS because the lungs are stiff, noncompliant, and do not collapse in the same way as an adult with a tension pneumothorax. In addition, it is common for neonates to have bilateral pneumothoraces, which makes it especially difficult to determine decreased breath sounds. If the pneumothorax is under tension, there may be a mediastinal shift and a shift in the point of maximal heart impulse.

Bradycardia, increased diastolic blood pressure followed by hypotension, increased central venous pressure, and distant heart sounds indicate very high intrathoracic pressures. Clinical findings of distended abdomen and palpable liver and spleen are useful signs of a tension

pneumothorax causing displacement of the diaphragm. Other findings include unequal chest wall movement (especially decreased on the affected side), increased anterior-posterior chest diameter, and hyper-resonance to percussion on the affected side.

Preliminary diagnosis of pneumothorax can be made by transillumination of the chest with a high-intensity fiberoptic light. This method has been successful in diagnosing a high percentage of pneumothoraces with a false positive rate of 5 percent.[26] The nursery should be darkened as much as is safely possible and the probe placed directly on the chest—initially superior to the nipple, then inferior to the nipple.[27] Air can be detected by illumination of the light on the affected side. Tape and monitor leads can obscure the light beam.

As with all forms of air leak, the diagnosis is confirmed radiographically. Anterior-posterior and lateral films are necessary to document air that has risen to the anterior part of the thorax or for smaller pneumothoraces. A pneumothorax is identified as a pocket of air impinging on the lung. A mediastinal shift toward the opposite side indicates the pneumothorax is under tension, and immediate intervention is indicated. Other radiographic findings of a pneumothorax include widened intercostal spaces and a depressed diaphragm (Figure 6-5).

Treatment

The infant in severe respiratory distress with a tension pneumothorax requires immediate emergency treatment. Needle aspiration is necessary to decrease mortality and morbidity. A 23–25 gauge needle or a 18–20 gauge angiocatheter is attached to a three-way stopcock and a 20–50 ml syringe. Following sterile preparation of the chest, the needle is inserted into the second or third intercostal space in the anterior axillary or midclavicular line.[28] These sites are most often recommended as air generally is anterior and in the apex of the pleural space.[29] Air is aspirated out through the syringe, then vented out the stopcock. The needle should be used to continue to remove air until a chest tube can be inserted and connected to a chest drainage system.

The insertion of a chest tube is performed using sterile technique. The neonate should be positioned with the affected side up. The chest wall is prepped with an iodine solution and injected with 1 percent xylocaine to provide local anesthesia. Analgesia, such as fentanyl or morphine, should be given because chest tube placement is a painful procedure.

Using the traditional superior approach, the tube is inserted into the first to third intercostal space on or just lateral to the midclavicular line. The lateral approach uses the fourth to sixth intercostal space just lateral to the anterior axillary line. Care must be taken not to pierce the pectoralis muscle, lacerate the intercostal artery, or injure the nipple or breast tissue.

There are several techniques of chest tube placement: the blunt dissection, modified blunt dissection, and trocar methods. Once the chest tube enters the pleural space, the catheter "steams up." The tube should immediately be connected to a chest drainage system and tube placement verified radiographically. Complications following chest tube insertion involve improper placement of the tube causing injury to the heart, liver, spleen, and kidney. The most serious complications include hemorrhage, lung perforation, infarction, phrenic nerve injury with eventration of the diaphragm, and cardiac tamponade.[30–33]

Nursing Care

The following nursing measures are important for neonates on mechanical ventilation who develop a pneumothorax:

1. Carefully monitor vital signs, including heart rate, respiratory rate, and blood pressure. Tachypnea and tachycardia followed by bradycardia and hypotension may indicate development of a pneumothorax.

2. Auscultate heart and breath sounds hourly. Diminished breath sounds may indicate inadequate functioning of the chest tube or development of a pneumothorax. A shift in the point of maximal impulse may indicate a tension pneumothorax.

3. Closely evaluate arterial blood gas and oxygen saturation levels to determine appropriate oxygen and ventilator settings. The goal is to reduce mean airway pressure, but often the severely compromised patient requires higher ventilator settings.

4. Ensure the safety of the infant with chest tubes.
   - If chest tubes are inserted, set up the three-bottle chest drainage system properly and evaluate it hourly.
   - Immediately after chest tube insertion, check the water seal for oscillations and bubbling—indications of evacuation of air.
   - Set or fill the suction chamber to the prescribed level—usually between 5 and 25 cm H_2O, the average being 10–15 cm H_2O.
   - Check the collection chamber hourly and mark it every shift. If chest tubes have been inserted for a pneumothorax, there should be minimal drainage. Stripping of chest tubes is contraindicated, and milking remains controversial.[2,34]
   - Observe the insertion site for drainage or signs of infection. An antibiotic ointment is usually applied to the insertion site. If a dressing is used, it should be changed daily. For additional discussion of nursing care of the infant with chest tubes, see Chapter 3.

5. Tape all connector sites securely. Because of the weight of the connecting tubing, it

is helpful to pin the first part of the tubing to the bed with a tab of tape to prevent accidental dislodgement. Measure the length of the chest tube from the insertion site to connector every shift to assure that it has not slipped out.

6. Turn and position the neonate to facilitate the evacuation of air and fluid. Because air rises, positioning the neonate on the unaffected side will assist in its evacuation.

7. Monitor the neonate's tone and activity. Irritability and agitation can be early signs of pneumothorax.

8. Assess the neonate for signs of intraventricular hemorrhage. (Changes in cerebral blood flow can be caused by air leaks.) Clinical signs of a cerebral hemorrhage are similar to those of an air leak: respiratory distress, bradycardia, hypoxia, hypercarbia, and acidosis. Any premature neonate with pneumothorax should have serial cerebral sonograms.

9. Consider the use of medications to enhance cardiac output. Cardiac output may be compromised because of high intrathoracic pressures. Insertion of chest tubes may help, but volume expanders or vasopressor drugs may be necessary as well.

10. Evaluate the level of agitation and pain in the neonate, and comfort or medicate as necessary. In the past, neonates were paralyzed if they were fighting mechanical ventilation. Recent work has shown that sedation and analgesia are extremely important in caring for these critically ill neonates. Continuous fentanyl or morphine infusions may be helpful. Chest tube insertion and having the actual chest tube in place are quite painful.

11. Provide parents with accurate, honest, and understandable information regarding the complications of mechanical

FIGURE 6-6 ▲ Pneumopericardium.

Air fills the pericardial sac causing a tamponade of the heart.

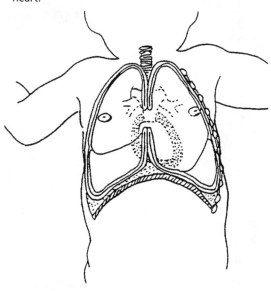

From: Oellrich RG. 1991. *Understanding Chest Drainage in the Neonate.* Fall River, Massachusetts: Pfizer Hospital Products Group, 9. Reprinted by permission.

ventilation and treatment of the air leak. Reassure them that the chest tube will help their baby to breathe more comfortably.

PNEUMOPERICARDIUM

Pneumopericardium is a rare complication of mechanical ventilation seen particularly in preterm neonates. Pulmonary interstitial emphysema and pneumomediastinum often precede the entry of air into the pericardial sac (Figure 6-6). It usually occurs during the first few days of life.

Cardiac tamponade as a result of pneumopericardium can develop very quickly. Death can occur if this is not diagnosed and treated promptly. Clinical signs of pneumopericardium include bradycardia, cyanosis, muffled heart sounds, and hypotension. Chest films using anterior and lateral views reveal decreased heart size and air surrounding the heart (Figure 6-7).

FIGURE 6-7 ▲ Pneumopericardium.

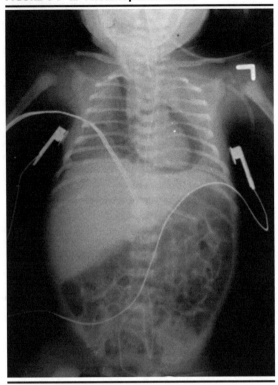

Uncompromised neonates with pneumopericardium have been managed with 100 percent oxygen therapy.[35] Emergency treatment for tamponade includes needling the pericardial space. Starting under the xiphoid, the angiocath is advanced at a 30- to 40-degree angle aiming at the left shoulder. A thoracotomy tube may be connected to a closed drainage system usually for two to three days. Nursing care is similar to that for the infant with pneumothorax with specific attention to cardiac output.

PNEUMOPERITONEUM

Another rare complication of mechanical ventilation is pneumoperitoneum. Air dissects through the diaphragm into the retroperitoneal space. Clinical signs of pneumoperitoneum include a firm, shiny, and distended abdomen. The cause of the pneumoperitoneum should be investigated because it is also associated with necrotizing enterocolitis, gastric rupture, and a perforated ulcer that may require surgery.

The x-ray shows a dark layer of air over the abdomen that blurs the normal bowel pattern. A right lateral view demonstrates the liver clearly defined from the anterior abdominal wall.

Medical treatment is indicated if the neonate's respiratory status is severely compromised or if venous return to the heart is impeded. A soft catheter may be inserted into the peritoneum.

AIRWAY INJURY

Subglottic stenosis, tracheobronchomalacia, tracheomegaly, necrotizing tracheobronchitis, and vocal cord injuries have been reported in infants requiring mechanical intubation and positive pressure ventilation.

Factors that appear to place intubated infants at risk for these complications include prolonged intubation, lack of an air leak around the endotracheal tube, repeated intubation, mechanical trauma from suctioning, gastroesophageal reflux, respiratory infection, hypoxia, hyperoxia, positive pressure ventilation, excessive movement of the endotracheal tube, and inadequate humidification of the endotracheal tube.[35,36] These complications are more common in infants with BPD but can develop in those who have required only short-term intubation and ventilation.

At a minimum, any infant who is intubated will develop edema in the airway followed by acute inflammation if intubation continues for more than a few hours. Pressure from the endotracheal tube reduces mucosal capillary perfusion, leading to ischemia, irritation, congestion, edema, and eventually ulceration.[37,38] Progressive ulceration can lead to perichondritis, chondritis, and necrosis of the cricoid cartilage.[39] Granulation tissue grows at the margins of the injured area and can persist as thick tissue leading to narrowing of the airways. These extensive changes can lead to fibrotic, firm scar tissue, which can cause subglottic stenosis and narrowing of the airways.[40] As a result, atelectasis and/or emphysema can develop. Many of these airway lesions contribute to the development of BPD.

Infants who have been intubated and ventilated for less than a week will have some edema, but their cries are normal within 24 hours after extubation. Infants who are extubated after one week to one month may have mild inspiratory and expiratory stridor lasting for a year or more. Extubation after one to several months, as in the infants with BPD, may result in stridor and a hoarse cry for months to years because of the airway damage.[39]

Diagnosis of upper airway obstruction is often difficult to make in premature infants. Following extubation, the infant may have decreased bilateral breath sounds, mild retractions, and apnea. The premature infant may not always develop stridor. If the infant develops respiratory failure, he will require reintubation, and if the respiratory distress immediately disappears, upper airway injuries are suspected.

Damage to the larynx can be caused by necrosis over the arytenoid cartilage and vocal cords. Necrosis occurs because the endotracheal tube is in contact with the area. As a result, there may be persistent ulceration and/or erosion of the vocal cords. Significant damage may affect vocalization and respirations.[36]

SUBGLOTTIC STENOSIS

Subglottic stenosis ranges from mild to severe in the intubated infant. The overall incidence of this acquired condition in preterm infants weighing <1,500 gm at birth is approximately 2 percent.[40] The lesion is usually associated with prolonged intubation and is diagnosed by bronchoscopy showing that the subglottic diameter (below the level of the glottic opening and above the level of the inferior margin of the cricoid cartilage) has become sufficiently narrow to cause symptoms of airway obstruction. The mildest form of subglottic stenosis is laryngeal edema.

Diagnosis of subglottic stenosis is made after physical examination, anterior-posterior and lateral neck and chest x-ray films, and direct or fiberoptic laryngoscopy and bronchoscopy. In addition to respiratory distress, the infant may have mild to severe respiratory stridor that is not positional.

Treatment of mild respiratory difficulty includes elevating the head of the bed, providing humidified air, and administering racemic epinephrine. Treatment with steroids before extubation has been shown to be quite effective in premature infants.[41] No significant side effects have been noted with the short-term use of dexamethasone.

The more severe form of acquired subglottic stenosis is a "hard" scar of fibrotic tissue. In order to extubate infants with this condition, an anterior cricoid split with or without immediate cartilage graft interposition may be required to increase the airway diameter.[42,43] Some surgeons prefer a tracheostomy because it provides a long-term secure airway, but it too has its complications. If a tracheostomy is performed, decannulation occurs when the subglottic region has grown, usually in infants over a year of age. Other treatments for subglottic stenosis include dilating the stenotic region, resecting the tissue with a laser through a bronchoscope, or performing a laryngotracheoplasty.[44,45]

TRACHEOMEGALY, TRACHEOMALACIA, AND BRONCHOMALACIA

Mechanical ventilation with positive pressure causing barotrauma can lead to dilation of the trachea and bronchi, resulting in tracheomegaly, tracheomalacia, or bronchomalacia. Tracheomegaly, diagnosed radiographically, results in an increase in the anatomic dead space, causing the infant to work harder at breathing to maintain normal carbon dioxide levels.[46] Tracheomalacia and bronchomalacia can develop when the cartilaginous rings fail to support the round shape of the trachea, allowing airway collapse. The infant can develop expiratory stridor, wheezing, and atelectasis when the airway collapses or becomes obstructed on expiration.[47]

There are multiple factors for the pathogenesis of tracheobronchomalacia, including barotrauma, immature airways, recurrent bacterial or viral infection, and pressure and irritation of the endotracheal tube.[47,48] Tracheobronchomalacia has been successfully treated with PEEP and ventilation or CPAP. Such treatment may place the infant at higher risk for BPD.

NECROTIZING TRACHEOBRONCHITIS

Necrotizing tracheobronchitis, a necrotic inflammatory process involving the mainstem bronchi and distal trachea, is characterized by replacement of normal tracheal mucosa with acute inflammatory cells, mostly neutrophils. This process leads to sloughing of the mucosa, which can occlude the distal trachea. As a result of granulation, there may be impaired gas exchange, airway obstruction, and atelectasis. This lesion has been seen in all sizes of neonates and has been identified after as little as one to five days of ventilation.[49]

Necrotizing tracheobronchitis has been associated with early work with high-frequency ventilation, but it has also been reported with conventional ventilation.[49,50] Problems with inadequate warmed humidification down the endotracheal tube, which result in mucus buildup and obstruction, have been reported in both conventional and high frequency ventilation.[50] There are various theories for the pathogenesis of necrotizing tracheobronchitis, including lack of humidification. The presence of the endotracheal tube has been suggested as a factor that causes damage by (1) direct pressure, (2) barotrauma due to the ventilator-transmitted piston effect, or (3) toxins from the plastic of the endotracheal tube. Bacterial or viral infection may play a role similar to that in infants with tracheobronchomalacia or subglottic stenosis. Infants with severe birth asphyxia and/or shock may develop necrotizing tracheobronchitis because of the ischemia to the airway mucosa. The practice of deep endotracheal suctioning as a causal factor for necrotizing tracheobronchitis is of major concern.[51,52]

Clinically, the infant may be asymptomatic, then suddenly deteriorate with carbon dioxide retention that fails to respond to ventilator changes, suctioning, and reintubation. This is caused by the sloughing of the mucosa, which may occlude the distal trachea. Treatments have included excision or cauterization of the lesions, but this is difficult because of the relatively small airways of preterm infants. Obstruction can lead to lobar atelectasis or death.

Two types of lesions have been found on autopsy. Type I lesions show necrosis, mucosal hemorrhage, and ulcerations. Type II lesions, more chronic, show mucosal fibrosis and extensive squamous metaplasia.[53] Long-term outcome is unknown, but follow-up is important because Type II lesions are considered to be premalignant in the area of the larynx and glottis.

NURSING CARE

Prevention of airway injury should be a priority for nurses caring for any mechanically intubated infant. The correct sized endotracheal tube should be used, and only experienced clinicians should intubate the extremely low birth weight infant or the infant who is known to be difficult to intubate. Following intubation, the tube should be stabilized to prevent excessive movement and accidental extubation.

A chest film should be taken to evaluate proper endotracheal tube placement. Once tube placement is confirmed, the length of the tube in relation to the infant's lip should be documented so that proper position can be checked every shift. When evaluating position by auscultating breath sounds, the caregiver should hear a slight air leak around the tube. Gas flow through the ventilator should be sufficiently warmed and humidified.

The nurse has a major role in preventing airway damage from suctioning. Prior to suctioning, the nurse should select the appropriately sized suction catheter and know the exact measurement of the endotracheal tube. Preoxygenation and hyperinflation have been recommended before suctioning.[54] The suction catheter should not be passed beyond the length of the endotracheal tube. No more than 50–80 cm H_2O pressure should be used when applying suction for five seconds. The frequency of suctioning should be individualized, based upon the infant's breath sounds, respiratory status, and clinical condition. Following suctioning, the infant should be given time for recovery, which often requires increased oxygen. Oxygen saturation and clinical status should be closely monitored while weaning the infant to appropriate ventilator settings (Chapter 5).

Mechanically ventilated infants require continuous monitoring to maintain the fine balance between hypoxia and hyperoxia. Assessment of changes in the infant's condition, oxygen saturations, and arterial blood gases is key to appropriate ventilator changes being made rapidly to prevent complications.

Prevention of infection is a major challenge to the NICU team. Initially, most infants are placed on broad-spectrum antibiotics. The endotracheal tube prevents the cilia in the airway from clearing airway debris and potentially pathogenic bacteria or viruses. As a result, infection may develop, leading to the previously described airway lesions. Maintaining sterile technique during intubation and endotracheal suctioning remains important. If infection is

suspected, antibiotics should be initiated and modified to specific organisms.

PULMONARY HEMORRHAGE

Pulmonary hemorrhage generally presents in the first week of life in neonates who require mechanical ventilation. A significant increase has been reported in infants receiving surfactant therapy. The extent of the hemorrhage may range from a focal disorder to a massive one that causes death. The mortality rate after a pulmonary hemorrhage is estimated to be as high as 75–90 percent.[3] The incidence of pulmonary hemorrhage ranges from 0.8 to 1.2 per 1,000 live births.[55] At autopsy, the incidence of hemorrhage in premature infants has been found to range from 55 to 84 percent.[56] A more correct name for this condition is hemorrhagic pulmonary edema because it is a form of fulminant lung edema with leakage of red cells and capillary filtrate into the lungs.[55]

PATHOPHYSIOLOGY

Pulmonary hemorrhage appears to be the extreme result of pulmonary edema in the neonate. The most common causes of pulmonary edema are increased pulmonary microvascular pressure, reduced intravascular oncotic pressure, reduced lymphatic drainage, and increased microvascular permeability.[57] All result in increased fluid leakage into the pulmonary interstitia, thus increasing pulmonary lymphatic fluid. Pulmonary edema occurs as lung interstitial fluid rises; the fluid leaks into the alveoli after damage to the alveolar epithelium or leakage caused by distention by the interstitial fluid.[12] Initially, only albumin leaks into the alveoli, but as the edema becomes more severe, capillary hemorrhage occurs.

Pulmonary hemorrhage has been divided into three categories according to autopsy findings: (1) Interstitial hemorrhages are characterized by hemorrhage in connective tissue spaces of the lung. (2) Lung hematomas are accumulations of fresh blood in the interstitium of alveolar spaces. (3) Intra-alveolar hemorrhages are characterized by fresh blood filling alveoli in areas not directly adjacent to the interstitium, often extending into the bronchioles and bronchi to produce massive hemorrhage.

The premature infant with severe RDS on mechanical ventilation or high oxygen concentration who has heart failure secondary to increased pulmonary blood flow is at high risk for developing pulmonary edema and hemorrhage even before receiving surfactant therapy. The pulmonary edema may inhibit surfactant function. Additional problems placing the neonate at risk include asphyxia, shock, hypoxia, and acidosis, which lead to left ventricular heart failure.

Other factors associated with pulmonary hemorrhage include intrauterine growth retardation, massive aspiration, hypothermia, infection, oxygen therapy, severe Rh hemolytic disease, congenital heart disease, fluid overload, and coagulopathies. Although disseminated intravascular coagulation may precede pulmonary hemorrhage, most infants do not have a coagulopathy, but may develop it after the hemorrhage.[3,12]

An analysis of five multicenter trials using Exosurf, a synthetic surfactant, revealed a 1.9 percent incidence of hemorrhage in the treated infants versus 1 percent in untreated infants. Birth weight was inversely related to hemorrhage in both groups. Pulmonary pathologic findings associated with hemorrhage included PIE and necrotizing laryngotracheitis in both groups. Other significant diagnoses among infants in both groups who developed hemorrhage were PDA, intraventricular hemorrhage (IVH), and pneumothorax.[56]

A thorough review of 33 treatment trials using exogenous surfactant from 1980 to 1992 focused on the association between exogenous surfactant therapy and pulmonary hemorrhage.

The natural surfactant trials reported an incidence of 5.87 percent in treated versus 5.36 percent in control infants; the synthetic trials reported an incidence of 2.51 percent in treated versus 1.04 percent in control infants. The relative risk for pulmonary hemorrhage with any surfactant product was 1.47 percent in these 33 trials. Analysis revealed that surfactant treatment and lower mean birth weight had a significant influence on the risk for a pulmonary hemorrhage. Interestingly, the patent ductus did not have an independent effect on the risk of a pulmonary bleed.[58]

The etiology of pulmonary hemorrhage following treatment with surfactant includes alterations in pulmonary hemodynamics because of a patent ductus arteriosus, fragile capillaries resulting from extreme prematurity, barotrauma caused by mechanical ventilation, and a localized coagulopathy caused by the surfactant.[59,60] Although a recent study showed no generalized coagulopathy or bleeding among premature infants receiving surfactant, a localized coagulopathy may cause the hemorrhage.[61]

SIGNS AND SYMPTOMS

Clinically, the infant may initially present with blood-tinged fluid from the endotracheal tube. With a massive hemorrhage, there may then be a sudden deterioration and simultaneous appearance of bloody secretions in the endotracheal tube and/or the infant's mouth. The fluid has the appearance of fresh blood, but the hematocrit of the fluid is 15 to 20 points lower than the circulating blood.[3]

Usually, the infant becomes pale, cyanotic, hypotensive, and hypotonic, but term infants may become agitated secondary to the hypoxemia and begin to "fight" the ventilator. Signs of heart failure may be present, including tachycardia, murmur (related to the PDA), hepatosplenomegaly, and edema. Hypotension results from the blood and fluid loss and heart failure caused by hypoxemia, and acidosis.

Auscultation of the chest reveals widespread crepitus and decreased air entry.

DIAGNOSIS

A few infants may deteriorate clinically without apparent cause for an hour or two before the hemorrhage begins. Once the frank blood becomes evident, the diagnosis is made. Chest radiographic findings depend on whether the hemorrhage was focal or massive. It is often difficult to differentiate a focal hemorrhage from atelectasis or pneumonia. Massive hemorrhage reveals a "whiteout" due to atelectasis and opacifications with some air bronchograms (Figure 6-8).

Blood gases rapidly deteriorate following a massive hemorrhage, resulting in severe hypoxia, hypercarbia, and a marked metabolic acidosis. Although the hematocrit of the lung fluid is diluted, considerable amounts of blood may be lost. There are no specific white blood cell changes unless sepsis is present. Drawing of blood cultures is recommended following the hemorrhage. Development of disseminated intravascular coagulation is not uncommon after the bleed occurs.

MANAGEMENT

Control of pulmonary edema and heart failure in addition to positive pressure ventilation and oxygenation are critical in preventing pulmonary hemorrhage. Following administration of surfactant, the nurse should closely monitor the infant for signs of heart failure, hypotension, decreased air entry, and wet or crepitus breath sounds.

Early detection and aggressive intervention are vital in the management of pulmonary hemorrhage. Infants experiencing pulmonary bleeding should be intubated and ventilated. They usually have severe lung diseases that require high PEEP and PIP. Initial settings of rates of 50–60/minute, inspiratory time of 0.4 to 0.5 second, and PEEP of 6–7 cm H_2O are

FIGURE 6-8 ▲ Pulmonary hemorrhage x-ray.

A. Infant with moderate respiratory distress.

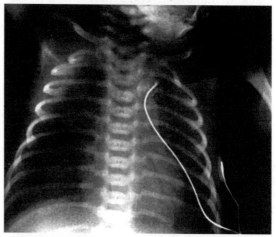

B. Three hours later, x-ray demonstrates a severe pulmonary hemorrhage.

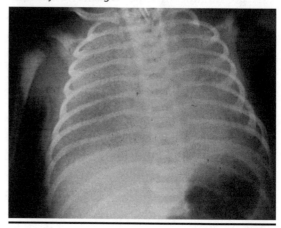

recommended.[12] This may help in redistributing lung fluid back into the interstitial space, improving ventilation and perfusion.[62]

Control of heart failure and of the amount of blood shunting through the PDA is crucial. Diuretics including furosemide can be given to reduce the left ventricular failure. The use of digoxin is controversial. Fluid balance is difficult because the infant is in congestive heart failure with pulmonary edema but at the same time is hypotensive with poor peripheral perfusion. The blood pressure needs to be closely monitored, and vasopressors may be necessary.

Transfusion of blood products, including packed red blood cells, may be necessary because of the acute blood loss. Infusions of fresh frozen plasma and administration of vitamin K may be successful to correct clotting deficiencies. Antibiotic therapy should be started if the infant is not currently being treated because sepsis is a major risk factor for pulmonary hemorrhage.

Treatment of the PDA with indomethacin is contraindicated immediately after a pulmonary hemorrhage because the drug inhibits platelet aggregation. It can be given 24–48 hours after the bleed if coagulation is normalized.[12]

Complications following pulmonary hemorrhage include air leaks and periventricular hemorrhage. Bronchopulmonary dysplasia is often a sequela because of the pulmonary edema and treatment with oxygen and mechanical ventilation.

NURSING CARE

Care of the infant with a pulmonary hemorrhage includes all aspects of neonatal intensive care nursing. Maintaining an open airway is a major priority. During the first few hours after the hemorrhage, the endotracheal tube may require suctioning every 10 to 15 minutes. There is significant risk of blockage of the tube from bloody secretions. Breath sounds must be evaluated frequently.

The infant is often placed on maximum ventilator settings requiring vigilant monitoring of arterial blood gases and vital signs. Monitoring for the development of air leaks is important because of high pressure settings. Based upon evaluation of blood gases, ventilator settings may be changed, and sodium bicarbonate may be ordered. If hypotension occurs, fluids will be recalculated. Blood products and vasopressors may also be necessary.

CARDIOVASCULAR COMPLICATIONS

The respiratory and cardiovascular systems work in close harmony to provide the body with adequate oxygen and to remove waste products from the cells. The respiratory system affects cardiovascular function by altering venous return and pulmonary vascular resistance. Cardiac output depends on venous return to the heart, which is determined in part by differences between extrathoracic and intrathoracic pressures. Subatmospheric intrapleural pressure establishes a favorable pressure gradient for blood to flow back to the right atrium.

The use of CPAP or positive pressures from mechanical ventilation can affect the cardiovascular system by causing an increase in intrathoracic pressure, which results in a decrease in venous return.[63] Cardiac output is then decreased by both the diminished venous return and compression of the ventricles as a result of the increased intrathoracic pressure.[63]

The impact of mechanical ventilation on cardiac output depends on the degree of pressure transmitted from the airway to the intrapleural space. This pressure is influenced by lung compliance. Neonates with RDS who have reduced lung compliance transmit significantly less pressure to the intrapleural space than those with normal compliance, and so ventilation in these compromised neonates exerts little effect on venous return and cardiac output. They can generally tolerate high levels of PIP and PEEP without significant decreases in cardiac output. However, the premature infant who develops a tension pneumothorax has a sudden rise in intrathoracic pressure, which increases central venous pressure. These changes can result in intraventricular hemorrhage.[22]

When neonates are recovering from RDS following surfactant therapy, compliance may increase rapidly along with increased intrapleural pressure. High ventilator pressures in these neonates can decrease cardiac output and increase venous pressure leading to possible systemic hypotension, altered perfusion, and intraventricular hemorrhage.

Another potential complication of positive pressure ventilation and CPAP is ventilation-to-perfusion mismatch ($\dot{V}_A/\dot{Q}_C$). This ratio describes the relationship between alveolar ventilation and capillary perfusion of the lung. In neonates with lung disease, even though CPAP or positive pressure is applied, areas that are atelectatic tend to remain so, while inflated regions tend to become further distended. The circulation responds by perfusing the areas of the lung that are distended and diminishing circulation in atelectatic portions.[62] A maximum ventilation-to-perfusion mismatch occurs in an infant with a tension pneumothorax: Ventilation escapes into the pleural space, where no gas exchange occurs, while perfusion remains only in the lung.

Mechanical ventilation increases airway pressure, which is also transmitted to the intraparenchymal pulmonary vessels. The effect is complex and depends on several factors, including the lung disease and compliance. In infants with RDS, there is a decrease in functional residual capacity (FRC), which can result in increased pulmonary vascular resistance. In infants with lung diseases treated with mechanical ventilation causing lung overdistention, the air spaces compress arterioles and capillaries causing ventilation/perfusion mismatch, leading to increased pulmonary vascular resistance.

Persistent pulmonary hypertension of the newborn (PPHN) is a well-known condition in which pulmonary vascular resistance remains elevated. During transition to extrauterine life, pulmonary vascular resistance normally decreases. In the infant with PPHN, the pulmonary vascular resistance remains higher than the systemic blood pressure, resulting in a right-to-left shunt across the ductus arteriosus and/or

foramen ovale, so blood bypasses the lungs. Clinically, these neonates present with severe cyanosis, high preductal oxygen saturations, and lower postductal oxygen saturations.

Hyperventilation with mechanical ventilation has been an important aspect of care because it has been shown to decrease pulmonary vascular resistance in infants with PPHN. Hyperventilation may not be necessary in treating milder cases and may result in complications, including air trapping. Moderate to severe PPHN may necessitate the use of high-frequency ventilation or ECMO (Chapters 13 and 14).

PATENT DUCTUS ARTERIOSUS

Patent ductus arteriosus is a condition in which the cardiovascular system has a direct effect upon ventilation and perfusion. The PDA is a challenging problem for the team caring for the premature neonate on mechanical ventilation. The large left-to-right shunt and resulting cardiac failure aggravate pre-existing pulmonary disease.

The ductus arteriosus arises from the distal dorsal sixth aortic arch and forms a bridge between the pulmonary artery and the dorsal aorta. During fetal life, its purpose is to direct blood away from the fetal lungs and toward the descending aorta and placenta.

In the term neonate, the ductus begins to constrict rapidly after delivery with the initiation of breathing and completely disappears during the first year of life. Muscle media indent into the lumen, and the intima increases in size to form intimal mounds or cushions that partially occlude the lumen.[64] These intimal changes occur in conjunction with extensive constriction and shortening of the ductus as well as migration of smooth muscle cells from the media into the intima. At birth, ductal constriction results from multiple factors, increased arterial oxygen tension being one of the most important.[65] The ductus responds better to oxygen with increasing gestational age.

The role of prostaglandin in relation to the ductus closure continues to be explored. Prostaglandin appears to play a significant role in keeping the ductus patent *in utero*. Fetal and neonatal ductal tissue produce prostaglandins, including PGE_2 and PGI_2, and metabolites of arachidonic acid.[66,67] During gestation, these endogenous prostaglandins inhibit the ability of the ductus to constrict in response to oxygen.

It has been proposed that high oxygen tension at birth initiates the synthesis of hydroperoxy fatty acid, which suppresses prostacyclin production. This exposes the ductus to the contractile effects of prostaglandin endoperoxide.[66] Other factors that may cause ductal constriction at birth include an increase of prostaglandin E receptors in the ductus and a rise in catecholamines, including epinephrine and norepinephrine.[68,69]

Incidence

The incidence of PDA is 12–15 percent in the total newborn population but increases with decreasing gestational age and birth weight and the occurrence of RDS.[70,71] Among infants less than 1,500 gm, the incidence rises to approximately 40–60 percent.[72,73]

An early study reported that surfactant therapy may increase the incidence of PDA in mechanically ventilated premature infants to as high as 90 percent.[74] Clinical and echocardiographic reports of these surfactant treated infants show the PDA is of greater diameter, has greater blood flow, and causes greater clinial deterioration.[75] Other studies report a low incidence of PDA after administration of exogenous surfactant.[76]

Pathophysiology

The persistent PDA in preterm infants appears to be related to incomplete or abnormal ductal structure, metabolic development, and a disturbed or immature interaction between the various mediators of ductal tone, including prostaglandin. Inflation and ventilation of the lungs at birth should cause a decrease in pulmonary vascular resistance and induce ductal constriction. The drop in pulmonary vascular resistance allows blood to flow from left to right (aorta to pulmonary artery) in the opposite direction from fetal circulation: If pulmonary resistance remains high as it does during the acute phase of RDS, a bidirectional shunt may occur across the ductus arteriosus.

The effects of the shunt through the PDA depend upon several factors: diameter of the ductus, ductal tone, systemic and pulmonary vascular resistance, and left ventricular output. Quite often in premature neonates, especially those with RDS, the pulmonary vascular resistance remains elevated. In addition, persistent hypoxia may prevent the ductus from closing.

Prior to the use of surfactant, the development of a significant PDA usually corresponded to the diuresis phase of RDS. Following surfactant therapy, improved pulmonary compliance causes pulmonary vascular resistance to drop below systemic vascular resistance, and so the amount of ductal flow becomes significantly larger.[77] Surfactant is thought to cause the release of circulating prostaglandins, which cause relaxation of the smooth muscles, including those of the patent ductus arteriosus.

Most shunting in the preterm infant is left to right, resulting in stress on the heart and lung. In the premature infant, the ventricles are less distensible and generate less force; this can result in left ventricular enlargement from the PDA. This produces elevated left ventricular end-diastolic pressures, which increase pulmonary venous pressures and cause pulmonary congestion. As a result, the infant develops right-sided heart failure.

Studies have shown that premature infants with a PDA increase left ventricular output by increasing stroke volume. Stroke volume increases as a result of a simultaneous decrease in afterload resistance on the heart and an increase in left ventricular preload. This may cause a redistribution of systemic blood flow to organs.

Very low birth weight infants with PDA have been found to have increased blood flow in the ascending aorta and decreased flow in the descending aorta, which have been associated with intraventricular hemorrhage and necrotizing enterocolitis.[78,79]

In addition, the infant with RDS frequently has a low plasma oncotic pressure and increased capillary permeability, which respond to the increased microvascular perfusion by allowing leakage of plasma proteins into the alveolar space. This leads to pulmonary edema. This leakage may inhibit surfactant function and increase surface tension, thereby worsening the disease. The pulmonary edema plus the continuous distention of pulmonary vessels during diastole may be factors in the development of bronchopulmonary dysplasia.[80]

Clinical Picture

Prior to the use of surfactant, clinical signs of PDA did not usually appear until the third or fourth day during the recovery phase of RDS. Although the ductus is patent, the elevated pulmonary vascular resistance secondary to lung disease diminishes left-to-right shunting. As pulmonary functioning and oxygenation improve, pulmonary vascular resistance decreases. With the early administration of surfactant to infants with RDS, significant shunting through the ductus is seen much earlier. Ninety percent of infants with severe RDS have evidence of a PDA by contrast echocardiogram within the first 24 hours of life, but only 40 percent develop hemodynamically significant shunts requiring intervention.[80]

Moderate to large amounts of shunting through the PDA in which there is left ventricular volume overload and increased left ventricular end-diastolic volume and pressure result in congestive heart failure. Clinical signs include tachypnea, tachycardia, decreased urine output, increased pulse amplitude, and widened pulse pressure (systolic and diastolic difference greater than 30 mmHg). Increased precordial activity and bounding pulses are caused by the increase in cardiac output and blood flow back to the left side of the heart. The classic continuous murmur is not always heard.

Preterm infants may have a patent ductus that is clinically silent but hemodynamically significant. The infant may have a reduction in systolic and diastolic blood pressures severe enough to require volume expanders and inotropic drugs.[81,82] Long-term effects of a patent ductus arteriosus include poor weight gain, recurrent respiratory infections (because of increased lung fluid and left sided heart failure), and the need for additional ventilator support.

Diagnosis

The diagnosis of PDA is based upon clinical findings plus color doppler and M-mode or, more currently, 2D echocardiography, which assesses for left-sided cardiac overload. With M-mode, if the ratio of the size of the aortic root to left atrium is greater than 1:1, the presence of a PDA is confirmed. Currently, doppler and 2D echocardiography are more accurate than M-mode. The pulsed color doppler permits analysis of blood flow in the pulmonary artery and aorta. Using echocardiography and doppler diagnosis on day 3 of life, one can predict PDAs that will later become symptomatic.[83]

Treatment

Definitive treatment of a PDA is closure of the ductus arteriosus. Conservative methods are implemented before indomethacin or surgical ligation. Fluid restriction has been recommended but is unlikely to close the PDA without other interventions. A combination of fluid restriction and diuretics may lead to electrolyte imbalances, dehydration, and reduced caloric intake. According to one study, furosemide (Lasix) is associated with an increased incidence of PDA.[84] Digoxin has been suggested to improve ventricular output but has been proven to be ineffective, and toxic levels can develop if indomethacin is given concurrently.

The use of PEEP has been shown to reduce the left-to-right shunt through the PDA.[85] Mechanical ventilation management of the infant with a PDA is an important issue. Infants without RDS but with a large left-to-right shunt may have increased interstitial and peribronchiolar edema. Because lung compliance is relatively normal, high inflating pressures should be avoided. These high pressures may impair venous return and cardiac output, and so alter pulmonary perfusion and the ventilation-to-perfusion ratio. Infants with RDS may benefit from higher pressures because lung compliance is decreased.

Indomethacin has been proven to be clinically effective in closing PDAs in premature infants within the first seven days of life, with successful closure in approximately 80 percent of cases.[86–88] Indomethacin is a potent inhibitor of the cyclo-oxygenase pathway, which forms the various prostaglandins.[72] It was originally developed as an anti-inflammatory agent. Oral suspensions were initially used to treat PDA in infants during the 1970s.

Currently, intravenous indomethacin, 0.1–0.3 mg/kg/dose, is given every 12 to 24 hours for a total of three doses. In most cases, a single dose has not resulted in persistent constriction of the ductus arteriosus.

One of the debates surrounding the use of indomethacin is over when treatment should begin. Some recommend that indomethacin be given to infants who weigh <1,000 gm only after the PDA becomes clinically apparent.[80] But a study published in 1994 reports that low-dose prophylactic indomethacin given to infants weighing between 600 and 1,250 gm at less than 12 hours of age resulted in a significantly lower incidence of IVH. The PDA closed with no significant adverse effects of the drug.[89]

Following administration of indomethacin, the infant should be monitored for success of the closure. Significant improvements in lung compliance have been noted.[90,91] Mechanical ventilation pressures and rates can be lowered, thus exposing infants to lower mean airway pressures. Ductus reopening is a common problem in the infant who weighs <1,000 gm.

Complications from indomethacin can be significant, so infants must be screened before therapy is initiated.[91] Renal dysfunction can be a major complication. Indomethacin may be contraindicated if the serum creatinine is above 1.2–1.8 mg/dl or if urine output is less than 1 ml/kg/hour. Indomethacin decreases renal blood flow and glomerular filtration rate, and it may potentiate vasopressor activity.[92] If urine output decreases in an infant who has received indomethacin, the administration of furosemide or low-dose dopamine has been suggested.[93,94]

Platelet function may be impaired for at least a week after indomethacin administration. For this reason, it is contraindicated in infants with renal or gastrointestinal bleeding or with necrotizing enterocolitis. Although the drug has been associated with occasional intestinal perforation, there has been no evidence of increased necrotizing enterocolitis. Because of its anti-inflammatory properties, indomethacin is contraindicated in proven sepsis.

Indomethacin has been shown to decrease cerebral blood flow by 12–40 percent in premature infants.[86] There is concern that rapid infusion, which has been the standard practice, might reduce cerebral blood flow to unsatisfactorily low levels, resulting in brain ischemia. Two studies have shown a significant decrease in cerebral blood flow velocities when the drug is given quickly over 5 minutes or slowly over 30 minutes. Therefore, further studies are necessary to determine the safest rate of administration.[95,96]

Indomethacin's ability to decrease cerebral blood flow may account for a possible additional benefit: It may prevent intraventricular hemorrhage.[95] The drug may decrease production of prostacyclin, which causes a vasodilation of cerebral microvasculature.

Another prostaglandin inhibitor, ethamsylate, has been shown to reduce the incidence of PDA in very low birth weight infants treated with exogenous surfactant.[97] Further studies are required to determine its benefits and risks.

Surgical ligation of the PDA is usually reserved for infants for whom indomethacin is contraindicated or who fail to respond to conservative and/or indomethacin therapy. Ligation through a left lateral thoracotomy can be done in a short time either in the operating room or at the bedside. Mortality and morbidity are relatively low, but the treatment does require a thoracotomy and chest tube drainage. Complications of ligation include laryngeal nerve paralysis and chylothorax.[98]

Nursing Care

Nursing care of the ventilated premature infant requires careful monitoring for signs of a patent ductus arteriosus—especially after administration of surfactant. Changes in vital signs suggesting heart failure should be reported. A low mean arterial blood pressure may be an early sign of a PDA in the infant weighing <1,000 gm. If possible, heart sounds should be auscultated while the infant is off the ventilator, and any murmurs or clicks should be noted. Increased precordial activity is an extremely reliable sign of a significant PDA. Infants who

require higher ventilatory support should be further evaluated for PDA.

Medical treatment is based upon echocardiography, clinical signs, and unit standards. Prior to administration of indomethacin, the infant should be evaluated for signs of renal and platelet dysfunction, necrotizing enterocolitis, and recent intraventricular hemorrhage. Laboratory studies should include complete blood count (CBC) with differential, platelet count, electrolytes, blood urea nitrogen (BUN), creatinine, and bilirubin levels.

Strict measurement of urine output before and during treatment with indomethacin will reflect renal dysfunction. Assessment for clinical bleeding includes heelstick sites, gastric drainage, and blood in the stools. Auscultation for the absence of a heart murmur during treatment is important. Even after the PDA has been determined to be closed, auscultation for recurrence of a murmur is important in the very low birth weight infant. Retreatment may be considered.

If the infant is unresponsive to indomethacin and requires increased ventilatory support, surgical ligation is recommended. Preoperative care includes stabilizing fluid and electrolyte levels, thermoregulation, and oxygenation and ventilation. Packed red blood cells may be ordered and held for possible transfusion. The surgeon and neonatologist should discuss the benefits and risks of the surgery with the parents and obtain surgical consent. The ligation is usually performed in the operating room. If the infant is extremely unstable, or is on ECMO or high-frequency ventilation, the surgery may be performed in the NICU.

Following surgical ligation, the nurse should assess vital signs and determine the need for pain medication. The thoracotomy site should be assessed for signs of bleeding or infection. The chest tube drainage system should be checked hourly for proper functioning and any drainage.

TABLE 6-3 ▲ Stages of Bronchopulmonary Dysplasia

Stages	Time	Pathology	Radiology	Clinical Features
Stage I (mild)	Two to three days	Patchy loss of cilia; bronchial epithelium intact; profuse hyaline membranes	Air bronchograms; diffuse reticulogranularity (identical to RDS)	Identical to RDS
Stage II (moderate)	Four to ten days	Loss of cilia; fewer hyaline membranes; necrosis of alveolar epithelium; regeneration of bronchial epithelium; ulceration in bronchioles	Opacification; coarse, irregularly shaped densities containing small vacuolar radiolucencies	Increased oxygen requirements and increasing ventilatory support when recovery is expected; rales, retractions
Stage III (severe)	Ten to 20 days	Advanced alveolar epithelial regeneration; extensive alveolar collapse; bronchiolar metaplasia and interstitial fibrosis; bronchial muscle hypertrophy	Small radiolucent cysts in generalized pattern	Prolonged oxygen dependency, CO_2 retention; retractions; early barrel chest; severe acute episodes of bronchospasm
Stage IV (advanced-chronic)	One month	Obliterative bronchiolitis; active epithelial proliferation; peribronchial and some interstitial fibrosis; severe bronchiolar metaplasia	Dense fibrotic strands; generalized cystic areas, large or small heart, hyperinflated lungs, hyperlucency at bases	Increased chest AP diameter, cor pulmonale; frequent respiratory infection; prolonged oxygen dependency; failure to thrive

From: Korones SB. 1996. *Assisted Ventilation of the Neonate,* 3rd ed. Goldsmith JP, and Karotkin EH, eds. Philadelphia: WB Saunders, 328. Reprinted by permission.

Parents can be brought to the bedside once the infant and equipment are stabilized.

BRONCHOPULMONARY DYSPLASIA

Bronchopulmonary dysplasia is a chronic lung disease that develops in neonates who are being treated for a lung disorder that requires oxygen and positive pressure ventilation. In 1967, Northway, Rosan, and Porter described BPD as a new type of chronic lung disease that developed in premature infants with severe RDS who were treated with positive pressure mechanical ventilation and oxygen.[99] Bronchopulmonary dysplasia is now known to occur in term and preterm neonates with a variety of neonatal conditions, including apnea, meconium aspiration, pneumonia, and congenital heart disease.[100] Originally, Northway's group postulated that oxygen toxicity caused BPD, but research has revealed that there are multiple complex mechanisms that cause the disease. The clinical severity of BPD varies from thriving infants requiring low levels of oxygen to sicker infants with multisystem effects who remain ventilator dependent.

Currently, there is no universally accepted definition of BPD. Northway's original definition, in 1967, included the radiologic, pathologic, and clinical criteria found in infants with advanced chronic disease (Stage IV) plus a requirement of ventilatory support (Table 6-3).[99]

Bancalari and associates, in 1979, further defined an infant with BPD as one who requires positive pressure ventilation for at least three days during the first week of life, has clinical signs of respiratory distress, requires supplemental oxygen to maintain an oxygen tension (PaO_2) of 50 torr for more than 28 days, and shows radiographic evidence of BPD.[101]

Tooley, also in 1979, considered infants to have BPD if they were older than 30 days of age, had radiologic abnormalities, plus any one of the following: PaO_2 <60 torr in room air, $PaCO_2$ >45 torr, or oxygen dependency.[102]

As smaller and sicker infants survive because of all the new technologies, including surfactant replacement therapy, high-frequency ventilation, prenatal and postnatal steroids, and ECMO, the clinical and radiographic findings that define BPD have changed. A 1988 definition by Shennan and associates, requires inclusion of infants with radiographic abnormalities who require oxygen support at 28 days and infants who require oxygen therapy at 36 weeks postconceptional age.[103] Davis and Rosenfeld's 1994 definition includes the requirement for oxygen supplementation after 28 days of life.[104]

Biochemical, histologic, and radiologic changes associated with the development of BPD can be recognized before 28 days of age. Because of these early recognizable characteristics and varying degrees of lung damage, the disease is often referred to as chronic lung disease, with BPD indicating the most severe form.

The incidence of BPD is difficult to report because it depends on the definition used. The overall approximation is 20 percent in premature infants with RDS and 2–3 per 1,000 live births.[100,105] The risk for BPD increases with decreasing birth weight and gestational age. The reported incidence is as high as 85 percent in infants weighing 500–699 gm but decreases to 5 percent in infants weighing >1,500 gm.[106,107] Investigators using exogenous surfactant have reported a decreased incidence of BPD, but it is estimated that the total number of infants with BPD will increase because of improved survival of infants less than 25 weeks gestation who continue to develop BPD despite surfactant administration. Approximately 7,000 new cases of BPD are reported each year, and approximately 10–15 percent of these infants will die by one year of age.[104]

PATHOGENESIS

Bronchopulmonary dysplasia has been attributed to oxygen toxicity, barotrauma, lung

FIGURE 6-9 ▲ **The pathogenesis of bronchopulmonary dysplasia.**

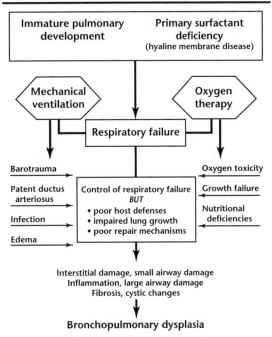

From: Knoppert DC, and Mackanjee HR. 1994. Current strategies in the management of bronchopulmonary dysplasia: The role of corticosteroids. *Neonatal Network* 13(3): 54. Reprinted by permission.

immaturity, inflammation, and infection (Figure 6-9). The causes are multifactorial and depend on the nature of the acute injury as well as abnormal repair processes that occur in the lung. Normal lung growth and development are disrupted by a premature birth. The immature lung, already deficient in surfactant, is then exposed to adverse stimuli.

Oxygen toxicity has been associated with BPD because of the delicate balance between free radicals (an atom or molecule that has an unpaired electron in its outer orbit, making it highly reactive) and antioxidant defenses, which protect pulmonary cells. Oxygen can rapidly accept free electrons generated by oxidative metabolism within the cell, producing free radicals. Imbalances occur when hyperoxia, reperfusion, or inflammation cause increased free radical production. Oxygen free radicals can damage cell membranes and unravel nucleic acids.[108]

Cells defend themselves against free radical damage by producing antioxidants.[108,109] If there are inadequate antioxidant defenses, free radicals can increase. Increased survival and prevention of lung damage from hyperoxia has been demonstrated in animal studies by increasing concentrations of lung antioxidants.[104]

Oxygen can directly injure epithelial and endothelial cells, leading to pulmonary edema.[110] As pulmonary edema progresses, proteins leak into the alveoli, inhibiting the surface tension properties of surfactant, thereby exacerbating the surfactant deficiency of prematurity.[111] Worsening atelectasis, decreased lung compliance, and increased ventilation-to-perfusion mismatch leads to the need for higher oxygen and ventilator settings, which in turn leads to worsening chronic lung disease.

Positive pressure ventilation also appears to be important in the pathogenesis of BPD because it causes barotrauma, which may induce a complex inflammatory cascade. It is often difficult to distinguish whether the injury is caused by oxygen or barotrauma alone. The role of barotrauma depends on the structure of the tracheobronchial tree and the physiologic effects of surfactant deficiency. Infants with surfactant deficiency and atelectasis will have decreased alveolar compliance and highly compliant upper airways, which causes distortion of distal airways.

Because of difficulty in obtaining adequate gas exchange, ventilator pressures are often increased, and this causes further airway damage. Early airway injury increases the need for ventilator support, which can cause distal air trapping and regional hyperinflation. Uneven ventilation due to airway injury and alveolar immaturity can result in pulmonary interstitial emphysema and air leaks. Both are strongly associated with increased risk for BPD.

Several infectious agents have been implicated in the development of BPD, among them cytomegalovirus and Chlamydia.[112] *Ureaplasma urealyticum* has been identified as a possible cause of chorioamnionitis, prematurity, and BPD.[113,114] Studies have demonstrated that this organism may cause a chronic subclinical pneumonia, resulting in increased ventilation and oxygen requirements. It has been suggested that infection may act as an additional stimulus in the inflammatory response, with recruitment of neutrophils and activation of the arachidonic cascade ultimately leading to BPD.

Inflammation may play an important role in the pathogenesis of BPD because it unifies many of the risk factors. Beginning as a cascade of destruction, BPD then proceeds to abnormal repair, and finally becomes chronic lung disease. Oxygen toxicity, pulmonary barotrauma, or infection results in attraction and activation of neutrophils. Activated neutrophils and macrophages can release inflammatory mediators that cause the release of toxic products from plasma membranes. These products include arachidonic acid, lysoplatelet activating factor, and oxygen free radicals which initiate an inflammatory cascade.[104] This cascade culminates in pulmonary damage including breakdown of capillary endothelial cells and leakage of plasma protein into the alveolar space. This leakage of protein causes pulmonary edema, which has been proposed as a major factor in the development of BPD.[115]

Compromised nutritional status in the premature infant may also exacerbate the development of BPD (Table 6-4).[116] Adequate caloric and protein intake is required for cell growth and division. Copper, zinc, iron, manganese, and selenium are required cofactors for antioxidant enzymes and may be necessary for repair of elastin and collagen. Vitamin E may provide antioxidant protection, but research findings are inconclusive. Vitamin A deficiency may also

TABLE 6-4 ▲ The Potential Effects of Undernutrition in Premature New- borns of Very Low Birth Weight

Condition	Result
Poor caloric/energy reserves	Early onset of catabolic state
Respiratory distress syndrome	Inhibited/delayed surfactant production; decrease in respiratory muscle function
Effects on protection from hyperoxia/ barotrauma	Decreases in epithelial integrity (vitamin A), defense against oxygen free radicals and lipid peroxidation (decreases in quantity of antioxidant enzymes, vitamin E stores, and polyunsaturated fatty acid in comparison with term infants), and lung biosynthesis/cell replication for repair of injury
Effects on lung repair and development of bronchopulmonary dysplasia	Decreases in lung biosynthesis, replacement of damaged cells, and replacement of damaged extracellular components (collagen, elastin)
Effects on lung growth	Decreases in lung biosynthesis/cell replication and lung structural maturation (alveolarization)
Effects on suscepti- bility to infection	Decreases in cellular, humoral defenses against pathogens, epithelial cell integrity, and clearance mechanisms

Adapted from: Frank L, and Sosenko IR. 1988. Undernutrition as a major con- tributing factor in the pathogenesis of bronchopulmonary dysplasia. *American Review of Respiratory Disease* 138(3): 725. Reprinted by permission.

play a significant role in pathogenesis because it is essential for differentiation, integrity, and repair of respiratory epithelial cells.[117] A defi- ciency of vitamin A results in loss of cilia and in squamous metaplasia.[118,119] Malnutrition in the premature infant may impair macrophages and neutrophil and lymphocyte function, which protect the lung against infection.[120]

Other factors that have been correlated with the pathogenesis of BPD include a genetic pre- disposition, PDA, fluid management, lipid infu- sion, and gas temperature and humid- ification.[121] Reports that infants are more like- ly to develop BPD if there is a family history of airway reactivity (including asthma) are inconclusive. Studies have shown that infants who develop airway obstruction early have increased airway reactivity, a possible con- tributing factor to BPD. Fluid overload may cause pulmonary edema. Early closure of the PDA has been associated with improvement of pulmonary function, but this treatment has not decreased BPD.

PATHOLOGY

The pathologic features of BPD first described by Northway and associates are divided into four stages (Table 6-3). This original four-stage radiographic pro- gression to the severe hyper- inflated cystic appearance in the chest films of infants with chronic BPD is seen in very severe cases. More common- ly, radiographic changes are more subtle, and the pro- gression may be more pro- longed. Stage II—originally described as complete opaci- fication—is now uncom- mon.[122] A radiographic scoring system developed in 1984 is based upon the four most prominent findings in BPD: lung expansion, emphysema, interstitial densities, and cardiovascular abnormalities.[123]

There are many acute and chronic lung changes that occur simultaneously within the spectrum of BPD. The disease begins with an exudative and early repair stage. It may progress to a chronic fibroproliferative phase in which there is obliterative airway disease, widespread parenchymal fibrosis with atelectasis and emphy- sema, and capillary vascular damage resulting in reduced alveolar development.

In infants with mild BPD, there is patchy loss of cilia accompanied by mucosal break- down of the airway lining. Edema develops in the interstitial spaces of the bronchi, blood vessels, and alveolar septa. Also common is the incorporation of fibrin into the alveolar septa.

Infants with moderate BPD experience extensive loss of cilia in the bronchial and bron- chiolar lining cells. Mucosal inflammatory cells are present; there is necrosis of alveolar lining cells and edema of the peribronchial and

FIGURE 6-10 ▲ Progression of bronchopulmonary dysplasia.

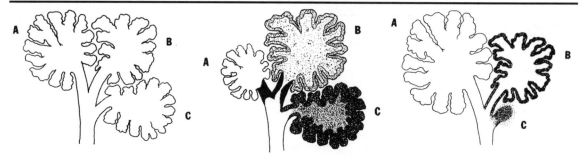

Left. Schematic drawing of normally expanded and aerated pulmonary lobules. *Center,* acute bronchopulmonary dysplasia. *A.* Necrotizing bronchiolitis occludes the bronchiolar lumen, "protecting" the parenchyma distal to it from the high oxygen tension and pressure used in maintaining adequate oxygenation. *B.* The bronchiole is narrowed by mucosal hyperplasia and muscular hypertrophy, thereby reducing the amount of pressure and oxygen tension in the lobule distal to it. Alveolar cell hyperplasia, septal fibroplasia, and alveolar macrophage dysplasia, however, occur to a mild to moderate degree. *C.* The bronchiole is widely patent, exposing the distal sublobule to the full ventilatory pressure and oxygen tension. The alveolar lumina are largely obliterated by alveolar macrophages, alveolar cell hyperplasia, and marked septal fibroplasia. *Right.* Long-standing "healed" bronchopulmonary dysplasia (LSHBPD). *A.* With resolution of the necrotizing bronchiolitis that occluded the lumen of the bronchiole, the uninjured sublobule overexpands to compensate for the less expansile injured portions of lung (*B* and *C*). *B.* With resolution of the mild to moderate injury incurred by the parenchyma during the acute stages of bronchopulmonary dysplasia, the sublobule displays the hallmark of LSHBPD: septal fibrosis. *C.* The sublobule is virtually obliterated by organization of the severe acute bronchopulmonary dysplasia.

From: Stocker JT. 1986. Pathologic features of long-standing healed bronchopulmonary dysplasia: A study of 28 3- to 40-month-old infants. *Human Pathology* 17(9): 943–961. Reprinted by permission.

perivascular spaces and alveolar septa. Small areas of atelectasis may be present. The cells lining the conductive airways develop squamous metaplasia.

In infants with severe BPD, marked necrosis of the airway lining results in excessive amounts of debris containing necrotic epithelial cells, mucus, and inflammatory cells. The alveolar structure is disturbed with areas of atelectasis and hyperinflated sacs, leading to severe ventilation-to-perfusion mismatch. In addition, there is patchy interstitial fibrosis and squamous metaplasia of bronchial and bronchiolar epithelia. In the most severe cases, there is fibrosis, obliterative bronchiolitis, severe disturbance of the alveoli, and severe vascular changes, with a reduction in the volume of the capillary beds (Figure 6-10).[124,125]

Pulmonary circulation in infants with BPD can be abnormal, leading to increased pulmonary vascular pressures and pulmonary hypertension, with the development of cor pul-

monale. Infants with severe BPD may have cor pulmonale, recurrent pulmonary edema, worsening ventilation-to-perfusion mismatch, and late morbidity from viral infection or sudden death.[126]

In the early stages of BPD, increased airway obstruction has been demonstrated, and as the disease progresses in severity, airway obstruction can become more significant. Airway constriction can occur secondary to hypoxia or airway damage. Upper airway damage in infants with BPD includes tracheal, subglottic, and bronchial stenosis; polyps; granulomas; and tracheobronchomalacia. Other mechanisms that can cause airway obstruction include marked hyperplasia of bronchial epithelium, increased mucus production, decreased mucociliary clearance, and mucosal edema.

Infants with BPD have upper airway damage, and significant changes occurring in the terminal bronchioles and alveolar ducts. The cellular debris, inflammatory cells, and exudate

TABLE 6-5 ▲ **Clinical Findings and the Associated Possible Causes in the Infant with Bronchopulmonary Dysplasia**

Signs or Symptoms	Possible Causes
Rapid respirations	Hypoxemia Increased secretions Inadequate support, rapid weaning Early signs of respiratory infections Airway hyperresponsiveness
Wheezing	Airway hyperresponsiveness Bronchomalacia Laryngeal webs Subglottic stenosis Congestive heart failure
Cough	Increased secretions Early signs of infection Tracheitis Airway hyperresponsiveness
Fever	Upper respiratory infection, lower respiratory infection Otitis media
Desaturation	All of above leading to hypoxemia
Bradycardia	Obstructive apneic episode Hypoxemia
Infiltrate on chest x-ray film	Residual changes of bronchopulmonary dysplasia Partial atelectasis Pneumonia

From: Bhutani VK, and Abbasi S. 1992. Long-term pulmonary consequences in survivors with bronchopulmonary dysplasia. *Clinics in Perinatology* 19(3): 653. Reprinted by permission.

may obstruct many of the terminal airways. This process may be beneficial because it may protect the distal alveolus from further damage from oxygen and barotrauma.[124] Increased airway resistance may cause increased work of breathing and abnormal ventilation and perfusion. Airway hyperactivity is commonly found in infants with BPD and can persist into childhood.[127] Pulmonary function studies are often performed at the bedside to determine the progress of the disease. Based on serial studies of pulmonary compliance and resistance, the progress of the disease can be evaluated and treated (Chapter 12).

SIGNS AND SYMPTOMS

Early clinical signs of BPD may begin within the first week of life when recovery from the initial disease (such as RDS) is anticipated, yet the infant requires increased oxygen and ventilatory support. Mild chronic lung disease is generally characterized by a need for mechanical ventilation for several days, followed by several weeks of supplemental oxygen. Clinically, the infant may have retractions, diminished breath sounds, and fine crackles (Table 6-5).

During the early phases of mild to moderate chronic lung disease, oxygen and ventilator

TABLE 6-6 ▲ **Bronchopulmonary Dysplasia Clinical Scoring System**

Variable	0 (Normal)	Score* 1 (Mild)	2 (Moderate)	3 (Severe)
Respiratory rate (average number/minute)	<40	40–60	61–80	>80
Dyspnea (retractions)	0	Mild	Moderate	Severe
FiO$_2$ (PaO$_2$ 50–70 torr)	0.21	0.22–0.30	0.31–0.50	>0.50
PaCO$_2$ (torr)	<45	46–55	56–70	>70
Growth rate (gm/day)	>25	15–24	5–14	<5

*Score at 28 days of age or at 36 weeks postconceptional age. Score is a mean of four measures for respiratory rate, dyspnea, and FiO$_2$ obtained at 6-hour intervals. Growth rate represents average daily weight gain over a 7-day period before the assignment of the score. Highest score is 15. A score of 15 is assigned if the patient is receiving mechanical ventilation.

From: Toce SS, et al. 1984. Clinical and roentgenographic scoring systems for assessing bronchopulmonary dysplasia. *American Journal of Diseases in Children* 138(6): 581–585. Copyright 1984, American Medical Association. Reprinted by permission.

TABLE 6-7 ▲ Long-Term Complications Associated with Bronchopulmonary Dysplasia

Respiratory	Cardiovascular
Chronic respiratory distress	Pulmonary hypertension
Respiratory acidosis	Right ventricular hypertrophy
Bronchospasm	Systemic hypertension
Recurrent pneumonia	Left ventricular hypertrophy
Ventilator dependency	Heart failure
Tracheostomy	Patent foramen ovale
Subglottic stenosis	Occult congenital heart disease
Tracheomegaly	Systemic-to-pulmonary arterial shunts
Tracheomalacia	**Renal**
Bronchomalacia	Nephrocalcinosis
Airway granulation tissue and pseudopolyps	**Neurologic**
Acquired lobar emphysema	Developmental delay
Laryngospasm	Static encephalopathy
Apnea	Progressive encephalopathy
Atelectasis	Movement disorders
Chronic hypoxemia	Seizures
Sleep hypoxemia	Visual impairment
Sudden death	Hearing impairment
Gastrointestinal	Oromotor feeding disorders
Gastroesophageal reflux	**Metabolic**
Aspiration	Metabolic alkalosis
Behavioral feeding disorders	Hypokalemia
Oral movement disorder	Hypochloremia
	Elevated metabolic rate
	Failure to thrive
	Rickets of prematurity

From: Alpert BA, Allen JL, and Schildlow DV. 1993. Bronchopulmonary dysplasia. In *Pediatric Respiratory Disease: Diagnosis and Treatment,* Hilman BC, ed. Philadelphia: WB Saunders, 448. Reprinted by permission.

settings need to be increased. Overdistention of the lung causes a barrel chest. Hypoxia, hypercarbia, and respiratory acidosis must be corrected by increasing ventilator settings.

If these infants are oxygen dependent after a month of life, hypoxia and cyanosis develop quickly when they are removed from oxygen. Bilateral breath sounds are diminished because of areas of atelectasis and hypoinflation. Signs of right-sided heart failure develop as a result of increased pulmonary vascular resistance.

A clinical scoring system has been developed to help evaluate the severity of BPD (Table 6-6).[123] The scoring helps determine response to treatment and progression of the disease.

Treatment

Just as the etiology and pathophysiology of BPD are multifactorial, treatment too is multifaceted. Management of the infant with BPD requires a multidisciplinary team in which all members are aware of the infant's response to various treatments. The goal is to promote growth and maintain homeostasis in all systems, while keeping the infant free from infection and gradually weaning him off the ventilator and oxygen. Prevention and early recognition of the many complications associated with BPD are essential (Table 6-7).

The clinician, knowing that oxygen therapy is necessary but also causes further damage to the infant with BPD, must strive for a fine balance. Although cumbersome, oxygen therapy remains the essential element of BPD care. In patients with BPD, PaO_2s should remain between 55 and 70 torr, and oxygen saturations (based on pulse oximetry) should be maintained between 90 and 95 percent.[104] Oxygen may be delivered via endotracheal tube, nasal prong CPAP, oxyhood, tent, or nasal cannula. Oxygen should be reduced gradually based upon the infant's tolerance. Because of the fears of toxicity, oxygen therapy is frequently underutilized and discontinued too early.[128] The resulting hypoxia can cause the development of feeding difficulty, slow growth, nutrient malabsorption, bronchoconstriction, pulmonary hypertension, and cor pulmonale.[128,129] The use of booster blood transfusions to increase oxygen-carrying capacity in infants with BPD is controversial. Hyperoxia may worsen the BPD and cause retinopathy of prematurity.

Using pulse oximetry and physical findings, the nurse should continuously assess the infant with BPD to determine oxygen requirements. During activities that may stress the infant—bathing; feeding; painful procedures, including laboratory work; and endotracheal tube suctioning—additional oxygen may be required. Following these periods, the infant should be given time to stabilize before the oxygen is returned to baseline levels.

Parents should be taught to maintain adequate oxygen saturations at all times; awake, feeding, and asleep. They need to be taught to observe for respiratory distress, cyanosis, irritability, and early signs of respiratory infections. Chest physiotherapy and suctioning of the endotracheal tube should be done based upon breath sounds in order to maintain a patent airway and prevent atelectasis.

Like oxygen, mechanical ventilation is a known risk factor for infants with BPD but is also commonly used in the treatment. Ventilators designed in the late 1970s were time-cycled, pressure-limited machines. Research has shown that there are differing time constants in different lung regions. Satisfactory gas flow rates and pressures generated by conventional ventilation for one area of the lung may be inappropriate or excessive for another area.[130]

Few prospective randomized trials have been conducted to determine the combination of ventilator settings that either limit the severity or prevent the development of BPD. One study showed no significant difference in long-term outcome between use of rapid rates as opposed to short inspiratory times.[131] Another study showed that an inspiratory time ≥ 0.6 seconds improved pulmonary function.[132]

In general, the goal is to decrease the $\overline{Paw}$ by decreasing the PIP, PEEP, and rate. Newer ventilation strategies for infants with BPD tolerate lower PaO_2 (50–60 torr) and higher $PaCO_2$ (50–60 torr). The appropriate amount of PEEP is variable. Infants with tracheobronchomalacia, a probable cause of intermittent cyanotic "spells," respond to higher levels of PEEP. However, increased PEEP leads to higher mean airway pressures, which can cause further lung injury.

Hot-wire anemometry and pneumotachography have been applied to current ventilators to measure inspiratory and expiratory tidal volume, minute ventilation, and air leak. It is hoped that this monitoring will permit ventilation at lower peak airway pressures, thereby reducing the incidence of pneumothorax and PIE, factors known to contribute to BPD.[133] Also being developed are computer-assisted feedback mechanisms for the ventilator. Based on end tidal carbon dioxide tensions and oxygen saturations, microprocessors can more accurately control FiO_2, PIP, and $\overline{Paw}$.[134]

Synchronized intermittent mandatory ventilation (SIMV) and pressure support ventilation (assist-control) are two of the newest commercially available methods to ventilate newborns (Chapter 5). They are designed to improve interaction and reduce antagonism between infant-generated and mechanically generated breaths. SIMV has been recommended for infants with BPD who have a more mature respiratory drive and often have difficulty with conventional intermittent mandatory ventilation. Also, the ability of SIMV to limit lung overdistension reduces the need for the neonate to fight the ventilator breaths.

Several infant ventilators have been developed or adapted to provide some form of SIMV, including the Infant Star Ventilator (Infrasonics), Bear Cub Infant Ventilator (Bear Medical Systems), Servo 900C and Model 300 (Siemens Elma, AB), Bird VIP (Bird Products Co.), and Babylog 8000 (Draeger, Inc.). Each ventilator works a little differently but is programmed to provide ventilation in synchrony with the infant's breathing pattern. The clinical responses of infants to these ventilators are being evaluated. SIMV may improve ventilation-to-perfusion matching, help wean patients from ventilation, and prevent BPD.

High-frequency ventilation (Chapter 13) has been evaluated to determine its impact on BPD. One high-frequency jet ventilator, Bunnell Life-Pulse (Bunnell, Inc.), has been shown to be more effective in treating and preventing neonatal air leak syndrome than conventional ventilation but has had no significant effect in reducing the incidence of BPD.

A multicenter trial using the Senko Hummingbird high-frequency oscillator (Senko Medical Institutional Manufacturing Co.) reported a similar incidence of BPD—approximately 40 percent—in both the high-frequency oscillator and the conventional ventilator groups.[135] A single-center group using the SensorMedics 3100 (SensorMedics Corp.), another form of high-frequency oscillation, reported a 30 percent incidence of BPD in the experimental group versus a 65 percent incidence in the conventionally ventilated neonates.[136]

Studies continue using high frequency ventilation in order to find better ways of ventilating infants and thus preventing BPD.

In some situations, methods of weaning the infant from mechanical ventilation may fail, and the infant may require a tracheostomy. This may reduce the risk for airway scarring from the endotracheal tube and decrease cyanotic spells, airway plugging, and irritability. Less noxious oral stimuli and enhanced interaction for the infant and family are other important advantages.

MEDICATIONS

Long-term management of infants with BPD often includes treatment with many drugs such as diuretics, bronchodilators, and steroids. Decisions to use each drug should be individualized. The addition of each drug to the infant's management plan should be closely monitored in order to prevent the "polypharmacy" phenomenon associated with BPD care (Table 6-8). For a detailed review of all medications used for the infant with BPD, see Chapter 10.

NUTRITION

Several studies have shown that infants with BPD have reduced rates of growth in terms of both weight and length.[137,138] Long-term studies have shown that infants with severe BPD requiring oxygen have increased metabolic rates and may have delayed growth up to eight years of age as compared to children of similar birth weight and gestational age.[139] A major cause for this delayed growth may be that infants with BPD have a metabolic rate approximately 25 percent higher than infants without BPD.[140] The increased work of breathing resulting from decreased lung compliance, increased airway resistance, and tachypnea is one of the factors interfering with normal growth.

Providing adequate nutrition to the very low birth weight neonate at risk for BPD is often

TABLE 6-8 ▲ **Commonly Used Medications for Bronchopulmonary Dysplasia**

Medication	Dosage
Diuretics	
Furosemide	0.5–2 mg/kg/dose IV or PO, bid (every day in infants <31 weeks postconceptional age)
Chlorthiazide	5–20 mg/kg/dose IV or PO, bid
Hydrochlorthiazide	1–2 mg/kg/dose PO, bid
Spironolactone	1.5 mg/kg/dose PO, bid
Inhaled Agents	
Albuterol	0.02–0.04 ml/kg/dose of a 0.5% solution diluted to 1–2 ml with half-normal or normal saline, every 4–6 hours
Metaproterenol	0.1–0.25 ml (5–12.5 mg) of a 5% solution diluted to 1–2 ml with half-normal or normal saline, every 6 hours
Isoetharine	0.1–0.25 ml (1–2.5 mg) of a 1% solution diluted to 1–2 ml with half-normal or normal saline, every 4–6 hours
Isoproterenol	0.1–0.25 ml (0.5–1.25 mg) of a 0.05% solution diluted to 1–2 ml with half-normal saline every 3–4 hours
Atropine, ipratropium bromide	0.025–0.08 mg/kg diluted to 1.5–2.5 ml in half-normal or normal saline, every 6 hours; doses of ipratropium up to 0.176 mg may be used
Cromolyn sodium	20 mg by inhalation, every 6–8 hours
Systemic Agents	
Aminophylline (IV), theophylline (PO)	Loading dose 5 mg/kg; maintenance dose 2 mg/kg/dose, every 8–12 hours; serum levels of 5–15 mg/liter
Caffeine citrate	Loading dose 20 mg/kg; maintenance dose 5 mg/kg IV or PO, every 24 hours
Terbutaline	SC 5 µg/kg, every 4–6 hours
Dexamethasone	0.5 mg/kg/day IV or PO every 12 hours for three days, decrease to 0.3 mg/kg/day for three days, then taper 10–20% every three days
Albuterol	0.15 mg/kg/dose PO, every 8 hours

From: Davis JM, and Rosenfeld WN. 1994. Chronic lung disease. In *Neonatology: Pathophysiology and Management of the Newborn*, 4th ed., Avery GB, Fletcher MA, and MacDonald MG, eds. Philadelphia: JB Lippincott, 466. Reprinted by permission.

quite challenging. Restricting fluids to 75–90 ml/kg/day during the acute phase of respiratory disease has been recommended in order to reduce pulmonary edema and improve cardiac output.[141] One recent study with a population of 100 infants weighing <1,750 gm started fluids at levels as low as 50 ml/kg/day; the control group started at 80 ml/kg/day. Eleven infants in the control group died versus only 1 in the "dry group." At day 28, 54 percent of infants in the dry group had no signs of BPD versus 30 percent in the control group. The results suggested that fluid restriction can reduce the mortality and morbidity of low birth weight infants.[142]

In order to support adequate growth and development, the infant requires appropriate nutrition from early admission. By 40 weeks gestational age, weight gain should be 20–30 gm/day. It is recommended that 70 parenteral or 95 enteral kcal/kg/day and 2 gm/kg/day of protein be initiated during early lung disease.[141,143] As the infant matures, 130–160 kcal/kg/day and 2.5–3.5 gm/kg/day of protein may be necessary to promote growth.

Initially, nutrition is provided in parenteral form via peripheral intravenous catheters. If full enteral feedings are not tolerated, percutaneous central venous catheters or Broviacs are used to administer parenteral nutrition. High concentrations of glucose can be given through these lines, but excessive loads (>4 mg/kg/minute) can result in increased oxygen consumption, increased carbon dioxide production, and increased metabolic rates in infants with BPD.[144] Amino acids are increased daily while the infant is closely monitored for acid-base imbalances.

Complete nutrition should include 2–3 gm/kg/day of an intravenous fat emulsion (20 percent). Intravenous fat emulsion administration should start within 24 hours after birth in infants greater than 28 weeks gestational age, or weighing more than 1,000 gm. Administration may be delayed until the second or third day in more immature infants.[145] Early administration of fat emulsion has been associated with hypoxia, pulmonary vascular lipid deposits, and more severe BPD.[146] Careful monitoring of serum triglyceride levels is important to minimize complications of lipid administration.

Electrolyte and mineral imbalances often accompany BPD as a result of fluid restriction, diuretics, dexamethasone, and other medications. Monitoring of serum electrolyte levels is important in order to determine appropriate amounts of supplementation. Calcium and phosphorous supplements are added to formulas, and fortifiers can be added to breast milk.

Multivitamin supplementation including vitamin D is indicated, especially when fluid volume is restricted. Vitamin A supplementation is recommended, especially for premature infants, because it plays an important role in epithelial tissue repair.[147] One study reports a lower incidence of BPD when supplemental vitamin A was given intramuscularly and then added to oral feedings.[148]

Vitamin E has been recommended as an antioxidant to be given when infants are receiving oxygen therapy, but reports regarding its effectiveness in preventing BPD are controversial.[149,150] Another concern is its possible toxic effect when large doses are given. It is suggested that serum levels of vitamin E (normal 1–3.5 mg/dl) be monitored if the infant is receiving supplements. Recommended supplementation

is 5 IU of vitamin E per day via parenteral vitamins, liquid vitamin supplementation, or in premature formula.[151]

Inositol, a component of membrane phospholipids and part of the vitamin B complex, may also play a role in prevention of BPD. One study giving infants intravenous inositol reported increased survival and decreased BPD.[152] Inositol is found in colostrum and is generally not added to parenteral nutrition.

Gastroesophageal reflux often leads to difficulties in providing adequate nutrition to infants with BPD. Reflux may alter lung function in these patients by causing aspiration of stomach contents and triggering bronchial reactivity. Conservative measures include thickening the feedings, decreasing the volume by increasing the number of feedings, and elevating the head of the bed to a 30-degree angle. Nipple feeding the infant with BPD can be problematic because of the negative oral stimulation from the endotracheal tube, gastric feeding tubes, and frequent oral suctioning.

INFECTION

Preventing and monitoring for infection are important for any infant at risk for BPD. Aseptic technique must be employed at all times, especially during invasive procedures. Early treatment with erythromycin as a means of reducing the incidence and severity of BPD has been suggested following recent studies showing the impact of *Ureaplasma urealyticum*.[112,113,153]

Recurrent bacterial and viral infections add to the problems of the infant with BPD. Intermittent cultures of tracheal secretions of chronically ventilated infants should be evaluated to determine types of colonizing organisms. Sepsis workups that include chest radiographs, complete blood count, cultures, and/or gram stains should be done whenever the infant's condition deteriorates, suggesting sepsis. Broad-spectrum antibiotics are used initially until specific sensitivities are identified. Multiple courses of broad-spectrum antibiotics substantially increase the risk of fungal infections among this population.

After discharge from the hospital, infants with BPD continue to be at risk for respiratory infections, including respiratory syncytial virus (RSV).[153] The prophylactic use of ribavirin at home in patients with BPD is being investigated as is the use of RSV immunoglobulins. Parents should understand that their infant is at risk for infection and should limit visitors and exposure to potential pathogens.

NURSING CARE

Caring for the infant with BPD can be a frustrating experience for even the most experienced nurse. The infant often becomes agitated before going into bronchospasm and frequently does not respond to the usual soothing techniques such as rocking, patting, holding, or talking.[143] Interpreting the infant's behavior is essential in supporting the infant and family. Two important studies have shown that individualized behavior assessment and intervention that reduces stress and helps the infant to organize self-regulating abilities have a significant impact on the infant's long-term outcome. Als and colleagues reported significantly shorter length of ventilation, decreased days on oxygen support, earlier establishment of feeding, improved daily weight gain, lower incidence of IVH, and decreased hospital stay with infant modulation.[154,155]

Als has developed a model of preterm development that describes early behavioral organization based upon the autonomic, motor, state, attention, and self-regulatory systems.[156] Major considerations in caring for the infant include limiting environmental demands when the infant loses control, identifying early signs of loss of control, understanding when intervention is needed, and knowing strategies to reduce stress. Individualized developmental plans should be constructed by the neonatal team.

The incidence of neurodevelopmental disorders in children with BPD is quite variable. Neurodevelopmental problems may not be any greater in infants with BPD than in premature infants. The risk for disabilities increases as the birth weight decreases and more complications develop. Factors that appear to place the BPD infant at higher risk include moderate to severe intraventricular hemorrhage and low socioeconomic and parent education levels.[157]

One study in 1987 reported approximately one-quarter of infants who weighed 500–999 gm at birth are likely to have major deficits at 5 years of age. Seventy-two percent had no functional handicap and thirty-three percent exhibited functional improvement since two years of age.[158] A more recent study reported approximately half of infants with BPD are free of any handicaps; cerebral palsy is the most common handicapping condition in the other 50 percent. Approximately 4 percent of infants with BPD are blind from ROP, and approximately 4 percent have sensorineural hearing loss.[157]

Maximizing neurodevelopmental outcome in infants with BPD requires a multidisciplinary team approach. A team consisting of developmental specialists, physical therapists, speech therapists, neonatologists, and nurses should develop a plan of care to maximize neurologic growth and development. Goals include maximizing the environmental conditions in the NICU, reducing stress, and maintaining normal oxygen levels. Proper positioning in natural flexion using rolls and blankets is helpful. Minimizing stimulation and evaluating the infant's response to procedures using oxygen saturation monitoring as a guide are important. Discharge planning should ensure that the family understands the plan of care, including handling, positioning, stimulation, and stress reactions.

Teaching and supporting the family who has an infant with BPD is a challenge for NICU nurses. The nurse is often coordinator of the various disciplines involved in the infant's care. Evaluation and reporting of the infant's responses to the various therapists help in developing an individualized plan of care. A more in-depth review of nursing can be found in several texts referenced, including *Bronchopulmonary Dysplasia: Strategies for Total Patient Care* by Lund.[159]

RETINOPATHY OF PREMATURITY

Improvements in medical technology, including mechanical ventilation, have resulted in the survival of greater numbers of premature infants, with a concomitant incidence of retinopathy of prematurity. Formerly known as retrolental fibroplasia, ROP is a disorder of retinal vascularization in the premature retina that causes a proliferation of abnormal vasculature leading to visual loss from cicatrization (scarring) and retinal detachment. Immature retinal vessels are a prerequisite for the development of ROP. Initiated by an injury, ROP represents the healing process.

ROP was first described by Terry in 1942, who called the disease "retrolental fibroplasia" because of the formation of scar tissue behind the lens of the eye in premature infants.[160] In the late 1940s and 1950s, the amount of blindness from this disorder was considered epidemic. Following a report of a controlled study by Patz and associates showing that high concentrations of oxygen contributed to the development of retrolental fibroplasia, the use of oxygen was greatly curtailed.[161] Although the incidence of blindness decreased significantly with decreased use of oxygen, there was an increase in morbidity and mortality including such conditions as cerebral palsy and lung disease.[162]

In the late 1960s, technology was available to measure arterial blood gases, which helped to justify the use of oxygen concentrations >40 percent. As survival improved because of mechanical ventilation and other technologies, smaller infants were surviving, and there was a resurgence of retrolental fibroplasia. The disorder was renamed retinopathy of prematurity in the 1980s because of its association with prematurity and its occurrence despite excellent oxygen monitoring and the absence of high oxygen blood levels.

The incidence of ROP is inversely related to birth weight and gestational age. It appears to be increasing as the limits of viability decrease. Infants weighing >1,500 gm have a 10 percent incidence of ROP.[163] Fortunately, approximately 90 percent of infants with acute Stage 1 and 2 ROP go on to spontaneous regression, healing with little or no visual loss.[164] Cicatricial sequelae, including blindness, occur in the other 10 percent, most commonly infants weighing <1,000 gm.[165]

In 1981, Phelps estimated that approximately 600 infants a year in the U.S. were considered at risk for blindness from ROP.[166] Results from a recent multicenter study involving 23 institutions in the U.S. following 4,009 infants reported the incidence of ROP to be 47 percent in infants weighing 1,000–1,250 gm, 78 percent in infants weighing 750–999 gm, and 90 percent in infants weighing less than 750 gm at birth. The overall rate of severe ROP—greater than threshold (Stage 3+ or greater)—was 22 percent. Multiple births and gender had no significant effect on the incidence. Caucasian infants had a higher chance of progressing to severe ROP than the African American infants.[167] Of the 291 infants who developed severe ROP and were enrolled in the cryotherapy trial, approximately 20 percent were found to be blind at 3 1/2 years of age.[168] In a recent study from Australia reviewing 1,001 infants, the overall rate of ROP was 40 percent for infants between 500 and 999 gm. Severe ROP was 20 percent, similar to the multicenter study in the U.S.[169] Four infants in this study were blind. We do not know the exact number of children being visually handicapped and blinded by ROP today in the U.S. because there is no specific registry.

A knowledge of the development of retinal vasculature will help the nurse understand the disease, diagnosis, and treatment of ROP. Normal ocular development occurs in the hypoxic intrauterine environment. At six weeks gestation, the hyaloid artery enters the eye and begins to fill the vitreous cavity with blood vessels. The retina remains avascular until approximately 16 weeks gestation, when capillary precursor cells (spindle cells) start branching out from the tissue around the fetal optic nerve and slowly grow centrifugally toward the ora serrata, the anterior edge of the retina. The network reaches the temporal ora serrata at approximately 40–44 weeks gestation. The blood vessels behind the leading edge of capillaries gradually form arteries and veins.

Retinopathy of prematurity can occur when the newly forming network of capillaries, which is progressing toward the ora serrata, is disrupted. Multiple factors can interfere with normal growth of these blood vessels, among them hyperoxia, septic shock, heart failure, and pneumothorax.[170]

During Stage 1, also called the acute phase, hyperoxia or an unidentified agent can produce vasoconstriction in the immature retinal vessels. This vasoconstriction may be reversible in its early stages, but if it continues, there is tissue ischemia. This acute phase starts usually from four to ten weeks after birth and may progress slowly or rapidly. An angiogenic response to the ischemia results in new vessel growth (neovascularization). If vascularization is able to re-establish circulation to the central retina and to the peripheral avascular retina, ROP regresses, and excess vessels are reabsorbed. If the process is aggravated, neovascularization erupts into the vitreous, and vessel growth is uncontrolled. These vessels may regress and heal, but residual scarring causing a neovascular ridge may result.

An international classification system for ROP has been developed by ophthalmologists from 11 countries. This system describes ROP in terms of three categories: retinal location of disease, extent of the developing vasculature involved, and the stages of the disease.[171,172]

Retinal vessel development occurs from the optic nerve in the posterior of the eye toward the periphery. The location of the disease in one of three zones is a measure of how the progression of blood vessels has developed.

- **Zone I** is a small area around the optic nerve and macula, the most vital areas of the retina. Zone I disease is the most dangerous because progression to extensive scar tissue and total retinal detachment is most likely in this location.
- **Zone II** extends from the edge of Zone I to the front of the retina on the nasal side of the eye and partway to the front of the retina on the temporal side.
- **Zone III** is the remainder of the temporal retina, the last to be vascularized during fetal development.

The extent of the disease is defined by how many clock hours of the eye's circumference are diseased. Figure 6-11 illustrates the zones and clock hours of ROP. Classification of ROP by stages of increasing severity is important because it is a progressive disease.

- **Stage 1** ROP is characterized by a sharp white line separating the vascular and avascular retina.
- **Stage 2** displays a rolled ridge of scar tissue in place of the white demarcation line. It may be limited to a small area of the retina or encircle the eye.

FIGURE 6-11 ▲ Zones and clock hours of retinopathy of prematurity.

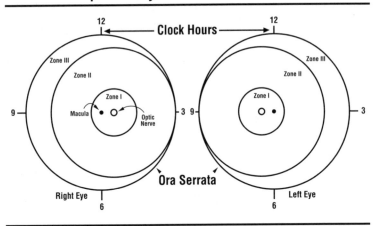

From: An international classification of retinopathy of prematurity. 1984. *Pediatrics* 74(1): 127–133. Reprinted by permission.

• **Stage 3** is characterized by neovascularization proliferating from the posterior aspect of the ridge out of the retina into the vitreous. Stage 3 is further subdivided into mild, moderate, or severe amounts of tissue into the vitreous.

• **Stage 4** is subtotal retinal detachment caused by the scar tissue formed in Stages 1–3. Stage 4a is a partial detachment in the periphery of the retina. Stage 4b is a subtotal or total detachment involving the macula and fovea, usually with a fold extending through Zones I, II and III.

• **Stage 5** involves a complete retinal detachment, with the retina assuming a closed or partially closed funnel from the optic nerve to the front of the eye.

If, at any of these stages, the posterior veins are enlarged and arterioles are tortuous, a designation of plus is added (for example, Stage 3+). The plus sign indicates extensive ROP changes that may signify a rapidly progressive course.

An unusually aggressive pattern of ROP development termed Rush disease has been reported in infants weighing <1,000 gm. The disease develops earlier than usual (three to five weeks after birth) and can progress rapidly to severe ROP with retinal detachment.[173]

The infant's visual outcome depends upon the stage of the disease, whether the macula is involved, and the results of treatment. Because Stages 1 to 3 generally occur in the peripheral retina, the macula is not affected. For most infants with Stage 1 and 2 ROP, the disease resolves spontaneously without scarring. Although these infants do not require treatment, they are at greater risk for developing myopia, amblyopia, astigmatism, strabismus, and glaucoma.[170] If they are not treated, infants with moderate to severe Stage 3 or 4 ROP are at risk for reduced vision because scar tissue shrinks and then exerts traction on the retina. Moderate traction results in the distortion of the macula. In severe cases of ROP (Stages 4b and 5) the retina and macula may be totally detached, resulting in blindness.

Any infant who has had ROP is at risk of functional or cosmetic disability. One study found that ophthalmologic problems developed in 55 percent of patients over six to ten years.[174] In addition, late peripheral retinal degeneration and late retinal detachment have been reported in teens and adults with regressive ROP.[174,175]

RISK FACTORS

Since the 1950s, investigators have been looking at the many factors that may be associated with the development of ROP. Prematurity and low birth weight appear to be the leading risk factors, although ROP has been reported in healthy term infants and in term infants with severe cyanotic heart disease.[176] The many factors leading to ROP appear to include immaturity, hyperoxia, blood transfusions, IVH, pneumothorax, mechanical ventilation, apnea, infection, hypercarbia, hypocarbia, PDA, administration of prostaglandin synthetase inhibitors (indomethacin), vitamin E deficiency, lactic acidosis, prenatal complications, and genetic factors.[177,178] After controlling for immaturity, the sicker the infant, the more likely it is that serious ROP will develop.

The role of oxygen in the development of ROP is complex and remains controversial. Early studies in the 1950s suggested that infants exposed to high levels of oxygen developed significant ROP. This theory, based on kitten and puppy research, proposed that elevated oxygen levels led to retinal vasoconstriction, which if prolonged led to permanent closure of vessels. After the patient was returned to room air, the endothelial cells adjacent to closed capillaries proliferated, leading to new vessel growth.[179] One problem with this vasoconstriction-vasoobliterative theory is its failure to explain the development of ROP in infants exposed to minimal or no oxygen. Also, the studies done on animals have not been replicated in infants.

A more recent theory proposes that high levels of oxygen damage spindle cells, the precursors of the vascular endothelial cells in the retina. These spindle cells are bombarded with oxygen free radicals when the premature infant is exposed to oxygen levels higher than those of the hypoxic intrauterine environment. The free radicals induce extensive plasma membrane peroxidation because the premature infant has reduced free radical scavenging capabilities. The injured spindle cells react by forming massive intercellular linkages via gap junctions. The gap junction–linked spindle cells lose their ability to migrate and become activated to secrete angiogenic factor that promotes neovascularization at the border between the vascular and avascular retina.[180,181]

A debate continues as to whether (or not) vascular ablation is caused by direct oxidant injury or lack of blood flow in vessels whose endothelial cells are constantly remodeling in a disconnected manner. If the disease is due to oxidant injury then antioxidants may be beneficial, whereas in the latter case they would have no effect.

PREVENTION

Based upon these theories, much research has been done in an effort to prevent ROP. Early studies demonstrated a correlation between the duration of oxygen therapy and the development of ROP. A multicenter study designed to assess the relationship between arterial oxygen levels and ROP failed to find any significant differences.[182] A 1980s study comparing transcutaneous oxygen ($TcPO_2$) levels demonstrated no difference in the incidence or severity of ROP for varying $TcPO_2$ levels in infants weighing <1,000 gm.[183] One 1992 study supports an association between the incidence and severity of ROP and the duration of exposure to transcutaneous oxygen levels of greater than 80 mmHg.[184]

Maintaining appropriate oxygen levels is important because hyperoxia has been suggested as a major risk factor for ROP. In the 1950s, Szewczyk theorized that infants developed ROP if they were removed from oxygen too quickly and that their retinas became hypoxic.[185] Currently, the National Institutes of Health are investigating premature infants with "prethreshold" ROP. The purpose of the study is to determine whether maintaining arterial oxygen saturations at 96–99 percent will reduce the number of infants who progress to threshold ROP as compared to those who receive more conventional oxygen saturations of 89–94 percent. Until researchers are able to establish a critical blood oxygen level, the duration of oxygen therapy that induces ROP, or a regimen to prevent development of ROP, the neonatal team must critically analyze the infant's oxygen requirements and maintain an optimal balance between hyperoxia and hypoxia.

Several clinical and experimental studies have indicated that vitamin E (tocopherol) deficiency may cause ROP.[186–188] It has been theorized that premature infants have a deficiency of vitamin E, a naturally occurring antioxidant. Without sufficient amounts of vitamin E to protect the spindle cells in the retina, the free oxygen radicals destroy the cells.[180] Several infant trials using vitamin E reported mixed results in terms of lowering the incidence and severity of ROP.[187–189]

Even though vitamin E has been effective, there are concerns about the risk of sepsis, necrotizing enterocolitis, intraventricular hemorrhage, and retinal hemorrhage.[189–192] Many of these problems were reported with the use of intravenous, pharmacologic megadoses or unapproved formulations of the vitamin. If vitamin E is administered, serum levels should be monitored to prevent overdose.

Exposure to high levels of ambient light has been suggested as a cause of possible progression of ROP. It is proposed that light can generate free radicals, thus damaging the developing retinal blood vessels.[193] Glass, Avery, and Subramanian, in 1985, reported a reduced incidence of ROP in neonates—especially those weighing <1,000 gm—exposed to reduced (150 lux) compared to standard (600 lux) lighting in the nursery.[194] Two studies reported in 1988 and 1989 conflict with these findings.[195,196] It was reported in 1994 that the fused eyelids of the very premature infant do not appear protective; the incidence of ROP was determined more by gestational age.[197]

Another finding reported in 1992, which may support the light theory, reveals that ROP begins in most immature neonates in the areas of the retina receiving the greatest light dose, and its onset is either retarded or inhibited in the darker areas. These regional variations could not be explained by vascular or neuroanatomic organization.[198] Although the light theory is controversial, dimming of lights in the NICU and protecting the infant from bright lights have become part of standard neonatal care.

A trial conducted in Hungary, reported in 1986, suggests that D-penicillamine, an antioxidant, may reduce the incidence of ROP.[199] A 1992 study reports beneficial effects of inositol, a dietary supplement.[152] Both of these drugs need to be further tested for safety and effectiveness. Reports suggest that treatment with steroids to prevent BPD may actually reduce the likelihood of ROP progressing to the threshold level.[200] The effect of artificial surfactant on the incidence of ROP is under investigation. One study reported in 1994 found no significant effect.[201]

Screening

Screening for ROP should be started four to six weeks after birth, which corresponds to 28 to 30 weeks gestation for the most high risk premature infants. The infants at highest risk for ROP include those weighing <1,800 gm, those <35 weeks gestation who require oxygen, and any infant who weighs <1,300 gm or is <30 weeks gestation, regardless of oxygen therapy.[202] Other authors recommend screening any premature or term infant who requires prolonged oxygen therapy and blood transfusions.[164,165]

Eyes are rarely examined during the first month of life because of the risks of disturbing the mechanically ventilated infant. In addition, during the first month, the pupil in premature infants does not dilate widely, and examination is difficult because of a hazy media and residual fetal pupillary membrane.[203]

The object of screening is to detect ROP before it reaches the point of requiring treatment. Early screening also allows time to educate the parents about ROP. The optimal age for performing the examination appears to be

32 weeks postconceptional age because 5 percent of infants develop moderate ROP by 32.4 weeks.[203] Follow-up examinations continue every one to two weeks until one of the following occurs: The retinal blood vessels are developing normally; two successive two-week examinations show Stage 2 in Zone III (infants are then examined in four to six weeks); ROP is regressing. If ROP requires treatment (prethreshold), then examinations will occur more frequently.[164] In general, retinal vascularization is considered complete at 40–44 weeks gestation. If ROP is going to develop, it is usually present by this time.

The nurse should identify infants who meet screening criteria and schedule eye examinations around the infants' feeding and care routines. The nurse administers mydriatic agents prescribed by the ophthalmologist, including either Cyclomydril (0.2–0.5 percent cyclopentolate and 1 percent phenylephrine) or 0.5 percent cyclopentolate (0.5–1 percent tropicamide) along with 2.5 percent phenylephrine. Phenylephrine should be used cautiously if the infant has hypertension.

Prior to and during the examination, a nurse should be at the bedside to monitor responses to the medication and examination. Resuscitative equipment should be available because neonates can react to the examination with apnea, bradycardia, increased blood pressure, and oxygen desaturations.

Using indirect ophthalmoscope with a lid speculum and scleral depressors, the ophthalmologist examines each eye, evaluating all zones to determine retinal vascularization. If the infant does not tolerate the exam, it should be stopped and the infant treated appropriately. Administering atropine to the unstable infant has been recommended—especially if the examination is critical.

TREATMENT

There are several new procedures available to treat infants with severe progressive ROP. Cryotherapy, currently used worldwide, involves freezing the avascular area of the retina anterior to the area of disease. Cryotherapy is recommended when ROP has progressed to the "threshold level"—Stage 3 in Zone I and Zone II—and involves at least five continuous clock hour sectors or at least eight cumulative interrupted clock hour sectors. At this threshold level, the risk for an unfavorable outcome, including retinal detachment, is close to 50 percent.[168]

In a multicenter trial of cryotherapy for ROP, 6 percent of infants weighing <1,250 gm developed threshold ROP, 90 percent of whom were between 33 and 42 weeks gestation. After the disease was detected, treatment with cryotherapy occurred within 72 hours. Cryotherapy was shown to improve visual outcome by 50 percent.[167,168]

Some observers have voiced the concern that by the time infants have reached the threshold level of ROP based upon the previous criteria, it may be too late for treatment. The 12-month follow-up of the multicenter trial previously described showed a 25.7 percent structural failure rate and a 35 percent functional failure rate. (Data were based upon grading visual acuity with Teller acuity cards in which eyes below 6.4 cycles per degree, approximately 80/20 vision, were classified as an unfavorable outcome.) At the three-and-one-half-year follow-up, many infants whose eyes had been functionally normal at one year did not show the improvement in visual acuity necessary to be in the normal range.[168]

Suggestions for improved outcome include changing the definition of threshold ROP for Zones I and II so that therapies are initiated before further damage occurs. Another recommendation is to use cryotherapy or photo-

FIGURE 6-12 ▲ Laser therapy.

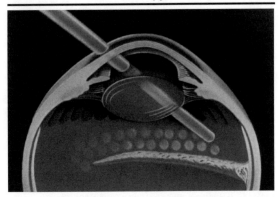

Courtesy of Coherent, Inc., Palo Alto, California.

coagulation in infants weighing <600 gm at birth when the disease is in the posterior part of Zone I before threshold is reached. Retinopathy of prematurity progresses rapidly in these infants, and they have had poor outcomes despite cryotherapy.[166]

Cryotherapy is often done at the bedside in the NICU or in a "short procedure" unit. Local anesthesia plus secobarbital or morphine are given for pain relief. The cryoprobe is placed on the external surface of the eye, freezing through the sclera and destroying the avascular retina. Ablation of the avascular tissue is presumed to eliminate the angiogenic factor that stimulates the extraretinal blood vessel growth.

Laser photocoagulation has been used to treat ROP (Figure 6-12). A prospective randomized trial using argon green laser photocoagulation found the outcome for laser-treated infants to be at least equal to that for cryotherapy-treated infants.[204] Laser therapy acts in the same way as cryotherapy in destroying avascular tissue. The advantages of this therapy include ease in treating more difficult locations, less trauma to the tissue, less discomfort for the infant, and fewer ocular and systemic complications such as intraocular hemorrhage and bradycardia.[178,205] Further investigation with laser therapy has been recommended.

If cryotherapy or laser therapy is unsuccessful in preventing retinal detachment, scleral buckling may be indicated. Under general anesthesia, a silicone band is placed around the eye. This reduces the circumference so that the retina can get close enough to the wall to attach itself. But if the scar continues to contract, the retina is pulled to the center of the eye. This technique has been reported to have a 50–100 percent anatomic success rate for patients with Stage 4a, and 4b ROP.[164] Favorable visual acuity of 20/60 to 18/400 has been reported with this technique, but if surgery is delayed, blindness may result.[206]

When retinal detachment progresses to Stage 5, a vitrectomy may be indicated. Two techniques, closed and open eye, have been reported with comparable results. During this three- to four-hour procedure, the lens and vitreous humor are removed from the eye. The scar tissue is removed, and the retina is laid back against the eye wall. Anatomic attachment is achieved in less than 50 percent of these infants, most of whom may have only perception of light.[206]

NURSING CARE

Caring for the mechanically ventilated infant who is at risk for ROP requires collaborative practice. Because of the multitude of current theories regarding the etiology of the disease, the NICU nurse needs to be aware of all the potential risk factors.

Until the role of oxygen is clearly defined, current recommendations are that PaO_2 levels should be maintained between 50 and 80 mmHg.[203] One 1992 study, which supports this recommendation, found that the longer the transcutaneous oxygen level exceeded 80 mmHg, the greater the risk of ROP.[184] As pulse oximetry has replaced transcutaneous monitoring, oxygen saturations are used instead of frequent blood gases. The nurse needs to be vigilant in maintaining oxygen saturations at the current acceptable levels of 89–92 percent. When the infant's oxygen saturations reflect changes in oxygenation and ventilation, adjustments in the oxygen and ventilator settings should be made to keep oxygen saturations within acceptable levels.

Nursing care for the infant requiring ocular surgery is similar to that for any preoperative patient. All systems should be stabilized and baseline laboratory values and vital signs documented. The parents should understand the reason for surgery, its potential risks, and its possible outcomes. Cryotherapy and laser therapy can be done in the NICU, but other surgeries may require general anesthesia.

Postoperatively, all vital signs should be assessed as the infant is recovering from anesthesia. Respiratory status should be carefully monitored, especially in premature infants and infants with bronchopulmonary dysplasia. Following cryotherapy, premature infants may require more oxygen and may have more apnea. This may be related to nasal obstruction from serosanguinous tears. Eyelid edema and nasal stuffiness usually resolve in a few days. The infant should be monitored for level of comfort even though ocular surgery causes only a small amount of pain.

Nurses should educate and support all parents of infants at risk for developing ROP. The neonatologist generally informs the parents of the possibility of ROP and prognosis based upon the infant's gestational age and early NICU course. Parents vary in their understanding of this complication. Following the initial ophthalmologic screening, parents are given information that may be difficult to understand. Often their infant has passed through the critical phase and is off the ventilator, so they are not prepared for new problems. The nurse should assist the parents in understanding the diagnosis and possible treatment by giving them written pamphlets and arranging meetings with the ophthalmologist and neonatologist.

Before discharge from the nursery, reinforcement for follow-up visits with the ophthalmologist is crucial. Parents need to understand that even after ROP regresses, continued ophthalmologic screening is required because the infant is at risk for visual problems.

SUMMARY

As nurses, we are aware of the many benefits of mechanical ventilation, but we must be diligent in monitoring for the adverse effects. Nurses play a key role in recognizing early signs of potential complications and alerting the neonatal team. Support of the family through this stressful time is important.

REFERENCES

1. Harris TR. 1988. Physiologic principles. In *Assisted Ventilation of the Neonate,* 2nd ed., Goldsmith JP, and Karotkin EH, eds. Philadelphia: WB Saunders, 22–69.

2. Carroll P. 1991. Pneumothorax in the newborn. *Neonatal Network* 10(2): 27–34.

3. Whitsett L, et al. 1994. Acute respiratory disorders. In *Neonatology: Pathophysiology and Management of the Newborn,* 4th ed., Avery GB, Fletcher MA, and MacDonald MG, eds. Philadelphia: JB Lippincott, 429–452.

4. Yu VY, et al. 1986. Pulmonary air leaks in extremely low birth weight infants. *Archives of Disease in Childhood* 61(3): 239–241.

5. Thibeault DW. 1986. Pulmonary barotrauma: Interstitial emphysema, pneumomediastinum and pneumothorax. In *Neonatal Pulmonary Care,* 2nd ed., Thibeault DW, and Gregory GA, eds. Norwalk, Connecticut: Appleton & Lange, 499–517.

6. Berg TJ, et al. 1975. Bronchopulmonary dysplasia and lung rupture in hyaline membrane disease: Influence of continuous distending pressure. *Pediatrics* 55(1): 51–53.

7. Tarnow-Mordi WO, Narang A, and Wilkinson AR. 1985. Lack of association between barotrauma and air leak in hyaline membrane disease. *Archives of Disease in Childhood* 60(6): 555–559.

8. Greenough A, et al. 1984. Pancuronium prevents pneumothoraces in ventilated premature babies who actively expire against positive pressure inflation. *Lancet* 1(8367):1–3.

9. Tarnow-Mordi WO, Sutton P, and Wilkinson AR. 1985. Inspiratory:expiratory ratio and pulmonary interstitial emphysema. *Archives of Disease in Childhood* 60(5): 496–497.

10. Yu VYH, et al. 1986. Pulmonary interstitial emphysema in infants less than 1,000 g at birth. *Australian Paediatric Journal* 22(3): 189–192.

11. Plenat F, et al. 1978. Pulmonary interstitial emphysema. *Clinics in Perinatology* 5(2): 351–375.

12. Greenough A, et al. 1992. Acute respiratory disease in the newborn. In *Textbook of Neonatology,* Roberton NRC, ed. Edinburgh: Churchill Livingstone, 385–504.

13. Sharp MJ, and Goldsmith JP. 1988. Ventilatory management casebook: Resolution of PIE using position therapy. *Journal of Perinatology* 8(1): 163–165.

14. Weintraub Z, and Oliven A. 1988. Successful resolution of unilateral pulmonary interstitial emphysema in a premature infant by selective bronchial balloon catheterization. *Journal of Pediatric Surgery* 23(11): 1005–1006.

15. Weintraub Z, et al. 1990. A new method for selective left main bronchus intubation in premature infants. *Journal of Pediatric Surgery* 25(6): 604–606.

16. Keszler M, et al. 1991. Multicenter controlled trial comparing high-frequency jet ventilation and conventional mechanical ventilation in newborn infants with pulmonary interstitial emphysema. Part I. *Journal of Pediatrics* 119(1): 85–93.

17. Madansky DL, et al. 1979. Pneumothorax and other forms of pulmonary air leaks in newborns. *American Review of Respiratory Disease* 120(4): 729–737.

18. Kendig JW, et al. 1988. Surfactant replacement therapy at birth: Final analysis of a clinical trial and comparisons with similar trials. *Pediatrics* 82(5): 756–762.

19. Collaborative European Multicenter Study Group. 1988. Surfactant replacement therapy for severe neonatal respiratory distress syndrome: An international randomized clinical trial. *Pediatrics* 82(5): 683–691.

20. Wiswell TE, Tuggle JM, and Turner BS. 1990. Meconium aspiration syndrome: Have we made a difference? *Pediatrics* 85(5): 715–721.

21. Hill A, Perlman JM, and Volpe JJ. 1982. Relationship of pneumothorax to occurrence of intraventricular hemorrhage in the premature newborn. *Pediatrics* 69(2): 144–149.

22. Hillman K. 1987. Intrathoracic pressure fluctuation and periventricular hemorrhage in the newborn. *Journal of Australian Pediatrics* 23(6): 343–346.

23. Mehrabani D, Gowen C, and Kopelman A. 1991. Association of pneumothorax and hypotension with intraventricular hemorrhage. *Archives of Disease in Childhood* 66(1 spec no): 48–51.

24. Ryan CA, Barrington KJ, and Phillips HJ. 1987. Contralateral pneumothoraces in the newborn: Incidence and predisposing factors. *Pediatrics* 79(3): 417–421.

25. Bashour BN, and Balfe JW. 1977. Urinary tract anomalies in neonates with spontaneous pneumothorax and/or pneumomediastinum. *Pediatrics* 59 (supplement 6 part 2): S1048–1049.

26. Wyman ML, and Kuhn LR. 1977. Accuracy of transillumination in the recognition of pneumothorax and pneumomediastinum in the neonate. *Clinical Pediatrics* 16(4): 323–327.

27. Kuhns LR, et al. 1975. Diagnosis of pneumothorax pneumomediastinum in the neonate by transillumination. *Pediatrics* 56(3): 355–362.

28. Hagedorn M, Garden S, and Abman S. 1993. Respiratory diseases. In *Handbook of Neonatal Intensive Care,* 3rd ed., Merenstein GB, and Gardner SL, eds. St. Louis: Mosby-Year Book, 334–338.

29. Gomella TL. 1994. Chest tube placement. 1994. In *Neonatology: Management, Procedures, On-Call Problems, Diseases and Drugs,* Gomella TL, Cunningham MD, and Eyal FG, eds. Stamford, Connecticut: Appleton & Lange, 144–146.

30. Marinelli PV, et al. 1981. Acquired eventration of the diaphragm: A complication of chest tube placement in neonatal pneumothorax. *Pediatrics* 67: 522–524.

31. Stahly TL, and Tench WD. 1977. Lung entrapment and infarction by chest tube suction. *Radiology* 122(2): 307–309.

32. Quak JM, et al. 1993. Cardiac tamponade in a preterm neonate secondary to a chest tube. *Acta Paediatrica* 82(5): 490–491.

33. Ary AH, et al. 1991. Neonatal paralysis caused by chest drains. *Archives of Disease in Childhood* 66(4): 441.

34. Gordon PA, Norton JM, and Merrell R. 1995. Refining chest tube management: Analysis of the state of practice. *Dimensions of Critical Care Nursing* 14(1): 6–12.

35. Thibeault DW. 1988. Pulmonary care of infants with endotracheal tubes. In *Neonatal Pulmonary Care,* 2nd ed., Thibeault D, and Gregory G, eds. Norwalk, Connecticut: Appleton & Lange, 393–399.

36. Benjamin B. 1993. Prolonged intubation injuries of the larynx: Endoscopic diagnosis, classification and treatment. *Annals of Otology, Rhinology and Laryngology* 160(supplement): 1–15.

37. McCulloch TM, and Bishop MR. 1991. Complications of translaryngeal intubation. *Clinics in Chest Medicine* 12(3): 507–522.

38. Gaynor EB, and Greenberg SB. 1985. Untoward sequelae of prolonged intubation. *Laryngoscope* 95(12): 1461–1467.

39. Donnelly WH. 1969. Histopathology of endotracheal intubation: An autopsy study. *Archives of Pathology* 88(5): 511–520.

40. Ratner I, and Whitfield J. 1983. Acquired subglottic stenosis in the very-low-birth-weight infant. *American Journal of Diseases of Children* 137(1): 40–43.

41. Couser RJ, and Ferrera B. 1992. Effectiveness of dexamethasone in preventing extubation failure in preterm infants at risk for airway edema. *Journal of Pediatrics* 121(4): 591–596.

42. Cotton RT, and Seid AB. 1980. Management of the extubation problem in the premature child: Anterior cricoid split as an alternative to tracheotomy. *Annals of Otology, Rhinology and Laryngology* 89(6 part 1): 508–511.

43. Richardson MA, and Inglis A. 1991. A comparison of anterior cricoid split with and without costal cartilage graft for acquired subglottic stenosis. *International Journal of Pediatric Otorhinolaryngology* 22(2): 187–195.

44. Myer CM. 1991. Current management of subglottic stenosis in infants and children. *Ear, Nose, and Throat Journal* 70(1): 6–11.

45. Seid AB, Pransky SM, and Kearns DB. 1991. One stage laryngotracheoplasty. *Archives of Otolaryngology—Head and Neck Surgery* 117(4): 408–410.

46. Bhutani VK, et al. 1986. Acquired tracheomegaly in very preterm neonates. *American Journal of Diseases of Children* 140(5): 449–452.

47. Sotomayor JL, and Godiney RI. 1986. Large-airway collapse due to acquired tracheobroncho malacia in infancy. *American Journal of Diseases of Children* 140(4): 367–371.

48. MacMahon HE, and Ruggieri J. 1969. Congenital segmental bronchomalacia. *American Journal of Diseases of Children* 118(6): 923–926.

49. Hanson JB, et al. 1988. Necrotizing tracheobronchitis: An ischemic lesion. *American Journal of Diseases of Children* 142(10): 1094–1098.

50. Carlo WA, and Chatburn RL. 1988. High frequency ventilation. In *Neonatal Respiratory Care*. Chicago: Year Book Medical Publishers, 383.

51. Miller R, et al. 1987. Tracheobronchial abnormalities in infant with bronchopulmonary dysplasia. *Journal of Pediatrics* 111(5): 779–782.

52. Pietsch JB, et al. 1985. Necrotizing tracheobronchitis: A new indication for emergency bronchoscopy in the neonate. *Journal of Pediatric Surgery* 20(4): 391–393.

53. Hwang WS, et al. 1988. The histopathology of upper airway in the neonate following mechanical ventilation. *Journal of Pathology* 156(3): 189–195.

54. Hodge D. 1991. Endotracheal suctioning and the infant: A nursing care protocol to decrease complications. *Neonatal Network* 9(5): 7–15.

55. Strang LB. 1977. Hemorrhagic lung edema and massive pulmonary hemorrhage. In *Neonatal Respiration,* Strang LB, ed. Oxford: Blackwell Scientific, 259.

56. van Houten J, et al. 1992. Pulmonary hemorrhage in premature infants after treatment with synthetic surfactant: An autopsy evaluation. *Journal of Pediatrics* 120(supplement 2 part 2): S40–44.

57. Bland RD. 1982. Edema formation in the newborn lung. *Clinics in Perinatology* 9(3): 593–611.

58. Raju TN, and Langenberg P. 1993. Pulmonary hemorrhage and exogenous surfactant therapy: A meta-analysis. *Journal of Pediatrics* 123(4): 603–610.

59. Pappin A, et al. 1994. Extensive intraalveolar pulmonary hemorrhage in infants dying after surfactant therapy. *Journal of Pediatrics* 124(4): 621–626.

60. Pramanik AK, et al. 1993 Surfactant replacement therapy for pulmonary diseases. *Pediatric Clinics of North America* 40(3): 913–936.

61. Long W, et al. 1992. Retrospective search for bleeding diathesis among premature newborn infants with pulmonary hemorrhage after synthetic surfactant treatment. *Journal of Pediatrics* 120(supplement 2 part 2): S45–48.

62. Malo J, Ali J, and Wood LD. 1984. How does positive end-expiratory pressure reduce intrapulmonary shunt in canine pulmonary edema? *Journal of Applied Physiology* 57(4): 1002–1010.

63. Spitzer AR, Shaffer TH, and Fox WW. 1992. Assisted ventilation: Physiologic implications and complications. In *Fetal and Neonatal Physiology,* Polin RA, and Fox WW, eds. Philadelphia: WB Saunders, 902, 910.

64. Heymann MA, and Rudolph AM. 1975. Control of ductus arteriosus. *Physiological Reviews* 55(1): 62–78.

65. Leffler CW, Hessler JR, and Green RS. 1984. The onset of breathing at birth stimulates pulmonary vascular prostacyclin synthesis. *Pediatric Research* 18(10): 938–942.

66. Needleman P, et al. 1981. Ductus arteriosus closure may result from suppression of prostacyclin synthetase by an intrinsic hydroperoxy fatty acid. *Prostaglandins* 22(4): 675–682.

67. Clyman RI. 1987. Ductus arteriosus: Current theories of prenatal and postnatal regulation. *Seminars in Perinatology* 11(1): 64–71.

68. Padbury JF, et al. 1981. Neonatal adaptation: Sympatho-adrenal response to umbilical cord cutting. *Pediatric Research* 15(12): 1483–1487.

69. Coceani F, et al. 1975. Lamb ductus arteriosus: Effect of prostaglandin synthesis inhibitors on the response to prostaglandin E$_2$. *Prostaglandins* 9(2): 299–308.

70. Kitterman JA, et al. 1972. Patent ductus arteriosus in premature infants. *New England Journal of Medicine* 287(10): 473–477.

71. Anthony CL, et al. 1979. *Pediatric Cardiology*. New York: Medical Examination, 226–242.

72. Douidar SM, Richardson J, and Snodgrass WR. 1988. Role of indomethacin in ductus closure: An update evaluation. *Developmental Pharmacology and Therapeutics* 11(4): 196–212.

73. Dudell GG, and Gersony M. 1984. Patent ductus arteriosus in neonates with severe respiratory disease. *Journal of Pediatrics* 104(6): 915–920.

74. Fujiwara T, et al. 1980. Artificial surfactant therapy in hyaline membrane disease. *Lancet* 1(8159): 55–57.

75. Heldt GP, et al. 1989. Closure of the ductus arteriosus and mechanics of breathing in preterm infants after surfactant replacement therapy. *Pediatric Research* 25(3): 305–310.

76. Kendig JW, and Sinkin R. 1988. The effect of surfactant replacement therapy on conditions associated with respiratory distress syndrome: Patent ductus arteriosus, intraventricular hemorrhage and bronchopulmonary dysplasia. *Seminars in Perinatology* 12(3): 255–258.

77. Clyman RI, et al. 1992. Increased shunt through the patent ductus arteriosus after surfactant replacement therapy. *Journal of Pediatrics* 100(1): 101–107.

78. Martin CG, Snider AR, and Katz SM. 1982. Abnormal cerebral blood flow patterns in preterm infants with a large patent ductus arteriosus. *Journal of Pediatrics* 101(4): 587–593.

79. Cotton RB, et al. 1981. Early prediction of symptomatic patent ductus arteriosus from perinatal risk factors. *Acta Paediatrica Scandinavica* 70(5): 723–727.

80. Clyman RI. 1991. Patent ductus arteriosus in diseases of the newborn. In *Diseases of the Newborn,* 6th ed., Taeusch HW, Ballard RA, and Avery ME, eds. Philadelphia: WB Saunders, 563–570.

81. Evans N, and Moorcraft J. 1992. Effect of patency of the ductus arteriosus in blood pressure on very preterm infants. *Archives of Disease in Childhood* 67(10 spec no): 1169–1173.

82. Ratner I, et al. 1985. Association of low systolic and diastolic blood pressure with significant patent ductus arteriosus in very low birthweight infants. *Critical Care Medicine* 13(6): 497–500.

83. Mellander M, et al. 1987. Prediction of symptomatic patent ductus arteriosus in preterm infants using Doppler and M-Mode echocardiography. *Acta Paediatrica Scandinavica* 76(4): 553–559.

84. Green TP, et al. 1983. Furosemide promotes patent ductus arteriosus in premature infants with RDS. *New England Journal of Medicine* 308(13): 743–748.

85. Cotton RB, et al. 1980. Effect of positive end-expiratory pressure on right ventricular output in lambs with hyaline membrane disease. *Acta Paediatrica Scandinavica* 69(5): 603–606.

86. Gersony WM, et al. 1983. Effects of indomethacin in premature infants with patent ductus arteriosus: Results of a national collaborative study. *Journal of Pediatrics* 102(6): 895–906.

87. Merritt TA, et al. 1981. Early closure of the patent ductus arteriosus in very low birth weight infants: A controlled trial. *Journal of Pediatrics* 99(2): 281–286.

88. Yanagi RM, et al. 1981. Indomethacin treatment for symptomatic patent ductus arteriosus: A double-blind control study. *Pediatrics* 67(5): 647–652.

89. Ment LR, et al. 1994. Low-dose indomethacin and prevention of intraventricular hemorrhage: A multicenter randomized trial. *Pediatrics* 93(4): 543–549.

90. Stefano J, et al. 1991. Closure of the ductus arteriosus with indomethacin in ventilated neonates with respiratory distress syndrome. *American Review of Respiratory Disease* 43(2): 236–239.

91. Noerr B. 1991. Indomethacin. *Neonatal Network* 10(4): 81–83.

92. Yeh T, et al. 1989. Indomethacin therapy in premature infants with patent ductus arteriosus—determination of therapeutic plasma levels. *Developmental Pharmacology and Therapeutics* 12(4): 169–178.

93. Seri I, et al. 1984. The use of dopamine for the prevention of renal side effects of indomethacin in premature infants with patent ductus arteriosus. *International Journal of Pediatric Nephrology* 5(3): 209–214.

94. Yeh TF, et al. 1982. Furosemide prevents the renal side effects of indomethacin therapy in premature infants with patent ductus arteriosus. *Journal of Pediatrics* 101(3): 433–437.

95. Mardoum R, et al. 1991. Controlled study of the effects of indomethacin on cerebral blood flow velocities in newborn infants. *Journal of Pediatrics* 118(1): 112–115.

96. Simko A, et al. 1994. Effects on cerebral blood flow velocities of slow and rapid infusions of indomethacin. *Journal of Perinatology* 14(1): 29–35.

97. Amato M, Huppi P, and Mackus D. 1993. Prevention of symptomatic patent ductus arteriosus with ethamsylate in babies treated with exogenous surfactant. *Journal of Perinatology* 8(1): 2–7.

98. Wilkinson JL, and Cooke RW. 1992. Cardiovascular disorders. In *Textbook of Neonatology,* Roberton NRC, ed. Edinburgh: Churchill Livingstone, 559–603.

99. Northway WH, Rosan RC, and Porter DY. 1967. Pulmonary disease following respirator therapy of hyaline membrane disease: Bronchopulmonary dysplasia. *New England Journal of Medicine* 276(7): 357–368.

100. Farrell PM, and Palta M. 1986. Bronchopulmonary dysplasia. In *Bronchopulmonary Dysplasia and Related Chronic Respiratory Disorders,* Farrell PM, and Taussig LM, eds. Columbus, Ohio: Ross Laboratories, 1–7.

101. Bancalari E, et al. 1979. Bronchopulmonary dysplasia: Clinical presentation. *Journal of Pediatrics* 95(5 part 2): 819–823.

102. Tooley WH. 1979. Epidemiology of bronchopulmonary dysplasia. *Journal of Pediatrics* 95(5 part 2): 851–858.

103. Shennan AT, et al. 1988. Abnormal pulmonary outcomes in premature infants: Prediction from oxygen requirement in the neonatal period. *Pediatrics* 82(4): 527–532.

104. Davis JM, and Rosenfeld W. 1994. Chronic lung disease. In *Neonatology: Pathophysiology and Management of the Newborn,* 4th ed., Avery GB, Fletcher MA, and MacDonald MG, eds. Philadelphia: JB Lippincott, 453–477.

105. Alpert B, Allen J, and Scheldow DV. 1993. Bronchopulmonary dysplasia. In *Pediatric Respiratory Disease,* Hilman BC, ed. Philadelphia: WB Saunders, 440–457.

106. Parker RA, Lindstrom DP, and Cotton RB. 1992. Improved survival accounts for most but not all of the increase in BPD. *Pediatrics* 90: 663–668.

107. Avery ME, et al. 1987. Is chronic lung disease in low birth weight infants preventable? A survey of eight centers. *Pediatrics* 79(1): 26–30.

108. Bryan CL, and Jenkinson SG. 1988. Oxygen toxicity. *Clinics in Chest Medicine* 9(1): 141–152.

109. Saugstad OD. 1985. Oxygen radicals and pulmonary damage. *Pediatric Pulmonology* 1(3): 167–175.

110. Jackson RM. 1985. Pulmonary oxygen toxicity. *Chest* 88(6): 900–905.

111. Hudak BB, and Egan EA. 1992. Impact of lung surfactant therapy on chronic lung disease in premature infants. *Clinics in Perinatology* 19(3): 591–602.

112. Wang EE, et al. 1993. *Ureaplasma urealyticum* and chronic lung disease of prematurity: Critical appraisal of the literature on causation. *Clinical Infectious Diseases* 17(supplement 1): S112–116.

113. Payne NR, et al. 1993. New prospective studies of the association of *ureaplasma urealyticum* colonization and chronic lung disease. *Clinical Infectious Diseases* 17(supplement 1): S117–121.

114. Sawyer MH, Edwards DK, and Spector SA. 1987. Cytomegalovirus infection and bronchopulmonary dysplasia in premature infants. *American Journal of Diseases of Children* 141(3): 303–305.

115. O'Brodovich HM, and Mellins RB. 1985. Bronchopulmonary dysplasia: Unresolved neonatal acute lung injury. *American Review of Respiratory Disease* 132(3): 694–709.

116. Frank L, and Sosenko IR. 1988. Undernutrition as a major contributing factor in the pathogenesis of bronchopulmonary dysplasia. *American Review of Respiratory Disease* 138(3): 725–729.

117. Bell EF. 1986. Prevention of bronchopulmonary dysplasia: Vitamin E and other antioxidants. In *Bronchopulmonary Dysplasia and Related Chronic Respiratory Disorders,* Farrell PM, and Taussig LM, eds. Columbus, Ohio: Ross Laboratories, 77–81.

118. Lawson EE, and Stiles AD. 1987. Vitamin A therapy for prevention of chronic lung disease in infants. *Journal of Pediatrics* 111(2): 247–248.

119. Shenai JP, et al. 1987. Clinical trial of vitamin A supplementation in infants susceptible to bronchopulmonary dysplasia. *Journal of Pediatrics* 111(2): 269–277.

120. Edelman NH, Rucker RB, and Peavy HH. 1986. NIH workshop summary: Nutrition and the respiratory system. *American Review of Respiratory Disease* 134(2): 347–352.

121. Abman SH, and Groothius JS. 1994. Pathophysiology and treatment of bronchopulmonary dysplasia. *Pediatric Clinics of North America* 41(2): 277.

122. Northway WH. 1992. Bronchopulmonary dysplasia: Twenty-five years later. *Pediatrics* 89(5 part 1): 969.

123. Toce SS, et al. 1984. Clinical and radiographic scoring systems for assessing bronchopulmonary dysplasia. *American Journal of Diseases of Children* 138(6): 581.

124. Stocker JT. 1986. Pathologic features of long-standing "healed" BPD: A study of 28 3–40 month old infants. *Human Pathology* 17(9): 943–961.

125. Bonikos DS, and Bensch KG. 1988. Pathogenesis of bronchopulmonary dysplasia. In *Bronchopulmonary Dysplasia,* Merritt TA, Northway WH, and Boynton BR, eds. Boston: Blackwell Scientific Publications, 33–58.

126. Abman SH. 1988. Pulmonary hypertension in infants with bronchopulmonary dysplasia: Clinical aspects. In *Bronchopulmonary Dysplasia,* Bancalari E, and Stocker JT, eds. Washington, DC: Hemisphere Publishing, 221.

127. Bader D, et al. 1987. Childhood sequelae of infant lung disease: Exercise and pulmonary function abnormalities after BPD. *Journal of Pediatrics* 110(5): 693–699.

128. Rush MG, and Hazinski TA. 1992. Current therapy of bronchopulmonary dysplasia. *Clinics in Perinatology* 19(3): 563–590.

129. Abman SH, et al. 1985. Pulmonary vascular response to oxygen in infants with bronchopulmonary dysplasia. *Pediatrics* 75: 80.

130. Troug WE, and Jackson C. 1992. Alternative mode of ventilation in the prevention and treatment of BPD. *Clinics in Perinatology* 19(3): 621–647.

131. Spahr RC, et al. 1980. Hyaline membrane disease: A controlled study of inspiratory and expiratory ratio in its management of ventilator. *American Journal of Diseases of Children* 134(4): 373.

132. Goldman SL, et al. 1991. Inspiratory time and pulmonary function in mechanically ventilated babies with chronic lung disease. *Pediatric Pulmonology* 11(3): 198–201.

133. Hodson WA, et al. 1979. Bronchopulmonary dysplasia: The need for epidemiologic studies. *Journal of Pediatrics* 95(5 part 2): 848–852.

134. Carlo WA, et al. 1986. Efficiency of computer-assisted management of respiratory failure in neonates. *Pediatrics* 78(1): 139–143.

135. Keszler M, et al. 1991. Multicenter controlled trial comparing high-frequency jet ventilation and conventional mechanical ventilation in newborn infants with pulmonary interstitial emphysema. *Journal of Pediatrics* 119(1 part 1): 85–93.

136. Clark RH, et al. 1990. High-frequency oscillatory ventilation reduces the incidence of severe chronic lung disease in respiratory distress syndrome. *American Review of Respiratory Disease* 141(4): 686A.

137. Davidson S, et al. 1990. Energy intake, growth, and development in ventilated very-low-birth-weight infants with and without bronchopulmonary dysplasia. *American Journal of Diseases of Children* 144(5): 553–559.

138. Yu VYH, et al. 1983. Growth and development of very low birthweight infants recovering from bronchopulmonary dysplasia. *Archives of Disease in Childhood* 58(10): 791.

139. Robertson CMT, et al. 1992. Eight-year school performance, neurodevelopmental, and growth outcome of neonates with bronchopulmonary dysplasia: A comparative study. *Pediatrics* 89(3): 365–372.

140. Weinstein MR, and Oh W. 1981. Oxygen consumption in infants with bronchopulmonary dysplasia. *Journal of Pediatrics* 99(6): 958–961.

141. Van Marter LJ, et al. 1990. Hydration during the first days of life and the risk of bronchopulmonary dysplasia in low birthweight infants. *Journal of Pediatrics* 116(6): 942–949.

142. Tammela OK, and Koivisto ME. 1993. Fluid restriction for preventing BPD. *Acta Paediatrica* 81(3): 207–212.

143. Lund CL, and Collier SB. 1990. Nutrition and bronchopulmonary dysplasia. In *Bronchopulmonary Dysplasia: Strategies for Total Patient Care,* Lund CH, ed. Petaluma, California: Neonatal Network, 75.

144. Yunis KA, and Oh W. 1989. Effects of intravenous glucose loading on oxygen consumption, carbon dioxide production, and resting energy expenditure in infants with bronchopulmonary dysplasia. *Journal of Pediatrics* 115(1): 127–132.

145. Innis S. 1993. Fat. In *Nutritional Needs of the Preterm Infant: Scientific Basis and Practical Guidelines,* Tsang RC, et al., eds. Baltimore: Williams & Wilkins, 65–86.

146. Pereira GR, et al. 1980. Decreased oxygenation and hyperlipemia during intravenous fat infusions in premature infants. *Pediatrics* 66(1): 26.

147. Shenai JP, et al. 1990. Plasma retinol-binding protein response to vitamin A administration in infants susceptible to bronchopulmonary dysplasia. *Journal of Pediatrics* 116(4): 607–614.

148. Lawson EE, and Stiles AD. 1987. Vitamin A therapy for prevention of chronic lung disease in infants. *Journal of Pediatrics* 111(2): 247–248.

149. Gutcher GR, and Farrell PM. 1985. Early intravenous correction of vitamin E deficiency in premature infants. *Journal of Pediatric Gastroenterology and Nutrition* 4(4): 604–609.

150. Gross SJ, and Gabriel E. 1985. Vitamin E status in preterm infants fed human mild or infant formula. *Journal of Pediatrics* 106(4): 635.

151. Cox JH. 1994. Bronchopulmonary dysplasia. In *Nutritional Care for Risk Newborns,* Groh-Wargo M, Thompson M, and Cox J, eds. Chicago: Precept Press, 245–261.

152. Hallman M, et al. 1992. Inositol supplementation in premature infants with respiratory distress syndrome. *New England Journal of Medicine* 326(19): 1233.

153. Tammela OK. 1992. First-year infections after initial hospitalization in low birth weight infants with and without bronchopulmonary dysplasia. *Scandinavian Journal of Infectious Diseases* 24(4): 515–524.

154. Als H, et al. 1986. Individualized behavioral and environmental care for the very low birth weight preterm infant at high risk for bronchopulmonary dysplasia: newborn intensive care unit and developmental outcome. *Pediatrics* 78(6): 1123–1132.

155. Als H, et al. 1986. Individualized behavioral and environmental care for the very low birth weight preterm infant at high risk for bronchopulmonary dysplasia and intraventricular hemorrhage. Study II: NICU outcome. Abstract. Woodstock, Vermont: New England Perinatal Association.

156. Als H, et al. 1982. Manual for assessment of preterm infant behavior (APIB). In *Theory and Research in Behavioral Pediatrics,* vol. 1, Fitzgerald HE, Lester BM, and Yogman MW, eds. New York: Plenum, 65–132.

157. Bregman J, and Farrell EE. 1992. Neurodevelopmental outcome in infants with bronchopulmonary dysplasia. *Clinics in Perinatology* 19(3): 673–694.

158. Kitchen W, et al. 1987. Outcome in infants of birth weight 500 to 999 g: A continuing regional study of 5-year-old survivors. *Journal of Pediatrics* 111(5): 761–766.

159. Lund C, ed. 1990. *Bronchopulmonary Dysplasia: Strategies for Total Patient Care,* Petaluma, California: Neonatal Network.

160. Terry TL. 1942. Extreme prematurity and fibroblastic overgrowth of persistent vascular sheath behind each crystalline lens. *American Journal of Ophthalmology* 25(2): 203–204.

161. Patz A, et al. 1952. Studies on the effect of high oxygen administration in retrolental fibroplasia: Nursery observations. *American Journal of Ophthalmology* 35(9): 1248–1253.

162. Cross KW. 1973. Cost of preventing retrolental fibroplasia? *Lancet* 2(835): 954–956.

163. Reisner SH, et al. 1985. Retinopathy of prematurity: Incidence and treatment. *Archives of Disease in Childhood* 60(8): 698–701.

164. Hunter DG, and Mukai S. 1992. Retinopathy of prematurity: Pathogenesis, diagnosis, and treatment. *International Ophthalmology Clinics* 32(1): 163–184.

165. Flynn JT, et al. 1987. Retinopathy of prematurity: Diagnosis, severity and natural history. *Ophthalmology* 94(6): 620–629.

166. Phelps DL. 1981. Retinopathy of prematurity: An estimate of visual loss in the United States. *Pediatrics* 67(6): 924–925.

167. Cryotherapy for Retinopathy of Prematurity Cooperative Group. 1990. Multicenter trial of cryotherapy for retinopathy of prematurity: One-year outcome—structure and function. *Archives of Ophthalmology* 108(10): 1408–1416.

168. Cryotherapy for Retinopathy of Prematurity Cooperative Group. 1993. Multicenter trial of cryotherapy for retinopathy of prematurity: 3 1/2 year outcome—structure and function. *Archives of Ophthalmology* 111(3): 339–344.

169. Keith CG, and Doyle LW. 1995. Retinopathy of prematurity in extremely low birth weight infants. *Pediatrics* 95(1): 42–45.

170. Phelps DL. 1992. Retinopathy of prematurity: Current problems in pediatrics. *Pediatrics* 22(8): 349–370.

171. Committee for the Classification of retinopathy of prematurity. 1984. An international classification of retinopathy of prematurity. *Archives of Ophthalmology* 102(8): 1130–1134.

172. International Committee for the Classification of Retinopathy of Prematurity. 1987. An international classification of the late stages of retinopathy of prematurity. Part II: The classification of retinal detachment. *Archives of Ophthalmology* 105(7): 906–912.

173. Nissenkorn I, et al. 1987. Rush type retinopathy of prematurity: Report of three cases. *British Journal of Ophthalmology* 71(7): 559–562.

174. Cats BP, and Tan K. 1989. Prematures with and without regressed retinopathy of prematurity: Comparison of long term (6–10 years) ophthalmological morbidity. *Journal of Pediatric Ophthalmology and Strabismus* 26(6): 271–275.

175. Tasman W, and Brown CC. 1988. Progressive visual loss in adults with retinopathy of prematurity. *Trans American Ophthalmologic Society* 86(1): 367–375.

176. Lucey JF, and Dangman B. 1984. Reexamination of the role of oxygen in retrolental fibroplasia. *Pediatrics* 73(1): 82–96.

177. Darlow BA, Horwood LJ, and Clemett RS. 1992. Retinopathy of prematurity: Risk factors in a prospective population-based study. *Paediatric and Perinatal Epidemiology* 6(1): 62–80.

178. Hunsucker K, et al. 1995. Laser surgery for retinopathy of prematurity. *Neonatal Network* 14(4): 21–26.

179. Ashton N, Ward B, and Serpelli G. 1954. Effect of oxygen on developing retinal vessels with particular reference to the problem of retrolental fibroplasia. *British Journal of Ophthalmology* 38(7): 397–432.

180. Kretzer FL, et al. 1983. Spindle cells as vasoformative elements in the developing human retina: Vitamin E modulation. In *Developing and Regenerating Vertebrate Nervous Systems,* Coates PW, Markwald RR, and Kenney AD, eds. New York: Alan R. Liss, 199–210.

181. Kretzer FL, and Hittner HM. 1988. Spindle cells and retinopathy of prematurity: Interpretations and predictions. *Birth Defects* 24(1): 147–168.

182. Kinsey VE, et al. 1977. PaO$_2$ levels and RLF: A report of the cooperative study. *Pediatrics* 60(5): 655–668.

183. Bancalari E, et al. 1987. Influence of transcutaneous monitoring on the incidence of ROP. *Pediatrics* 79(5): 663–669.

184. Flynn JT, et al. 1992. A cohort study of transcutaneous oxygen tension and the incidence and severity of ROP. *New England Journal of Medicine* 326(16): 1050–1054.

185. Szewczyk TS. 1953. Retrolental fibroplasia and related ocular diseases: Classification, etiology, and prophylaxis. *American Journal of Ophthalmology* 36(10): 1336–1361.

186. Finer NN, et al. 1982. Effect of intramuscular vitamin E on frequency and severity of retrolental fibroplasia: A controlled trial. *Lancet* 1(8281): 1087–1091.

187. Johnson L, et al. 1989. Effect of sustained pharmacologic vitamin E levels on incidence and severity of retinopathy of prematurity: A controlled clinical trial. *Journal of Pediatrics* 114(5): 827–838.

188. Milner RA, et al. 1981. Vitamin E supplement in under 1,500 gram neonates. Retinopathy of Prematurity Conference, Columbus, Ohio: Ross Laboratories, 703–716.

189. Ehrenkranz RA. 1989. Vitamin E and retinopathy of prematurity: Still controversial. *Journal of Pediatrics* 114(5): 801–803.

190. Johnson L, et al. 1985. Relationship of prolonged pharmacologic serum levels of vitamin E to incidence of sepsis and necrotizing enterocolitis in infants with birth weight 1,500 grams or less. *Pediatrics* 75(4): 619–638.

191. Phelps DL, et al. 1987. Tocopherol efficacy and safety for preventing retinopathy of prematurity: A randomized, controlled, double-masked trial. *Pediatrics* 79(4): 489–500.

192. Rosenbaum AL, et al. 1985. Retinal hemorrhage in retinopathy of prematurity associated with tocopherol treatment. *Ophthalmology* 92(8): 1012–1014.

193. Riley PA, and Slater TF. 1991. Retinopathy of prematurity (letter). *Lancet* 337(8739): 492–493.

194. Glass P, et al. 1985. Effect of bright light in the hospital nursery on the incidence of retinopathy of prematurity. *New England Journal of Medicine* 313(7): 401–404.

195. Hommura S, et al. 1988. Ophthalmologic care of very low birth weight infants: Clinical studies of the influence of light on the incidence of retinopathy of prematurity. *Nippon Ganka Gakkai Zasshi* 92(3): 456–460.

196. Ackerman B, Sherwonit E, and Williams J. 1989. Reduced incidental light exposure effect on the development of retinopathy of prematurity in low birth weight infants. *Pediatrics* 83(6): 958–962.

197. Deurksen K, et al. 1994. Fused eyelids in premature infants. *Ophthalmic Plastic and Reconstruction Surgery* 10(4): 234–240.

198. Fielder AR, et al. 1992. Light and ROP: Does retinal location offer a clue? *Pediatrics* 89(4): 648–653.

199. Lakatos L, et al. 1986. Controlled trial of D-penicillamine to prevent retinopathy of prematurity. *Acta Paediatrica Hungarica* 27(1): 47–56.

200. Ehrenkranz R. 1992. Steroids, chronic lung disease and retinopathy of prematurity. *Pediatrics* 90(4): 646–647.

201. Holmes JM, et al. 1994. Randomized clinical trial of surfactant prophylaxis in retinopathy of prematurity. *Journal of Pediatric Ophthalmology and Strabismus* 31(3): 189–191.

202. American Academy of Pediatrics and American College of Obstetricians and Gynecologists. 1992. *Guidelines for Perinatal Care,* 3rd ed. Elk Grove Village, Illinois: American Academy of Pediatrics, 201–203.

203. Palmer EA. 1993. Focal points: Clinical modules for ophthalmologists. *Current Management of ROP* 2(3): 1–8.

204. McNamara JA, et al. 1991. Laser photocoagulation for stage 3+ retinopathy of prematurity. *Ophthalmology* 98(5): 576–580.

205. Takayama S, Tachibana H, and Yamamoto M. 1991. Changes in the visual field after photocoagulation or cryotherapy in children with retinopathy of prematurity. *Journal of Pediatric Ophthalmology and Strabismus* 28(2): 96–100.

206. Topilow HW, and Ackerman AL. 1989. Cryotherapy for stage 3+ retinopathy of prematurity: Visual and anatomic results. *Ophthalmic Surgery* 20(12): 864–871.

NOTES

NOTES

7 Nursing Procedures

Barbara S. Turner, RN, DNSc, FAAN

Most infants are admitted to newborn intensive care units because of respiratory system immaturity or compromise. Caring for these critically ill infants requires refined observational and assessment skills, skilled nursing interventions, and a knowledge of the physiologic processes underlying the infant's admission to the unit.

This chapter reviews respiratory system assessment and discusses various nursing interventions used in treating infants with respiratory problems. Possible solutions to, and interventions for, common nursing problems are outlined. Both the nurse who is new to neonatal nursing and the more experienced nurse will find help with some of the most frequent and challenging aspects of caring for the newborn with respiratory compromise.

RESPIRATORY ASSESSMENT

Each infant admitted to the NICU receives a nursing assessment, including a physical examination. This examination is updated as needed during the current and following shifts and is an invaluable tool for assessing the impact of nursing interventions on the respiratory status of the infant. The initial physical assessment provides the baseline for gauging changes that occur over time and enables the nurse to relate those changes to the earlier status of the infant. Because this initial evaluation will be referred to frequently by the other caregivers, it must be documented immediately after a nurse assumes care of an infant.

A respiratory assessment begins with observation of the infant at rest. The respiratory rate is counted for a full minute, the chest is observed for symmetry of movement and retractions, and the nares are watched for signs of flaring. The nurse also listens to the infant for grunting, stridor, wheezing, or crying. The infant's color is assessed; signs of cyanosis must be evaluated as to their origin. Central cyanosis is evidenced by cyanotic gums and mucous membranes; peripheral cyanosis is usually confined to the hands and feet.

The chest is then auscultated along the anterior, posterior, and mid-axillary line. Sounds from each side of the chest are compared for equality of breath sounds and presence or absence of rales, rhonchi, and other abnormal sounds. Rales (fine crackles) are fine rustling noises that result from air passing fluid in the alveoli. Rhonchi (coarse crackles) are deeper, coarser, snoring sounds that result from air passing plugs of mucus or debris in the bronchi.

Problem: *How do I assess an infant who is breathing at a rate of 80 breaths per minute and has nasal flaring and audible grunting?*

This infant is exhibiting the classic signs of respiratory distress. Rapid respirations occur when the infant is unable to meet his oxygenation demands with a normal respiratory rate and thus must increase the respiratory rate in an effort to meet these needs. The normal respiratory rate for newborn infants is 40 to 60 breaths per minute.

Nasal flaring is the infant's attempt to bring additional air into the lungs. When the infant's nares flare with inspirations, the airway is enlarged. As a result, airway resistance is decreased, and the infant can improve ventilation.

Expiratory grunting occurs when the infant exhales against a partially closed glottis. This is the infant's attempt to maintain end-expiratory pressure in the lungs by increasing transpulmonary pressure. When the alveoli are partially expanded, as they normally are, further expansion consumes relatively little additional energy; when the alveoli are collapsed, it is more difficult to expand them with each breath. It is much the same as inflating a balloon: Initial expansion is difficult, but once the balloon has begun to inflate, it is easier to inflate the remainder.

By maintaining positive end-expiratory pressure (PEEP) in the lung, the infant overcomes the breath-to-breath problems of inflating the alveoli.

Problem: *What causes an infant's chest to appear depressed with each breath?*

This is a classic sign of respiratory distress in the premature infant. This phenomenon, known as retraction, occurs when the lungs are noncompliant (or stiff) and the chest wall is compliant. In adults, the lungs are compliant, and the chest wall is not as compliant; there-fore, with each inspiration, the lungs expand while the chest wall resists movement. In the premature infant, the stiff lungs resist movement while the compliant chest wall moves readily with the respiratory cycle, making the chest appear to be depressed with each breath.

Of all the signs of respiratory distress, chest retractions are the most disturbing for parents to witness. A careful explanation will ease some of their concerns.

INTUBATION

Intubation is the insertion of an endotracheal tube into the trachea for the purpose of supporting ventilation and oxygenation. Endotracheal tubes used for newborns are uncuffed straight tubes which have the same internal and external diameter throughout the length of the tube.[1] These tubes can have a single end-hole opening or side-hole opening(s). Some of the newer types of tubes include nonkinking tubes and tubes with side ports for monitoring or double lumen tubes for administering intratracheal medications.

Neonatal endotracheal tubes are uncuffed to prevent excessive pressure against the tracheal wall and to allow the largest endotracheal tube to be inserted. Cuffed tubes, because of the extension of the cuff, require relatively more room than uncuffed tubes. The advantage of cuffed endotracheal tubes is that inflation of the cuff limits tube movement.

Because neonatal endotracheal tubes are uncuffed, they move within the trachea. The respiratory cycle of the ventilator can account for up to 2 cm of tube movement; movement of the infant's head can result in 1 cm or more of tube movement.[2] Flexion of the infant's head moves the endotracheal tube toward the carina and beyond into a mainstem bronchus. Extension of the head moves the tip of the tube toward the glottis and away from the carina.[3] Nasotracheal tubes have been reported to result

Baby:	Jones, J
Weight:	2,200 gm
GA:	34 weeks
ET tube size:	3.5 mm
Inserted:	8 cm at the lips
Suction catheter size:	6½ Fr
Suction depth:	12 cm

in more intratracheal movement than orotracheal tubes.[4]

Keeping the infant's head in a neutral position maximizes the position of a correctly placed tube. An infant positioned on a radiant warmer or in an incubator with the head elevated deserves particular attention to ensure that his head does not become extended as gravity pulls his body toward the end of the bed. Recent literature has focused on the role of head position in the interruption of airflow and pulmonary mechanics in low birth weight infants.[5]

Nurses are responsible for assessing the integrity of the airway as well as determining when the endotracheal tube is incorrectly positioned. If the tube is positioned too low, it may be in one bronchus, resulting in single-lung ventilation, or it may impinge on the carina, resulting in granuloma formation.

A correctly placed endotracheal tube, as shown on x-ray examination, is positioned below the clavicles and above the carina. Because the term newborn's trachea is approximately 4 cm in length, the endotracheal tube should be positioned 1–2 cm below the vocal cords and approximately 2–3 cm above the carina.[6] Endotracheal tube placement can also be determined by sonography.[7] When the tip of the endotracheal tube is visualized 1 cm above the aortic arch, the tube is correctly positioned.

Once the tube is determined to be in the correct position, it is secured by tape or other methods. Insertion depth should be noted and posted on the infant's incubator or radiant warmer. For endotracheal tubes that have centimeter markings, the mark located at the infant's lips is the depth that is recorded. For those tubes that do not have depth markings, the lettering on the tube can be used as a marker. Figure 7-1 is an example of a bedside card used to document the depth of insertion.

Recording insertion depth helps nurses determine if the tube has moved from the correct position. Because excessive secretions may loosen tape or other securing mechanisms and movement of the infant's head and neck may move the endotracheal tube, assessing endotracheal tube position is an ongoing process.

The 1-2-3, 7-8-9 rule can generally be used for determining tube depth for orotracheal intubation: An infant weighing 1 kg would have the endotracheal tube placed at a depth of approximately 7 cm, a 2 kg infant would have the endotracheal tube inserted to 8 cm, and a 3 kg infant would have it inserted to 9 cm. For nasotracheal intubation, 1 cm is added to the 7-8-9 rule to compensate for the increased distance that nasotracheal intubation requires. This additional depth changes the 1-2-3, 7-8-9 rule to the 1-2-3, 8-9-10 rule.

Intubation is not a benign procedure and should be carried out with care. In the premature infant, intubation has been associated with cardiac rhythm changes, apnea, increased blood pressure, and decreased heart rate and transcutaneous oxygen tension.[8] Other complications of intubation are noted in Table 7-1. Thermal support, adequate ventilation, oxygenation, and physiologic monitoring, as well as necessary equipment and supplies, should be in place before intubation is begun.

The inadvertent or accidental displacement of an endotracheal tube out of the trachea is an emergency that occurs in an estimated 2 to 40 percent of all intubated neonates.[9] Nurses are responsible for assessing and maintaining correct endotracheal tube position.

Assessing the position of the endotracheal tube takes only a few minutes and is noninvasive; it is therefore imperative that this be done frequently enough to assure that effective ventilation is not impeded by an incorrectly positioned tube. The tip of the endotracheal tube should be situated approximately 1.5 cm below the glottis. Radiographically, this corresponds to the tip lying at T2–4.

Problem: *How can I determine whether the endotracheal tube is in the correct position?*

Four methods can be used to determine the relative position of the endotracheal tube:

1. **Auscultation of the chest.** Auscultation of the infant's chest will provide clues to the relative position of the endotracheal tube. The nurse should routinely auscultate the chest along the mid-axillary line, comparing the right and left breath sounds. Endotracheal tubes that are positioned too low may enter the right mainstem bronchus instead of the left because of the degree of angulation of each bronchus from the trachea.

   It was believed previously that, in the infant, the angulation of each bronchus from the trachea was 55 degrees and that with growth and development, it gradually assumed the adult angulation of 25 degrees

TABLE 7-1 ▲ Complications Associated with Intubation

Complication	Reason
Palatal grooves[98–100]	Pressure of tube on palate
Nasal erosion and stricture[101–103]	Pressure of nasal tube on nares
Defective dentition[104,105]	Pressure of tube on gums
Subglottic stenosis[106,107]	Irritation from tube
Esophageal perforation[108–110]	Insertion trauma
Aspiration[111]	No cuff on the tube
Bacterial colonization[2,112]	Presence of endotracheal tube
Tracheal granuloma[113]	Irritation from tip of endotracheal tube

for the right bronchus and 45 degrees for the left.[10] It is now known that the angulation of each bronchus from the trachea in newborns and infants is approximately equal to that of the adult.[11,12]

With a right mainstem bronchus intubation, there will be hyperinflation of the right lung and collapse of the left because only the right side of the chest will be ventilated. However, breath sounds may not always be decreased on the left because some breath sounds from the right may be referred to the left side of the chest.

An infant with a left-sided pneumothorax presents with many of the same clinical signs as one with a right mainstem bronchus intubation. The electrocardiogram (EKG) complex is often used to distinguish between the two conditions. With a pneumothorax, the R-S voltage may be decreased because the extrapulmonary air does not transmit electrical activity as well as fluid.

The treatment for a right mainstem bronchus intubation is to pull the endotracheal tube back until bilateral breath sounds are heard. The distance the tube is pulled back can be measured from a recent radiograph, if one is available. If the cause of the decreased breath sounds is a pneumothorax rather than a misplaced endotracheal tube, pulling the tube back may result in accidental extubation. So if a pneumothorax has not been ruled out and there is no radiographic confirmation of a misplaced endotracheal tube, the tube should *not* be pulled back.

2. **Observation of chest movement**. With accidental extubation or intubation of the right mainstem bronchus, chest movement may not be observable or may be unequal. In a right mainstem bronchus intubation, the inflated lung will cause the chest to rise higher on the right side than on the left.

3. **Auscultation of the chest and abdomen.** Breath sounds should be heard better in the chest than in the abdomen. Breath sounds clearly heard in the abdomen accompanied by distention of the abdomen may indicate that the endotracheal tube has slipped out of the trachea and into the esophagus. If this occurs, the endotracheal tube is removed, and the infant is reintubated. An oral gastric tube is placed for decompression.

4. **Observation of the endotracheal tube** for fogging or condensation upon exhalation. When the infant exhales, the endotracheal tube will fog or show evidence of condensation if it is placed in the trachea. Condensation upon exhalation will not be found in endotracheal tubes positioned in the oral pharynx or the esophagus.

If it is difficult to see the fogging in the endotracheal tube during ventilation and if the infant has some spontaneous respirations, the ventilator can be momentarily disconnected while the flat end of the laryngoscope is placed near the end of the endotracheal tube. Fogging of the laryngoscope should be evident.

Problem: *How can the endotracheal tube be secured in position?*

Endotracheal tubes can be secured using a variety of methods, including adhesive tape, "pink tape," suture and tape, locking mechanisms, Velcro, umbilical clamps, Logan's bow, and cloth ties. Descriptions of step-by-step

methods of securing endotracheal tubes in position can be found in the literature.[13,14] Securing the tube requires two persons: one to hold it in the correct position while simultaneously ventilating the infant, another to anchor the tube. For those methods of securing endotracheal tubes that require adhesive tape, "tagging" the end of the tape by folding it over on itself to create a "flag" or "tag" facilitates tape removal and repositioning of the endotracheal tube.

Problem: *What causes the movement of the endotracheal tube once it is in place?*

It is not uncommon to find that the endotracheal tube will be positioned too high on one radiograph and in perfect position on the next without any caregiver intervention. Every uncuffed endotracheal tube has a certain amount of "play" or tube movement. Flexion or extension of the head and neck, body position, and position and tension of the ventilator tubing may affect endotracheal tube position. For radiographic interpretation, it is most convenient if the infant is positioned on the x-ray plate with his head in a neutral position to help radiologists, neonatologists, and nurses assess tube position.

Another cause of endotracheal tube movement is what is loosely called the "sliding tube syndrome," in which the infant's oral secretions loosen the securing tape or devices used to hold the tube in place. This allows for increased tube movement with movement of the infant's head or the ventilator tubing. There may be sufficient tube movement to allow the infant to become extubated. In these instances, the tube must be resecured in the correct position, which requires either replacing or reinforcing the old securing tape or device.

Accidental extubation requires immediate recognition and intervention. Because any infant may become extubated at any time, each intubated infant should have at his bedside the equipment necessary to reintubate: laryngoscope, appropriate sized blade, endotracheal tubes in one size smaller and the current size, oxygen, and equipment needed to provide bag and mask ventilation.

Posting the correct endotracheal tube size and insertion depth prominently at the bedside facilitates reintubation. The bag and mask at the bedside should be tested at the beginning of each shift and set up to deliver the appropriate oxygen concentration and positive end-expiratory pressure. Oxygen blenders at the bedside and manometers connected to the manual resuscitation bag allow the nurse to ventilate the infant with appropriate levels of oxygen (FiO_2) and safe positive inspiratory and end-expiratory pressures.

Problem: *How can I determine if the infant is extubated?*

Indicators of possible extubation are:

- Audible crying
- Absent breath sounds
- Visible struggling or extreme agitation
- Absence of condensation in the endotracheal tube on exhalation
- Increased abdominal distention
- Cyanosis
- Bradycardia
- Hypoxemia

The most definitive sign is an audible cry. Intubated infants have silent cries; the endotracheal tube passes through the vocal cords, precluding their ability to make any sound.

FIGURE 7-2 ▲ Steps to assess the position of the artificial airway.

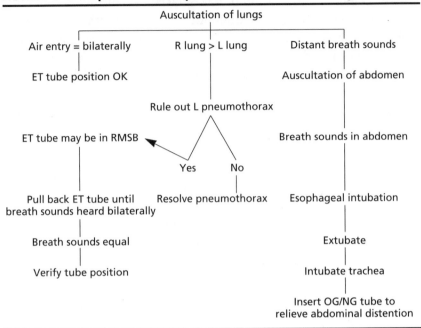

When an infant is correctly intubated, breath sounds can be heard equally well on both sides of the chest. Absent breath sounds may indicate extubation. Breath sounds will not be audible in an extubated infant who is hand or mechanically ventilated; however, breath sounds may be heard bilaterally when the infant initiates a breath because the air is not entering the lungs through the endotracheal tube.

Any infant who is visibly struggling or very agitated should be assessed for potential extubation or blocked endotracheal tube. The endotracheal tube may be blocked with secretions or kinked, or it may have slipped into the esophagus or oropharynx.

Failure to see condensation in the endotracheal tube on exhalation suggests extubation. Because exhaled air is fully saturated with water, there will be condensation in the endotracheal tube on exhalation. Placing the end of the laryngoscope handle near the endotracheal tube adapter will also result in fogging of the laryngoscope on exhalation; however, infants who are apneic or chemically restrained will not have the respiratory effort needed to fog the laryngoscope.

Infants who have increasing abdominal distention and who do not have a nasogastric or orogastric tube in place may be extubated. If the esophagus is intubated, the volume of air will be delivered to the stomach, resulting in abdominal distention. The presence of a nasogastric or an orogastric tube may mask the distention because it will allow excess air to escape from the stomach. The steps to assess the position of the endotracheal tube are summarized in Figure 7-2.

Problem: *What causes excessive water collection in the endotracheal tube adapter, and how can I prevent it?*

Ventilator tubing circuits have two sides: inspiratory and expiratory. Depending upon the type of tubing, the inspiratory and expiratory circuits may be of different colors. By consistently using one color for the inspiratory circuit, the health care team can determine at a glance which tubing is inspiratory and which is expiratory. This is helpful if there is a problem with excessive water accumulation at the site of the endotracheal tube adapter.

When the infant is positioned on his side, the inspiratory tubing should be on the top and the expiratory tubing on the bottom to prevent excessive water buildup in the adapter.

When the fully water-saturated and warmed gases are propelled toward the infant, they cool, and the water condenses in the tubing as it travels to the infant. This condensation travels by gravity toward the water traps in the ventilator circuit. Excessive "rain out" can also occur at the endotracheal tube adapter site.

When the inspiratory tube is in the superior position, the excess water drops down into the

FIGURE 7-3 ▲ Ventilator tubing with in-line thermometer at the proximal airway.

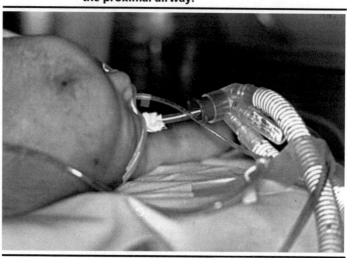

expiratory circuit and is removed. In contrast, when the inspiratory tube is in the inferior position, the excess water cannot get into the expiratory circuit and thus pools at the end of the inspiratory circuit. Excessive water collected at this point can then run down the endotracheal tube into the infant.

Heated ventilator circuits have been used to combat rain out. Inspired gas temperatures should be regulated and monitored at the proximal airway site with an in-line thermometer. Safe temperature ranges are 32° to 36°C. Temperature settings of 36°C require the use of a heated wire in the ventilator circuit to control rain out. An example of in-line temperature monitoring is shown in Figure 7-3.

All ventilators have in-line water traps to collect the excess water on both the inspiratory and expiratory circuits. These traps must be drained or emptied to remove any water they collect. Some traps must be removed from the ventilator in order to be drained; these have valves that allow ventilation to continue uninterrupted while the traps are removed.

There is a relationship between the temperature of ventilator humidifiers and the humidity of the inspired gases: As the temperature rises, the humidity of the gases increases. The ideal temperature is that which adequately humidifies the inspired gases. Too much humidity results in rain out in the ventilator tubing, increased airway resistance, and inadvertent tracheal lavage. Too little humidity inhibits mucociliary function, dries the tracheal epithelium, and is associated with plugged endotracheal tubes.

It has been suggested in the literature that lower inspired gas temperatures and humidity are associated with a higher incidence of pneumothoraces in infants weighing <1,500 gm.[15]

Recommended humidity for inspired gases is 30 mg H_2O/liter. At 36°C, the inspired gas humidity ranges from 167 to 43 mg H_2O/liter.[16] An interesting issue that needs further investigation is the impact of different ventilator temperatures on the tracheal epithelium. Loan found that inspired gas temperatures of 36°C and 37°C in an animal model were associated with more damage to the tracheal epithelium than temperatures of 32° to 35°C.[17]

NEW TECHNIQUES

Two new types of endotracheal tubes that help the health care professional ensure correct tube placement have been developed. Both involve noninvasive methods that can be carried out at the infant's bedside:

1. The indwelling fiberoptic light tube, when connected to a high-intensity light source, illuminates the tip of the endotracheal tube. The light is visible through the skin and thus allows the caretaker to assess tube position as often as necessary without disturbing the infant or subjecting him to excessive radiographs. When the light is visible at the suprasternal notch, the tube is correctly positioned below the larynx and above the carina (T2–T4).[18] Infant skin color does not appear to impede visualization of the light. However, this type of tube does not allow the

practitioner to differentiate an esophageal from a tracheal intubation.

The fiberoptic filament alters the outer to inner diameter ratio of the endotracheal tube. The inner diameter of a tube with the fiberoptic strand is 0.5 mm smaller than that of a conventional endotracheal tube. Although investigators state that no excess heat was transmitted to the infant's trachea, the temperature at the tip of the light was not reported.[18,19]

2. A metallic ring embedded in the endotracheal tube wall, which does not alter the tube's inner diameter, is the basis for the other new tube.[20,21] When a handheld monitoring device is placed at the infant's suprasternal notch, a green light and audible alarm indicate that the tube is in the correct position. The monitoring device does not discriminate between tracheal and esophageal intubation. This type of noninvasive endotracheal tube position monitor is useful during transport of the critically ill infant when more traditional methods of assessing tube position are not available or are difficult because of ambient noise or vibration.

Some practitioners have used a "light wand" inserted into the endotracheal tube as a method of assessing endotracheal tube position.[22,23] The usefulness of this technique in the neonatal population awaits the results of further research.

OXYGEN HOOD

Oxygen hoods or "head boxes" are designed to concentrate the gas mixture around the infant's head. The hoods are Plexiglas with openings for the head and neck; some are designed with side access doors and openings for intravenous lines and monitoring cables. Noise that results from the delivery of gas to the hood can be muffled by placing a foam baffle inside. A thermometer is used to monitor the ambient temperature of the air in the hood. Oxygen delivered via a hood may be all the oxygen support needed by infants who have mild transient tachypnea of the newborn, respiratory distress syndrome, or aspiration syndrome.

The hood size used is based on the size of the infant. A box that is too small may result in pressure areas around the infant's neck or shoulders; one that is too large may allow the infant's head to slip out of the oxygen-enriched environment. Hoods can be used for infants cared for on radiant warmer beds or in incubators. An infant in an incubator who requires >30 percent FiO_2 should have a hood in the incubator as opposed to having the gas mixture delivered to the incubator itself. This will concentrate the oxygen around his face and thus prevent wide fluctuations of FiO_2 when incubator doors or ports are opened.

The percentage of oxygen in the hood is continuously monitored while the infant is inside by an oxygen analyzer placed near the infant's nose. The inspired oxygen percentage is recorded hourly on the infant's flow sheet. Because of drifts in the calibration, the oxygen analyzer should be calibrated at least every eight hours to both high and low FiO_2. The calibration process requires removing the analyzer from the oxygen hood for a few minutes. The probe is placed in room air until the reading has stabilized.

If the analyzer does not read 21 percent, it is adjusted to bring the reading to 21 percent. The probe is then exposed to 100 percent oxygen by placing it in a glove along with a source of 100 percent oxygen. If the reading is not 100 percent, the calibrating mechanism is used to bring it to 100 percent. The probe is then re-exposed to room air, and a check is made to ensure that the reading is 21 percent. Linearity of the analyzer can be assessed by placing the probe in a glove containing 50 percent oxygen.

The oxygen/air mixture delivered to the hood should be both warmed and humidified. The temperature probe in the hood is checked with vital signs to ensure that the hood temperature is within the recommended range of 32° to 35°C.

To prevent carbon dioxide accumulation, the gas flow into the hood should be at least 5 to 7 liters/minute. When there is excessive condensation from the humidified air on the inside of the hood, it can be wiped with a soft cloth so that the infant's head is clearly visible.

NASAL CONTINUOUS POSITIVE AIRWAY PRESSURE

Nasal prongs are used to administer continuous positive airway pressure (CPAP) to neonates. Because infants are obligate nose breathers, the application of continuous distending pressure may help increase end-expiratory pressure. The prongs, made of molded soft plastic and available in sizes to fit the premature as well as the term newborn, fit inside the infant's nares and are attached to the ventilator. Selecting the correct size prongs is important: If too large, they create trauma to the nares from erosion and pressure; if too small, they may not be effective in providing sufficient oxygenation and ventilation to the infant.

The disadvantages of using nasal prongs include nasal trauma and the variability of end-expiratory pressure. End-expiratory pressure is lost whenever the infant opens his mouth. Taping the infant's mouth shut, even with a gastric tube in place, is not recommended because of the risk of aspiration.

As with the delivery of any gas to an infant, the air must be both warmed and humidified. Body temperature regulation is difficult in the small infant but becomes even more problematic if the inspired gases are not warmed. Unwarmed gases dry out the nasal membranes and create generalized chilling of the infant.

Problem: *How do I keep the prongs in position?*

The initial positioning of the nasal prongs is not difficult. They can be positioned in the nares using securing devices of Velcro or surgical masks with tie strings.

Maintaining the prongs in the correct position is more difficult. Nasal prongs irritate the nares and result in increased nasal secretions. Patience and creativity are required to maintain proper positioning of the nasal prongs. The goal should be to keep the infant in a quiet awake state, asleep, or at least calm and not struggling. Stroking, creating a quiet environment, and/or playing soft music often help quiet the infant and keep him from fighting the prongs. At times, nothing seems to help quiet the infant, and the nurse may spend much time repositioning the prongs.

Frames that will hold ventilator tubing in position are available. Use of these frames with soft linen rolls or intravenous bags positioned on either side of the head will help maintain the infant in position and limit head movement, thus helping to keep the prongs in position.

Care must be taken to change the infant's position frequently to prevent skin breakdown on the head. Use of sheepskin, a water mattress, or foam bedding will help preserve skin integrity. All linen under the infant needs to be free of wrinkles and folds because these can contribute to skin breakdown.

NONINVASIVE OXYGEN AND CARBON DIOXIDE MONITORING

The advent of noninvasive oxygen and carbon dioxide tension monitoring heralded a new frontier for nursing management of the infant with respiratory distress. Previously, nurses relied on intermittent arterial or capillary blood samples to determine the degree of hypoxia, hyperoxia, and hyper- and hypocarbia.

For years, nurses have recognized that the values from arterial blood gases were often not in concert with their assessment of the infant's oxygenation status. The infant who has had multiple arterial blood gases drawn often becomes hypoxemic when his arm is straightened to draw blood; thus, timing of the intermittent samples is important. Nurses who attempt to obtain blood when the child is quiet and appears normoxic find that touching him or making noises associated with gathering and arranging supplies for drawing a blood sample can be enough to upset the infant and change his oxygenation status.

Prior to the advent of noninvasive monitoring, decisions to change oxygen therapy and mechanical ventilation therapy were based on isolated blood gas values. Because noninvasive monitoring provides a continuous reflection of the oxygenation status of the infant, health care team members are able directly to observe the infant's responses to different aspects of therapy.

Even parents have become involved in the use of monitors. They may notice the positive response on the noninvasive monitor when they touch or speak to their infant. This helps reinforce their importance in his care. Conversely, parents may notice that touch causes the infant to become agitated and upset, thereby decreasing the oxygenation readings. For these parents, counseling by the nurse is of utmost importance to convey their vital role in their infant's care.

TRANSCUTANEOUS OXYGEN MONITORING

In the 1970s, transcutaneous oxygen monitoring appeared to be the "silver bullet" that solved the problems associated with basing ventilator changes on intermittent blood gas samples. We finally had continuous output of the infant's oxygenation status that resulted in a decrease in the number of blood gas samples drawn and a better understanding of the infant's physiologic response to interventions.

Transcutaneous oxygen monitoring is the measurement of skin oxygen tension rather than arterial oxygen tension. Given an accurate instrument with a specific temperature range under specified conditions, the correlation between skin oxygen tension and arterial oxygen tension is excellent.[24,25] Normally, skin oxygen tension ranges from 1 to 3 mmHg, and arterial oxygen tension ranges from 60 to 90 mmHg. Although skin oxygen tension may be elevated in the extremely premature infant, it does not equal arterial oxygen tension.[24]

For skin oxygen tension to approximate arterial oxygen tension, heat must be applied to the skin. Transcutaneous oxygen tension relies on the application of an external heat source to a small area of the skin. The heat produces a hyperemia or increased blood supply to the area. This alters skin oxygen tension and makes the skin more permeable to oxygen by altering the lipid layer under the skin and by shifting the oxygen dissociation curve to the right. When the oxygen dissociation curve is shifted to the right, oxygen is not bound as tightly to the hemoglobin molecule and is released more readily in the tissues.

These changes alter skin oxygen tension so that it correlates closely with arterial oxygen tension.[24–27] The correlation between skin and arterial oxygen tensions is best when the infant has normal perfusion to the monitoring site, normal body temperature, and normal blood pressure.

For best results, the monitor must be calibrated frequently, usually every four hours. With time, transcutaneous oxygen monitors are subject to drifts from their calibration points. Frequent calibration will help improve the correlation between transcutaneous and arterial oxygen tensions. Transcutaneous oxygen monitors have a limited range of accuracy: Hypoxia (<40 mmHg) and hyperoxia (>120 mmHg) may not be accurately reflected by the transcutaneous oxygen tension (TcPO$_2$) monitor.

As with any new technology, transcutaneous oxygen monitoring soon showed its "warts." The monitor was accurate and reliable only under certain circumstances, given that it had been calibrated and applied appropriately. Problems with probe positioning, pressure on the probe, thermal injuries, the 30- to 40-second delay in response time, and the drifts from calibration were all accepted as inconveniences that came with the monitor. The benefit clearly outweighed the problems for several years, but when pulse oximetry became available, most institutions readily changed over to it as the standard monitoring instrument.

A recent article questions the reliance on pulse oximetry and advocates the use of transcutaneous oxygen monitoring as an adjunct to pulse oximetry in monitoring very low birth weight infants. The rationale is this: Each monitor has both strengths and weaknesses; by using both monitors, we can compensate for the shortcomings of one with the other.[28] For those units that continue to use the transcutaneous oxygen monitor, the following are the most frequently asked questions.

Problem: *The reading of the TcPO$_2$ monitor is 159 after I reposition either the baby or the probe. What does this mean?*

Readings of 159 on the transcutaneous monitor may reflect the oxygen tension of the ambient room air rather than that of the infant (21 percent oxygen × 760 mmHg barometric pressure = 159 mmHg ambient oxygen tension). This reading occurs when air is trapped under the probe because it is not in proper contact with the skin. Removing the probe, reapplying the contact liquid and adhesive ring, and reapplying the probe are required. The reading may be substantially higher if the infant is in an oxygen-enriched environment such as 35 percent FiO$_2$ (35 percent FiO$_2$ × 760 mmHg barometric pressure = 266 mmHg).

Problem: *During a procedure, the infant is lying on the transcutaneous probe for a short time, and the readings do not appear to be accurate. Why does this occur?*

Placing the probe under the infant alters the blood supply to the probe site because the tissue between the probe and the infant is compressed, so the readings may be inaccurate. Repositioning either the infant or the probe will rectify the problem.

Problem: *When the probe is removed, I notice small reddened areas on the skin under it. How do I assess this?*

Because the transcutaneous monitor requires heat (44–45°C) to increase the blood supply to the skin site, these are local erythematous areas. They will fade, usually within 60 hours, and require no intervention other than not reusing the site until it has healed.[29] The severity of the burns depends on skin sensitivity, probe temperatures, and the length of time the probe is left in position. If there are blisters from the monitor, the probe position needs to be changed more frequently (every two hours) or the temperature of the probe reduced. Reducing the probe temperature, however, reduces the accuracy of the readings. Skin craters have been reported as a complication of transcutaneous monitoring.[30]

Problem: *When drawing arterial blood gas samples, when do I take the reading from the monitor?*

The $TcPO_2$ monitor generally has a 30- to 40-second delay in responding to changes in arterial oxygenation; therefore, the value on the monitor should be recorded approximately 20 seconds after the blood is drawn. Crying, agitation, and handling will cause the values to change.

Problem: *Why is it that the longer the monitor is on an infant, the less accurate the reading becomes?*

Transcutaneous monitors, like many instruments, are subject to "drifts" from their calibration. With transcutaneous monitors, the drift will increase with time since calibration. To correct and/or control the drift, calibrate the monitors every three to four hours while in use. Calibration requires that the probe be removed from the infant for approximately five to ten minutes, depending on the type of monitor used.

Once the monitor has been calibrated and the probe position changed, approximately 15–20 minutes are required for "warm up." The warm-up period allows the probe and the skin to be heated to the correct temperature so that the alteration in skin oxygen tension can begin. During the calibration and warm-up time, the monitor will not accurately reflect the partial pressure of oxygen in arterial blood (PaO_2).

Problem: *What if the $TcPO_2$ does not accurately reflect the PaO_2 of the infant?*

As part of the troubleshooting process, the membrane is routinely checked for air bubbles, wrinkles, and collected debris, which can contribute to inaccurate readings. Readings that do not reflect PaO_2 accurately, despite troubleshooting the equipment and probe, can still be used to follow trends in oxygenation.

If an infant has significant shunting through the ductus, close attention must be given to the site of the transcutaneous monitor and the source of the arterial blood sample. Preductal blood is sampled from the right arm and postductal blood from the lower body. The left arm may contain mixed preductal and postductal blood. Therefore, if the $TcPO_2$ probe is on the right chest wall (preductal) and the blood is drawn from the umbilical artery catheter (postductal), there will be poor correlation between $TcPO_2$ and PaO_2 during significant shunting.[31]

In cases of right-to-left shunting, both the $TcPO_2$ probe and the arterial blood should be

FIGURE 7-4 ▲ Pulse oximeter probe on an infant's foot.

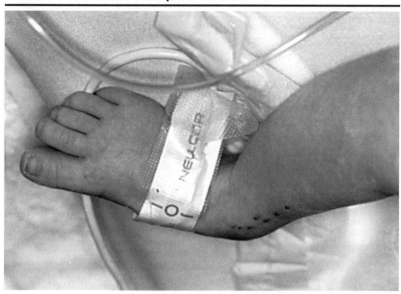

sampled preductally because the goal is to prevent hypoxia to the lungs, brain, and eyes.[25] Transcutaneous readings are recorded at least every hour and each time an arterial blood sample is drawn for gas analysis.

PULSE OXIMETRY

Pulse oximetry is a method of continuously and noninvasively monitoring the oxygen saturation of the hemoglobin molecule. Unlike $TcPO_2$, which measures skin oxygen through the use of a heated probe, oximetry measures oxygen saturation using spectrophotometric principles. Oxygen saturation is measured by placing a probe emitting red spectrum light on one side of a pulsating vessel and a receptor on the opposite side of the vessel. Figure 7-4 illustrates a pulse oximeter probe on an infant's foot.

The oxygen saturation monitor consists of a monitor, a patient probe, and a cable connecting the two. The monitor produces two different wavelengths of red and infrared light, which are transmitted to the patient probe, which contains a photodetector. The light and the photodetector are placed opposite each other in such a position that a pulsating arterial bed is between them.[32] Light absorption is measured as the light passes through the tissue. The response time is near instantaneous. The equipment requires no calibration or warm-up time prior to use.

Pulse oximetry requires adequate perfusion of the tissues and near-normal body temperature. The light must be able to detect arterial pulsations in order to differentiate arterial from venous and capillary blood. Advantages of the oxygen saturation monitor include instantaneous detection of changes in oxygen saturation, no required calibration, and digitally displayed output within seconds of probe application.

There are no reported complications associated with the use of the pulse oximeter. The adhesive on the skin probe has the potential to cause some interruption of the infant's skin integrity, but neonatal probes held in place with gentle pressure using an elastic band will circumvent this problem.

Because the probe is not heated and the light source does not produce burns, there is no thermal injury to the infant. Oxygen saturation monitoring is indicated for use in the extremely small immature infant who may experience serious thermal injury with the $TcPO_2$ monitor. Infants with bronchopulmonary dysplasia (BPD) have been reported as having increased and unpredictable gradients between arterial and transcutaneous oxygen tension. Pulse oximetry has been shown to be a reliable method of measuring oxygen saturation in these infants who have greater than 50 percent adult hemoglobin.[33–36]

TABLE 7-2 ▲ Comparison of Transcutaneous Oxygen Tension and Pulse Oximetry Monitors

Factor	Transcutaneous Oxygen Tension Monitor	Pulse Oximetry Monitor
Calibration	8–10 minutes every 4 hours	None (Some pulse oximeters have a pocket tester to test the calibration of the internal mechanics.)
Warm-up time	Approximately 15 minutes after probe application for the skin to reach 43–44°C and capillary bed to "arterialize"	None (displays oxygen saturation level instantly once a pulse is located)
Lag time (time from the change in oxygenation status to its reflection on the monitor)	30–40 seconds	None (instantaneous)
Complications	Thermal injuries resulting in first- and second-degree burns due to heat generated from probe	Compromised skin integrity under the probe (may go unnoticed because the probe does not need repositioning at set intervals)
Artifact (factors causing inaccurate readings)	Membrane wrinkles, air between the membrane and skin, pressure on the probe	Movement of extremity with probe, inflated blood pressure cuff proximal to probe, light with red spectrum reaching an unshielded probe

Problem: *Can ambient light interfere with pulse oximetry readings?*

Ambient light containing the red spectrum may interfere with accurate readings from the oxygen saturation monitor. Light from heat lamps and phototherapy lights has been reported to skew readings.[37] The high intensity of light emitted from these sources masks the small changes in light transmission from the probe. The remedy is to shield the probe from the ambient light. Current probes on the market, designed for use in the newborn population, contain a light shield.

Problem: *How can I determine monitor accuracy?*

Most pulse oximeters have a visual representation of the pulse intensity as well as a digital display of the pulse. The pulse display should be within three beats per minute of the display on the cardiac monitor.[38] Differences greater than this will not reflect accurate oxygen saturation values because the probe is not detecting the arterial pulsations accurately. Some

newer monitors have integrated the EKG complex with the oxygen saturation probe.

Problem: *What if the readings from the pulse oximeter are inaccurate or do not register?*

This can be caused by an incorrectly positioned probe resulting in a lack of opposition between the light source and sensor or a probe that is partially occluded with debris from the skin or adhesive. These problems can be easily corrected by replacing, repositioning, or cleaning the probe.

Placing the probe distal to a blood pressure cuff will result in an inaccurate or absent reading when the blood pressure cuff is inflated because the blood supply to the probe site has been interrupted.

The monitors are sensitive to motion and will display inaccurate readings when the extremity with the probe is moving. One group of investigators has reported that monitors were unreliable from 11.9 to 29 percent of the time because of movement artifact.[37] Soft restraints for the very active infant will preclude this. In infants with severe hypotension, the monitor may not be able to detect and display the heart rate and saturation because of difficulty in detecting a pulsating arterial bed.

Problem: *Which infants can be monitored using the oxygen saturation monitor?*

The oxygen saturation monitor is reliable, practical, and accurate for use in detecting hypoxemia in infants with a wide range of birth

TABLE 7-3 ▲ Nursing Care Responsibilities for Infants with Transcutaneous and Oxygen Saturation Monitors

Transcutaneous Oxygen and Carbon Dioxide Monitors

Calibrate the monitor prior to use and every 4 hours thereafter.

Change the position of the probe at least every 4 hours, more often if the infant has blistering of the skin.

Document the monitor readings at least every hour and with each blood sample taken for gas analysis. Document the current FiO_2 reading.

Note the infant's response to nursing procedures by monitoring $TcPO_2$ and $TcPCO_2$ readings. Alter the nursing care plan accordingly.

Position the probe on a flat, well-perfused area of the infant.

Document on the infant's flow sheet when the probe position is changed.

Set monitor alarms in accordance with unit policy.

Pulse Oximetry Monitors

Calibrate the monitor, if applicable, for the model and brand.

Select the appropriate sized probe, and locate a position for monitoring.

Place the probe so that the light source and the photodetector are opposite each other.

Set monitor alarms in accordance with unit policy.

Document monitor readings and FiO_2 every hour and with each blood sample drawn for gas analysis.

Change probe site as necessary to avoid skin breakdown.

---

weights, postnatal ages, and heart rates.[24,33–42] There is one report in the literature of an infant with yellow-stained skin from heavy meconium in whom pulse oximetry produced false low readings because the meconium staining absorbed more red, thereby filtering the infrared light.[43]

Another report in the literature suggests that, for infants with severe arterial desaturation (65 percent), pulse oximetry overestimates oxygen saturation; this author recommends reliance on arterial sampling for the severely compromised infant.[41]

Problem: *Are there any complications from using the oxygen saturation monitor?*

In the newborn population, there are no known complications from oxygen saturation monitoring when the neonatal probes are used as indicated.

Problem: *What are the comparative advantages and disadvantages of the transcutaneous oxygen monitor and the oxygen saturation monitor?*

A comparison of the two monitoring systems is outlined in Table 7-2.

Problem: *How do the nursing responsibilities compare for infants with transcutaneous as opposed to oxygen saturation monitors?*

The nursing care responsibilities for the two types of monitors are compared in Table 7-3.

Problem: *Because there is no calibration for the monitor, how do I know it is accurate?*

Current pulse oximetry monitors do not require external calibration. One model has a handheld calibrating device that emits a known wavelength of light at a set pulsation. Connecting this to the monitor will result in a given saturation and pulse reading. Should this not match the numbers on the calibrating device, it is an indication that the monitor is not calibrated internally and needs to be returned to the manufacturer.

Problem: *What are the normal values for pulse oximetry?*

In general, pulse oximetry values should be maintained between 87 and 93 percent for neonates.[42] In premature infants with respiratory disease, pulse oximetry values up to 95 percent may be accepted. An oxygen saturation of 90 to 95 percent corresponds to an oxygen tension of 50 to 100 mmHg at sea level. Because of the shape of the oxygen dissociation curve, oxygen saturation values in the 98 to 100 percent range may reflect PaO_2s that range from 100 to 400 mmHg. Therefore, in order to keep PaO_2 <100 mmHg, a pulse oximeter reading in the low 90s should be sought.

TRANSCUTANEOUS CARBON DIOXIDE MONITORING

Transcutaneous carbon dioxide pressure ($TcPCO_2$) monitoring may be carried out either separately from or in conjunction with transcutaneous oxygen monitoring. There may be two probes and one monitor, two probes and two monitors, or a single probe and monitor. Although $TcPCO_2$ monitoring depends less on arterialization of the capillary bed, better correlation is obtained using a heated probe.[24,44-50]

As with pulse oximetry and transcutaneous oxygen monitoring, $TcPCO_2$ is an alternative to frequent arterial sampling of the neonate. As with $TcPO_2$ monitoring, $TcPCO_2$ monitoring requires calibration of the probe and monitor at selected intervals, usually every four hours. The calibration process requires 5–10 percent carbon dioxide gases, which corresponds to 20–60 mmHg partial pressure of carbon dioxide in arterial blood ($PaCO_2$). Positioning of the probe is similar to that of the $TcPO_2$ probe.[25]

New probes that extend the calibration time are under investigation. Reports have indicated that an iridium oxide sensor can both reduce the temperature required for monitoring and increase the duration of monitoring one site without changing probe location or compromising monitor accuracy.[51]

In general, $TcPCO_2$ overestimates arterial carbon dioxide because it measures skin carbon dioxide tension. This may or may not be electronically corrected by the monitor; therefore, it is important to refer to manufacturer's instructions to determine which type of monitor is in use.[45]

The $TcPCO_2$ monitor is useful in infants with BPD, apnea, those requiring mechanical ventilation, and infants with problems related to hypercapnia. Problems reported with using this monitor during surgery include the need for recalibration, the long calibration time, and limited sites for placement that will not interfere with the operative site.

END-TIDAL CARBON DIOXIDE MONITORING

End-tidal carbon dioxide ($PetCO_2$) monitoring is, as the name implies, the measurement of carbon dioxide tension through gas analysis during respiration. The basis of monitoring carbon dioxide during respiration is the understanding of carbon dioxide as a product of cellular respiration, the transport of carbon dioxide via the circulatory system to the lungs, and the exhalation of carbon dioxide from the lungs during ventilation. The carbon dioxide content of gases during ventilation varies from minimal during inspiration to maximal at the end of exhalation.

Initially, this monitor was used in the adult population. Transferring the technology to neonates was problematic because of the fast respiratory rate and small tidal volume (6 ml/kg) of the prematurely born infant. Nonetheless, $PetCO_2$ monitoring is now available for use in the neonatal population.

In the infant with a significant ventilation-to-perfusion mismatch, at least one scenario can be presented in which the $PetCO_2$ will not correlate with arterial carbon dioxide and yet each measurement is valid. In this instance, the alveoli may be well ventilated but poorly perfused, resulting in little or no exchange of gases across the alveolar membrane. Thus, the $PetCO_2$ would show that there are low carbon dioxide levels in the expired gas because it would be reflecting the inspiratory gas remaining in the alveoli, but arterial blood analysis would demonstrate elevated carbon dioxide levels because the gases were not eliminated.

In a second scenario, the alveoli may be well perfused, but no gases are reaching the alveoli because of obstruction or atelectasis. Although one would postulate that this would result in a large discrepancy between $PaCO_2$ and $PetCO_2$, in reality, there is correlation between the two measurements.

PetCO$_2$ is the most accurate measure of PaCO$_2$ when infants have normal lung function and a normal ventilation-to-perfusion ratio. The correlation has been reported as $r = .79$ in infants with moderate lung disease, dropping to $r = .39$ in those with severe lung disease characterized by a large alveolar-arterial (A-a) gradient.[46]

End-tidal carbon dioxide can be monitored using sidestream or mainstream analysis:

1. Sidestream analysis is accomplished by using a narrow lumen tube to sample gas at the distal end of the endotracheal tube. The advantages are obvious: no increased dead space in the ventilator circuit and less chance of inspiratory gases contaminating the sample. The disadvantages are the potential for the narrow lumen tube to become occluded by pulmonary secretions and the relatively slow response time when compared to mainstream sampling.

2. Mainstream analysis is accomplished by sampling the expired gases from the ventilator circuit. This requires a separate chamber on the circuit, adding dead space and weight to the ventilator circuit.

A comparison of distal PetCO$_2$ with proximal PetCO$_2$ measurements showed that (1) distal values were higher than proximal values and (2) distal PetCO$_2$ values correlated more closely with PaCO$_2$ values. The variation was postulated to be due to the mixing of end-tidal and fresh gases.

In the infant with a large A-a gradient, PetCO$_2$ monitoring cannot be relied upon for accuracy.[46,48] It may be useful in premature infants with mild to moderate lung disease and is reliable in infants with normal lung function. Transcutaneous carbon dioxide tension monitoring is of more value than PetCO$_2$ in the infant with severe lung disease.

An interesting area for nursing is use of the end-tidal carbon dioxide waveform for clinical interpretation. The capnographic waveform

FIGURE 7-5 ▲ Waveform of capnogram.

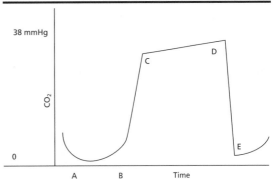

A - End of inspiration
B - Beginning of exhalation
C - End of mixed gases washout (dead space and alveolar gases)
D - End of expiration of alveolar gases
E - Inspiration

typically has a sharp, rapid rise on expiration, reflecting the mixture of dead space and alveolar gases, followed by a plateau that reflects the cessation of dead space gases and the measurement of alveolar gas (Figure 7-5).[49,50] At the end of the plateau phase is a sharp drop that reflects inspiration with fresh gases that have minimal carbon dioxide content.

Changes in the capnogram can be used in clinical decision making. If you understand and recognize a normal capnogram, then you can interpret variations in the slope of the rise or drop of the waveform or the height of the plateau.

The sharp rise characteristic of the capnogram will be altered by any factor that compromises exhalation. Partially plugged or displaced endotracheal tubes will alter the angle of the rise. Severe hypotension or decreased cardiac output will alter the height of the plateau. Leaks around the endotracheal tube will alter the slope of the drop of the capnogram because of entrainment of tracheal carbon dioxide gases.

ENDOTRACHEAL SUCTIONING

Endotracheal suctioning is a nursing procedure that removes accumulated secretions and

TABLE 7-4 ▲ Components of Endotracheal Suctioning

Component	Recommendation
Oxygen	Increase 10–15 percent over baseline
Pressure	Baseline
Rate	Additional breaths prior to and following suctioning
Irrigant	Normal saline, 0.25–0.5 ml
Catheter size	6 French for ET size 3.0 or less 8 French for ET size 3.5 and 4.0
Negative pressure	75–80 mmHg
Suction duration	5 seconds applied intermittently only during withdrawal of catheter
Suction depth	Length of endotracheal tube or length of endotracheal tube plus 1 cm

debris from the tracheobronchial tree of intubated infants through mechanical aspiration. Because the presence of an endotracheal tube does not allow the glottis to close, the infant is unable to cough. This, in conjunction with the inhibition of ciliary activity that results from the tube in the trachea, inhibits the infant's ability to remove secretions from the pharynx.

In the newborn infant, endotracheal tube suctioning is not without complications, such as hypoxia, bradycardia, atelectasis, tissue trauma, bacteremia, perforation, pneumothorax, and increased intracranial pressure.[52–64] Endotracheal suctioning consists of inserting a sterile catheter into the trachea and applying negative pressure while withdrawing it through the endotracheal tube. In an effort to ameliorate or lessen the complications associated with the procedure, additional components have been added, including increasing FiO_2 prior to, during, and following suctioning, which may help decrease the degree of suction-induced hypoxemia; hyperventilating; maintaining a set ratio between catheter and endotracheal tube; and regulating the negative pressures used (Table 7-4).[52,65–67]

The amount of supplemental oxygen depends on the infant's response to endotracheal suctioning. A reasonable estimate of the supplemental oxygen required is 10 to 15 percent above baseline followed by careful monitoring

of $TcPO_2$ and/or pulse oximetry during the procedure. If the infant has minimal drops in oxygenation during the procedure, then use of that amount of supplemental oxygen is appropriate. Larger drops indicate poorer tolerance of the procedure and the need for additional supplemental oxygen.

Normal saline solution (0.25–0.5 ml) may be used as an irrigant during endotracheal suctioning. Routine use of saline irrigation has been debated because it is recognized that bolus normal saline will not in and of itself liquefy secretions.[65,68] The saline will lubricate the tube and perhaps enhance the ability of the plastic catheter to slide against the plastic endotracheal tube. This practice has not been thoroughly investigated, and its efficacy has not been established. It has been practiced as a matter of tradition. Further research is warranted to verify the necessity of this procedure. The optimal temperature of the saline has not been researched; most units use room temperature normal saline, but some heat the saline to body temperature.

If normal saline is used, the volume should be premeasured to assure delivery of the desired amount, and care should be taken to prevent contaminating the solution.[68] Normal saline is administered through the endotracheal tube, and the infant is ventilated two or three times to disperse the saline. The infant is then removed from the ventilator and bagged with a manual resuscitation bag or left on the ventilator and given additional breaths using the manual inspiration mode.

The suction catheter is premeasured according to the length of the endotracheal tube. The catheter is advanced only the length of the endotracheal tube or the length plus 1 cm.[65] This practice decreases the risk of tissue trauma yet still removes secretions pooled at the end of the tube.

The suction catheter is inserted through the endotracheal tube, and a negative pressure of 75–80 mmHg is applied as the catheter is withdrawn.[66] The infant is placed back on the manual resuscitation bag or the ventilator and given 20–30 seconds of additional ventilation or sufficient ventilation to return the oxygen saturation/transcutaneous monitors to baseline.

Pass the catheter only once or twice unless the amount of secretions warrants additional passes. Do not rotate the infant's head. The routine practice of passing the suction catheter three times (once to remove the majority of secretions, once to remove the residual secretions, and once to ensure that all secretions have been removed) results in oxygen desaturation. The suction catheter should be inserted only to remove accumulated secretions.

Rotating the infant's head with suctioning was once commonplace and originated when deep endotracheal suctioning was practiced. In the past, the head was rotated to the right to enhance the nurse's ability to suction the left mainstem bronchus, and then the infant's head was turned to the left to facilitate right mainstem bronchus entry. With the passing of routine deep suctioning of infants, head rotation during suctioning should also have disappeared.

The amount and type of secretions recovered are recorded along with the infant's response to the procedure. After suctioning, the chest is assessed for changes in breath sounds. The secretions recovered from suctioning may vary from thin and watery to thick and viscous. The color may be clear, white, yellow, green, blood tinged, or bloody.

Problem: *While the suction catheter is being withdrawn from the endotracheal tube, should the finger port of the suction catheter be occluded the entire time, or should it be covered intermittently?*

In theory, if the finger port is occluded for the duration of the application of negative pressure, there would be more secretions removed because there is a longer period of time for negative pressure to capture and aspirate the secretions. However, continuous negative pressure may cause increased trauma because secretions or tracheal epithelial tissue caught by the negative pressure will be shorn off and removed.

In contrast, using intermittent negative pressure would, in theory, remove fewer secretions, remove less lung gas, and cause less trauma than continuous pressure because negative pressure is applied to the trachea for a shorter period of time. A concern that has been voiced about intermittent negative pressure is that secretions, once caught at the tip or at the eyehole openings of the suction catheter, should fall off and drop back down into the trachea when negative pressure is released. To date, no studies in the premature infant population have evaluated the efficacy of the two procedures.

Problem: *Is it better to use a manual resuscitation bag or the manual inspiration mode on the ventilator during suctioning?*

The purpose of ventilating the infant prior to, during, and following suctioning is to prevent some of the complications associated with endotracheal suctioning by providing the infant with additional oxygen and ventilation.

Both the manual resuscitation bag and the ventilator are used to ventilate the infant while suctioning. There are advantages and disadvantages to each, and the health care practitioner's decision will be based on personal preference as well as unit policy.

Using the manual resuscitation bag during suctioning requires both skill and experience. This method allows the caregiver to control the parameters of ventilation: FiO_2, positive inspiratory pressure (PIP), PEEP, inspiratory time, and rate. If this method is used, an in-line manometer is essential for monitoring the pressures used during ventilation. An extensive review of the existing manual resuscitation bags is available in the literature.[45]

Skill is required to match the controlled waveform of the ventilator breaths. In times of crisis, the caregiver may become anxious and transmit this to the patient by an increased rate and/or pressure. New NICU nurses are often most comfortable giving additional breaths through the ventilator. Experienced NICU nurses may prefer the bag because it gives them an opportunity to "feel" the compliance of the lung.

Using the ventilator to give additional breaths or to ventilate the infant during suctioning allows the caregiver to control the FiO_2 and the rate while the ventilator administers the pre-established PIP and PEEP. Using the ventilator thus prevents inadvertent increases in PIP or PEEP from reaching the infant. Even in inexperienced hands, the manual ventilator breaths given in this manner are nearly indistinguishable from controlled ventilator breaths.

Problem: *How long after I increase the oxygen on the ventilator do I wait to suction?*

Additional oxygen is given to the infant prior to suctioning to help reduce the suction-induced hypoxemia that can occur with endotracheal suctioning. Increasing the oxygen on the ventilator and immediately suctioning the infant does not allow sufficient time for the infant to benefit from the increased oxygen levels; therefore, suctioning should be delayed until the infant has a chance to benefit from the hyperoxygenation breaths.

The time needed is based on the "washout time" of the ventilator. This is the time it takes for the increase in oxygen to reach the end of the ventilator's inspiratory circuit. The time will be based on the ventilator; the type, length, and diameter of tubing; the flow rate; and the settings. Some ventilators will reflect the change in oxygen as quickly as 18 seconds; others will require a considerably longer time. The washout time can be measured using a second ventilator, by placing a calibrated oxygen analyzer at

the end of the ventilation tubing and measuring the time required for the analyzer to detect the increase in oxygen.

Problem: *When I suction the infant, I have to remove him from the ventilator, and the ventilatory cycle is lost. Can this be prevented?*

In some units, modified endotracheal tube adapters are used to help prevent the loss of both oxygenation and ventilation during suctioning. The modified adapters have side-port openings that allow the suction catheter to be inserted while the infant remains on the ventilator, so that only minor disruptions occur in the ventilatory cycle.[69,70]

Although this is advantageous, some nurses have observed that it is more difficult to suction the infant using the modified adapters because the opening is small, and maintaining sterile technique becomes difficult. It is imperative to close the side-port openings following suctioning so that the infant receives the full benefit of the ventilatory cycle.

Problem: *With the concern over infections and AIDS, what protection should I use when suctioning?*

Health care professionals must be cognizant of the potential danger of contamination from respiratory secretions as well as other body fluids. Current recommendations include wearing goggles and gloves on both hands while suctioning. There have been case reports of cross-transmission of infectious secretions from health care workers not using proper endotracheal suctioning techniques.[71,72]

New in-line catheters that are enclosed in plastic and remain attached to the endotracheal tube adapters are one answer to compliance with universal precautions. These catheters, which are changed once every 24 hours, protect the health care professional from the infant's respiratory secretions. The other advantage is that the catheter is inserted into the endotracheal tube without removing the infant from the ventilator, ameliorating some of the problems associated with loss of PIP, PEEP, and FiO_2 during endotracheal suctioning. Currently, the catheters are relatively expensive, and their use in the NICU, in my experience, has received mixed reviews by nurses.

CHEST PHYSIOTHERAPY

The 1979 Conference on the Scientific Basis of In-Hospital Respiratory Therapy sponsored by the National Heart, Lung, and Blood Institute defined chest physiotherapy as "consisting of physical maneuvers such as cough, forced expiration, chest wall percussion and vibration, and postural drainage to improve respiratory function and treat atelectasis and pneumonia."[73]

Cough and forced expiration are not used in newborns as part of chest physiotherapy because they are difficult to elicit. In this population, chest physiotherapy consists of external chest percussion and/or vibration and postural drainage followed by suctioning.

Chest percussion is generally believed to alter the pressure in the airways of the newborn, which helps dislodge mucus plugs. Externally administered chest percussion generally ranges from 4 to 5 Hz. In contrast, vibration is administered at up to 41 Hz and is believed to help propel mucus from the smaller bronchi to the larger airways.

It has been postulated that mucus is cleared by chest percussion or vibration by the following mechanisms: improving mucociliary interaction, simulating the ciliary beat frequency, stimulating active substances in the lung, or releasing chemical mediators in the airways.

Percussion, vibration, and positioning are used to move secretions from the periphery of the lungs to the bronchi and up toward the pharynx. Cilia movement is responsible for transporting the secretions from the lower trachea to the pharynx. In the intubated infant, the presence of an endotracheal tube inhibits ciliary activity in the area around the end of the endotracheal tube; thus, the secretions may pool at the distal end of the tube, where they are removed by suctioning.

There has been considerable interest in the role of chest physiotherapy in the neonatal population. The methods of chest physiotherapy may vary, but the procedure generally includes the gentle percussion and/or vibration of the chest and back in a variety of positions to loosen and drain secretions.[74–76]

Before chest physiotherapy is initiated, it should be determined that there is sufficient volume of secretions to be loosened and moved. Murphy termed this concept the "ketchup bottle effect: The bottle must contain some ketchup before it can be turned upside down, thumped on the back... and a splash... appears."[77]

Chest physiotherapy is used with newborns who have pneumonia, meconium aspiration, or other conditions resulting in atelectasis and hypercapnia. It is generally believed that there will be an improvement in pulmonary function after chest physiotherapy. Infants with respiratory distress syndrome have few secretions in the early phase of the disease process and probably would not derive benefit from chest percussion until they reach the later stages of the disease.

Percussion is given for three to five minutes over the right and left sides of the infant's chest and back. The atelectatic area of the lung is emphasized, and care must be taken not to percuss over the liver or spleen. Devices used for percussion include face masks, pediatric percussors, nipples, padded medicine cups, a bulb syringe cut in half with padded edges, and the nurse's fingers. The percussion device should deliver a column of air under pressure to the chest wall, ideally at 40 compressions per minute. Percussion is administered every two to eight hours, depending on the infant's condition and ability to tolerate the procedure.

TABLE 7-5 ▲ Postural Drainage[49,50,52]

Position	Lung Area
Sitting	Upper lobe
Supine	Anterior segment of upper lobe
Side, 30 degrees upright	Posterior segment of upper lobe
Flat, prone	Superior segment of upper lobe
Head down, supine	Anterior basal segment of lower lobe
Head down, side rotated forward	Lateral basal segment
Head down, prone	Posterior basal segment
Head down, left side	Right middle lobe

Vibration may be used in conjunction with or in place of percussion. A padded electric toothbrush or vibrator can be used. Most infants seem to tolerate vibration better than percussion. Throughout the administration of percussion and vibration, the infant should be monitored for signs of distress.

Postural drainage is used to move the loosened secretions to the larger airways so they can be transported toward the pharynx, where they are removed by suctioning. The infant is positioned so that the bronchus supplying the larger airways is in a dependent position during percussion. The head-down position may be difficult for many infants to tolerate because it increases the work of breathing.

In general, infants weighing <1,250 gm or with known or suspected intracranial bleeds should not be placed in the head-down position. Infants with abdominal surgery, abdominal wall defects, or umbilical artery catheters should not be placed in the prone position unless the hips and abdomen are supported so that pressure over the abdomen is avoided.[14]

The research on chest physiotherapy in neonates is confusing, primarily because of methodological issues and the nonstandardization of chest physiotherapy across protocols. For the infant with respiratory distress syndrome, physiotherapy within the first 24 hours of life appears not to enhance secretion removal or improve oxygenation and is associated with a higher incidence of intraventricular hemor-rhage.[78] An excellent review of the research on chest physiotherapy published in 1991 is available in the literature.[76]

If chest physiotherapy is indicated, the procedure should be carried out with ongoing monitoring of oxygen saturation, heart rate, and respiratory rate. The nurse should also monitor the infant for signs of distress. Following the procedure, documentation should include the infant's response to the procedure, the amount and type of secretions obtained, and assessment of the respiratory status, including retractions, nasal flaring, and breath sounds.

There are conflicting reports in the literature concerning the efficacy of chest physiotherapy.[79-83] The goal is to facilitate the removal of secretions to promote better oxygenation and ventilation; but the procedure is not without complications, such as hypoxia, rib fractures, bruising, and dislodged tubes.[14,84] The advantages of using chest physiotherapy must be weighed against the disadvantages associated with the procedure.

Problem: *What position is used to drain which lung segment during postural drainage?*

The position of the infant and the corresponding lung segment to be drained are identified in Table 7-5. For practical purposes, the infant's condition and tolerance will dictate the amount of time and the positions used for postural drainage.

AIR LEAKS AND CHEST TUBES

It has been estimated that 2 to 10 percent of normal newborns will have a spontaneous pneumothorax. The majority of these infants will be asymptomatic. In the distressed newborn who is subjected to mechanical ventilation, incidence of air leaks is significantly higher, ranging from 16 to 40 percent, with the highest incidence seen in infants with meconium aspiration syndrome.[85] Although there has been a dramatic decrease in the incidence of meconium aspiration over the past 14 years because of good airway management in the delivery room, the incidence of pneumothorax in infants with meconium aspiration syndrome (12 percent) has remained unchanged.[86]

Air leaks are caused by alveolar rupture, usually at the base of the alveoli. This can result from a number of factors, including positive pressure ventilation and ball-valve obstruction with distal air trapping. Hand ventilating an infant with a manual resuscitation bag without an in-line manometer to measure inspiratory pressure can result in inadvertent administration of high inspiratory pressure, leading to rupture.[87] Infants who require high inspiratory pressure on the ventilator in order to ventilate the lung adequately are at an increased risk for pneumothorax because the high pressure may only marginally expand some alveoli while overexpanding and rupturing others.

Secretions and debris in the lung may cause a ball-valve phenomenon leading to pneumothorax. Air is able to enter the alveoli around the debris, but is unable to be exhaled around the debris because the airways narrow during exhalation. This results in air retention in the alveoli during exhalation and the resultant addition of air to the alveoli during the next inhalation, causing overdistention and the potential for rupture.

Infants with atelectasis are particularly prone to air leaks because of the presence of both normally expanded and nonexpanded alveoli. The pressure required to ventilate the infant is often sufficient to overexpand the normally expanded alveoli, causing them to rupture. When the alveoli rupture, air escapes into the interstitium and travels along the perivascular spaces to the hilum, where it may rupture into the pleural space, causing a pneumothorax; into the mediastinum, resulting in a pneumomediastinum; or into the pericardium, causing a pneumopericardium. A more in-depth discussion of these conditions can be found in Chapter 6.

The iatrogenic causes of air leaks are often overlooked. A pneumothorax will occur during thoracic surgery when the chest is opened. Other iatrogenic causes are related to aggressive endotracheal suctioning or a malpositioned endotracheal tube. In each of these instances, the catheter or endotracheal tube may have entered the right mainstem bronchus, eroding through the bronchial wall and creating an air leak.

One study found that infants with respiratory distress syndrome (RDS) and pulmonary interstitial emphysema (PIE) who had one pneumothroax were at high risk of developing a contralateral pneumothorax. In contrast, 90 percent of infants with RDS and one pneumothorax who did not have PIE did not have a contralateral pneumothorax.[88]

SIGNS AND SYMPTOMS

The signs and symptoms of tension pneumothorax in an infant on the ventilator may be overt or subtle, and the condition is often first suspected by the nurse at the bedside. Rapid detection and treatment of a pneumothorax are imperative in the critically ill infant. The presence of a pneumothorax causes swings in blood pressure that result in changes in cerebral blood flow. An increase in the cerebral blood flow causes increased intracranial pressure and in preterm infants may cause rupture of the very fragile vessels of the germinal matrix.

The infant may show a sudden deterioration in color, increasing agitation, hypoxia, and ineffective ventilation. Auscultation may demonstrate decreased breath sounds on the affected side and asymmetry of chest movement. A thorough discussion of the common presenting signs of pneumothorax can be found in Chapter 6.

FIGURE 7-6 ▲ Anterior chest tube with purse-string suture.

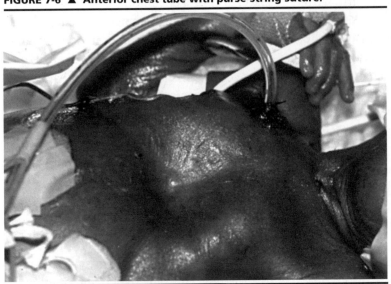

The voltage change in the R-S wave on the EKG complex results from the accumulated air in the extrapleural space not conducting the electrical voltage as well as fluid. This causes a decrease in the R-S wave that can be seen on the bedside monitor.

DIAGNOSIS

Radiographs, transillumination, and echocardiography are used to diagnose air leaks. The radiograph remains the gold standard for the diagnosis of air leaks. When reviewing any radiograph, it is vital to evaluate the x-ray film in its entirety to avoid a misinterpretation.

Transillumination is used as a quick, noninvasive tool for immediate interpretation. This method has been used in nurseries for almost 20 years and is well accepted as a first-line diagnostic tool. The fiberoptic probe with a high-intensity light is placed against the infant's chest wall, and the diameters of the circles of light are compared as it is moved from right to left.

The area with the increased diameter of light should be suspect for an air leak. Dimming the ambient light in the room facilitates interpretation. If an air leak is suspected based on transillumination, chest radiography should follow.

As with most noninvasive measures, the possibility exists for false positive or false negative results. A false positive finding (you believe there is an air leak when in fact there is not) can occur in infants with subcutaneous air and/or subcutaneous edema. A false negative finding (you believe there is no air leak when in fact there is one) can occur in infants with a thick chest wall or dark skin and when the high-intensity light is weak or the infant's chest is heavily bandaged.

The first reports of echocardiograms used to diagnose pneumothorax were made in 1991 by

FIGURE 7-7 ▲ Chest tube with bulky dressing covering insertion site.

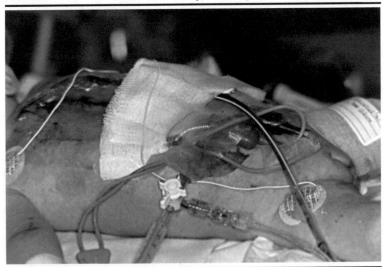

FIGURE 7-8 ▲ Chest tubes secured with purse-string sutures and tape.

FIGURE 7-9 ▲ A one-bottle chest tube drainage system.

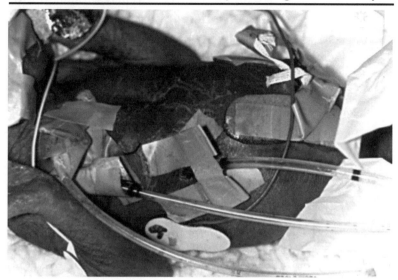

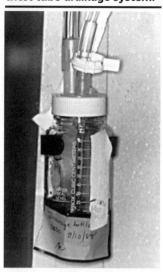

a British group.[89] In the normal course of conducting routine echocardiograms in the NICU, they identified four cases of pneumothorax that were previously unrecognized. On the echocardiogram, there was difficult visualization and lateral displacement of the heart.

TREATMENT

The treatment of choice for excess air in the pleural space is removal of the air using needle aspiration or indwelling chest tubes. Needle aspiration is a single procedure in which a scalp vein needle (23–25 gauge) or angiocatheter, attached to a stopcock and syringe, is inserted through the chest wall to remove excess air. Air is evacuated by the syringe and then vented to the room by turning the stopcock. Because of its potential complications, this procedure is performed by a physician or by a nurse certified to perform needle aspiration. If this procedure is done and there is no pneumothorax, needling the chest in error seldom produces a pneumothorax.

A chest tube is placed for the continual removal of fluid or air from the pleural space. Using sterile procedures, the chest tube is inserted through a small skin incision at the mid-axillary line at the level of the fifth to sixth rib. The tube is threaded over the rib and into the pleural space. Using the first and third intercostal space at the mid-clavicular line has the potential to injure the internal mammary artery.[90] The tip of the chest tube is placed anteriorly for air removal (air rises) and posteriorly for fluid removal (fluid falls). The tube is held in position with purse-string sutures (Figure 7-6), bulky dressing (Figure 7-7) and/or tape (Figure 7-8).

The tube may be connected to a Heimlich valve (Bard-Parker) or to underwater sealed vacuum using a one-bottle (Figure 7-9) system or a commercially available chest tube drainage set (Figure 7-10). If a one-bottle system is used, the negative pressure must be able to be regulated to prevent trauma to the infant. The negative pressure (10 cm H_2O) connected to the drainage set may be continual or intermittent. The drainage collection system used must be able to be secured to prevent accidental breakage or other mishaps.

Two new types of chest tubes have been discussed in the literature. The "pigtail catheter" is a tightly curled catheter (hence the name

FIGURE 7-10 ▲ A commercially available chest tube drainage set.

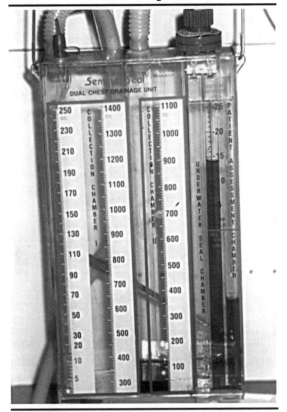

pigtail) with side openings. A needle is inserted into the chest and a guide wire advanced. The catheter is then threaded over the guide wire. The reported advantage is the decreased depth of insertion required and the relatively atraumatic insertion technique. No complications were reported with 19 catheter insertions.[91]

The second catheter is a "J" tube, which is similar to the pigtail catheter. This catheter's advantage is also a decreased depth required for insertion, thus minimizing the risk of lung trauma. The catheter is placed so that its curve lies parallel to the chest wall. In one sample of 38 neonates in whom the "J" tube was used, 92 percent of the pneumothoraces were completely resolved.[92]

Problem: *What are the complications associated with chest tube insertion?*

Complications associated with chest tube insertion include hemorrhage of the intercostal or pulmonary vessels, phrenic nerve paralysis, bronchopleural fistula, and lung perforation.[93–96] One study reported a 35 percent incidence of lung perforation when a trocar was used to insert the chest tube.[97]

Problem: *How do I prevent tension on the chest tube at the insertion site?*

Secure the chest tube to the bed with pins or hemostats to prevent tension on the insertion site.

Problem: *What precautions can I take against inadvertent disconnection of the chest tube connections with ensuing respiratory compromise?*

Securely tape all chest tube connections with adhesive tape. Keep rubber-protected clamps at the bedside for clamping the tubing should it become disconnected. Keep the bottles below the level of the patient at all times.

Problem: *How can I quantify the drainage of fluid from the chest tube?*

In general, chest tubes placed after surgery will have greater fluid drainage than those placed to relieve a tension pneumothorax. Fluid output can be quantified by using a tape strip to mark the fluid level in the container at the beginning of the shift and again four to eight hours later. If there is a significant fluid output, the drainage is measured more frequently. If small collection bottles (90 ml) are used, it may be necessary to replace or empty the bottle if it becomes more than half filled. The fluid accumulated is measured and then documented on the infant's flow sheet.

The negative pressure setting is based on the initial fluid level in the bottle and the diameter of the chest tube; additional fluid alters the negative pressure, as does the addition of another chest tube or changing a chest tube for one of a different diameter.

Assessing chest tube drainage also includes evaluating the degree of bubbling or fluctuation of the fluid in the bottle or tubing. Bubbling or fluctuation of the fluid in the tubing indicates that the chest tube is patent and removing air/fluid. Although tube position is evaluated radiographically, one indicator that it may be outside the chest wall is active continual bubbling. This may also indicate an air leak in the collection tubing.

No bubbling or fluctuations may indicate either that the air leak is resolved or that the tube is no longer patent. Chest tubes that are not patent when the pneumothorax is unresolved are removed and replaced with new ones.

If the bubbling or fluctuation of the fluid has stopped for 24 hours, the tube is clamped and a chest film obtained to rule out reaccumulation of air, which would indicate that the air leak has not resolved. Many hospitals do not clamp chest tubes prior to removal if the infant remains on positive pressure ventilation. Leaving the tube unclamped provides an outlet for any air which may reaccumulate in the pleural space after suction is stopped.

The chest tube is removed under aseptic conditions, and an occlusive dressing is applied using petroleum jelly or a similar substance to prevent air from entering through the incision site. A chest film is taken after the tube has been removed to rule out reaccumulation of air.

Problem: *What is the relationship of pneumothorax to the incidence of intraventricular hemorrhage?*

There are conflicting reports in the literature on the relationship between pneumothorax and cerebral hemorrhage.[114-117] The proposed mechanism relating these two conditions is as follows: The increase in intrathoracic pressure that occurs with a pneumothorax causes a dramatic rise in cerebral capillary pressure, which causes the capillaries to rupture.

One study using puppies found that the rate of removal of the air in reducing the pneumothorax was related to cerebral blood flow velo-city. Rapid air removal resulted in increased arterial blood pressure and cerebral blood flow velocity; slow evacuation led to a gradual normalization of mean arterial pressure and cerebral blood flow velocity.[115]

Problem: *What precautions should be observed when an infant with a chest tube is transported?*

The tube can be clamped for a short time while the bottle is elevated and repositioned for transport. During transport, the bottle must be kept below the level of the infant's chest unless the tubing is clamped. An alternative is to use a Heimlich valve placed in-line, which negates the need for the bottle collection system during transport. The Heimlich flutter valve is connected to the chest tube with the distal end connected to a specimen trap.

SUMMARY

Caring for the infant with respiratory compromise requires integrating information from multiple sources: clinical assessment of the infant, data from invasive and noninvasive monitors, and interpretation of clinical cues. Understanding the physiologic concepts that underlie nursing procedures enables the nurse to provide appropriate, planned, and individualized care to this vulnerable population.

REFERENCES

1. Thibeault DW. 1986. Pulmonary care of infants with endotracheal tubes. In *Neonatal Pulmonary Care*, Thibeault DW, and Gregory GA, eds. Menlo Park, California: Addison-Wesley, 388.

2. Kuhns LR, and Poznanski AK. 1971. Endotracheal tube position in the infant. *Journal of Pediatrics* 78(6): 991–996.

3. Tordes D, et al. 1976. Endotracheal tube displacement in the newborn infant. *Journal of Pediatrics* 89(1): 126–127.

4. Donn SM, and Blane CE. 1985. Endotracheal tube movement in the preterm neonate: Oral versus nasal intubation. *Annals of Otology, Rhinology, and Laryngology* 94(1): 18–20.

5. Reiterer F, Abbasi S, and Bhutani VK. 1994. Influence of head-neck posture on airflow and pulmonary mechanics in preterm neonates. *Pediatric Pulmonology* 17(3): 149–154.

6. Cohen MD. 1980. Tubes, wires and the neonate. *Clinical Radiology* 31(3): 249–256.

7. Slovis TL, and Poland RL. 1986. Endotracheal tubes in neonates: Sonographic positioning. *Radiology* 160(1): 262–263.

8. Marshall TA, et al. 1984. Physiologic changes associated with endotracheal intubation in premature infants. *Critical Care Medicine* 12(6): 501–503.

9. Martin RJ, Fanaroff AA, and Skalina M. 1983. The respiratory distress syndrome and its management. In *Behrman's Neonatal-Perinatal Medicine,* Fanaroff AA, and Martin RJ, eds. St. Louis: Mosby-Year Book, 438.

10. Andriani J, and Griggs T. 1954. An improved endotracheal tube for pediatric use. *Anesthesiology* 15(5): 466–470.

11. Kubota V, et al. 1986. Tracheo-bronchial angles in infants and children. *Anesthesiology* 64(3): 374–376.

12. Fewell J, Arrington R, and Seibert J. 1979. The effect of head position and angle of tracheal bifurcation on bronchus catheterization in the intubated neonate. *Pediatrics* 64(3): 192–194.

13. Richards SD. 1981. A method for securing pediatric endotracheal tubes. *Anesthesia and Analgesia* 60(4): 224–225.

14. Fletcher MA. 1983. Tracheal intubation. In *Atlas of Procedures in Neonatology,* Fletcher MA, MacDonald MG, and Avery GB, eds. Philadelphia: JB Lippincott, 220–223.

15. Tarnow-Mordi WO, et al. 1989. Low inspired gas humidity and respiratory complications in very low birth weight infants. *Journal of Pediatrics* 114(3): 438–442.

16. O'Hagan M, Reid E, and Tarnow-Mordi WO. 1991. Is neonatal inspired gas humidity accurately controlled by humidifier temperature? *Critical Care Medicine* 19(11): 1370–1373.

17. Loan L. 1992. Neonatal implications of ventilator inspired gas temperatures. Unpublished master's thesis, University of Washington, Seattle.

18. Heller RM, and Heller TW. 1994. Experience with the illuminated endotracheal tube in the prevention of unsafe intubations in the premature and full-term newborn. *Pediatrics* 93(3): 389–391.

19. Heller RM, and Cotton RB. 1985. Early experience with illuminated endotracheal tube in premature and term infants. *Pediatrics* 75(4): 664–666.

20. Hauser G, et al. 1990. Prospective evaluation of a non-radiographic device for determination of endotracheal tube position in children. *Critical Care Medicine* 18(7): 760–763.

21. Blaney M, et al. 1991. A new system approach for location of endotracheal tube in preterm and term neonates. *Pediatrics* 87(1): 44–47.

22. Weis FR, and Holton MN. 1989. Intubation by use of the light wand: Experience in 253 patients. *Journal of Oral Maxillofacial Surgery* 47(6): 577–581.

23. Stone DJ, et al. 1984. A complication of light wand-guided nasotracheal intubation. *Anesthesiology* 61(6): 780–781.

24. Cassady G. 1983. Transcutaneous monitoring in the newborn infant. *Journal of Pediatrics* 103(6): 837–848.

25. Rooth G, Huch A, and Huch R. 1987. Transcutaneous oxygen monitors are reliable indicators of arterial oxygen tension (if used correctly). *Pediatrics* 79(2): 283–286.

26. Peabody JL. 1987. Historical perspective of noninvasive monitoring. *Journal of Perinatology* 7(4): 306–308.

27. Gunderson LP, and Kenner C. 1988. Transcutaneous oxygen monitoring: Description and clinical application. *Neonatal Network* 6(6): 7–14.

28. Poets CF, and Southall DP. 1994. Noninvasive monitoring of oxygenation in infants and children: Practical consideration and areas of concern. *Pediatrics* 93(5): 737–746.

29. Boyle RJ, and Oh W. 1980. Erythema following transcutaneous PO_2 monitoring. *Pediatrics* 65(2): 333–334.

30. Golden SM. 1981. Skin craters—a complication of transcutaneous oxygen monitoring. *Pediatrics* 67(4): 514–516.

31. Pierce JR, and Turner BS. 1993. Physiologic monitoring. In *Handbook of Neonatal Intensive Care,* 3rd ed., Merenstein GB, and Gardner SL, eds. St. Louis: Mosby-Year Book, 115–126.

32. Turner BS. 1989. Noninvasive monitoring of the newborn. Part I. *NAACOG Update Series* 6(10): 5.

33. Anderson JV. 1987. The accuracy of pulse oximetry in neonates: Effects of fetal hemoglobin and bilirubin. *Journal of Perinatology* 7(4): 309–319.

34. Fanconi S. 1988. Reliability of pulse oximetry in hypoxic infants. *Journal of Pediatrics* 112(3): 424–427.

35. Ramanathan R, Durand M, and Larrazabal C. 1987. Pulse oximetry in very low birth weight infants with acute and chronic lung disease. *Pediatrics* 79(4): 612–617.

36. Jennis MS, and Peabody JL. 1987. Pulse oximetry: An alternative method for the assessment of oxygenation in newborn infants. *Pediatrics* 79(4): 524–528.

37. Barrington KJ, Finer NN, and Ryan CA. 1988. Evaluation of pulse oximetry as a continuous monitoring technique in the neonatal intensive care unit. *Critical Care Medicine* 16(11): 1147–1153.

38. Hay WW. 1987. Physiology of oxygenation and its relation to pulse oximetry. *Journal of Perinatology* 7(4): 309–319.

39. Cunningham MD, Shook LA, and Tomazic T. 1987. Clinical experience with pulse oximetry in managing oxygen therapy in neonatal intensive care. *Journal of Perinatology* 7(4): 333–335.

40. Emery JR. 1987. Skin pigmentation as an influence on the accuracy of pulse oximetry. *Journal of Perinatology* 7(4): 329–330.

41. Fanconi S. 1988. Reliability of pulse oximetry in hypoxic infants. *Journal of Pediatrics* 112(3): 424–427.

42. Comer DM. 1992. Pulse oximetry implications for practice. *Journal of Obstetric, Gynecologic, and Neonatal Nursing* 21(1): 35–41.

43. Johnson N, et al. 1990. The effect of meconium on neonatal and fetal reflectance pulse oximetry. *Journal of Perinatal Medicine* 18(5): 351–355.

44. Brunstler I, Enders A, and Versmold HT. 1982. Skin surface PCO_2 monitoring in newborn infants in shock: Effect of hypotension and electrode temperature. *Journal of Pediatrics* 100(3): 454–457.

45. Gerhardt T, and Jensen LP. 1988. Physiologic monitoring and pulmonary function. In *Neonatal Respiratory Care,* Carlo WA, and Chatburn RL, eds. Chicago: Year Book Medical Publishers, 78.

46. Watkins AMC, and Weindling AM. 1987. Monitoring of end tidal CO_2 in neonatal intensive care. *Archives of Disease in Childhood* 62(8): 837–839.

47. Paige PL. 1990. Noninvasive monitoring of the neonatal respiratory system. *Clinical Issues in Critical Care Nursing* 1(2): 416–417.

48. McEvedy BAB, et al. 1988. End tidal, transcutaneous, and arterial PCO_2 measurements in critically ill neonates: A comparative study. *Anesthesiology* 69(1): 112–116.

49. Weingarten M. 1990. Respiratory monitoring of carbon dioxide and oxygen: A ten year perspective. *Journal of Clinical Monitoring* 6(3): 217–225.

50. VonRuden KT. 1990. Noninvasive assessment of gas exchange in the critically ill patient. *Clinical Issues in Critical Care Nursing* 1(2): 239–247.

51. Bucher HU, et al. 1986. Transcutaneous carbon dioxide tension in newborn infants: Reliability and safety of continuous 24 hour measurement at 42°C. *Pediatrics* 78(4): 631–635.

52. Turner BS. 1983. Current concepts in endotracheal suctioning. *Journal of the California Perinatal Association* 3(1): 104–106.

53. Cunningham ML, Baun MM, and Nelson RM. 1984. Endotracheal suctioning of premature neonates. *Journal of the California Perinatal Association* 4(1): 49–52.

54. Raval D, et al. 1980. Changes in transcutaneous PO_2 during tracheobronchial hygiene in neonates. *Perinatology-Neonatology* 4(4): 41–46.

55. Cabal LA, et al. 1984. Cardiac rate and rhythm changes during airway suctioning in premature infants with RDS. *Journal of the California Perinatal Association* 4(1): 45–48.

56. Brandstater B, and Muallem M. 1969. Atelectasis following tracheal suction in infants. *Anesthesiology* 31(5): 468–473.

57. Kuzenski BM. 1978. Effect of negative pressure on tracheobronchial trauma. *Nursing Research* 27(4): 260–263.

58. Storm W. 1980. Transient bacteremia following endotracheal suctioning in ventilated newborns. *Pediatrics* 65(3): 487–490.

59. Vaughan RS, Menke JA, and Giocoia GP. 1978. Pneumothorax: A complication of endotracheal tube suctioning. *Journal of Pediatrics* 92(4): 633–634.

60. Rudy EB, et al. 1986. The relationship between endotracheal suctioning and changes in intracranial pressure: A review of the literature. *Heart and Lung* 15(5): 488–494.

61. Perlman JM, and Volpe JJ. 1983. Suctioning in the preterm infant: Effects on cerebral blood flow velocity, intracranial pressure, and arterial blood pressure. *Pediatrics* 72(3): 329.

62. Fanconi S, and Duc G. 1987. Intratracheal suctioning in sick preterm infants: Prevention of intracranial hypertension and cerebral hypoperfusion by muscle paralysis. *Pediatrics* 79(4): 538–543.

63. Anderson KD, and Chandra R. 1976. Pneumothorax secondary to perforation of sequential bronchi by suction catheters. *Journal of Pediatric Surgery* 11(5): 687–693.

64. Skov L, et al. 1992. Changes in cerebral oxygenation and cerebral blood volume during endotracheal suctioning in ventilated neonates. *Acta Paediatrica* 81(5): 389–393.

65. Hodge D. 1991. Endotracheal suctioning and the infant: A nursing care protocol to decrease complications. *Neonatal Network* 9(5): 7–15.

66. Turner BS. 1990. Maintaining the artificial airway: Current concepts. *Pediatric Nursing* 16(5): 487–493.

67. Stone K, and Turner BS. 1989. Endotracheal suctioning. *Annual Review of Nursing Research* 7: 27–49.

68. Ackerman MH. 1985. The use of bolus normal saline instillations in artificial airways: Is it useful or necessary? *Heart and Lung* 14(5): 505–506.

69. Cabal L, et al. 1979. New endotracheal tube adaptor reduces cardiopulmonary effects of suctioning. *Critical Care Medicine* 7(12): 552–555.

70. Zmora E, and Merritt TA. 1980. Use of side-hole endotracheal tube adaptor for tracheal aspiration. *American Journal of Diseases of Children* 134(3): 250–253.

71. Ballard JL, Musia MJ, and Myers MG. 1986. Hazards of delivery room resuscitation using oral methods of endotracheal suctioning. *Pediatric Infectious Disease Journal* 5(2): 198–200.

72. Van Dyke RB, and Spector SA. 1984. Transmission of herpes simplex virus type 1 to a newborn infant during endotracheal suctioning for mechanical aspiration. *Critical Care Medicine* 3(2): 153–156.

73. Proceedings of the Conference on the Scientific Basis of In-Hospital Respiratory Therapy. 1980. Atlanta, Georgia, November 14–16, 1979. *American Review of Respiratory Disease* 122(1): 1–161.

74. Meyers C. 1982. Pulmonary physiotherapy. In *Practical Neonatal Respiratory Care,* Schreiner R, and Kisling JA, eds. New York: Raven Press, 384.

75. Nugent J, Hanks H, and Goldsmith JP. 1988. Pulmonary care. In *Assisted Ventilation of the Neonate,* Goldsmith JP, and Karotkin A, eds. Philadelphia: WB Saunders, 97–102.

76. Dulock HL. 1991. Chest physiotherapy in neonates. *Clinical Issues in Critical Care Nursing* 2(3): 446–450.

77. Murphy JF. 1979. The ketchup bottle method. *New England Journal of Medicine* 300(20): 1155–1157.

78. Ravel D, et al. 1987. Chest physiotherapy in preterm infants with RDS in the first 24 hours of life. *Journal of Perinatology* 7(4): 301–304.

79. Etches PC, and Scott B. 1978. Chest physiotherapy in the newborn: Effect on secretions removed. *Pediatrics* 62(5): 713–715.

80. Finer NN, and Boyd J. 1978. Chest physiotherapy in the neonate: A controlled study. *Pediatrics* 61(2): 282–285.

81. Fox WW, Schwartz JG, and Shaffer TH. 1978. Pulmonary physiotherapy in neonates: Physiologic changes and respiratory management. *Journal of Pediatrics* 92(6): 977–981.

82. Holloway R, et al. 1969. Effect of chest physiotherapy in blood gases of neonates treated by intermittent positive pressure respiration. *Thorax* 24(4): 421–426.

83. Curran CL, and Kachoyeanos MK. 1979. The effects on neonates of two methods of chest physical therapy. *American Journal of Maternal Child Nursing* 4(5): 309–313.

84. Purohit DM, Caldwell C, and Levkoff AH. 1975. Multiple rib fractures due to physiotherapy in a neonate with hyaline membrane disease. *American Journal of Diseases of Children* 129(9): 1103.

85. Hagedorn MI, Gardner SL, and Abman SH. 1993. Respiratory disease. In *Handbook of Neonatal Intensive Care*, 3rd ed., Merenstein GB, and Gardner SL, eds. St. Louis: Mosby-Year Book, 334.

86. Wiswell TE, Tuggle J, and Turner BS. 1990. Meconium aspiration syndrome: Have we made a difference? *Pediatrics* 85(5): 715–721.

87. Carroll P. 1991. Pneumothorax in the newborn. *Neonatal Network* 10(2): 27–34.

88. Ryan CA, et al. 1987. Contralateral pneumothoraces in the newborn: Incidence and predisposing factors. *Pediatrics* 79(3): 417–421.

89. Skinner JR, Milligan DWA, and Hunter S. 1991. Diagnosis of pneumothorax by echocardiography. *Archives of Disease in Childhood* 66(8): 1001–1002.

90. Fletcher MA, and Eichelberger MR. 1983. Thoracostomy tubes. In *Atlas of Procedures in Neonatology*, Fletcher MA, MacDonald MG, and Avery GB, eds. Philadelphia: JB Lippincott, 264.

91. Lawless S, et al. 1989. New pigtail catheter for pleural drainage in pediatric patients. *Critical Care Medicine* 17(2): 173–175.

92. Jung AL, et al. 1991. Clinical evaluation of a new chest tube used in neonates. *Clinical Pediatrics* 30(2): 85–87.

93. Lester PD, and Jung AL. 1981. Complications of intubation and catheterization in the neonatal intensive care unit. *Radiographics* 1(1): 35–38.

94. Odita JC, et al. 1992. Neonatal phrenic nerve paralysis resulting from intercostal drainage of pneumothorax. *Pediatric Radiology* 22(5): 379–381.

95. Berger JT, and Gilhooly J. 1993. Fibrin glue treatment of persistent pneumothorax in a premature infant. *Journal of Pediatrics* 122(6): 958–960.

96. Martin RJ, and Fanaroff AA. 1988. Complications of neonatal respiratory care. In *Neonatal Respiratory Care*, Carlo WA, and Chatburn RL, eds. Chicago: Year Book Medical Publishers, 351.

97. Moessinger AC, Driscoll JM Jr, and Wigger HJ. 1978. High incidence of lung perforation by chest tube in neonatal pneumothorax. *Journal of Pediatrics* 92(4): 635–637.

98. Carillo PJ. 1985. Palatal groove formation and oral endotracheal intubation. *American Journal of Diseases of Children* 139(9): 859–860.

99. Saunders BS, Easa D, and Slaughter RJ. 1976. Acquired palatal groove in neonates. *Journal of Pediatrics* 89(6): 988–989.

100. Duke PM, et al. 1976. Cleft palate associated with prolonged orotracheal intubation in infancy. *Journal of Pediatrics* 89(6): 990–991.

101. Gowdar K, et al. 1980. Nasal deformities in neonates. *American Journal of Diseases of Children* 134(10): 954–957.

102. Pettett G, and Merenstein GB. 1976. Nasal erosion with nasotracheal intubation. *Journal of Pediatrics* 87(1): 149.

103. Jung AL, and Thomas GK. 1984. Stricture of the nasal vestibule: A complication of nasotracheal intubation in newborn infants. *Journal of Pediatrics* 85(3): 412–414.

104. Boice KB, Krous HF, and Foley JM. 1976. Gingival and dental complications of orotracheal intubation. *Journal of the American Medical Association* 236(8): 957–958.

105. Moylan FMB, et al. 1980. Defective primary dentition in survivors of neonatal mechanical ventilation. *Journal of Pediatrics* 96(1): 106–108.

106. Marshak G, and Grundfast KM. 1981. Subglottic stenosis. *Pediatric Clinics of North America* 28(4): 941–948.

107. Strong RM, and Passy V. 1977. Complications in neonates. *Archives of Otolaryngology* 103(6): 329–335.

108. Johnson DE, et al. 1982. Management of esophageal and pharyngeal perforation in the newborn infant. *Pediatrics* 70(4): 592–596.

109. Clarke TA, et al. 1980. Esophageal perforations in premature infants and comments on the diagnosis. *American Journal of Diseases of Children* 134(4): 367–368.

110. Talbert JL, et al. 1977. Traumatic perforation of the hypopharynx in infants. *Journal of Thoracic and Cardiovascular Surgery* 74(1): 152–156.

111. Goodwin SR, Graves SA, and Haberkern CM. 1985. Aspiration in intubated premature infants. *Pediatrics* 75(1): 85–88.

112. Harris H, Wirtschafter D, and Cassady G. 1976. Endotracheal intubation and its relationship to bacterial colonization and systemic infection of newborn infants. *Pediatrics* 56(6): 816–823.

113. Grylack LJ, and Anderson KD. 1984. Diagnosis and treatment of traumatic granuloma in tracheobronchial tree of newborn with history of chronic intubation. *Journal of Pediatric Surgery* 19(2): 200–201.

114. Hill A, Perlman JM, and Volpe JJ. 1982. Relationship of pneumothorax to occurrence of intraventricular hemorrhage in the premature newborn. *Pediatrics* 69(2): 144–149.

115. Baton DG, Hellman J, and Nardis EE. 1984. Effect of pneumothorax-induced systemic blood pressure alteration on the cerebral circulation in newborn dogs. *Pediatrics* 74(3): 350–353.

116. Hillman K. 1987. Intrathoracic pressure fluctuations and periventricular haemorrhage in the newborn. *Australian Paediatric Journal* 23(6): 343–346.

117. Mehrabani D, Gowen CW, and Kopelman AE. 1991. Association of pneumothorax and hypotension with intraventricular hemorrhage. *Archives of Disease in Childhood* 66(1 spec no): 48–51.

NOTES

8 Blood Gas Analysis

Debbie Fraser Askin, RNC, MN

Blood gas analysis is one of the major tools in assessing the respiratory status of the newborn. To adequately use this information, one must have a basic understanding of gas transportation and acid-base physiology. This chapter reviews these topics and provides a basis for applying these principles to the interpretation of neonatal blood gases. Common terminology used in this chapter is listed in Table 8-1.

TRANSPORT OF OXYGEN AND CARBON DIOXIDE

OXYGEN

Oxygen is used in metabolic reactions throughout the human body and is supplied to the tissues through the efforts of the respiratory and cardiovascular systems. The lungs are responsible for bringing an adequate supply of oxygen to the blood. Control of this process occurs mainly in response to the effect of carbon dioxide levels on receptors in the large arteries and the brain. At moderate to severe levels of hypoxemia, peripheral chemoreceptors may also be stimulated to increase ventilation, resulting in increased oxygen intake and lower than normal partial pressure of carbon dioxide in arterial blood ($PaCO_2$).[1]

The cardiovascular system regulates the oxygen supply by altering cardiac output in response to the metabolic rate of peripheral tissues. Distribution to specific tissues is set by local metabolic activity. Oxygen transport is affected by:[4]

- partial pressure of oxygen in inspired air
- alveolar ventilation
- ventilation-to-perfusion matching
- arterial pH and temperature
- cardiac output
- blood volume
- hemoglobin
- hemoglobin's affinity for oxygen

Oxygen transport to the tissues can be divided into a three-part process that involves oxygen diffusion from the alveoli to the pulmonary capillaries (external respiration) (phase 1), gas transport in the bloodstream (phase 2), and diffusion of oxygen from the capillaries to the cells (internal respiration) (phase 3). Phases 1 and 2 are discussed here.

Oxygen diffusion is from the alveoli to the pulmonary capillaries (external respiration). Oxygen enters the lung during inspiration and

TABLE 8-1 ▲ Terminology Associated with Blood Gas Analysis

Term	Definition
Acid	Donator of H^+ ions
Base	Acceptor of H^+ ions
Buffer	Weak acid and strong base pair that accept or donate hydrogen ions to maintain a balanced pH
pH	Negative logarithm of hydrogen ion
↑ H^+	pH more acid
↓ H^+	pH more alkaline
Acidemia	Blood pH below 7.35
Alkalemia	Blood pH above 7.45
Acidosis	Process causing acidemia
Alkalosis	Process causing alkalemia

FIGURE 8-1 ▲ Oxygen diffusion across the alveolar-capillary membrane.

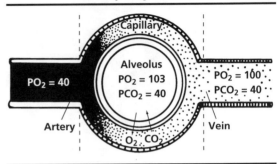

From: Cherniack RM. 1972. *Respiration in Health and Disease*, 2nd ed. Philadelphia: WB Saunders. Reprinted by permission.

diffuses across the alveolar-capillary membrane according to the concentration gradient of oxygen in the alveolus and the capillary (Figure 8-1). Factors that interfere with oxygenation at this point include a decrease in minute ventilation, ventilation-perfusion mismatch, and alterations in the alveolar-capillary membrane.[1]

Once into the blood, oxygen must be transported to the tissues. A small amount of oxygen (about 5 percent) is dissolved in the plasma; 95 percent is bound to hemoglobin. The total volume of oxygen carried in the blood is termed the "arterial oxygen content" and reflects both the oxygen dissolved in the plasma and the amount combined with hemoglobin.

Each hemoglobin molecule contains four atoms of iron and therefore can combine with four molecules of oxygen. The amount of oxygen bound to hemoglobin depends on several factors, the most important being the partial pressure of oxygen in the blood (PaO_2). The combination of oxygen and hemoglobin is expressed as "oxygen saturation": a measure of the hemoglobin sites filled divided by the sites available (Figure 8-2).

The oxygen-hemoglobin saturation is plotted on an S-shaped curve known as oxyhemoglobin dissociation curve which is based on adult hemoglobin at normal temperature and blood pH (Figure 8-3). Normal adult hemoglobin is 50 percent saturated at a PaO_2 of 27 mmHg, 75 percent saturated at a PaO_2 of 40 mmHg, and 90 percent saturated at a PaO_2 of 60 mmHg.[2] At a PaO_2 of 100 mmHg, 95–97 percent of hemoglobin is saturated with oxygen.

At low PaO_2 values seen on the steep slope of the curve in Figure 8-3, a small increase in PaO_2 results in a large increase in oxygen saturation. Conversely, on the flat upper portion of the curve, a large increase in PaO_2 results in only a small increase in saturation. Hemoglobin cannot be more than 100 percent saturated but PaO_2 can exceed 100 mmHg. At a PaO_2 of >100 mmHg O_2, saturation cannot reflect PaO_2. For this reason, PaO_2 is a more sensitive indicator of high oxygen levels in the blood.[3]

Several factors change the affinity of hemoglobin for oxygen, shifting the curve to the left or to the right (Figure 8-3). Alkalosis, hypocarbia, hypothermia, decreased amounts of 2,3-diphosphoglycerate (2,3-DPG), and the presence of fetal hemoglobin (HgbF) all shift the curve to the left.[1] 2,3-DPG is an organic phosphate produced as a by-product of red cell metabolism. It binds with hemoglobin and decreases hemoglobin's oxygen affinity.

FIGURE 8-2 ▲ Oxygen saturation.

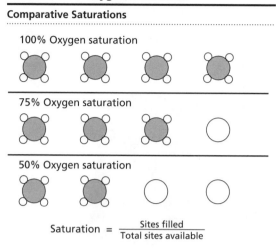

Comparative Saturations

100% Oxygen saturation

75% Oxygen saturation

50% Oxygen saturation

$$Saturation = \frac{Sites\ filled}{Total\ sites\ available}$$

From: Oxygen Transport Physiology Slide Series. 1987. Pleasanton, California: Nellcor, Inc. Reprinted by permission.

FIGURE 8-3 ▲ Oxyhemoglobin dissociation curve.

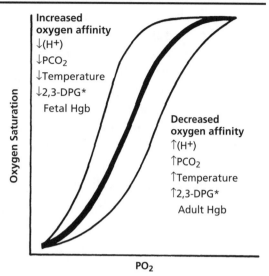

* 2,3-DPG = 2,3-diphosphoglycerate

From: Hay WW. 1987. Physiology of oxygenation and its relation to pulse oximetry in neonates. *Journal of Perinatology* 7(4): 309–319. Reprinted by permission.

With a shift to the left, there is an increased affinity between oxygen and hemoglobin; therefore, hemoglobin more easily picks up oxygen and doesn't release it until a lower PaO_2 level is reached. This can impede oxygen release to the tissues but enhances the uptake of oxygen in the lungs.[4]

Acidosis, hypercapnia, hyperthermia, increased 2,3-DPG, and the presence of mature or adult hemoglobin (HgbA) move the curve to the right.[1] A shift to the right causes oxygen to bind less tightly to hemoglobin and to release from hemoglobin at higher levels of PaO_2, thereby enhancing oxygen unloading at the tissue level.[4]

Tip: An easy way to remember how shifts in the curve affect oxygen delivery is to think of it this way: left on the hemoglobin, right into the tissues.

Carbon Dioxide

Body cells produce carbon dioxide as a by-product of metabolism. Carbon dioxide diffuses from the cells across a concentration gradient from areas of high partial pressure to areas of low partial pressure. A small amount of carbon dioxide (5 percent) travels dissolved in the plasma while 95 percent is transported within the red blood cells.

In the red blood cells, about one-third of the carbon dioxide forms carbo-amino compounds by combining with amino acids contained in the globin portion of hemoglobin. The remaining two-thirds is acted upon by carbonic anhydrase, which speeds the conversion of carbon dioxide and water to carbonic acid.

The transport of carbon dioxide is illustrated in Figure 8-4. As oxygen is unloaded from hemoglobin along the peripheral capillaries, more carbon dioxide can be transported because of the enhanced ability of deoxygenated hemoglobin to form carbo-amino compounds.[5]

Acid-Base Homeostasis

Normal function of the body's cells depends on a biochemical balance maintained within a narrow range of free hydrogen ion (H+) concentration. Free hydrogen ions are constantly released in the body as waste products from the metabolism of proteins and fats. The measurement of free hydrogen ions, present in the body in very low concentrations, is expressed as "pH," which is the negative logarithm of the hydrogen ion concentration—that is, the more hydrogen ions present in a solution, the lower the pH or the more acidic the solution. Conversely, the fewer hydrogen ions present, the higher the pH or the more alkalotic the solution. A pH of 7 is neutral, that is, neither alkaline or acidic; a range of 7.35 to 7.45 is the normal range for cellular reactions.

Most of the acids formed by metabolism come from the interaction of carbon dioxide and water, which forms carbonic acid (H_2CO_3), as illustrated in the following equation:

$$CO_2 + H_2O \leftrightarrow H_2CO_3 \leftrightarrow H^+ + HCO_3^-$$

Carbonic acid is able to exist either as a liquid (nonvolatile acid) or a gas (volatile acid). It is transformed back into carbon dioxide in the lungs and exhaled, allowing the respiratory system to control the majority of acid-base regulation.

Changes in carbon dioxide affect the pH by altering the amount of carbonic acid in the body. Changes in pH caused by changes in carbon dioxide tension are therefore termed *respiratory*. Hyperventilation causes a lower partial pressure of carbon dioxide (PCO_2), lower carbonic acid concentration, and increased pH. Hypoventilation has the opposite effect. Remember that concentrations of carbon dioxide, carbonic acid, and hydrogen move in the opposite direction of pH:

$$\uparrow PCO_2 \rightarrow \uparrow H_2CO_3 \rightarrow \uparrow H^+ \rightarrow \downarrow pH$$

$$\downarrow PCO_2 \rightarrow \downarrow H_2CO_3 \rightarrow \downarrow H^+ \rightarrow \uparrow pH$$

Metabolic acids are formed in the body during the metabolism of protein, anaerobic metabolism resulting in the formation of lac-

FIGURE 8-4 ▲ Carbon dioxide transport.

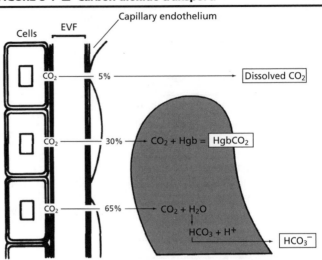

From: Shapiro BA, Peruzzi WT, and Kozelowski-Templin R. 1994. Respiratory acid-base balance. In *Clinical Application of Blood Gases*. St. Louis: Mosby-Year Book, 26. Reprinted by permission.

tic acid, and keto acids which are formed when glucose is unavailable as a fuel source.

The kidneys provide the most important route by which metabolic acids can be excreted and buffered. Hydrogen excretion takes place through the active exchange of sodium ions (Na^+) for H^+. The enzyme carbonic anhydrase accelerates the formation of carbonic acid from hydrogen and carbon dioxide. The kidneys are also responsible for the plasma levels of bicarbonate (HCO_3^-), the most important buffer of hydrogen ions (discussion follows). Therefore, pH changes that occur because of changes in bicarbonate concentrations are termed *metabolic*.

Tip: Remember the following equations:

$$\uparrow HCO_3^- \rightarrow \uparrow pH$$

$$\downarrow HCO_3^- \rightarrow \downarrow pH$$

THE HENDERSON-HASSELBALCH EQUATION

The concentration of hydrogen ions resulting from the dissociation of carbonic acid is

FIGURE 8-5 ▲ Mechanisms of renal bicarbonate excretion/retention.

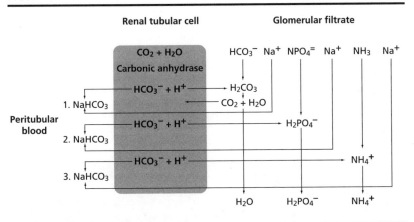

From: Shapiro BA, Peruzzi WT, and Kozelowski-Templin R. 1994. Metabolic acid-base balance. In *Clinical Application of Blood Gases*. St. Louis: Mosby-Year Book, 7. Reprinted by permission.

determined by an interrelationship between bases, buffers, and blood acids. In blood gas analysis, the Henderson-Hasselbalch equation is used to calculate bicarbonate if pH and PCO_2 are known.[6] This equation describes the fixed relationship between carbonic acid, bicarbonate, and hydrogen ion concentration. When the equation is used in the clinical situation, carbonic acid is replaced by the amount of dissolved carbon dioxide in the blood as shown in the following equation:[7]

$$pH = pK + log \frac{[HCO_3^-]}{[s \times PCO_2]}$$

in which pK (a constant) = 6.1 and s (solubility of CO_2) = 0.0301. It is important to remember that this is a calculated bicarbonate value, not one that is measured.

BUFFER SYSTEMS

Buffer systems are a combination of a weak acid and a strong base, which work by accepting or releasing hydrogen ions to maintain acid-base balance. The body has three primary buffers: plasma proteins, hemoglobin, and bicarbonate.[6] Of these, bicarbonate is the most important system and is regulated by the kidney. Bicarbonate ions are formed from the

hydroxylation of carbon dioxide by water inside the red blood cells. This reaction is tremendously accelerated by carbonic anhydrase. Once formed, bicarbonate enters the plasma in exchange for chloride ions through an active transport mechanism known as the "chloride shift."

In blood gas analysis, bicarbonate and base deficit/excess are used in determining the nonrespiratory portion of the acid-base equation. Some centers provide both values in blood gas results; others report either bicarbonate levels or base excess/deficit.

Bicarbonate is expressed in milliequivalents per liter. The normal range is 22 to 26.[1,8] Base excess or base deficit is reported in mEq/liter with a normal range of −2 to +2.[9] Negative values indicate a deficiency of base or an excess of acid (metabolic acidosis); positive values indicate alkalosis. Clinically, the base excess or deficit is calculated from the Siggard Anderson nomogram (Appendix A).

The kidney has several mechanisms for controlling the excretion of hydrogen ions and the retention of bicarbonate. These are illustrated in Figure 8-5 and include the following:[2]

- Reabsorption of filtered bicarbonate (H^+ is excreted in the renal tubular cells in exchange for Na^+. The sodium combines with bicarbonate to form sodium bicarbonate, which enters the blood.)

- Excretion of acids such as phosphoric acid formed from the combination of H^+ and HPO_4^{--}

- Formation of ammonia (Elevated acid levels in the body will result in the formation of ammonia [NH_3], which combines with

FIGURE 8-6 ▲ **Normal 20:1 bicarbonate:carbon dioxide ratio.**

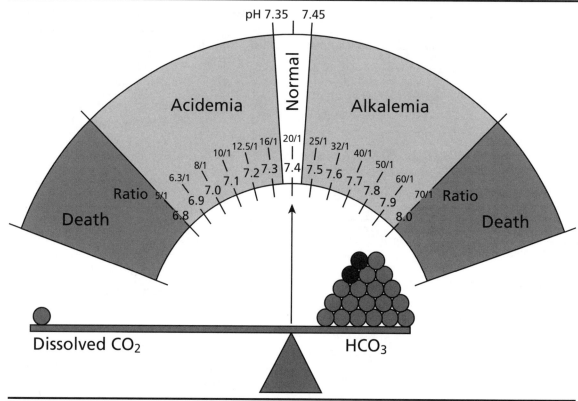

From: Jacob SW, and Francone CA. 1970. *Structure and Function in Man,* 2nd ed. Philadelphia: WB Saunders.
    Reprinted by permission.

H^+ to form NH_4^+, which is excreted in the urine.)

An acid:base ratio of 1:20 is needed to maintain a pH of 7.4—that is, 1 part carbonic acid to 20 parts bicarbonate.[10] Because it is the ratio of PCO_2 to HCO_3^- that determines the pH, abnormalities can be compensated for by adding or subtracting on one side of the scale or the other. This is demonstrated in Figure 8-6.

If buffers cannot normalize the pH, compensatory mechanisms are activated. Healthy lungs are able to compensate for acid-base imbalances within minutes by altering the respiratory rate or volume to regulate carbon dioxide levels. The kidneys have a slower but sustained response and either retain or excrete bicarbonate in response to changes in the blood

TABLE 8-2 ▲ **Renal Response to Acid-Base Imbalance**

Imbalance	Response
Metabolic acidosis	Phosphate and ammonia buffers are used to increase H^+ excretion.
Respiratory acidosis	H^+ excretion and HCO_3^- reabsorption are increased.
Metabolic alkalosis	HCO_3^- reclamation from the urine is decreased. H^+ excretion decreases when serum Na^+ and K^+ are normal. If hyponatremia is present, Na^+ is reabsorbed, requiring H^+ excretion and HCO_3^- retention. If hypokalemia is present, K^+ is reabsorbed in place of H^+.
Respiratory alkalosis	H^+ excretion and HCO_3^- reabsorption decrease.

Adapted from: Shapiro BA, Peruzzi WT, and Kozelowski-Templin R. 1994. *Clinical Application of Blood Gases.* St. Louis: Mosby-Year Book, 8–9.

TABLE 8-3 ▲ Normal Arterial Blood Gas Values

Value	Normal Range
pH	7.35–7.45
$PaCO_2$	35–45 mmHg
PaO_2 (term infant)	50–70 mmHg
(preterm infant)	45–65 mmHg
HCO_3^-	22–26 mEq/liter
Base excess	−2 to +2 mEq/liter
O_2 saturation	92–94%

Adapted from: Malley WJ. 1990. *Clinical Blood Gases.* Philadelphia: WB Saunders; and Phillips BL, McQuitty J, and Durand DJ. 1988. Blood gases: Technical aspects and interpretation. In *Assisted Ventilation of the Neonate*, Goldsmith JP, and Karotkin EH, eds. Philadelphia: WB Saunders. Reprinted by permission.

pH. The kidneys are also able to excrete additional hydrogen ions in combination with phosphate and ammonia. Renal compensatory responses are outlined in Table 8-2. In the neonate, compensatory mechanisms may be limited by respiratory disease and the inability of the immature neonatal kidney to conserve bicarbonate.

DISORDERS OF ACID-BASE BALANCE

The classification and interpretation of blood gases are based on a set of normal values such as the ones shown in Table 8-3. Because of immaturity and the presence of fetal hemoglobin, values for the term and preterm infant differ from those of the adult. In addition, the exact values accepted as normal vary from institution to institution and in the literature.[7,11,12]

The terms applied to acid-base disorders can be a source of confusion and should be examined. Alkalemia and acidemia refer to measurements of blood pH; acidosis and alkalosis refer to the underlying pathologic process.

As previously discussed, a blood pH less than 7.35 is said to be acidemic; a pH greater than 7.45 is alkalemic. The PCO_2 and bicarbonate levels, respectively, determine the respiratory and metabolic contributions to the acid-base equation.

During a disturbance of acid-base balance, the body can attempt to return the pH to a normal level in one of two ways:[13]

1. Correction occurs when the body alters the component responsible for the abnormality. If carbon dioxide levels are increased, the body attempts to correct the problem by increasing the excretion of carbon dioxide. The neonate is often unable to correct an acid-base disturbance because of the limitations of immaturity (such as diminished response of chemoreceptors and decreased lung compliance).

2. Compensation occurs when the body normalizes the pH by altering the blood gas component not responsible for the abnormality. If metabolic acidosis is present, the lungs will excrete more carbon dioxide in order to normalize the pH. If respiratory acidosis is present, the kidneys will excrete more H^+ and conserve bicarbonate in an attempt to compensate for the respiratory problem. Compensation is also limited in the neonate because of immaturity.

Respiratory acidosis results from the formation of excess carbonic acid because of increased PCO_2 ($\uparrow PCO_2 \rightarrow \uparrow H_2CO_3 \rightarrow \uparrow H^+ \rightarrow \downarrow pH$). Blood gas findings are low pH, high PCO_2, and normal bicarbonate.

Respiratory acidosis is caused by insufficient alveolar ventilation secondary to lung disease. Compensation occurs over three to four days as the kidneys increase the rates of hydrogen excretion and bicarbonate reabsorption. Compensated respiratory acidosis is characterized by a low-normal pH (7.35–7.40), with increased carbon dioxide and bicarbonate as a result of the kidney retaining bicarbonate to compensate for elevated carbon dioxide levels.[9]

Respiratory alkalosis results from alveolar hyperventilation, leading to a deficiency of carbonic acid. Blood gas findings are high pH, low PCO_2, and normal bicarbonate.

TABLE 8-4 ▲ Causes of Acid-Base Imbalances in Neonates

↑ PaCO₂	
Respiratory Acidosis	**Metabolic Alkalosis**
Hypoventilation	Gain of bases
Asphyxia	Bicarbonate administration
Apnea	Acetate administration
Upper airway obstruction	Loss of acids
Decreased lung tissue	Vomiting, gastric suctioning
Respiratory distress syndrome	Diuretic therapy
Pneumothorax	Hypokalemia, hypochloremia
Pulmonary interstitial emphysema	
Ventilation-to-perfusion mismatching	
Meconium aspiration	
Pneumonia	
Pulmonary edema	
Transient tachypnea	
Persistent pulmonary hypertension of the newborn	
Cardiac disease	
↓ pH ———————————————————————————— ↑ pH	
Metabolic Acidosis	**Respiratory Alkalosis**
Increased acid formation	Hyperventilation
Hypoxia due to lactic acidosis	Iatrogenic mechanical hyperventilation
Inborn errors of metabolism	
Hyperalimentation	Central nervous system response to:
Loss of bases	
Diarrhea	Hypoxia
Renal tubular acidosis	Maternal heroin addiction
Acetazolamide administration	
↓ PaCO₂	

Respiratory alkalosis is caused by hyperventilation, usually iatrogenic.[9] To compensate, the kidneys decrease hydrogen secretion by retaining chloride and excreting fewer acid salts. Bicarbonate reabsorption is also decreased. The pH will be high normal (7.40–7.45), with low carbon dioxide and bicarbonate levels.

Metabolic acidosis results from a deficiency in the concentration of bicarbonate in the extracellular fluid. It also occurs when there is an excess of acids other than carbonic acid. Blood gas findings are low pH, low bicarbonate, and normal PCO_2.

This condition can be caused by any systemic disease that increases acid production or retention or by problems leading to excessive base losses. Examples are hypoxia leading to lactic acid production, renal disease, or loss of bases through diarrhea.[9,10] If healthy, the lungs will compensate by blowing off additional carbon dioxide through hyperventilation. If renal disease is not a problem, the kidneys will respond by increasing the excretion of acid salts and the reabsorption of bicarbonate. The pH will be low normal (7.35–7.40), with low levels of carbon dioxide and bicarbonate ions.

Metabolic alkalosis results from excess concentration of bicarbonate in the extracellular fluid. Blood gas findings are high pH, high bicarbonate, and normal PCO_2.

This condition is caused by problems leading to increased loss of acids, such as severe vomiting, gastric suctioning, or increased retention or intake of bases, such as occurs with excessive administration of sodium bicarbonate. The lungs compensate by retaining carbon dioxide through hypoventilation. The pH will be high normal (7.40–7.45), with high levels of carbon dioxide and bicarbonate ions.

Table 8-4 lists common causes of acid-base disturbances in the neonate.

BLOOD GAS SAMPLING

Blood gas analysis provides the basis for determining the adequacy of alveolar ventilation and perfusion. According to the National Committee for Clinical Laboratory Standards, blood gas analysis has a more immediate and potentially larger impact on patient care than any other laboratory determination.[14] It is therefore crucial that this test be done with

TABLE 8-5 ▲ Normal Fetal Blood Gas Values

Value	Umbilical Artery	Umbilical Vein	Fetal Scalp
pH	≥7.20	≥7.25	≥7.25
PCO_2 (mmHg)	40–50	≤40	≤50
PO_2 (mmHg)	18 ± 2	30 ± 2	≥20
Base excess (mEq/liter)	0 to ⁻10	0 to ⁻5	<⁻6

From: Martin RW, and McColgin SG. 1990. Evaluation of fetal and neo-natal acid-base status. *Obstetrics and Gynecology Clinics of North America* 17(1): 225. Reprinted by permission.

an understanding of appropriate techniques and potential sources of error.

Regardless of the type of sample obtained, attention should be given to the following factors:

1. Infection control/universal precautions. All types of blood gas sampling carry the risk of transmission of infection to the infant through the introduction of organisms into the bloodstream. In addition, the potential exposure of the clinician to the infant's blood demands the use of appropriate precautions.

2. Bleeding disorders. The potential for bruising and excessive bleeding should be considered, particularly if an arterial puncture is being considered.

3. Steady state. Ideally, blood gases should measure the infant's condition in a state of equilibrium. A period of 20 to 30 minutes after changing ventilator settings or disturbing the infant should be allowed for the arterial blood to reach a steady state.[1] The length of time to reach steady state will vary from infant to infant.

INTRAPARTUM TESTING

Fetal Scalp Sampling

Scalp pH sampling in the fetus has been shown to be a useful tool for evaluating fetal well-being in the presence of suspect fetal heart tracings.[6] Values are similar to umbilical cord gases obtained at delivery.

A pH value of 7.25 or greater is classified as normal. Values of 7.2 to 7.25 are borderline and should be repeated in 30 minutes, and

those below 7.2 are considered indicative of fetal acidosis.[15]

Cord Blood Gases

Cord blood gases provide an accurate assessment of the condition of the fetus at the time of delivery but do not predict long-term outcomes.[16] Table 8-5 lists normal umbilical cord blood gas values.

Blood from the umbilical artery represents fetal status because this is blood returning from the fetus. Umbilical venous blood provides a measure of placental status. For example, in cases of cord compression, the placenta is functioning normally. Therefore, the venous gas would be normal, and the arterial gas would reflect a lower pH and increased PCO_2. With decreased placental perfusion, the pH in the venous gas would drop, as would the arterial pH.[6]

ARTERIAL SAMPLING

Arterial blood can be obtained either from an indwelling line or through intermittent sampling of a peripheral artery. The choice of sample site will depend on the clinical situation. An indwelling arterial catheter should be placed when it is anticipated that the neonate will require frequent arterial blood sampling. Many criteria are used to determine the need for an indwelling line. These include gestational age, disease process, and the percentage of oxygen required. Common sites for neonatal arterial sampling include the following:

1. Umbilical artery. The umbilical artery is usually readily accessible for line placement for three to four days and often useable for up to two weeks after birth.[12] The umbilical arterial catheter can be positioned either between T6 and T10 or between L3 and L4. The higher positioning offers the advantage of fewer complications, but complications that do occur may be more severe.[17–19]

Umbilical arterial catheter placement is unsuccessful in 10 to 15 percent of infants.[12] Complications include hemorrhage, ischemic organ damage, infection, and thrombus formation.[20–23]

2. **Peripheral arterial lines** (radial, posterior tibial, temporal, and dorsalis pedis). These vessels can be accessed at any time beyond delivery with a small-gauge intravascular catheter. Risks for these lines include tissue necrosis, thrombus formation, infection, and hemorrhage.[24]

3. **Intermittent arterial samples**. These can be obtained from the radial, posterior tibial, dorsalis pedis, or temporal arteries. The femoral and brachial arteries are not recommended for sampling because of poor collateral circulation, close proximity of nerves, and the risk of complications.[12,25] Figure 8-7 illustrates the radial site for peripheral sampling.

CAPILLARY SAMPLING

Capillary blood can be "arterialized" by warming the skin to increase local blood flow. Samples can then be obtained from the outer aspects of the heel (Figure 8-8) or from the sides of a finger or toe. When perfusion is normal, capillary pH and PCO_2 correlate well with arterial values.[1,12,26,27]

Transitional events during the first few hours of life and poor perfusion at any time will diminish the accuracy of capillary gas measurements. Partial pressure of oxygen (PO_2) and PaO_2 do not correlate well; therefore, treatment decisions are not normally based on capillary PO_2 alone.

ERRORS IN BLOOD GAS MEASUREMENT

In examining blood gases, the clinician should be aware of potential sources of error that may affect the quality of the results:[12,28,29]

FIGURE 8-7 ▲ Radial artery location.

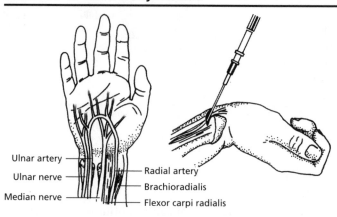

Ulnar artery
Ulnar nerve
Median nerve
Radial artery
Brachioradialis
Flexor carpi radialis

Redrawn from: Durand DJ, and Phillips BL. 1996. Blood gases: Technical aspects and interpretation. In *Assisted Ventilation of the Neonate*, Goldsmith JP, and Karotkin EH, eds. Philadelphia: WB Saunders, 262. Reprinted by permission.

• **Temperature**. Most blood gas machines report results for 37°C. Hypothermia or hyperthermia can alter true arterial gas values.

• **Hemoglobin**. Calculated oxygen saturations are based on adult hemoglobin, not on fetal or mixed hemoglobins.

* **Dilution**. Heparin in a gas sample will lower the PCO_2 and increase the base deficit without altering the pH.

• **Air bubbles**. Room air has PCO_2 close to 0 and a PO_2 of 150; therefore, air bubbles in the sample will decrease the $PaCO_2$ and increase the PaO_2 unless the PaO_2 is greater than 150.

INTERPRETING BLOOD GASES

The blood gas report contains a number of pieces of information that must be examined and interpreted. Although oxygenation and acid-base status are inter-related, it is usually easier to consider these in separate steps. The order in which to evaluate these parameters is a matter of personal preference, but it is important to use an organized, step-by-step approach to simplify the process and ensure that nothing is overlooked.

FIGURE 8-8 ▲ Heel sample technique.

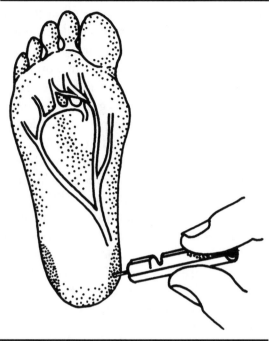

Redrawn from: Durand DJ, and Phillips BL. 1996. Blood gases: Technical aspects and interpretation. In *Assisted Ventilation of the Neonate,* Goldsmith JP, and Karotkin EH, eds. Philadelphia: WB Saunders, 263. Reprinted by permission.

The following steps can be used as a systematic way of evaluating neonatal blood gases. Figure 8-9 illustrates the first five of these steps and is a useful way of visualizing the decision-making process.

1. **Assess the pH**. A pH >7.45 is alkalotic and a pH <7.35 is acidotic. When pH and either PCO_2 or bicarbonate are abnormal, the abnormal factor defines the origin of the imbalance. A normal pH should be further evaluated because compensation can normalize the pH while primary acid-base imbalances are present.

2. **Assess the respiratory component**. A PCO_2 >45 lowers the pH. A PCO_2 <35 raises the pH.

3. **Assess the metabolic component**. A bicarbonate value <22 lowers the pH. A bicarbonate value >26 raises the pH.

Tip: For primary abnormalities, remember the following:

Abnormal pH and PCO_2 = respiratory alkalosis ($PaCO_2$ <35) or acidosis ($PaCO_2$ >45)

FIGURE 8-9 ▲ Blood gas algorithm.

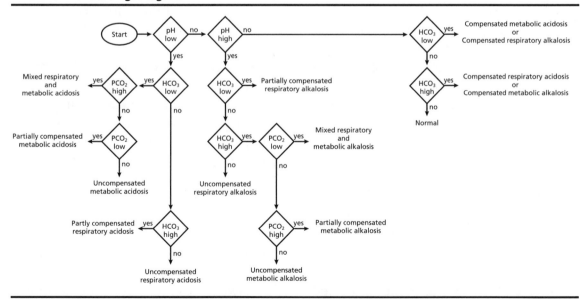

From: Chatburn RL, and Carlo WA. 1988. Assessment of neonatal gas exchange. In *Neonatal Respiratory Care,* Carlo WA, and Chatburn RL, eds. St. Louis: Mosby-Year Book, 56. (Modified from: Hess D. 1984. The hand-held computer as a teaching tool for acid-base interpretation. *Respiratory Care* 29[4]: 375–379.) Reprinted by permission.

TABLE 8-6 ▲ Compensated Acid-Base Imbalances

Primary Problem	pH	PCO$_2$	HCO$_3^-$
Respiratory acidosis	Low normal	High	High
Respiratory alkalosis	High normal	Low	Low
Metabolic acidosis	Low normal	Low	Low
Metabolic alkalosis	High normal	High	High

Abnormal pH and HCO$_3^-$ = metabolic acidosis (HCO$_3^-$ <22) or alkalosis (HCO$_3^-$ >26)

Mixed problems: In some cases, abnormalities in both the metabolic and respiratory systems may be present. This is more common in acidosis than alkalosis. If both PCO$_2$ and HCO$_3^-$ are abnormal, consider the patient's history to determine which problem came first or is more severe.[10]

4. **Assess the compensation status.** When the pH is abnormal, with one of the acid-base components (PCO$_2$/HCO$_3^-$) being abnormal and the other normal, the gas is said to be uncompensated.[1] When both acid-base parameters are abnormal in opposite directions, the body is beginning to compensate for the primary abnormality. When the pH reaches the normal range, the gas is compensated.

   When the pH is normal and respiratory and metabolic parameters are abnormal in opposite directions (e.g., one is acidotic and one alkalotic), it may be unclear which is the primary abnormality. Because the body does not normally compensate beyond the minimum acceptable pH, the pH usually leans in the direction of the primary problem. A pH of <7.4 in a compensated gas would result from a primary acidosis with an alkalotic compensation, and a pH >7.4 would result from a primary alkalosis with an acidotic compensation.[1] Table 8-6 outlines the common findings in compensated gases.

5. **Complete the acid-base classification.** Add the information from the blood gas analysis to the clinical assessment of the infant's con-dition and knowledge of the pathophysiology of the infant's disease process to determine a course of action. Remember, a gas that is abnormal on paper may be quite acceptable given the infant's gestational age or disease process. For example, a pH as low as 7.25 may be considered acceptable in a preterm infant. A pH of 7.50 may be desirable if a term infant has persistent pulmonary hypertension of the newborn (PPHN).

6. **Evaluate the oxygenation.** Three pieces of information are routinely used to determine oxygenation: PaO$_2$, oxygen saturation, and the presence of cyanosis. The arterial blood gas value provides information about the pulmonary component of oxygenation, specifically the PaO$_2$.

   • **PaO$_2$.** Normal values for PaO$_2$ in the term infant are 50 to 70 mmHg; in the preterm infant, they are 45 to 65 (fetal hemoglobin results in higher saturations at lower oxygen levels).[12]

   Hypoxia (inadequate tissue oxygen supply) may result from a number of factors, including heart failure, anemia, abnormal hemoglobin affinity for oxygen, and a decreased PaO$_2$. Hypoxemia (low PaO$_2$) results from lung disease or cyanotic congenital heart disease.[7] A PaO$_2$ value <45–50 mmHg is associated with vasoconstriction of pulmonary vasculature and vasodilation of the ductus arteriosus.[3] Low PaO$_2$ levels are implicated in the etiology of PPHN. Hyperoxemia (PaO$_2$ >90–100 mmHg) should also be avoided, especially in the preterm infant, in whom high levels of oxygen in the blood are associated with retinal injury.[3,10]

   Note: When interpreting neonatal PaO$_2$ values, identify whether the sample is preductal or postductal in origin. (See Chapter

2 for a discussion of preductal and postductal gases.)

• **Oxygen saturation.** Oxygen saturation levels may be reported as part of an arterial blood gas result, or they may be obtained from an oximeter (Chapter 7). Saturations described as part of the blood gas report may be measured or calculated from a nomogram. Calculated saturations predict saturation based on the pH and PaO_2 and have limited clinical value.[1]

Measured oxygen saturation is usually a good indicator of the arterial oxygen content. Because of the shape of the oxyhemoglobin dissociation curve, saturation is not a good indicator of hyperoxemia or pulmonary deterioration.[1] PaO_2 readings of >100 occur on the flat upper portion of the curve; therefore, there is little change in oxygen saturation. Normal oxygen saturations of 92 to 96 percent will avoid both hypoxemia and hyperoxemia in most (96 percent) infants.[30]

• **Cyanosis.** Peripheral cyanosis is defined as a blue discoloration of the skin. It may be difficult to assess in dark-skinned infants. Central cyanosis is a blue discoloration of mucous membranes.

Cyanosis results from an increased amount of uncombined or desaturated hemoglobin. It is normally seen when the quantity of desaturated hemoglobin in the capillaries exceeds 5 gm/100 ml or 5 gm percent.[1] This corresponds to a PaO_2 of about 40 mmHg. Because cyanosis depends on the quantity of desaturated hemoglobin, an anemic infant may not look cyanotic despite poor PO_2 readings, and an infant with polycythemia may appear cyanotic despite adequate oxygenation because of an increase in total hemoglobin.

7. **Formulate a plan.** Based on the interpretation of blood gas readings achieved in steps 1–6, a plan should be formulated to accomplish the following:

• **Correct acid-base imbalances**. Correction of acid-base imbalances is achieved, where possible, through treatment of the underlying cause.

Respiratory acidosis. Increase alveolar ventilation to remove carbon dioxide by applying nasal continuous positive airway pressure (CPAP) or mechanical ventilation. For infants already on mechanical ventilation, carbon dioxide removal can be facilitated by increasing the rate, peak inspiratory pressure (PIP), or positive end-expiratory pressure (PEEP) (Chapter 5). Sodium bicarbonate is not recommended for treating respiratory acidosis because it reacts with acids to form carbon dioxide.

Respiratory alkalosis. For mechanically ventilated infants, reduce the rate or pressure on the ventilator.

Metabolic acidosis. Where possible, treat the cause of the acidosis (correct hypovolemia, decrease the protein load in total parenteral nutrition). If the acidosis is severe, sodium bicarbonate can be administered at a dose of 2 mEq/kg or according to the following formula:[10]

$$\textit{Base deficit} \times \textit{(weight in kg)} \times \textit{(0.3)}$$

The amount of bicarbonate calculated by this formula should theoretically correct half of the base deficit and should be administered slowly over 30–60 minutes. Fluid replacement may also be of benefit in treating metabolic acidosis by helping the infant metabolize lactic acid.[12]

Note: After fluid replacement, the infant may show a transient deterioration in acid-base status resulting from improved transport of acid from the peripheral to the central circulation.

Metabolic alkalosis. Treat the cause by removing acetate from IV fluids, reducing diuretic doses, and replacing gastrointestinal secretions. Treat hyponatremia, hypokalemia, and hypochloremia.

- **Correct hypoxemia.** Hypoxemia secondary to ventilation-to-perfusion mismatching can be improved by administering supplemental oxygen. In addition, oxygenation can be improved by increasing the mean airway pressure in an infant receiving mechanical ventilation. Chapter 5 contains a discussion of mean airway pressure.

CASE STUDIES

The following case studies illustrate how the steps for interpreting blood gases might be applied in various infants.

CASE 1

An infant born at 34 weeks gestation is two hours old with the following physical findings: respiratory rate 84, heart rate 162, temperature 36.5°C, and grunting with moderate retractions.

Capillary blood gas results are as follows:
- pH   7.30
- PCO_2 56 mmHg
- HCO_3^- 26 mEq/liter
- PO_2 40 mmHg

Using the steps for analysis, one can see the following:
1. The pH is low, indicating acidosis.
2. The PCO_2 is high, indicating a respiratory problem.
3. The metabolic component (HCO_3^-) is normal.
4. No compensation is present (pH is not normal).
5. This is uncompensated respiratory acidosis.
6. Oxygenation is adequate.
7. Treatment should be aimed at improving alveolar ventilation. Depending on the infant's clinical status and chest x-ray find-

ings, treatment could consist of nasal CPAP or intermittent positive pressure ventilation.

CASE 2

A 26-week gestational age infant is receiving total parenteral nutrition with 3 gm/kg of protein and 15 gm/kg of glucose. The infant's urine output is 7 ml/kg/hour, and the weight has dropped 30 gm over the past 24 hours. Capillary refill is sluggish.

Capillary blood gas results are as follows:
- pH   7.27
- PCO_2 36 mmHg
- HCO_3^- 17 mEq/liter
- PO_2 50 mmHg

The steps for analysis indicate the following:
1. The pH is low, indicating acidosis.
2. The respiratory component (PCO_2) is normal.
3. The HCO_3^- is low, indicating a metabolic problem.
4. There is no compensation (pH is not normal).
5. This is uncompensated metabolic acidosis.
6. Oxygenation is adequate.
7. Consider giving volume to help metabolize lactic acids, or reduce the amount of protein in the total parenteral nutrition feedings to lower the metabolic acid load.

CASE 3

A 28-week gestational age infant is receiving mechanical ventilation for respiratory distress syndrome. Settings are rate 40, PIP 18, PEEP +4, fractional concentration of oxygen in inspired gas (FiO_2) 0.50.

Arterial blood gas results are as follows:
- pH   7.48
- $PaCO_2$ 27 mmHg
- HCO_3^- 22 mEq/liter
- PaO_2 95 mmHg

The steps for analysis indicate the following:
1. The pH is high and shows an alkalemia.

2. The PCO_2 is low, indicating respiratory alkalosis.

3. The metabolic component (HCO_3^-) is normal.

4. There is no compensation (pH is not normal).

5. This is uncompensated respiratory alkalosis.

6. The PO_2 is too high.

7. Reduce alveolar ventilation. Assess the infant's chest expansion and spontaneous respirations to determine whether the PIP or the ventilator rate should be lowered. Reduce the FiO_2, ensuring that the oxygen saturation remains within the desired range. Repeat the blood gas analysis after 15–20 minutes.

CASE 4

A three-week-old infant underwent bowel surgery three days ago. On continuous gastric suction, the infant is receiving total parenteral nutrition with sodium and potassium acetate.

Capillary blood gas results are as follows:

- pH   7.51
- PCO_2 43 mmHg
- HCO_3^- 34 mEq/liter
- PO_2 52 mmHg

Analysis indicates the following:

1. The pH is high, showing an alkalemia.

2. The respiratory component (PCO_2) is high normal.

3. The HCO_3^- is high, leading to metabolic alkalosis.

4. There is no compensation.

5. This is uncompensated metabolic alkalosis.

6. The PO_2 is adequate.

7. Consider eliminating the acetate in favor of chloride salts. Ensure that the serum sodium and potassium are adequate.

CASE 5

An infant born at 26 weeks gestation is now three weeks old and receiving mechanical ventilation for chronic lung disease. The infant is on full nasogastric feeds.

Capillary blood gas results are as follows:

- pH   7.37
- PCO_2 49 mmHg
- HCO_3^- 34 mEq/liter
- PO_2 52 mmHg

Analysis indicates the following:

1. The pH is normal.

2. The PCO_2 is high, suggesting respiratory acidosis.

3. The HCO_3^- is high, suggesting a metabolic alkalosis.

4. The pH is normal with abnormal carbon dioxide and HCO_3^-; therefore, there is compensation. The pH is low normal; therefore, it is compensated acidosis. The high HCO_3^- does not fit with acidosis, but the high PCO_2 does.

5. This is compensated respiratory acidosis that fits with the clinical history of chronic lung disease.

6. Oxygen levels are satisfactory.

7. This infant's kidneys have become efficient at conserving bicarbonate and excreting hydrogen ions, so treatment is not necessary. Keep in mind that further changes in the infant's condition (atelectasis, pneumonia, or metabolic causes of acidosis) will likely exceed the infant's ability to compensate and cause acidosis.

CASE 6

A term infant, with Apgars of 4 at one minute and 6 at five minutes and born through thick meconium, is pale, with retractions and grunting respirations. Temperature is 35.8°C.

Capillary blood gas results are as follows:

- pH   7.25
- PCO_2 49 mmHg
- HCO_3^- 16 mEq/liter
- PO_2 35 mmHg

Analysis indicates the following:

1. The pH is low, indicating an acidosis.

2. The PCO_2 is high, suggesting a respiratory acidosis.

3. The HCO_3^- is low, suggesting a metabolic acidosis.

4. No compensation is present.

5. This is a mixed respiratory and metabolic acidosis that is uncompensated.

6. The PO_2 is low.

7. Warm the infant slowly. Improve the alveolar ventilation and provide supplemental oxygen. Do not administer bicarbonate unless ventilation is improved.

SUMMARY

Interpretation of a blood gas requires a systematic approach based on an understanding of the physiology of gas transport and acid-base balance. Such an approach will allow timely and appropriate interventions aimed at providing optimal care for the compromised infant.

REFERENCES

1. Malley WJ. 1990. *Clinical Blood Gases.* Philadelphia: WB Saunders.

2. Shapiro BA, Peruzzi WT, and Kozelowski-Templin R. 1994. *Clinical Application of Blood Gases.* St. Louis: Mosby-Year Book.

3. Hay WW, Thilo E, and Curlander JB. 1991. Pulse oximetry in neonatal medicine. *Clinics in Perinatology* 18(3): 441–471.

4. Delivoria-Papadopoulos M, and Digiacomo JE. 1992. Oxygen transport and delivery. In *Fetal and Neonatal Physiology,* Polin RA, and Fox WW, eds. Philadelphia: WB Saunders, 801–813.

5. Leff A, and Schumacker PT. 1993. *Respiratory Physiology: Basics and Application.* Philadelphia: WB Saunders, 71–81.

6. Martin RW, and McColgin SG. 1990. Evaluation of fetal and neonatal acid-base status. *Obstetrics and Gynecology Clinics of North America* 17(1): 223–233.

7. Parry WH, and O'Rear GA. 1993. Acid-base homeostasis and oxygenation. In *Handbook of Neonatal Intensive Care,* 3rd ed., Merenstein GB, and Gardner SL, eds. St. Louis: Mosby-Year Book, 141–152.

8. Clancy G. 1987. Blood gas monitoring and management of neonates with respiratory distress. *Journal of Perinatal and Neonatal Nursing* 1(1): 72–83.

9. Brenner M, and Welliver J. 1990. Pulmonary acid-base assessment. *Nursing Clinics of North America* 25(4): 761–770.

10. Chatburn RL, and Carlo WA. 1988. Assessment of neonatal gas exchange. In *Neonatal Respiratory Care,* Carlo WA, and Chatburn RL, eds. Chicago: Year Book Medical Publishers, 40–60.

11. Koch G, and Wendel H. 1968. Adjustment of arterial blood gases and acid-base balance in the normal newborn infant during the first week of life. *Biology of the Neonate* 12(3): 136–161.

12. Phillips BL, McQuitty J, and Durand DJ. 1988. Blood gases: Technical aspects and interpretation. In *Assisted Ventilation of the Neonate,* Goldsmith JP, and Karotkin EH, eds. Philadelphia: WB Saunders, 213–232.

13. Koszarek K. 1991. Nursing assessment and care for the neonate in acute respiratory distress. In *Acute Respiratory Care of the Neonate,* Nugent J, ed. Petaluma, California: NICU INK, 59–60.

14. National Committee for Clinical Laboratory Standards. 1985. *Blood Gas Pre-Analytical Considerations: Specimen Collection, Calibration and Controls.* NCCLS Publication C27-P. Villanova, Pennsylvania: National Committee for Clinical Laboratory Standards.

15. Clark SL, and Miller FC. 1984. Scalp blood sampling—FHR patterns tell you when to do it. *Contemporary OB/GYN* 23: 47.

16. Aarnoudse YG, Yspeert-Gerards J, and Huisjes HJ. 1985. Neurological follow-up in infants with severe acidemia. Abstract No 297. Presented at Society for Gynecologic Investigation, Phoenix, Arizona, March. Cited in Martin RW, and McColgin SG. 1990. Evaluation of fetal and neonatal acid-base status. *Obstetrics and Gynecology Clinics of North America* 17(1): 223–233.

17. Mokrohisky ST, Levine RL, and Blumhagen JD. 1978. Low positioning of umbilical arterial catheters increases associated complications in newborn infants. *New England Journal of Medicine* 299(11): 561–564.

18. Harris MS, and Little GA. 1978. Umbilical artery catheters: High low or no. *Journal of Perinatal Medicine* 6(1):15–21.

19. Pierce JR, and Turner BS. 1993. Physiologic monitoring. In *Handbook of Neonatal Intensive Care,* 3rd ed., Merenstein GB, and Gardner SL, eds. St. Louis: Mosby-Year Book, 115–126.

20. Butt WW, et al. 1985. Complications resulting from the use of arterial catheters: Retrograde flow and rapid elevation in blood pressure. *Pediatrics* 76(2): 250–254.

21. Schmidt B, and Zipursky A. 1984. Thrombotic disease in newborn infants. *Clinics in Perinatology* 11(2): 461–488.

22. Cochran WD, Davis HT, and Smith CA. 1968. Advantages and complications of umbilical artery catheterization in the newborn. *Pediatrics* 42(5): 769–777.

23. Goetzman BW, et al. 1975. Thrombotic complications of umbilical artery catheters: A clinical and radiographic study. *Pediatrics* 56(3): 374–379.

24. Barr PA, et al. 1977. Percutaneous peripheral arterial cannulation in the neonate. *Pediatrics* 59 (supplement, 6 part 2): S1058–S1062.

25. Pape KE, Armstrong DL, and Fitzhardinge PM. 1978. Peripheral median nerve damage secondary to brachial arterial blood gas sampling. *Journal of Pediatrics* 93(5): 852–856.

26. Gandy G, et al. 1964. The validity of pH and PCO_2 measurement in capillary samples of sick and healthy newborn infants. *Pediatrics* 34: 192.

27. Bannister A. 1969. Comparison of arterial and arterialized capillary blood in infants with respiratory distress. *Archives of Disease in Childhood* 44: 726.

28. Fan LL, et al. 1980. Potential errors in neonatal blood gas measurements. *Journal of Pediatrics* 97(4): 650–652.

29. Drake MD, Peters J, and Teague R. 1984. The effect of heparin dilution on arterial blood gas analysis. *Western Journal of Medicine* 140(5): 792–793.

30. Blanchette T, Dziodzio J, and Harris K. 1991. Pulse oximetry and normoxemia in neonatal intensive care. *Respiratory Care* 36(1): 25–31.

NOTES

NOTES

9 Surfactant Replacement Therapy

Judith D. Polak, RNC, MSN, NNP
Barbara J. Nightengale, RNC, MSN, NNP

Surfactant replacement therapy, now a standard of care for the treatment of respiratory distress syndrome (RDS), is a true milestone in the progression of neonatal care. Unlike many other neonatal therapies that have been adopted without scientific confirmation, surfactant replacement therapy has been researched for roughly 30 years, since surfactant deficiency was first implicated as the cause of RDS.

This chapter reviews RDS and its relationship to surfactant deficiency. It discusses the biochemistry of natural surfactant and its physiologic properties, highlights the history of surfactant replacement therapy, describes the currently available preparations of surfactant (both those that are FDA approved and those currently under clinical investigation), and outlines recommendations for use and complications of therapy as currently understood. This chapter also discusses surfactant replacement therapy's impact on neonatal nursing.

NATURAL SURFACTANT

COMPOSITION

Surfactant is a complex, multicomponent substance that lines the terminal air spaces in the mature lung. It is synthesized in the highly differentiated Type II alveolar cells and stored in the lamellar bodies of these cells. Natural surfactant is composed of up to 90 percent phospholipids and 10 to 15 percent protein. Also present are some neutral lipids such as cholesterol. Phosphatidylcholine (PC) molecules make up about 80 percent of the surfactant phospholipids, and dipalmitoylphosphatidylcholine (DPPC) makes up about 70–75 percent of the PC fraction.[1] Although DPPC is the most abundant component of natural surfactant, it does not have all the biophysical properties of an active lung surfactant. Another phospholipid—phosphatidylglycerol (PG)—appears late in gestation and has proved useful as a specific marker of the presence of functional lung maturity.[2]

Much of the protein associated with surfactant consists of albumin and at least one unique class of glycoproteins called surfactant apoproteins. The most plentiful, surfactant apoprotein A (SP-A) is present in a ratio of 3 gm protein per 100 gm phospholipid and is synthesized in the Type II cell.[3] A second hydrophilic surfactant apoprotein, apoprotein D (SP-D), is also synthesized in the Type II cell.

TABLE 9-1 ▲ Physiologic Properties of Surfactant

Modifies surface tension
   Increases lung compliance
   Provides alveolar stability
   Allows different-sized alveoli to coexist
   Decreases opening pressure of the alveoli
   Decreases work of breathing
Enhances alveolar fluid clearance
Decreases precapillary tone, preventing vasoconstriction
Protects epithelial cell surface

It differs from SP-A in its interactions with phospholipids.[4] Surfactant apoproteins B (SP-B) and C (SP-C) are small, extremely lipophilic proteins present in a ratio of 1 gm per 100 gm phospholipid and are synthesized in the Type II cell. The synthesis of each apoprotein is developmentally regulated and is glucocorticoid responsive.[5]

METABOLISM

Pulmonary surfactant is synthesized in the Type II cell of the alveolar lining layer. Surfactant apoproteins play several roles in this process. SP-A and SP-B are required for the formation of tubular myelin, the lattice-shaped structure of surfactant necessary for spreadability and adsorption.[6] Surfactant replacement preparations function well physiologically despite their lack of SP-A. Therefore, the formation of tubular myelin may not be absolutely necessary for the function of these therapeutic agents, or there may be sufficient SP-A present even in the very immature lung to obviate the need for an exogenous source.[7]

SP-A apparently also participates in regulation of lung surfactant production. It is an inhibitor of lung surfactant synthesis *in vitro,* and it accelerates uptake of phospholipids into the Type II cell.[8] Surfactant apoprotein D appears to counter the effect of SP-A.[9] Thus, regulation of surfactant secretion responds in part to signals from beneath the alveolar surface layer.

Although SP-B and SP-C comprise less than 1 percent of lung surfactant, these quantitatively minor components play an extremely important role in surfactant function. Specifically, they accelerate the integration of phospholipids from the alveolar subphase into the surface layer.[3] SP-B appears to be more effective in this role than SP-C and also plays a direct role in stabilizing the alveolar surface layer.[10]

PHYSIOLOGIC PROPERTIES

Physiologic properties of surfactant are listed in Table 9-1. The principal function of surfactant is to modify surface tension. Surface tension at the alveolar surface of the lung is created by the greater attractions between liquid molecules than between liquid and gas molecules. These intermolecular force differences result in the fluid assuming a shape that minimizes the amount of surface area in contact with the gas molecules (the beading of a water droplet).

According to Laplace's Law, the pressure within a sphere is directly proportional to the surface tension and inversely proportional to the radius of the curvature. Thus, in a surfactant deficient lung different-sized alveolar sacs would have different pressures, leading to collapse or atelectasis of the smaller airways. This loss of smaller air spaces would reduce the surface area available for gas exchange.[11]

During inspiration, the surfactant is secreted and adsorbs to the water layer that lines the alveoli, becoming the air-liquid interface.[11] During expiration, surfactant lowers surface tension at low lung volumes and, during full inspiration, increases surface tension at high lung volumes.[12] This prevents alveolar collapse at low lung volumes and helps to limit overexpansion of the alveoli at high lung volumes. By modifying surface tension, surfactant (1) increases lung compliance, (2) provides alveolar stability, allowing different sized alveoli to coexist, and (3) decreases the opening pressure of the alveoli.

RESPIRATORY DISTRESS SYNDROME AND SURFACTANT DEFICIENCY

Basically a disease afflicting premature infants, RDS represents a phenomenon of developmental immaturity. The pathophysiology is not completely understood. Respiratory distress syndrome has been characterized as occurring secondary to surfactant deficiency; however, it is a more complex problem than can be explained by this deficiency alone. Rather, RDS represents a combination of (1) anatomic immaturity of the lung parenchyma, capillary endothelium, and the chest wall; (2) a decrease in the total amount of pulmonary surfactant and a qualitative alteration of the surfactant present; (3) the presence of a patent ductus arteriosus (PDA) with a left-to-right systemic-to-pulmonary shunt, resulting in pulmonary overcirculation; and (4) an increase in the interstitial and alveolar lung water.[13]

Surfactant deficiency does play a primary role in the pathogenesis of this disease. In general, the deficiency of surfactant leads to alveolar collapse, progressive atelectasis, and poor lung compliance. The clearance of pulmonary interstitial fluid is diminished because of alveolar collapse and increased surface tension.

Along with the quantitative deficiency of surfactant, there is an infiltration of protein-rich material—largely composed of fibrin and other plasma proteins—into the alveoli (hyaline membranes).[1] This material may trap or inactivate the surfactant that is present. Hypoxemia and hypercarbia develop, leading to the clinical manifestation of cyanosis and subsequent respiratory and metabolic acidosis. Without proper intervention, there continues to be a worsening cycle of events.

SURFACTANT REPLACEMENT THERAPY

HISTORY

In 1959, Avery and Mead discovered that saline lavaged from the lungs of infants who died from RDS had very high surface tension properties. Since these initial observations, RDS has been considered to result primarily from surfactant deficiency.[14] Subsequently, Klaus, Clements, and Havel identified DPPC as the principal surface-active component of surfactant, and Adams and coworkers showed that infants with RDS were deficient in quantity of surfactant.[15,16] Since that time, much of the research has centered around the pathophysiology of surfactant deficiency, identification of infants at risk, and replacement of the deficient surfactant.

Early attempts at surfactant component replacement met with little success. Dipalmitoylphosphatidylcholine, aerosolized into the trachea, could not adequately reach the distal alveoli or effectively alter the alveolar surface tension.[17,18] However, during the 1970s, using animal models, a sound experimental basis for the concept that RDS could be treated with exogenously administered surfactant was developed.[19–22]

Changes were made in the method of administration (surfactant in liquid suspension instilled as a bolus into the trachea) and the compounds administered (total surfactant rather than components). The results of these studies in animal RDS models were quite promising. These variations dramatically changed the efficacy of surfactant replacement therapy.

TERMINOLOGY

The terminology used to describe various surfactant replacement agents is inconsistent. Today there are four categories of surfactant preparations that have been evaluated for clinical use (Table 9-2).

TABLE 9-2 ▲ Surfactant Replacement Preparations

Type of Surfactant Preparation	Name	Source
Natural surfactants	Human	Recovered from amniotic fluid
	Infasurf	Calf lung extract
	Curosurf	Porcine lung extract
Modified natural surfactants	Survanta	Bovine lung extract "spiked" with DPPC and lipids
Synthetic surfactants	Exosurf Neonatal	DPPC plus hexadecanol and tyloxapol
	ALEC	DPPC and PG
Synthetic biologic surfactants	None at present	Reconstructed *in vitro* from synthesized surfactant components

Natural surfactant, which can be species homologous or heterologous, is surfactant that is recovered from fresh alveolar washes or from amniotic fluid by centrifugation or filtration procedures. Infasurf is prepared by extraction of lavage fluid from calf lungs. It contains the full range of surfactant phospholipids as well as SP-B and SP-C, but SP-A is removed by the extraction process. This preparation has been extensively studied and has been shown to be safe and effective. It remains under investigational protocols in the U.S. At this time, human surfactant is not commercially viable because the treatment of a single infant requires surfactant from the amniotic fluid of ten pregnant mothers at term.

Modified natural surfactants are obtained in the same manner as natural surfactants, followed by a selective addition or removal of compounds, sterilization, and suspension procedures used to restore the desired surface properties.[23] Survanta (Ross Laboratories) is the only modified natural surfactant approved in the U.S. It is made from bovine lung extract that has been supplemented with DPPC and other lipids to improve the characteristics of the natural surfactant.[24] SP-B and SP-C are present, but SP-A is removed by the extraction process. Survanta has undergone extensive clinical testing and has been shown to be clinically effective, reducing mortality and morbidity. FDA approval was granted in 1991.

Synthetic surfactants are made from a mixture of synthetic compounds that may or may not be normal components of natural surfactant. Exosurf Neonatal (Glaxo Wellcome), the first to receive FDA approval in 1990, is considered a synthetic or artifical surfactant, consisting of DPPC as the formulation's major constituent. This has been combined with hexadecanol and tyloxapol. These latter components facilitate rapid spreading at the air-liquid interface and adsorption of the DPPC.[25] There is substantial documentation of the clinical efficacy of this surfactant in terms of reducing both the morbidity and mortality of RDS.

Synthetic biologic surfactants are just beginning to be a possibility. These would be constructed *in vitro* and synthesized using molecular biologic techniques.

CLINICAL TRIALS

There have been two types of clinical trials involving surfactant replacement therapy: (1) rescue treatment, in which surfactant or placebo has been given to infants with documented RDS who have met some type of respiratory or ventilatory criteria and are usually more than two hours of age, and (2) prophylaxis treatment, in which surfactant or placebo has been given within the first few breaths to infants weighing less than a specific amount.

In 1980, Fujiwara and colleagues reported one of the first successful applications of surfactant therapy in amelioration of RDS in humans. Ten consecutive premature infants with severe RDS were treated with surfactant derived from bovine lung reconstituted with DPPC and PG. Within hours of treatment, all infants showed improvement in blood gases, lowered mean airway pressures, and lowered inspired oxygen concentrations. Radiographic changes were quite dramatic: Chest x-rays showed clearing of RDS changes.[26]

Though this was an uncontrolled study with a small sample size, the results were promising. After this success, an effective surfactant that could be produced on a large scale with minimal batch-to-batch variability was developed. It consisted of surfactant extracted from minced bovine lungs that was then "spiked" with DPPC, palmitic acid, and tripalmitin. This modified natural surfactant was designated as "Surfactant TA"; the lyophilized version of this is now known as Survanta. Subsequent trials using Surfactant TA documented similar improvements in oxygenation and reduction in ventilatory support to those reported in the earlier trials.[27,28]

Collaborative, multicenter studies examining the efficacy of Survanta both for the treatment of established RDS and the prevention of the disease have been completed. In 1990, Fujiwara and associates randomized 100 infants with documented RDS and birth weights between 750 gm and 1,750 gm to receive a single dose of either surfactant or air within eight hours of birth. Treatment with surfactant resulted in a significant reduction in the severity of RDS with a concomitant increase in the proportion of neonates with mild disease as measured by fraction of inspired oxygen (FiO_2) and mean airway pressure. Complications of RDS, including pulmonary air leaks, intracranial hemorrhage, and bronchopulmonary dysplasia (BPD) were also significantly decreased.[29]

Gunkel and collaborators reported the results of the prevention and rescue multidosing trials in which 770 infants with birth weights between 600 gm and 1,750 gm were randomized to receive either surfactant (Survanta) or air within 6 hours of birth. From 6 hours after the first dose through 48 hours of age, the infants received up to three additional treatments no more frequently than every 6 hours if they remained intubated, had radiographic evidence of RDS, and required $FiO_2 \geq 0.30$ to produce a $PaO_2 \leq 80$ mmHg. These trials demonstrated a reduced incidence of RDS as well as reduced mortality. There was also a significant improvement in arterial:alveolar oxygen tension ratio, and reduction in FiO_2 requirements, and mean airway pressure at 1, 6, and 72 hours.[30]

As with Survanta, Exosurf has undergone collaborative, controlled, multicenter studies examining its effectiveness in prevention of RDS and treatment of the established disease. The first multicenter study demonstrated significant improvement in the mortality and morbidity associated with RDS.

Bose and associates randomized 385 infants with birth weights between 700 gm and 1,750 gm to receive either Exosurf or air soon after delivery. The incidence of RDS was unchanged by treatment with Exosurf, but the severity of the disease was decreased, as evidenced by the treated infants requiring less oxygen and lower mean airway pressure during the first three days of life than the controls. Other complications associated with prematurity and RDS such as intraventricular hemorrhage, necrotizing enterocolitis, and sepsis were unchanged. Among the treated infants, there was a significant reduction in the combined outcome of neonatal death or survival with BPD and a significant enhancement of survival without BPD.[31]

Two large multidose trials have been reported. One study included infants whose birth weights ranged from 700 gm to 1,350 gm; the other included only infants whose birth weight exceeded 1,250 gm. Mortality from RDS was significantly reduced in both studies. The data also demonstrated an approximate 50 percent reduction in mortality from any cause at 28 days. In addition, there was a significant decrease in the incidence of pneumothorax and other forms of pulmonary air leak and, in those infants weighing 1,250 gm or more, a 50 percent reduction in the occurrence of BPD. There were also decreases in many of the nonpulmonary complications associated with prematurity.[32,33]

Three controlled, randomized clinical trials reported success with the use of calf lung surfactant extract, now marketed as Infasurf. Enhorning and colleagues randomized 72 infants of less than 30 weeks gestation to receive either surfactant or air as soon as possible after delivery. Efficacy of treatment was evaluated by the ventilatory requirements and the blood gas values of the two groups of infants for the initial 72 hours after birth. Surfactant treatment resulted in significant decreases in the amount of ventilation and oxygen required by the treated infants relative to the controls at all times. Clinical and radiologic scores of incidence and severity of disease also showed significant decreases with surfactant treatment.[34]

Two smaller trials using essentially the same surfactant administered in the delivery room to infants of less than 29 weeks gestation showed significant decreases in respiratory distress. Kwong and coworkers randomized 27 infants who had not been exposed to corticosteroids before birth. The surfactant treatment significantly decreased ventilatory requirements, oxygen need, and the frequency of diagnosis of RDS.[35]

The second study, by Shapiro and associates, randomized 32 infants in the delivery room. Though no actual respiratory variables or blood gas values were reported, the surfactant treat-ment did decrease the incidence and severity of RDS at 12 and 24 hours after birth as evaluated by a scoring system.[36]

In another study, Shapiro demonstrated that significantly improved results could be obtained if multiple-dose therapy was used in infants who met specific clinical respiratory criteria. Multidose therapy showed an improvement in survival in infants between 24 and 29 weeks gestation.[37]

Using calf lung surfactant extract, Kendig and colleagues studied 479 infants born at 30 weeks gestation or less. Infants were randomly assigned to prophylactic or rescue therapy. Rescue therapy was given if RDS developed and certain respiratory criteria were met. Prophylactic therapy was found to be superior to rescue therapy in many ways. Infants receiving prophylactic surfactant showed significantly improved oxygenation and a reduced need for ventilatory support for 72 hours. There was also a significant reduction in pulmonary air leaks and mortality in the prophylactic group, particularly among those infants less than 26 weeks gestation.[38] Infasurf is currently undergoing multicenter, controlled studies.

It is difficult to compare the previous studies' results because the treatment variables, populations, and surfactant preparations were different. There are several direct comparison trials under way at the present time. The results of the clinical studies generally have shown that although surfactant replacement therapy is not a cure-all, it does increase survival. There is a reduction of time on ventilatory support as well as a reduction in the incidence of pulmonary air leaks. Also, at least in the larger infant, there is a reduction in the incidence of chronic lung disease.[29,32]

COMPLICATIONS

Adverse effects of surfactant therapy can be divided into those that occur acutely during administration of the drug and those that may

TABLE 9-3 ▲ Complications of Surfactant Replacement Therapy

Increased incidence of hemodynamically significant patent ductus arteriosus

Pulmonary hemorrhage

Apnea

Plugging of endotracheal tube

Sepsis

Intradosing effects

    Reflux into endotracheal tube

    Desaturations

    Bradycardia

be related to the effects of the drug (Table 9-3). The adverse effects occurring during administration are discussed later in this chapter.

Early reports in the literature described an increased incidence of PDA in babies who received surfactant replacement therapy. The Oxford Perinatal Database continues to support this observation.[39]

A recent study, however, does not support these findings. Reller and associates routinely performed serial echocardiograms on all infants participating in a controlled trial of surfactant replacement therapy. The incidence of a PDA and the timing of ductal closure were about the same in surfactant-treated and control infants.[40] It can be speculated that significant improvement in lung compliance with surfactant therapy makes the PDA clinically apparent.

Pulmonary hemorrhage has been another reported complication. Although 1–6 percent of surfactant-treated infants develop pulmonary hemorrhage, these are generally very small infants (weighing less than 700 gm) with a PDA.[24,25] Early detection and treatment of a PDA should be considered.

Exosurf Neonatal has in some studies, but not others, been associated with a modest increase in apnea of prematurity.[25] The development of apnea following surfactant replacement therapy has been termed a "marker of health." For apnea to be detected, the infant must be extubated or on low ventilator settings.

There has been evidence of a slight increase in mucus plugging of the endotracheal tube following surfactant administration.[24,25] It is not clear whether surfactant replacement therapy increases the likelihood of mucus plugging; however, it is possible that because of the mucolytic effect of surfactants, secretions may be mobilized and obstruct the tube following dosing. Clinicians using surfactant have found that suctioning before dosing decreases this incidence. If plugging should occur, replacement of the endotracheal tube may be necessary.

Both Exosurf Neonatal and Survanta have, in some studies but not others, been associated with an increase in the incidence of sepsis or nonserious nosocomial infections.[24,25] These authors' experiences have shown that as the smaller infants live longer, the likelihood of sepsis increases. This increased incidence of sepsis might result from saving or prolonging the lives of smaller infants who presumably require invasive management and have immature immune systems.

RECOMMENDATIONS FOR USE

TREATMENT CRITERIA

Surfactant replacement is recommended for use in both the prevention and treatment of RDS. Prophylaxis or prevention involves the administration of surfactant at the time of delivery, immediately following resuscitation—usually within the first 15 minutes of life. This method of treatment occurs before the onset of symptoms and is the treatment of choice in many institutions for infants who are delivered prior to 30 weeks gestation, weigh less than 1,100 gm, or have proven pulmonary immaturity (via amniotic fluid sampling).

Prophylactic treatment potentially may overtreat a population of infants who would not develop RDS, but the benefits of treatment are proven to outweigh the risks—especially in the extremely low birth weight infant.

Immediate instillation of surfactant via the endotracheal tube after delivery is the ideal method for distribution of the drug into the lungs.

Rescue treatment is the administration of surfactant to infants who require mechanical ventilation and have respiratory distress not inconsistent with RDS clinically or radiologically. Treatment is recommended as soon as possible after the onset of clinical symptoms and intubation.[24,25]

The criteria for retreatment and the optimum total number of doses remain controversial. Although routine retreatment regimes were built into some protocols, only a few studies have addressed the necessity of retreatment because of persisting or worsening disease after initial surfactant treatment. These studies suggest that a single dose of surfactant may be insufficient in many cases and that babies who relapse may benefit from multiple doses.[38,41–43]

On the other hand, in a study of infants weighing 600–1,700 gm, Blackwell, Noguchi, and Devaskar found no additional benefit in the oxygen index, which was measured six hours after a third or fourth dose of Survanta, 4 ml/kg. In infants weighing <1,000 gm, an increase in FiO_2 requirements beginning on day 10 was associated with administration of four doses, but not with administration of fewer than four doses.[44]

Armsby and coworkers found that lung compliance may increase earlier with the administration of four doses of Exosurf, 5 ml/kg, at 6-hour minimal intervals for up to 48 hours as compared with two doses at a 12-hour interval. The number of days intubated and FiO_2, however, were not significantly different between the two groups.[45] Measurement of lung compliance alone appears to be an incomplete assessment of the effectiveness of additional doses of surfactant.

The need for repeated administration of surfactant should be determined by continuing evidence of respiratory distress. Infants receiving Survanta should be considered for repeat dosing no sooner than 6 hours after the preceding dose. Infants receiving Exosurf Neonatal should be assessed at 6- to 12-hour intervals. The infant's oxygen requirement, ventilator settings, and entire clinical status should be evaluated in the decision to redose. The commercial preparation, type of treatment, and decision to repeat doses should be made only by a clinician skilled in the care of infants with RDS.

ADMINISTRATION GUIDELINES

Current surfactant replacement therapy requires that the infant be intubated and the drug given as a liquid bolus into the upper airway. The volume of the bolus is divided into aliquots and each portion given with the infant's body in a different position to enhance even distribution of the drug throughout the lungs.

Each manufacturer developed a technique for instillation used during the FDA trials for drug efficacy and safety. To date, there has been little research on the actual techniques used for instillation. The package insert accompanying each drug provides instructions for use, preparation of the product, and administration. Instructional material and videotapes demonstrating the method of administration are available from the product manufacturers.

Exosurf Neonatal is supplied as a sterile, lyophilized powder that can be stored at room temperature. The recommended shelf life is two years. The powder is reconstituted with 8 ml of sterile water prior to dosing. Once reconstituted, Exosurf Neonatal is chemically and physically stable for up to 12 hours at room temperature, but the vial should not be reentered. The dose is 5 ml/kg, based on the infant's birth weight. Various sized Luer-Lok, side-port adapters are supplied with this surfactant and used for administration.

Exosurf Neonatal is administered through the side-port adapter, so there is no interruption of ventilation. Beginning with the infant in midline position, the volume of drug administered is two 2.5 ml/kg aliquots slowly, in small pulses, timed with inspiration. The infant is turned 45 degrees to the right for 30 seconds after the first aliquot is instilled, then to the midline position for the second aliquot, and finally repositioned to the left 45 degrees for 30 seconds after the second aliquot is instilled.

Survanta is supplied as a liquid suspension and must be refrigerated at between 2° and 8°C. The current recommended shelf life is one year. Before administration, the drug must be warmed at room temperature for at least 20 minutes or warmed in the hand for at least 8 minutes. Survanta should not be out of refrigeration for more than eight hours. Once warmed, unused, unopened vials of the drug may be returned to refrigeration within eight hours and subsequently rewarmed for use; however, the drug should not be warmed and returned to refrigeration more than once. Re-entry of the vial is not recommended.

The dose of Survanta is 4 ml/kg, based on birth weight. Survanta is instilled in four equal aliquots via a precut #5 French end-hole catheter inserted into the endotracheal tube, with the tip just beyond the end of the tube. Each quarter-dose is instilled with the infant in a different position to ensure homogenous distribution throughout the lungs. Ventilation is discontinued briefly during instillation of each aliquot.

Infasurf is currently an experimental drug. It may be used only under approved protocols. Infasurf is supplied as a liquid suspension and must be refrigerated at between 2° and 8°C. It has been administered at temperatures from 2°C to ambient room temperature. It may be warmed in the hand or at room temperature prior to use. Unopened, unused vials may be returned to the refrigerator for future use. The time of nonrefrigeration should not exceed 24 hours.

The dose of Infasurf is 3 ml/kg based on birth weight. It is an unstable suspension, and settling during storage will occur. Infasurf should be resuspended by a gentle wrist action swirl and/or vial inversion.

For prophylaxis treatment, Infasurf is instilled as a single bolus via a precut #5 French end-hole catheter inserted into the endotracheal tube, with the tip 1 cm shorter than the tube. For rescue treatment, it is instilled in four equal aliquots via a #5 French catheter precut in the same manner. Each quarter-dose is instilled with the infant in a different position to ensure homogenous distribution throughout the lungs. Ventilation is discontinued briefly during instillation of each aliquot.

A standard method of administration has not been established for surfactant therapy in general. The composition of the various products may require a specific technique to assure even distribution into the lungs. Future research will need to address these issues.

NURSING IMPLICATIONS

ADMINISTRATION OF SURFACTANT

Administration of surfactant therapy should be done by a clinician skilled in the respiratory management of premature infants. Preferably, two health care professionals—nurses, physicians, or respiratory therapists—should be present when the surfactant is instilled. Responsibilities include instillation of the surfactant, intervention in response to adverse reactions, and assessment and documentation of response to therapy.

Care that there is proper positioning (placement) of the endotracheal tube, enabling an even distribution of the drug, needs to be taken prior to administration of the surfactant. The tube should be in the trachea, slightly above the carina, and not in the right or left mainstem bronchus. Breath sounds should be equal and chest movements symmetrical with ventilation. Auscultation can be used to confirm endotracheal tube placement, but at least one chest x-ray examination should be done to confirm proper placement of the tube prior to future dosing.

Airway patency should be assessed and suctioning done prior to dosing (at the discretion of the clinician). To prevent evacuation of the drug, avoid suctioning for at least two hours postadministration unless it is clinically necessary.

Constant monitoring and assessment should occur prior to, during, and after administration of surfactant. Continuous heart rate and oxygen saturation monitoring is essential. The instillation of surfactant can be stressful to infants. Adverse reactions have been noted, the most common being a drop in oxygen saturation and/or bradycardia.[24,25] This is especially true if the infant is on low ventilator settings or requires minimal manual ventilation.

These adverse reactions are usually transient and can be overcome by increasing the FiO_2 or the peak inspiratory pressure. For infants receiving an initial rescue dose or a repeat dose, it is suggested that the ventilator rate be 35 breaths per minute or greater during the instillation procedure. During administration, ventilation should be adjusted at the discretion of the clinician to maintain oxygenation and ventilation. Ventilator settings can usually be returned to prior levels once dosing is complete.

Reflux of the drug into the endotracheal tube may occur. Slowing administration or increasing the ventilator rate should alleviate this. Reflux into the nasopharynx or oropharynx may affect how much of the prescribed amount reaches the lungs. If this occurs, dosing should be suspended and the airway checked for position and patency. It may be necessary to

FIGURE 9-1 ▲ Dosing record.

Patient:		Birth Weight	
Dose: 1 2 3 4		Prophylaxis	Rescue
Drug:			
ETT placement:		X-ray	Auscultation
Chest wall expansion:		Minimal	Good
Suctioned:	Yes	No	Time:
Ventilator:	Prior	During	Post
FiO_2			
PIP			
PEEP			
Rate			
$P\overline{aw}$			
Heart rate			
O_2 saturation			
Adverse reactions			
Bradycardia ≤80			
Desaturation ≥20 percent			
Intervention			
ABG postinstillation			

reposition the tube or reintubate the infant before dosing can resume.

After administration is completed, constant bedside attention is still required. Treatment with surfactant may result in rapid improvement in pulmonary compliance. The infant's color, oxygen saturation, and chest expansion may show dramatic improvement, requiring the ventilator setting to be decreased immediately to prevent overdistention of the lung and the occurrence of pulmonary air leaks. Vital signs should be monitored and blood gases obtained to assess adequate gas exchange.

Vigilant attention before, during, and after surfactant administration must be maintained to avoid any of these adverse reactions. Documentation should detail the treatment, responses to treatment, and any necessary intervention. Figure 9-1 provides an example of a detailed dosing record to be kept at the bedside or placed in the infant's chart.

IMPACT ON STAFFING PATTERNS

A key factor in addressing the quality of care of the premature infant is the nurse-to-patient ratio. In most institutions, the NICU policy is to have a nurse:patient ratio of one to two or even one to one if ventilation is required. When infants are not ventilated, the ratio may be one nurse to four or more infants. Because of surfactant therapy, many infants—including those weighing <1,000 gm—now come off the ventilator earlier, so there may be greater use of convalescent beds. This can lead to a situation in which traditional staffing patterns may be unsafe because they do not reflect the actual acuity of the infants.

Because there is a high degree of judgment, monitoring, and skill involved in caring for very small, high-risk infants, the nurse:patient ratio should not be determined by traditional markers of neonatal acuity alone. Optimal ratios in these new circumstances will take time to establish. Nursing administration should collaborate with the nursing and medical staffs to define patient acuity systems that meet patient care needs and provide adequate staffing.

REDEFINING CARE OF THE VERY LOW BIRTH WEIGHT INFANT

Although surfactant replacement therapy has improved survival rates of infants with RDS and decreased ventilatory support and its associated complications, this therapy does not cure prematurity. Other problems associated with prematurity remain. As the respiratory status of infants improves, nursing will continue to focus on the developmental aspects of care and provide a nurturing environment that will meet the needs of growing premature infants, enabling them to develop and grow to their optimal potential. Invasive and intensive care may be replaced with kinder and gentler care.

With the decreased need for ventilatory support, apnea of prematurity may increase. Monitoring and treatment of apnea must therefore be improved as necessary. Acceptance of some apnea may be required. Populations of smaller infants with prolonged hospitalizations may

also increase the risk of nosocomial infections. Nursing staff must be alert to prevent incidental contact in order to decrease this risk.

Nutritional aspects of care must also be evaluated. In the case of very low birth weight infants, poor digestive tract function makes it difficult to achieve adequate caloric intake needed for growth. Initiation of enteral feedings and timing of increase to full feedings vary in different units, depending on the size of the infant, the level of respiratory support, and the severity of illness. Surfactant therapy will impact future feeding methods. Parenteral feedings and methods of enteral feedings must be improved to provide sustenance for growth and to decrease nutritional complications.

As the care of the very low birth weight infant is redesigned, the nurse must also continue to meet the needs of the family. Education of the family regarding surfactant replacement therapy and its possible outcomes is essential. Parents will need to understand the continuing care needed for the infant once the respiratory component of prematurity is resolved. It is often very frustrating for parents to watch their infant "hurry up and grow." As early as possible, parents should be educated in the care of the premature infant to ease anxiety and to facilitate discharge.

On a larger scale, the neonatal health care team must also meet the needs of society. With less time on ventilatory support, the cost of hospitalization should be decreased for more mature infants. However, increased rates of survival among very low birth weight infants should increase the overall cost of caring for this specific group. In 1990, Tubman, Halliday, and Normand examined this issue and found that the costs per extra survivor in the treated group (the estimated cost per quality adjusted life year) are comparable to those of other established treatments in adults. They concluded that surfactant replacement therapy is therefore "fairly inexpensive and cost effective."[46]

Treatment of all babies less than 31 weeks gestation would increase overall net costs for newborn intensive care but would decrease costs per survivor.[47,48] This is not to suggest that all infants weighing under 600 gm should be treated. As providers and consumers face the future of health care, ethical considerations concerning treatment, survival, cost, and outcome of the premature infant must be addressed. The impact of surfactant replacement therapy will be examined as the future of health care evolves.

FUTURE CONSIDERATIONS

Surfactant replacement therapy is a welcome addition to the complex care of premature infants with RDS. Though it cannot solve all the problems of prematurity, it has simplified overall care by dramatically improving respiratory status and decreasing the need for ventilatory support.

However, surfactant replacement therapy is still relatively new, and there is much ongoing research to determine how to optimize its therapeutic effect. The optimal dose and frequency of dosing has yet to be determined. The current surfactant preparations must be viewed as first-generation drugs. The optimal surfactant preparation would need to include not only the phospholipid components, but all the apoproteins as well. The absence or the low amount of the proteins in current preparations may account for the failure of some infants to respond to surfactant.

Future preparations will most likely contain human surfactant proteins produced by recombinant DNA technology. This may protect against inhibition of surfactant by protein in pulmonary fluid. This approach has the potential to minimize the risk of sensitization while maximizing surfactant function.

Surfactant replacement therapy may be a useful adjunct with other therapies. A national collaborative trial studying the use of maternal corticosteroids given prenatally to prevent RDS found that there was a modest decrease in the incidence of the disease.[49] The combined use of prenatal steroids and postnatal surfactant therapy might ultimately be shown to provide the optimal outcome for the premature infant with RDS. Data from 1989 suggest that prenatal steroid treatment should and does improve pulmonary responses to lung surfactant in animals.[50]

Surfactant replacement therapy for the prevention and treatment of RDS may be only the tip of the iceberg. There has been some suggestion that surfactant may be useful in the treatment of lung injury accompanying nonRDS disease processes such as meconium aspiration, congenital pneumonia, asphyxia, and persistent pulmonary hypertension.[51] Experiential data have also shown surfactant to be a useful ventilatory adjunct for infants with these conditions.

Although the mechanism in each of these disease processes may be a little different, they all involve surfactant deficiency caused by damaged Type II cells. Surfactant administration will not cure the primary problem, but it may reduce the ventilatory requirements as the infant's primary problem is being treated. Surfactant treatment for nonRDS conditions should be investigated in multicenter trials before it is generally recommended.

As the natural course of RDS has changed with the advent of surfactant replacement, so has the style of ventilation. Surfactant has minimized the level of support needed regardless of the style of ventilation selected. It is possible that a particular ventilatory strategy will prove superior in surfactant-treated infants because of the possible effect of ventilation on lung volumes and/or surfactant metabolism and function. Although studies of clinical surfactant replacement and style of ventilation are now independent, they may be superimposed in the future. For the present, ventilator management will remain a bedside clinical skill.

SUMMARY

The success of surfactant replacement therapy in the treatment of infants with RDS in large clinical trials has led to its widespread acceptance in the field of neonatology. Although in its infancy, it has become a standard of care for the treatment of RDS. In spite of improved outcomes in premature infants resulting from surfactant replacement therapy, such infants are still at risk for other complications of prematurity. Nurses must understand the risks and benefits of surfactant replacement therapy not only to provide adequate daily care to the infants, but also to anticipate changes in neonatal nursing and to adapt care practices as needed.

REFERENCES

1. Robertson B. 1984. Pathology and pathophysiology of neonatal surfactant deficiency in pulmonary surfactant. In *Pulmonary Surfactant,* Robertson B, Van Golde LMG, and Batenburg JJ, eds. Amsterdam: Elsevier, 383–418.

2. Kulovich MV, Hallman MB, and Gluck L. 1979. The lung profile: Normal pregnancy. *American Journal of Obstetrics and Gynecology* 135(1): 57–64.

3. Hawgood S, and Clements JA. 1990. Pulmonary surfactant and its apoproteins. *Journal of Clinical Investigation* 86(1): 1–6.

4. Possmayer F. 1990. The role of surfactant-associated proteins. *American Review of Respiratory Disease* 142(4): 749–752.

5. Phelps DS, and Floros J. 1988. Localization of surfactant protein synthesis in human lung by *in situ* hybridization. *American Review of Respiratory Disease* 137(4): 939–942.

6. Suzuki Y, Fuita Y, and Kogishi K. 1989. Reconstitution of tubular myelin from synthetic lipids and proteins associated with pig pulmonary surfactant. *American Review of Respiratory Disease* 140(1): 75–81.

7. Coulter DM. 1993. The current status of replacement therapy with exogenous pulmonary surfactant for hyaline membrane disease. *Neonatal Pharmacology Quarterly* 1(1): 5–8.

8. Stevens PA, Wright JR, and Clements JA. 1989. Surfactant secretion and clearance in the newborn. *Journal of Applied Physiology* 67(4): 1597–1605.

9. Kuroki Y. 1991. Surfactant protein D (SP-D) counters the inhibitory effect of surfactant protein A (SP-A) on phospholipid secretion by alveolar Type II cells. *Biochemical Journal* 279(1): 115–119.

10. Cochrane CG, and Revak SD. 1991. Pulmonary surfactant protein B (SP-B): Structure-function relationships. *Science* 254(5031): 566–568.

11. Jobe A. 1988. Metabolism of endogenous surfactant therapy and exogenous surfactants for replacement therapy. *Seminars in Perinatology* 12(3): 231–244.

12. Gluck L. 1978. Fetal lung development. In *The Surfactant System and the Neonatal Lung,* vol. 14, Bloom RS, Sinclair JC, and Warsaw JB, eds. Evansville, Indiana: Mead Johnson, 40–51.

13. Mannino FL, and Merritt TA. 1986. The management of respiratory distress syndrome. In *Neonatal Pulmonary Care,* Thibeault DW, and Gregory GA, eds. Norwalk, Connecticut: Appleton & Lange, 427–457.

14. Avery ME, and Mead J. 1959. Surfactant properties in relation to atelectasis and hyaline membrane disease. *American Journal of Diseases of Children* 97(5): 517–523.

15. Klaus MH, Clements J, and Havel RJ. 1961. Composition of surface-active material isolated from beef lungs. *Proceedings of the National Academy of Sciences of the United States of America* 47(11): 1858–1859.

16. Adams FH, et al. 1965. Surface properties and lipids from lungs of infants with hyaline membrane disease. *Journal of Pediatrics* 66(2): 357–364.

17. Chu J, et al. 1967. Neonatal pulmonary ischemia: Clinical and physiological studies. *Pediatrics* 40(4): 709–728.

18. Robillard E, et al. 1964. Microaerosol administration of synthetic dipalmitoyl-lecithin in respiratory distress syndrome: A preliminary report. *Canadian Medical Association Journal* 90(1): 55–57.

19. Enhorning G, Grossman G, and Robertson B. 1973. Tracheal deposition of surfactant before the first breath. *American Review of Respiratory Disease* 107(6): 921–927.

20. Enhorning G, et al. 1978. Improved ventilation of prematurely delivered primates following tracheal deposition of surfactant. *American Journal of Obstetrics and Gynecology* 132(5): 529–536.

21. Enhorning G, and Robertson B. 1972. Lung expansion of the premature rabbit fetus after tracheal deposition of surfactant. *Pediatrics* 50(1): 58–66.

22. Enhorning G, et al. 1975. Radiologic evaluation of the premature newborn rabbit after pharyngeal deposition of surfactant. *American Journal of Obstetrics and Gynecology* 121(4): 475–480.

23. Taeusch WH, et al. 1986. Characterization of bovine surfactant for infants with respiratory distress syndrome. *Pediatrics* 77(4): 572–581.

24. Ross Laboratories. 1991. *Neonatal Respiratory Distress Syndrome: Survanta Beractant Intratracheal Suspension.* Columbus, Ohio: Ross Laboratories, 1–42.

25. Burroughs Wellcome Company. 1990. Synthetic surfactant for the treatment of respiratory distress syndrome. In *Product Monograph.* Research Triangle Park, North Carolina: Burroughs Wellcome, 1–43.

26. Fujiwara T, et al. 1980. Artifical surfactant therapy in hyaline membrane disease. *Lancet* 1(8159): 55–59.

27. Fujiwara T, et al. 1985. Exogenous surfactant therapy in infants with RDS: Comparison of early versus late treatment. *Pediatric Research* 18(4): 353A.

28. Gitlin JD, et al. 1987. Randomized control trial of exogenous surfactant for the treatment of hyaline membrane disease. *Pediatrics* 79(1): 31–37.

29. Fujiwara T, et al. 1990. Surfactant replacement therapy with a single postventilatory dose of a reconstituted bovine surfactant in preterm neonates with respiratory distress syndrome: Final analysis of a multicenter, double-blind, randomized trial and comparison with similar trials. *Pediatrics* 86(5): 753–764.

30. Gunkel JH, et al. 1990. A summary of clinical experience with Survanta. In *Proceedings of the Ross Laboratories Special Conference: Hot Topics '90 in Neonatology,* Lucey JF, chair. Columbus, Ohio: Ross Laboratories, 182–204.

31. Bose C, et al. 1990. Improved outcome at 28 days of age for very low birth weight infants treated with a single dose of synthetic surfactant. *Journal of Pediatrics* 117(6): 947–953.

32. Long W, et al. 1991. Effects of two rescue doses of a synthetic surfactant on mortality rate and survival without bronchopulmonary dysplasia in 700 to 1,350 gm infants with respiratory distress syndrome. *Journal of Pediatrics* 118(4): 595–605.

33. Long W, et al. 1991. A controlled trial of synthetic surfactant in infants weighing 1,250 gm or more with respiratory distress syndrome. *New England Journal of Medicine* 325(24): 1696–1703.

34. Enhorning G, et al. 1985. Prevention of neonatal respiratory distress syndrome by tracheal instillation of surfactant: A randomized clinical trial. *Pediatrics* 76(2): 145–153.

35. Kwong MS, et al. 1985. Double-blind clinical trial of calf lung surfactant extract for prevention of hyaline membrane disease in extremely premature infants. *Pediatrics* 76(4): 585–592.

36. Shapiro DL, et al. 1985. Double-blind, randomized trial of a calf lung surfactant extract administered at birth to very premature infants for the prevention of respiratory distress syndrome. *Pediatrics* 76(4): 593–599.

37. Shapiro DL. 1990. Surfactant replacement therapy. In *Current Therapy in Neonatal-Perinatal Medicine,* Nelson NM, ed. Philadelphia: BC Decker, 477–480.

38. Kendig JW, et al. 1991. A comparison of surfactant as immediate prophylaxis and as rescue therapy in newborns of less than 30 weeks gestation. *New England Journal of Medicine* 324(13): 865–871.

39. Halliday HL. 1991. Surfactant replacement. In *Yearbook of Neonatal and Perinatal Medicine,* Klaus MH, and Fanaroff AA, eds. St. Louis: Mosby-Year Book, 57–66.

40. Reller MD, et al. 1991. Ductal patency in neonates with respiratory distress syndrome. *American Journal of Diseases of Children* 145(8): 1017–1020.

41. Collaborative European Multicenter Study Group. 1992. Randomized European multicenter trial of surfactant replacement therapy for severe neonatal respiratory distress syndrome: Single versus multiple doses of Curosurf. *Pediatrics* 89(1): 13–20.

42. Corbet A. 1992. Prophylaxis versus rescue surfactant: How many doses and at what interval? In *Proceedings of the Exosurf Neonatal Investigators Meeting,* Long WA, and Tilson HH, eds. Langhorne, Pennsylvania: Adis International, 1–57.

43. Hoekstra RE, et al. 1991. Improved neonatal survival following multiple doses of bovine surfactant in very premature neonates at risk for respiratory distress syndrome. *Pediatrics* 88(1): 10–18.

44. Blackwell M, Noguchi A, and Devaskar U. 1992. How many doses for optimal multi-dose surfactant rescue therapy? *Pediatric Research* 31(4): 196A.

45. Armsby H, et al. 1992. Effect of two vs four doses of Exosurf on respiratory system static lung compliance in preterm infants. *Pediatric Research* 31(4): 299A.

46. Tubman TRJ, Halliday H, and Normand C. 1990. Cost of surfactant replacement treatment for severe neonatal respiratory distress syndrome: A randomized-controlled trial. *British Medical Journal* 301(6754): 842–845.

47. Mugford MJ, Piercy J, and Chalmers I. 1991. Cost implications of different approaches to the prevention of respiratory distress syndrome. *Archives of Disease in Childhood* 66(7): 757–764.

48. Maniscalco WM, Kendig JW, and Shapiro DL. 1989. Surfactant replacement therapy: Impact on hospital charges for premature infants with respiratory distress syndrome. *Pediatrics* 83(1): 1–6.

49. National Institutes of Health. 1985. Collaborative group on antenatal steroid therapy, effect of antenatal dexamethasone administration. In *Prevention of Respiratory Distress Syndrome.* Washington, DC: U.S. Government Printing Office, NIH Publication No. 85-2695.

50. Jobe A. 1989. Lung maturational agents and surfactant treatments: Are they complementary in preterm infants? *Journal of Perinatology* 9(1): 14–18.

51. Auten RL, Notter RH, and Kendig JW. 1991. Surfactant treatment of full term newborns with respiratory failure. *Pediatrics* 87(1): 101–107.

NOTES

10 Neonatal Respiratory Pharmacotherapy

Todd L. Wandstrat, PharmD

Neonates, infants, and children have been described as "therapeutic orphans" because of the paucity of clinical trials data and other information concerning neonatal/pediatric drug pharmacotherapy.[1] Few drugs carry federal Food and Drug Administration (FDA) indications for neonatal patients, and clinical trials data are lacking for many medications. In addition to the lack of neonatal pharmacokinetic and pharmacodynamic trial data, drug delivery systems to allow for adequate and dependable delivery of therapeutic agents to this population have only recently been developed.[2]

Monitoring the efficacy of certain medications is further complicated by lack of microassays for drug serum determinations as well as lack of readily available pulmonary function tests. Many medications that may be efficacious in the neonatal patient are not available in suitable dosage forms.[2]

Adult pharmacokinetic and pharmacodynamics studies cannot be used to extrapolate information for the neonatal patient. Neonatal patients are not "small adults"; they require specialized dosing, drug delivery, and monitoring methods to minimize toxicity and maximize efficacy.

NEONATAL PHARMACOKINETICS AND PHARMACODYNAMICS

During the intrauterine period, the fetus undergoes the most rapid development of drug transformation and metabolism pathways that will ever occur. Clinicians who care for premature neonates are faced with a rapidly developing patient whose drug dosing requirements can change daily. An understanding of pharmacokinetics and pharmacodynamics in the neonate is essential for proper drug regimen design.

ABSORPTION

Many factors affect drug absorption from gastrointestinal, intramuscular, and topical sites. These factors are age dependent and can profoundly affect drug concentrations and adversely affect the therapeutic outcomes of drug regimens.

Oral Route

Absorption in the premature and term neonate is affected by gastric pH, gastric motility, and gastric emptying time.[3,4] Drugs will be absorbed from the gastrointestinal tract only if they are nonionized. When gastric pH is low, drugs with a high ionization constant (pKa) (alkaline drugs such as theophylline) will not be absorbed very well because of ionization in the acidic pH of the gut. When little or no gastric acid is present (achlorhydria), the pH of the gut is increased, thereby decreasing absorption of acidic drugs such as phenobarbital.[3] The gastric pH can theoretically play a role in reduction of drug absorption and, hence, reduction in peak drug concentration.

Gastric acid production may begin shortly after birth or may be delayed for 1 to 4 weeks.[5] This relative achlorhydria may theoretically affect drug absorption. In the fetal stomach, gastric acid is rarely present before 32 weeks gestation.[6]

If gastric emptying time is slowed, peak drug concentrations may be reduced as a result of decreased intestinal absorption because of less drug presented to the GI tract per unit time. Peak drug concentrations also may be reduced when intestinal transit time is hastened, because of decreased contact time of the drug with the absorption surface of the intestine.[7] Diseases and factors that can slow gastric emptying time in the neonate include prematurity, gastroesophageal reflux, respiratory distress syndrome, congenital heart disease, and an increased number of long-chain fatty acids.[8–11] Factors that hasten gastric emptying time include human milk and hypocaloric feedings.[11]

The reduced bile salt pool in neonates may reduce the absorption of fat-soluble drugs and nutrients such as vitamins D and E.[12] Theoretically, changes in bacterial flora also may affect drug absorption and metabolism.

Intramuscular Route

Intramuscular administration of some drugs may be a viable option if the intravenous route is not available. Factors affecting the extent of intramuscular absorption of medications include physiochemical factors (drug pH), blood flow at the injection site, and muscular function.[13–15]

Drugs with a pH similar to physiologic pH, such as phenobarbital and benzathine penicillin, are absorbed well from the muscle.[14,15] Drugs with a pH that differs greatly from physiologic pH, such as phenytoin, will precipitate in the muscle and not be absorbed.[13] In general, regardless of the pH of a particular drug, intramuscularly administered drugs have lower peak concentrations than intravenously administered drugs.

Topical Route

The development of the integument system in the neonate proceeds throughout the fetal and neonatal periods. Previous reports have documented inadvertent poisoning in the neonate from topical administration of substances such as hexachlorophene, pentachlorophenol-containing laundry detergents, and aniline-containing disinfectant solutions.[16–18]

Researchers who investigated the possibility of delivering theophylline topically found serum concentrations comparable to orally administered regimens.[19] As the infant matures, the absorption of topically administered drugs is decreased and more erratic, making this route of administration undesirable.

DISTRIBUTION

Distribution is defined as the dynamic movement of a drug in and out of various body compartments: organs, such as the kidney or lung, or tissues, such as adipose or lymph. There are millions of compartments in the body, and, for simplification, distribution of drugs into the body is often said to follow a one- or two-compartment model.

Before distribution takes place, absorption has to occur. Poor vascular perfusion of a tissue or organ can delay distribution of a drug and conceivably reduce peak blood concentrations. Other factors that affect drug distribution include compartment fluid composition and protein binding.[20]

FIGURE 10-1 ▲ Maturation of hepatic metabolism pathways in the neonate and infant.

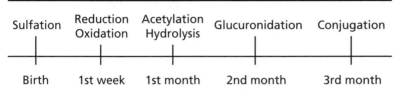

Sulfation	Reduction Oxidation	Acetylation Hydrolysis	Glucuronidation	Conjugation
Birth	1st week	1st month	2nd month	3rd month

Adapted from: Ritschel WA. 1992. Drug metabolism. In *Handbook of Basic Pharmacokinetics,* 4th ed. Hamilton, Illinois: American Pharmaceutical Association, 169. Reprinted by permission.

The majority of a premature neonate's body weight is composed of water. Therefore, most drugs have a greater volume of distribution in neonates than in adults.[20] A larger dose per kilogram is usually needed in the neonate than in the adult. Body water comprises approximately 85 percent of the premature neonate's total body weight, whereas in the term neonate, the water compartment accounts for 75 percent of total body weight.[21,22]

Therapeutic and adverse drug effects result from free (unbound) drugs only. Protein binding in the neonate is influenced by various factors:[23,24]

- Hypothermia
- Acidosis
- Hypoglycemia
- Sepsis
- Birth asphyxia
- Hypercapnia
- Presence of 2-hydroxbenzoylglycine

Substances that bind drugs include albumin and α_1 acid-glycoprotein. Albumin binds acidic drugs and α_1 acid-glycoprotein binds alkaline drugs.[25,26] The ability of these substances to bind drugs is reduced in the neonate. Therefore, free drug concentrations are increased, bound drug concentration decreases, and total drug concentration remain unchanged. Total drug concentrations may not truly reflect free concentrations.[23,24] It may be more beneficial to monitor free rather than total concentrations

of drugs that are highly protein bound, such as phenytoin.[23]

Nondrugs can also bind to albumin. Nonesterified fatty acids are reversibly bound to albumin.[27] At high levels, these fatty acids could displace drugs that are highly protein bound (>90 percent) and cause an increase in free concentrations. Although the clinical importance of this effect is still not well known, bilirubin can also displace drugs from albumin-binding sites. Sulfonamide antibiotics have been shown to displace bilirubin from albumin *in vitro,* thus possibly increasing the risk of kernicterus.[28]

METABOLISM

Biotransformation of drugs occurs primarily in the liver. Four metabolic pathways (oxidation, reduction, hydrolysis, and conjugation) are responsible for most hepatic drug metabolism.[29] In the developing premature neonate, these pathways mature at different rates (Figure 10-1).[30] Usually, metabolism of drugs makes them inactive and easier to excrete from the body. Of notable exception is theophylline, which is metabolized to caffeine, a pharmacologically active compound.[31]

Hepatic metabolism is divided into two phases:

- Phase I (nonsynthetic) reactions such as oxidation, reduction, and hydrolysis usually inactivate drugs.
- Phase II (synthetic) reactions such as conjugation usually make a drug more water soluble and easier to excrete.[32]

Drugs utilized during the newborn period may be metabolized by multiple pathways. These pathways may become saturated and cause an accumulation of drug in the blood, increasing the likelihood of toxicity. Saturation of metabolism pathways (dose-dependent metabolism) can lead to greatly increased drug concentrations in the blood with relatively small increases in dose. Drugs that exhibit this dose-dependent or enzyme capacity–limited metabolism include theophylline and phenytoin.[33,34]

EXCRETION

Most drugs utilized during the neonatal period are eliminated from the body through the kidneys. A variety of renal mechanisms exists to excrete drugs: glomerular filtration, active tubular transport, and passive tubular resorption. The amount of drug excreted depends on renal blood flow and protein binding.[35] These aforementioned processes develop at various rates throughout fetal life and postnatally.

Glomerular filtration refers to the passive transport of drugs or metabolites across the glomerulus. Protein-bound drugs are not filtered across the glomerulus. Prior to 34 weeks gestational age, the glomerular filtration rate remains relatively low; after that, it increases in direct proportion to gestational age.[36] Previous investigations with renally excreted drugs suggest that elimination processes mature at the same rate whether the fetus is still *in utero* or the infant has been born. Therefore, preterm and term neonates of the same postconceptional age will probably have the same renal drug excretion capabilities.[37] The clinical effects of developing glomerular filtration rate on the dosing for drugs that are renally filtered (such as vancomycin and gentamicin) are quite apparent. Neonates who are <30–32 weeks postconceptional age may require vancomycin and gentamicin only every 18–24 hours to maintain therapeutic blood concentrations, whereas neonates of >32 weeks postconceptional age may need administration of vancomycin and gentamicin every 6–8 hours.[38,39]

Tubular resorption and transport take place almost exclusively in the proximal tubule of the kidney. The tubular transport (secretion) func-

tion develops over the first 30 weeks of postnatal life and matures more slowly than glomerular filtration.[40] Drugs that depend on tubular transport for excretion include penicillin, ampicillin, ticarcillin, methicillin, and furosemide.[41–43]

In general, renal clearance of drugs is slower in the premature and term neonate than in the child or adult, necessitating a longer dosing interval for the neonate.

PHARMACODYNAMICS

For a drug to exert its therapeutic affects, it usually interacts with a specific receptor in the body. An adrenergic agonist (albuterol), for example, reacts with a β_2 receptor in the body to produce its effects. The interaction of the drug and its receptor can be defined in many ways, including serum concentration-effect relationships. Erroneous conclusions have been drawn concerning the similarities between neonatal, child, and adult serum concentration-effects relationships.[2] In neonates, differences in receptor drug concentrations and receptor sensitivities can contribute to alteration of "therapeutic" serum concentrations. For example, phenobarbital's brain-to-plasma ratio increases with increasing age. This would suggest a difference in receptor concentrations between neonates/children and adults.

Previously, phenobarbital blood concentrations in neonates were considered therapeutic at 10–30 µg/ml. Currently, multiple drug seizure regimens can be avoided, greater efficacy observed, and no increased adverse effects noted with the use of higher "therapeutic" blood concentration ranges (15–40 µg/ml).[44] The recognition and integration of pharmacodynamic and pharmacokinetic principles have also led to the more efficacious use of other drugs such as indomethacin and theophylline.[45,46]

In addition to differences in receptor concentrations and serum concentration-effect between the neonate and the adult, modulation of the pharmacologic response is related to immaturity of the neonatal nervous system. Data suggest that newborn and fetal animals have a decreased vascular response to sympathetic stimulation.[47] Specifically, the concentration of adrenergic transmitters is reduced in various species during the first one to two months of life, which affects the response of drugs whose effects are mediated through such adrenergic receptors as β_1 and β_2.[48]

DRUG CONCENTRATIONS

One of the methods used to determine drug dosing appropriateness is blood concentration monitoring. However, the measurement and use of drug concentrations without skilled interpretation are often misleading. Therapeutic drug monitoring can be defined as the achievement of increased efficacy and decreased adverse effects and cost of therapy by interpretation of blood concentrations and the application of pharmacokinetic and pharmacodynamic principles to the patient. To be successful, application of therapeutic drug monitoring in neonates requires a unified effort within the interdisciplinary health care team.

Many situations make therapeutic drug monitoring in neonates a challenging endeavor. Type and rate of drug administration, limited blood for sampling, changing pharmacokinetic and pharmacodynamic parameters, and lack of understanding concerning therapeutic blood ranges of drugs in neonates may make some blood concentration data useless.[49,50] (Drug delivery devices and their influence on drug concentrations are discussed later in this chapter.)

To accurately determine pharmacokinetic parameters of drugs, multiple blood sampling is necessary.[50] Unfortunately, phlebotomy has to be kept to a minimum in premature neonates because of its contribution to the development of anemia of prematurity and the need for erythrocyte transfusions.[51] In addition, the pharmacokinetic parameters in a neonate change over time and render previously gathered data useless. Therefore, multiple blood sampling may affect the neonate adversely and may not give meaningful data.[50]

Because it is sometimes difficult to obtain meaningful clinical direction from blood drug concentrations, therapeutic drug monitoring in neonates should be used only as a guide or as part of the decision-making process for dosage adjustment of drugs. Interpretation of the clinical status of the neonate in conjunction with therapeutic drug monitoring is the most appropriate method for optimization of neonatal drug therapy.

PULMONARY FUNCTION MONITORING

Several pulmonary function tests may be useful in monitoring the efficacy of various drugs, including β_2-agonists, diuretics, and steroids. Pre- and post-treatment pulmonary function tests, by assessing pulmonary resistance, compliance, and work of breathing, can indicate whether or not β_2-agonists are efficacious.[52] The long-term efficacy of steroids and diuretics can also be assessed with the use of pulmonary function tests before and at various times during therapy. As with drug concentrations, pulmonary function tests should be used only as a part of the overall clinical evaluation of drug efficacy.[52]

FACTORS IN CHOOSING PRODUCTS FOR NEONATES

Various brand-name and generic drug products may or may not be suitable for administration to neonates. Decisions should be based on the product's concentration, osmolality, excipient content, and pharmacokinetic behavior.

The concentration of the product should be such that the dose needed does not require a large amount of fluid. In a low birth weight neonate, a 10 ml dose every eight hours may account for 5–10 percent of daily fluid require-

TABLE 10-1 ▲ Osmolalities of Aminophylline/Theophylline Brands

Brand Name (Generic)	Concentration	Osmolality by Freezing Point Depression
Theostat-80 (theophylline)	80 mg/15 ml	4,985
Somophyllin (aminophylline)	105 mg/5 ml	171
Theophylline generic (Roxane)	80 mg/15 ml	301

Adapted from: Ernst JA, et al. 1983. Osmolality of substances used in the intensive care nursery. *Pediatrics* 72(3): 347–352.

ments, thus reducing the amount of nutrient volume that can be given.

The osmolality (mOsm/kg H_2O) of a drug can greatly affect the neonate's tolerance of the preparation. High osmolality in the neonatal gastrointestinal tract can cause a delay in gastric emptying and feeding intolerance and contribute to necrotizing enterocolitis (NEC).[53-55] Although neonatal enteral nutrition formulas are manufactured to maintain an osmolality of <400 mOsm/kg H_2O, oral medications are rarely screened before administration to neonates.[53]

The osmolality of drug preparations can vary greatly according to brand (Table 10-1).[56] Hypertonic medications are often added to enteral formulas, greatly increasing the total osmolality and decreasing tolerability.[57] Because many medications are not available in a neonatal peroral dosage form, intravenous and extemporaneously prepared preparations have become the mainstay of the expanding peroral neonatal formulary. Intravenous dosage forms usually have an osmolality much higher than desired for peroral use.[57] In peroral medications, additives or inert ingredients seem to account for the majority of the product's hypertonicity.[53] Osmolality data are usually not available for either extemporaneously prepared or commercial preparations. This leaves the clinician with a paucity of data concerning the "best" drug preparation to give to neonates.

Excipients or "inert ingredients" of drug products such as benzyl alcohol, propylene glycol, and methylparabens may cause adverse effects in the neonate and should be avoided if possible. Benzyl alcohol has been shown to cause a cluster of symptoms—gasping respirations, metabolic acidosis, neurologic deterioration, hematologic abnormalities, and death—that has been termed the "fetal gasping syndrome."[58] In 1982, when the syndrome was first described, the FDA and the American Academy of Pediatrics urged pediatricians not to use intravenous flush solutions preserved with benzyl alcohol.[59] Another study has linked the use of benzyl alcohol with the development of kernicterus.[60] Unfortunately, many medications that are used frequently in the critically ill neonate (parenteral benzodiazepines) still contain benzyl alcohol.[61] A recent study has shown that the toxicity of benzyl alcohol may be caused in part by the accumulation of its metabolite, benzoic acid, which results from the immaturity of hepatic pathways.[62]

The dose of benzyl alcohol needed to cause gasping syndrome is approximately 99–234 mg/kg/day.[58] To put this amount in perspective, a 1 kg neonate would have to receive 9.9 mg/kg/day of midazolam to be exposed to 99 mg/kg/day of benzyl alcohol. The therapeutic dose of midazolam in neonates is 0.1 mg/kg/dose every two to four hours, which would correspond to a dose of 1.2 ml/kg/day if it were used every two hours. In addition, most neonates do not receive continuous infusions of medications containing benzyl alcohol, thus lessening the chance of toxicity. The clinician should be aware of what medications contain benzyl alcohol and attempt to avoid this additive or minimize the neonate's exposure if possible. Other investigations have raised the question of parabens (preservatives) causing adverse effects similar to those seen with benzyl alcohol.[63]

Propylene glycol is another common additive to intravenous medications. The injection of Dilantin (phenytoin [a product containing propylene glycol]) at a rate in excess of 50 mg/minute can cause hypotension or cardiac instability.[64] The osmolality of a medication is greatly increased when propylene glycol is used as an inert ingredient.[65]

Careful attention to the differences and variability of the pharmacokinetics and pharmacodynamics in the neonatal population is essential for appropriate pharmacotherapy. Using therapeutic drug monitoring and pulmonary function tests, in addition to monitoring the patient's clinical status, will help the clinician reduce adverse effects and increase efficacy. Choosing the most appropriate intravenous or peroral brand name or generic medication with due consideration to "inert" ingredients is also essential in ensuring appropriate pharmacotherapy for the neonatal population.

DRUG DELIVERY SYSTEMS

INTRAVENOUS SYSTEMS

The delivery of medications to the neonate by the intravenous route has greatly increased the clinician's ability to treat and prevent disease states in patients who often cannot tolerate oral medications. For efficacious pharmacotherapy, the chosen intravenous infusion device must deliver the medication reliably and accurately to the patient.

Among the various types of intravenous delivery devices and systems currently available are the minibag, volumetric chamber (Figure 10-2), syringe pump (Figure 10-3), vented infusion syringe system (Accusave), retrograde administration (Figure 10-4), controlled-release infusion system (CRIS), and membrane intravenous controlled-release optimization system (MICROS). In the NICU, the syringe pump and volumetric chamber are often used in delivery of neonatal intravenous medications.

FIGURE 10-2 ▲ Volumetric chamber.

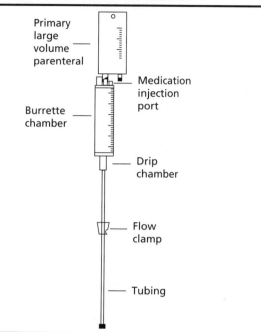

From: Pleasants RA. 1989. Intravenous delivery systems: Overview of systems and patient care implications. Glaxo, Inc., 15. Reprinted by permission.

FIGURE 10-3 ▲ Syringe pump.

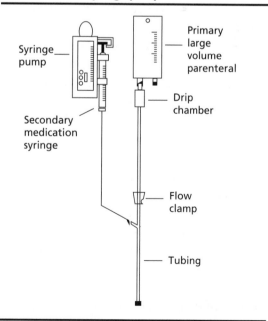

From: Pleasants RA. 1989. Intravenous delivery systems: Overview of systems and patient care implications. Glaxo, Inc., 16. Reprinted by permission.

FIGURE 10-4 ▲ **Retrograde setup.**

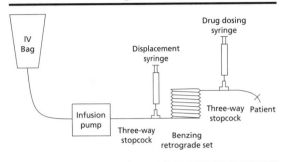

Courtesy of Medex Inc, Duluth, Georgia.

In the near future, the MICROS may be available for neonatal drug delivery. In the past, retrograde drug delivery was used in many neonatal units.

Drip or volumetric chamber sets have the advantage of reusability. Drip chambers do have many disadvantages: incompatibilities when multiple drugs are added, inability to identify the drug after addition, potential bacterial contamination, and possible decreased peak blood concentrations because of delayed drug delivery.[66,67] As with volumetric chambers, retrograde infusion has been shown to delay the delivery of antibiotics.[68]

Syringe pump medication delivery is a recent addition to intravenous drug therapy. Syringe pumps offer the advantages of accurate and reliable delivery of small or large drug dosages (0.1–60 ml) as well as low costs of syringes.[67] The disadvantage is the large initial cost of the device, but institutions have shown that, even with the increased initial costs of syringe pumps, the devices prove to be cost-effective in the first year of operation.[69] A potential disadvantage of the syringe pumps in pediatric units is that they are limited to a maximum of 60 ml delivery capacity. This may not be a problem for neonates, who require less fluid volume because of small total dose requirements.

The MICROS may prove to be an alternative delivery device for neonatal drug administration. Drug delivery is accomplished using the principle of electrodiffusion. Electrodiffusion is an energy-generating process that can move drugs across the membrane of the controlled-release device into the main intravenous solution flow. Potential advantages of MICROS include delivery of multiple drugs concurrently, delivery independent of flow rate of the primary intravenous fluid, and the capability of filtering bacterial, endotoxin, and particulate matter. One potential disadvantage is the possible inconsistency of drug delivery rate due to the variability of membrane size. Currently, few data exist concerning the use of this system in neonatal patients.[66]

PERORAL DELIVERY

Peroral medications are delivered to the oral cavity or directly into the stomach or intestine through naso- or orogastric or duodenal tubes. As already discussed, the osmolality and concentration of drugs are important considerations for their effective delivery by the gastrointestinal route. Of particular concern is the delivery of medications through feeding tubes. Medications may be incompatible with certain formulas or may cause obstruction or complete occlusion of the feeding tube.

This may happen because of the large particle size of the medication preparation. A way to avoid this complication is to flush the tube with sterile water in an amount to completely fill the volume of the feeding tube before and after delivery of the drug.[70]

Various investigations have been performed with adult enteral formulas, but no data exist concerning infant formulas and commonly administered medications in the neonate.[70,71]

Medications administered to neonates by the orogastric tube route have been reported to cause bezoar formation (a concretion) and perforation of the intestine by the bezoar.[54]

FIGURE 10-5 ▲ Modified metered-dose inhaler.

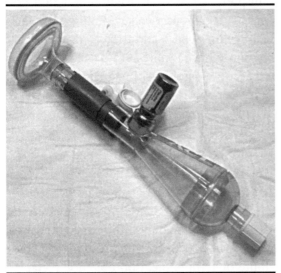

Courtesy of Matthew Mills, Biomedical Photographer, Robert C. Byrd Health Sciences Center, West Virginia University, Charleston, West Virginia.

FIGURE 10-6 ▲ In-line metered-dose inhaler.

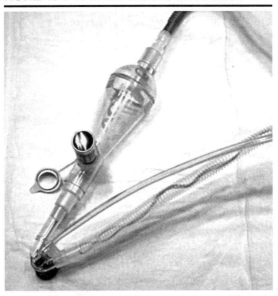

Courtesy of Matthew Mills, Biomedical Photographer, Robert C. Byrd Health Sciences Center, West Virginia University, Charleston, West Virginia.

INHALATION

Respiratory disease in the newborn encompasses various types of acute and chronic problems such as hyaline membrane disease and bronchopulmonary dysplasia (BPD). With the increased survival of premature neonates, respiratory disease of the neonate has become a significant cause of morbidity and mortality. With this increased respiratory disease incidence, delivery of medications by the inhalation or pulmonary route has become more important.

Medications can be delivered directly to the pulmonary system by the use of metered-dose inhaler (Figures 10-5 and 10-6) and jet or ultrasonic nebulizer (Figure 10-7). Such devices have been used to deliver steroids, β_2-agonists, and other medications. Ultrasonic nebulizers have the advantage of a shorter nebulization time and do not require an external gas supply. Larger particles and variability of particle size may limit the effectiveness of this type of nebulizer.[72]

Jet nebulizers are easy to use and can nebulize large amounts of fluid.[73] The disadvantages of this type of nebulizer are that it requires more nebulization time, leads to a high percentage of medication loss in the atmosphere and circuit, and results in lower inspired air temperatures.[73,74] Metered-dose inhalers can be modified with a spacer device and mask

FIGURE 10-7 ▲ Nebulizer.

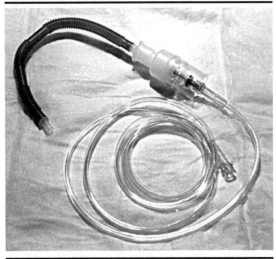

Courtesy of Matthew Mills, Biomedical Photographer, Robert C. Byrd Health Sciences Center, West Virginia University, Charleston, West Virginia.

attachment or modified for in-line ventilator delivery of medications to the neonate.[75]

There are few data concerning the use of metered-dose inhalers to deliver medications in neonates. Inert ingredients found in these devices may damage ciliated respiratory epithelium.[76] In addition, chlorofluorocarbon gas used as a propellant in metered-dose inhalers may result in a hypoxic gas mixture being delivered to the neonate. A recent consensus statement from the American Association for Respiratory Care and American Respiratory Care Foundation recommends that in-line metered-dose inhalers not be used in ventilated infants with a tidal volume of less than 100 ml because of the possible hypoxic mixture that may be delivered.[77]

PULMONARY THERAPEUTIC AGENTS

BRONCHODILATORS (β_2-ADRENERGIC AGONISTS)

A variety of β-adrenergic agonists is utilized in the treatment of acute and chronic conditions in the newborn. Generally, these agents are classified according to their ability to stimulate subtypes of β-receptors such as type 1 (β_1) or 2 (β_2).

Agents that stimulate β_2 receptors include albuterol (Ventolin), terbutaline (Brethaire), metaproterenol (Alupent), isoetharine (Bronkosol), and isoproterenol (Isuprel). Generally, in therapeutic doses, these agents stimulate only β_2 receptors, causing bronchorelaxation. The exception is isoproterenol, which also stimulates β_1 receptors at therapeutic dosages.[78] At higher doses still in the therapeutic range, all of these drugs become unselective and stimulate β_1 receptors, causing adverse effects such as tachycardia.

Mechanism of Action

β_2-agonists exert various physiologic effects such as bronchodilation, enhanced mucociliary

transport, increased surfactant production, and decreased pulmonary edema. Improved dynamic lung compliance and decreased pulmonary resistance have resulted from the physiologic effects of β_2-agonists in neonates. It has been suggested that the observed improvement in dynamic lung compliance is secondary to the beneficial decrease in pulmonary resistance.[74,79]

Uses and Comparisons

Many β_2-agonists have been utilized to treat existing and developing BPD and nonspecific wheezing in the neonate.[78,80] All have similar efficacy, but they may differ in their adverse effects. Reports in the literature indicate that albuterol, terbutaline, isoproterenol, metaproterenol, and isoetharine have been used in the treatment of neonates.[78,81] Isoproterenol, a mixed β_1- and β_2-agonist, appears to have a greater propensity to cause tachycardia than other more selective β_2-agonists.[78] Older agents, such as metaproterenol and isoetharine, usually cause fewer cardiogenic adverse effects than isoproterenol.[74,82,83]

Albuterol probably has the fewest cardiac side effects, but it has a slower onset of activity than isoproterenol, metaproterenol, and isoetharine.[78] Albuterol has a longer half-life than other β_2-agonists, allowing the drug to be used less often in nonacute patients.[78] Terbutaline-treated patients exhibit more tremor and possibly more tachycardia than albuterol-treated patients.[81]

In neonates, controversy has surrounded the use of β_2-agonists because of the presumed lack of bronchiole smooth muscle present in neonates to produce bronchoconstriction. Yet neonates and infants with BPD have bronchiolar smooth muscle hypertrophy.[84] One study reports that wheezing neonates had no response to inhaled albuterol; another investigation reports metaproterenol reversal of methacholine-induced pulmonary reactivity, which would indicate bronchodilation.[85,86]

In infants at 43 weeks postconceptional age with BPD, isoproterenol significantly decreased airway resistance and thus improved specific airway conductance.[74] Tachycardia was observed in this population after the administration of isoproterenol. Albuterol given orally to infants with BPD was shown to improve lung function acutely.[80]

When patients recovering from hyaline membrane disease were given inhaled isoetharine, pulmonary resistance decreased and dynamic compliance increased.[87] Another investigation also showed similar results with the use of isoetharine.[88]

Doses of β_2-agonists vary greatly, and clear dose-response relationships have not been established. Not only does controversy exist about the use and dose of β_2-agonists, but the preferred route of administration is also in question. Although perorally administered albuterol has been shown to be efficacious, the osmolality of the commercially available product may be inappropriately high for neonates.[89] For reasons already discussed, the use of the metered-dose inhaler for the delivery may also not be desirable in certain neonates. When nebulization is used to deliver β_2-agonists, it is very difficult to discern exactly how much aerosol is being delivered to the lung. Inhaled delivery methods may be preferred over peroral methods because of possible avoidance of systemic adverse effects, although peroral delivery of albuterol has been shown to be effective in short-term therapy of infants with BPD without major cardiovascular adverse effects.[80,90] Even with local delivery of β_2-agonists, neonates can experience adverse effects with repeated frequent dosing.[78]

Dosing, Monitoring, and Adverse Effects

As mentioned, there is a lack of controlled trials demonstrating the dose-response relationships of β_2-agonists in neonates. Repeated dosing with these agents may cause tachyphy-laxis, necessitating an increased dose for therapeutic effect.[78] Investigations in adults have shown that this escalation of dose can increase adverse effects while not increasing efficacy. Corticosteroids have been shown to eliminate the decreased responsiveness of β receptors from continued use of β-agonists by increasing the number of β receptors.[91,92]

Doses for albuterol in neonates have ranged from 0.02 to 0.2 mg/kg delivered by nebulizer or metered-dose inhaler.[78,93] Terbutaline has been used in doses of 0.2–0.5 mg/kg, isoetharine in doses of 1–2.5 mg/kg, metaproterenol in doses of 1 mg/kg, and isoproterenol in doses of 0.5–1.25 mg/kg.[94]

In addition to observing the drug's effect on clinical symptoms of wheezing, the clinician can use pulmonary function tests to determine if β_2-agonists are efficacious in a particular patient. Repeated pulmonary function tests can assess the need for prolonged β_2-agonist therapy (Chapter 12).

Rigorous evaluation for the development of adverse effects from β_2-agonist therapy is important—especially in the premature infant. The most common adverse effects associated with the use of β_2-agonists are tachycardia, tremor, hypertension, and gastrointestinal disturbances.[78] With continuous or high-dose β_2-agonist therapy, hypokalemia has been reported.[93]

ANTICHOLINERGICS

Mechanism of Action

Parasympathetic (cholinergic) stimulation of the lung leading to bronchospasm can be prevented by anticholinergic (antimuscarinic) agents such as atropine and ipratropium bromide. Although β receptors are plentiful even in premature neonates, data concerning muscarinic receptors exist only for adults. Therefore, the pharmacologic data justifying the use of ipratropium bromide are scarce.

Uses and Comparisons

Atropine and, more recently, ipratropium bromide have been used in infants with BPD.[94-97] Atropine has been used in combination with metaproterenol in infants with BPD. These agents were found to be equally efficacious in improving airway resistance and functional residual capacity.[96] Although they had a short duration of activity (three hours), their onset was rapid, within 15–30 minutes. Atropine's effect is mainly on the central airway, whereas β-agonists exert activity predominantly on peripheral airways, but no synergistic effect has been recognized with this combination.[96]

Three reports document the use of ipratropium alone or in combination with a β-agonist. All of the reports note improved pulmonary function tests with the use of ipratropium, but no long-term benefits have been reported with the use of this drug in neonates. Various doses of ipratropium were used in all reports to date.[94,95,97] Brundage recommends the use of a β-agonist with ipratropium bromide to ensure longer lasting bronchodilation.[97] No data are available concerning the beneficial effects of atropine or ipratropium bromide on the progression or resolution of BPD.

Dosing and Monitoring

Ipratropium bromide doses vary from 25 to 175 μg/kg in neonates and infants.[94,95,97] Both metered-dose inhalers with spacer devices and nebulizers have been used to deliver ipratropium, making it very difficult to compare studies because the amount of drug delivered to the lungs varies with administration method. Either method of delivery could be used, but the lack of data makes it difficult to recommend one delivery method over the other. Atropine has been given in single nebulized doses of 0.08 mg/kg.[96]

Adverse Effects

Data concerning the adverse effects of both atropine and ipratropium bromide after pulmonary administration are lacking. Atropine could conceivably be absorbed systemically and cause anticholinergic effects such as tachycardia, tremor, agitation, and confusion. Ipratropium, because of its quaternary ammonium structure, may have fewer central nervous system effects than atropine.

Studies document minimal adverse effects associated with the use of either inhaled ipratropium or atropine.[94-97] Paradoxical bronchoconstriction has been reported with the use of ipratropium bromide. This adverse effect is probably due to inert excipients contained within the preparation.[98]

DIURETICS

Mechanism of Action

Diuretics inhibit the reabsorption of water and electrolytes in various parts of the neonatal kidney. Loop diuretics exert their effect by blocking the transportation of sodium and potassium into the thick ascending limb of Henle's loop.[99] Loop diuretics (furosemide, bumetanide) produce rapid diuresis in the neonate when administered parenterally.[100]

Thiazide diuretics (hydrochlorothiazide and chlorothiazide) probably work by blocking sodium chloride reabsorption in the distal convoluted tubule. They are less potent than the loop diuretics.[100] Metolazone, a diuretic structurally similar to the thiazides, is a quinazolone type agent that acts in the same fashion as thiazide diuretics.[101]

Spironolactone, a competitive inhibitor of the mineralocorticoid aldosterone, exerts its diuretic effects in the collecting ducts of the nephron. Aldosterone augments the tubular reabsorption of sodium and chloride and increases the excretion of potassium. Spironolactone therefore is considered a potassium-sparing diuretic.[101]

In adults, methylxanthines also possess a weak diuretic effect through inhibition of solute reabsorption in the distal and proximal tubules of the kidney. The data concerning whether a diuretic effect is evident or not in preterm neonates are controversial.[100] (Methylxanthines are discussed later in this chapter.)

Uses and Comparisons

Furosemide and to a lesser extent bumetanide have been used in the neonate to treat pulmonary edema and fluid overload and as an adjunct treatment modality in infants with BPD.[101] In addition to its diuretic effects, furosemide causes a net decrease of fluid filtration into the pulmonary interstitium and also decreases vasopressin (antidiuretic hormone) in infants. In neonates with BPD, vasopressin may be elevated and interstitial edema is usually present.[102]

In acute fluid overload, loop diuretics can help to rapidly remove excess body fluid. Vigilant management of fluid and electrolyte therapy may decrease the need for diuretics. If utilized, diuretics such as furosemide should be given only once for the treatment of fluid overload.[103] Reassessment of the infant should guide further dosing. Significant diuresis, natriuresis, and kaliuresis have been observed when bumetanide was used to treat volume overload associated with extracorporeal membrane oxygenation.[104]

Favorable results on pulmonary function in neonates with BPD have been shown following single and multiple doses of furosemide.[78,104] Airway resistance decreased and dynamic pulmonary compliance increased.[105] Short-term studies (one week) have shown significant improvement in infants with BPD treated with furosemide.[104] Long-term therapy with furosemide has been shown to be effective in improving pulmonary function in infants with BPD, but adverse effects have limited its usefulness.[106] Furosemide has also shown effectiveness in improving pulmonary function after

erythrocyte transfusion by creating a forced diuresis and eliminating excess water load.[107]

Spironolactone and chlorothiazide have been used in infants with BPD for a one-week period and have resulted in decreased airway resistance and increased dynamic pulmonary compliance.[108] Albersheim and Solimano utilized spironolactone and hydrochlorothiazide in the long-term treatment of patients with BPD. They found that total respiratory system compliance was higher in the spironolactone/hydrochlorothiazide-treated patients than placebo-treated patients ($p = .016$). The survival rate for the diuretic-treated patients was also significantly higher than for the placebo group ($p = .025$). No significant adverse effects were noted in the diuretic group.[109]

Because furosemide has been associated in neonates with more adverse effects than other diuretics, alternate dosing regimens have been researched. Alternate-day dosing of peroral furosemide has been shown to significantly increase dynamic lung compliance and decrease total pulmonary resistance in neonates with BPD as compared to those treated with placebo ($p = .032$, for both variables).[110] This regimen did not result in urinary or serum electrolyte abnormalities or an increase in urinary output. Metolazone, in combination with furosemide, has been used to treat severe furosemide-resistant edema associated with surgery and nephrotic syndrome.[111,112]

Based on recent literature, furosemide should be the diuretic of choice for acute management of fluid overload or pulmonary edema because more data exist for its use in neonates than for other loop diuretics. It should be given once and the need for future doses closely scrutinized. Daily therapy for BPD may require the use of spironolactone in combination with a thiazide diuretic, although alternate-day dosing of furosemide may be an alternative diuretic regimen. Little data exist documenting the use of bumetanide and metolazone for the treatment of edema in the neonatal patient.

Dosing and Monitoring

For the management of acute fluid overload, furosemide should be given as a dose of 1 mg/kg by slow intravenous push.[113] For long-term treatment of infants with BPD, the recommended oral dose is 4 mg/kg/day divided twice daily every other day.[109] Individual doses of furosemide should not exceed 2 mg/kg in preterm neonatal patients.[74] In term neonates, furosemide dosing may be repeated every six to eight hours.

Because the preterm neonate has a limited ability to excrete furosemide, the intravenous dose (1 mg/kg) should not be repeated more often than every 12 hours. Some investigators recommend repeating the dose no more often than every 24 hours in preterm neonates.[114]

Chlorothiazide dosing for the treatment of patients with BPD ranges from 20 to 40 mg/kg/day divided into 2 doses. Aldactone (1–3.3 mg/kg/day) and hydrochlorothiazide (2–3 mg/kg/day) divided into 2 doses can be used in combination for infants with BPD.[109] An oral combination suspension product is not available and has to be extemporaneously prepared.

Bumetanide has been utilized in single doses or chronic dosing of 0.1 mg/kg/day and metolazone at a dose of 0.2 mg/kg/day.[104,111]

Adverse Effects

In previous studies, extended furosemide and bumetanide use has been shown to cause hyponatremia, hypokalemia, volume contraction, and possibly hypomagnesemia. Hypochloremic metabolic alkalosis has also been reported with both drugs.[101] Giacoia and Pineda found that moderate hypochloremia (less than 80 mEq/liter) and bicarbonate concentration greater than 30 mEq/liter was more likely in infants with BPD who died than in those who survived.[106]

Calciuria, nephrocalcinosis, and calcium nephrolithiasis have been reported with chronic use of furosemide.[115,116] The use of chlorothiazide, a calcium-sparing diuretic, may help to reverse the complications of furosemide-induced hypercalciuria.[101] Secondary hyperparathyroidism and pathologic fractures have been reported with the use of furosemide in infants with BPD.[116] The use of twice daily furosemide in very low birth weight (VLBW) neonates can cause toxicity because of the long plasma half-life exhibited in this population. In these neonates, furosemide should be given only once daily.[114]

The ototoxicity observed with the use of furosemide may be related to total dose and rate of infusion.[117] Previous investigations have concluded that bumetanide may be less ototoxic than furosemide when given concurrently with other ototoxic drugs (aminoglycosides).[118] Data from *in vitro* trials suggest that bumetanide has the ability to displace bilirubin from its protein-binding sites and should be used with caution in critically ill or jaundiced neonates.[119] Another report also documents the binding of furosemide to albumin.[120] The clinical significance of the displacement of bilirubin by either furosemide or bumetanide is still unknown.

Thiazide diuretics can cause some of the same adverse effects as loop diuretics: hyponatremia, hypokalemia, and volume depletion.[101] In contrast to furosemide, chlorothiazide and hydrochlorothiazide exhibit a calcium-sparing effect.[109] Although serum lipid profiles can be adversely affected by thiazides, this effect is probably not important in neonates because of the short duration of therapy.[101] In adults, thiazide diuretics have caused hyperglycemia resulting from impaired glucose tolerance.[78] Metolazone generally exhibits the same adverse effects as thiazide diuretics.[101]

Spironolactone is a potassium-sparing diuretic; therefore, hyperkalemia can develop with its use.[78] Hypernatremia does not develop unless spironolactone is used in combination with a thiazide or loop diuretic. In adults, spironolactone has rarely been reported to cause agranulocytosis, eosinophilia, and thrombocytopenia.[101]

CORTICOSTEROIDS

Mechanism of Action

Glucocorticoids have highly complicated mechanisms of action involving various organs and systems in the body. In the treatment of pulmonary disease of the neonate, multiple pharmacologic activities play a suspected role in the observed or perceived therapeutic effects of these agents. Acute effects of glucocorticoids in the neonatal lung include reduction in pulmonary edema, inhibition of prostaglandin and leukotriene synthesis, and increased surfactant production.[121] Ongoing pulmonary fibrosis could be minimized by glucocorticoid-induced reduction in pulmonary fibronectin and albumin and by stabilization of cell and lysosomal membranes.[122] Glucocorticoids have effects on organs and systems of the body other than the lung, discussed in "Adverse Effects."

Uses and Comparisons

Corticosteroids (dexamethasone, beclomethasone, and flunisolide) have been used to prevent or treat BPD as well as prenatally to reduce respiratory distress syndrome (RDS) in the premature neonate.[123-133] Dexamethasone has also been used as an adjunctive pharmacotherapy to prevent extubation failure in preterm infants. Beclomethasone has been used in an attempt to reduce infants' dependency on peroral steroid regimens.[134]

Maternal corticosteroids given 24 hours to seven days before anticipated delivery (prenatal administration) of 29–34-week gestation neonates have been shown to significantly reduce mortality and the incidence of RDS in

these patients.[123,124] The administration of corticosteroids to mothers of infants born at 24–28 weeks gestation has been shown to reduce the severity but not the incidence of RDS in these infants and to reduce the mortality and incidence of intraventricular hemorrhage (IVH).[123]

Additional benefits reported from the use of prenatal corticosteroids include improved circulatory stability and reduced requirements for oxygen and mechanical ventilatory support. Based on current reports, prenatally administered corticosteroids are an important pharmacotherapy for the treatment of patients who may develop RDS and BPD after birth.[123]

The use of dexamethasone for the prevention of extubation failure has been compared to placebo in neonates, infants, and children.[135-138] Studies involving older infants and children with a single, uncomplicated endotracheal intubation have shown dexamethasone to be ineffective in preventing extubation respiratory distress or stridor.[137,138] In an investigation of premature neonates who underwent multiple or long-term endotracheal intubations, a short course of dexamethasone has been shown to be significantly effective in decreasing $PaCO_2$ ($p \leq .006$) and resistance ($p \leq .006$) and increasing tidal volume ($p < .05$) and compliance ($p \leq .006$) as compared to placebo-treated controls 24 hours after extubation.[136] Based on such data and reports of limited adverse effects, short courses (three doses) of dexamethasone may be helpful in preventing extubation failure in small premature infants who have undergone multiple or long-term (≥ 14 days) endotracheal intubation.

Controversy exists concerning the efficacy and best route of administration of corticosteroids in the treatment of infants with BPD. In the 1970s, hydrocortisone was the first corticosteroid used in the treatment of lung disease in newborns. Then, reports of short-term administration of dexamethasone (two to three days) to infants documented decreased ventilator requirements.[136]

Numerous controlled trials have examined the short-term efficacy of dexamethasone in the treatment of patients with BPD.[139–149] With the exception of one study, these trials have reported improved pulmonary function tests, decreased respiratory support, shorter duration of ventilation, or suppression of pulmonary inflammation with the use of dexamethasone.[150] Dexamethasone is used and has been used in the treatment of infants with BPD in preference over other corticosteroids because of longer half-life and lack of comparative mineralocorticoid effects.[139]

Long-term (one year) outcome studies have shown no improved outcomes in patients who received dexamethasone for the treatment of BPD. O'Shea and colleagues did not find differences in mental development index, psychomotor development, incidence of cerebral palsy, anthropometric data, or death before or after discharge from the hospital in a dexamethasone-treated group as compared to controls.[127] Nor did the rate of rehospitalization because of respiratory infection differ significantly between the control and treatment groups. As with other investigators, O'Shea and colleagues did observe a significant reduction in days of ventilation in the dexamethasone-treated group as compared to the control group ($p = .0008$) after entry into the study.[127] As in O'Shea's study, Ferrara, Couser and Hoekstra found that one-year outcomes did not differ between the dexamethasone-treated group and the controls.[151]

Cummings and D'Eugenio compared an 18- and 42-day course of dexamethasone to placebo. Although both treatment regimens resulted in decreased ventilator rates and mean airway pressures, only the infants treated with 42 days of dexamethasone showed better neurologic outcome at 6 and 15 months than those treated with placebo ($p < .05$).[128] Although there are conflicting reports concerning the long-term improvement in outcomes of dexamethasone-treated infants, its short-term efficacy is well established. Infants in the previously mentioned studies were at least two weeks postnatal age.

Yeh and Torre have investigated the early (≤ 12 hours) postnatal use of dexamethasone compared to placebo in neonates with severe RDS. These researchers found that dexamethasone-treated neonates were extubated successfully more often ($p < .025$), had better pulmonary function tests ($p < .05$), and had less incidence of lung injury ($p < .05$) than the placebo group. These results are based on response criteria and tests obtained during the study or immediately after the two-week investigation period.[133]

Inhaled corticosteroids have been used to reduce peroral steroid requirements or as initial treatment in neonates and infants with BPD.[132,134] It is hoped that by using inhaled corticosteroids, the efficacy of the drug may be maintained with less potential for systemic adverse effects.

LaForce and Brudno utilized nebulized beclomethasone as an initial treatment of oxygen and ventilator-dependent infants starting at 14 days postnatal age. Airway resistance decreased significantly in the beclomethasone group during week 2 ($p < .05$), 3 ($p < .02$), and 4 ($p < .001$) of treatment as compared to the placebo group.[132] Dynamic compliance increased significantly in the beclomethasone group during week 3 ($p < .01$) and 4 ($p < .05$) of treatment as compared to the placebo group. In older infants with a mean gestational age of 28 weeks and postnatal age of 10.5 months, beclomethasone was shown to decrease the need for β-agonists and ipratropium bromide ($p < .001$) and decrease wheeze and cough compared to the placebo group.[132]

In this investigation, two six-week treatment periods were separated by a two-week washout period. Functional residual capacity increased in beclomethasone-treated infants as compared to placebo-treated controls (*p* <.002) only during the treatment periods and not during the washout period.[132] Currently, there are no data to justify the use of a second course of corticosteroid therapy in a neonate or infant with BPD.

Cloutier was able to wean infants with BPD from peroral prednisone within four to five months of institution of inhaled beclomethasone therapy. Although pulmonary function tests did not improve more with beclomethasone therapy than with prednisone therapy, the rate of linear growth and weight gain increased markedly.[134] Finally, Konig and Shatley reported a decrease in hospital admissions for infants with BPD when nebulized flunisolide was administered.[130]

Dosing and Monitoring

Initial doses of intravenous dexamethasone range from 0.25 to 0.5 mg/kg/day with various weaning schedules.[136] Duration of therapy varies from three doses for the prevention of extubation failure to 18 and 42 days for the treatment of BPD.[129] From existing evidence, it would seem that a three-dose dexamethasone regimen is appropriate for extubation adjunctive therapy, whereas 42 days of a tapering schedule is appropriate for the treatment of BPD.

Dosages of inhaled corticosteroid for efficacious therapy of BPD or for reducing peroral corticosteroid dependency are less well elucidated. Beclomethasone doses varying from 25 µg/kg/day divided into 3 doses to 400 µg/day divided into 2 doses have been delivered by metered-dose inhaler or nebulizer.[131,132,134] Flunisolide has been administered in doses of 187–250 µg/day divided into 4 doses.[130]

Adverse Effects

The occurrence and incidence of adverse effects of corticosteroids have not been studied as extensively in neonates as in adults and children. Many of the adverse effects in adults and children have not been reported in neonates to date. Many of the reported adverse effects associated with corticosteroid use in neonates include:[121]

Gross motor development retardation
Abnormalities of electroencephalography
Ultrasonographically diagnosed echodensities
Irritability
Retinopathy of prematurity
Cardiac hypertrophy
Hypertension
Bradycardia
Pneumothorax
Gastrointestinal perforations
Hyperglycemia
Nephrocalcinosis
Calciuria
Myopathy and muscle wasting
Increased white blood cell count and
    neutrophilia
Infections
Growth failure
Proteolysis
Hypothalamic-pituitary-adrenal axis
    suppression

The positive or negative effects that corticosteroids may have on neurologic development are not well known because of a lack of long-term follow-up studies. However, the literature reports no evidence that neurodevelopmental outcome is affected adversely by the use of corticosteroids in the neonatal period.[121]

One animal and two human studies suggest that the incidence of retinopathy of prematurity (ROP) may be increased with the use of corticosteroids because of rapid changes in oxygen requirements.[150,152,153] Other human investigations failed to show an increased incidence of ROP.[128,151,154,155]

Cardiac hypertrophy and hypertension associated with the use of corticosteroids are reversible and usually require no treatment.[156] If hypertension is persistent during therapy with corticosteroids, reduction in dose or specific pharmacotherapy for hypertension may be of benefit.[121] Sinus bradycardia associated with dexamethasone use has been reported,[121] but this is unsubstantiated by other investigators.[135]

Although recent investigations have not shown an increased number of infections associated with the use of corticosteroids, previous reports have noted more infections in corticosteroid-treated patients than in control or placebo groups.[129,155] One case report describes cytomegalovirus disease acquired during steroid therapy in a premature neonate.[157]

Neutrophil function has not been shown to be affected by corticosteroid therapy.[158] The inhibition of neutrophil function has been noted in neonates with infections and probably plays an important role in the morbidity and mortality in neonates with infectious causes of disease.

Corticosteroids have been shown to induce in the infant a catabolic effect, which may inhibit linear growth and weight gain.[159] This observation is supported by the fact that when infants have been weaned from systemic corticosteroids with the institution of inhaled corticosteroids, linear growth and weight gain have increased dramatically.[134] Therefore, this adverse effect seems to be reversible with cessation of systemic corticosteroid treatment.

Gastrointestinal hemorrhage and perforation have been reported as adverse effects of corticosteroids.[160] Patients in the NICU are stressed in various ways and may therefore be at higher risk for gastrointestinal bleeding. Few data exist concerning the prevention of drug-induced or stress-induced ulcers in the neonate.

Nevertheless, because the gastrointestinal complications that have been associated with the use of corticosteroids may be deadly, appropriate monitoring for prevention is indicated.

For patients not receiving gastric feeds, gastric pH monitoring should be done. If the gastric pH is below 4, intravenous therapy with histamine-receptor type 2 (H_2) antagonists such as cimetidine (10–20 mg/kg/day) or ranitidine (1–2 mg/kg/day) is indicated.[161–165] These agents can be compounded into hyperalimentation or given as an intermittent infusion divided twice or three times daily and given slowly over five to ten minutes. All H_2 antagonists can block hepatic enzyme function and increase concentrations of hepatically metabolized drugs such as theophylline, although such an interaction is rarely documented.

Antacids should not be used in the neonate because of the possibility of gastrointestinal complications and aspiration.[54] Although very few data exist, H_2 antagonist therapy may be warranted in all neonatal patients receiving dexamethasone therapy.

Endogenous steroid suppression due to the use of exogenous corticosteroids has been reported in adults and children. Short courses of corticosteroids for asthma have not been shown to suppress the hypothalamic-pituitary-adrenal axis. Longer courses of therapy, as in the treatment of BPD, may suppress adrenal responsiveness in VLBW infants.[121] This effect does not seem to be dose related and may be acute in nature or take up to six months to resolve.[166] In any case, this potentially serious adverse effect deserves further study.

Investigations documenting inhaled corticosteroid use have not reported any adverse effects.[130–132,134] This may be because steroids delivered directly to the lung may not be appreciably absorbed systemically, or not enough patients have been treated by this route to observe adverse effects. In terms of adverse effects unique to the inhaled route of corticosteroid administration, there are concerns about the use of in-line metered-dose inhalers in infants with a tidal volume of less than 100 ml.[77] So-called inert ingredients contained within inhaled corticosteroid preparations may cause adverse effects not currently reported in the literature.[76] The use of various delivery devices with few data documenting the amount of drug delivered to the lung makes the determination between a therapeutic dose and toxic inhaled dose difficult.

Short-term adverse effects have not been attributed to prenatal corticosteroid therapy. No long-term neurodevelopmental adverse effects have been observed, as data concerning the effect of prenatal corticosteroids on the onset of puberty and growth have not been reported.

Place in Therapy

Prenatal maternal corticosteroids seem to benefit the neonate and to have minimal adverse effects. Because of their beneficial effects on neonatal RDS, these agents should be used prenatally 24 hours to seven days before the anticipated delivery of a neonate of 29–32 weeks gestation. The use of prenatal steroids in pregnancies of less than 29 weeks is being examined.[123]

A three-dose regimen of dexamethasone seems to be an effective adjunctive pharmacotherapy for preventing extubation failure in infants with a history of prolonged or repeated endotracheal intubation. Although no current data exist, theophylline and dexamethasone may prove to be effective when given in combination to VLBW infants with multiple or prolonged endotracheal intubations.

Inhaled corticosteroids may someday be a useful method to decrease or eliminate peroral or intravenous regimens. Before general use is advocated, however, further studies documenting the differences and efficacy and adverse effects of various delivery methods are needed.

Controversy concerning the routine use of corticosteroids in neonates and infants still exists. Although short-term efficacy has been documented, no clear long-term benefit has been documented justifying the use of corticosteroids in patients with BPD. The long-term efficacy and adverse effects of corticosteroids in these patients need further study before corticosteroids become the standard of care in the NICU.

METHYLXANTHINES

Methylxanthine compounds (aminophylline, theophylline, and caffeine) have been used in the neonate to treat or prevent apnea and bradycardia, bronchoconstriction associated with BPD, and diaphragmatic fatigue.[167–171] Although classic pharmacologic studies were performed a century ago, only recently have we begun to understand the utility of these compounds in the neonate.

Mechanism of Action

In preventing or treating apnea and bradycardia, methylxanthines probably stimulate the central nervous system directly as well as increase the sensitivity of central carbon dioxide receptors.[169,172] Additionally, caffeine has been shown to increase intracellular calcium stores, thus affecting smooth muscle tone. This physiologic effect could make caffeine effective in infants with obstructive as well as central apnea.[172] Because most apnea is mixed (central and obstructive), methylxanthines have been shown to be efficacious in the treatment of this disorder. The bronchorelaxation observed with the use of theophylline is probably the result of adenosine antagonism.[173] Methylxanthines may be effective in weaning infants from the ventilator because of their stimulatory effect on the central respiratory center, intercostal muscles, and diaphragm.[170]

TABLE 10-2 ▲ Extemporaneously Prepared Caffeine Citrate Solution

Formulation is caffeine citrate 20 mg/ml (10 mg/ml caffeine base) (500 ml)

Compounding:
1. Dissolve 10 gm citrated caffeine powder (purified) in 250 ml sterile water for irrigation, and stir until clear.
2. Pour into an amber glass bottle, and add an amount to make 500 ml with 2:1 simple/cherry syrup mixture. Shake well.

Stability:
90 days at room temperature

From: Eisenberg MG, and Kang N. 1984. Stability of citrated caffeine solutions for injectable and enteral use. *American Journal of Hospital Pharmacy* 41(11): 2405–2406. Reprinted by permission (R9682).

Uses and Comparisons

Aminophylline and theophylline have shown equal efficacy in the treatment of apnea and bradycardia. Both drugs are available for intravenous and peroral use. Previously, it was recommended that the dosage be reduced when converting from aminophylline to theophylline (aminophylline × 0.8 = theophylline) to account for different pharmacologic activities of these two methylxanthine salts. A recent investigation shows that this conversion is not necessary and no decrease in efficacy or increase in adverse effects occurs when a one-to-one conversion is used.[174]

Caffeine is not commercially available as a medication and has to be extemporaneously prepared (Table 10-2). Despite this disadvantage, many clinicians feel caffeine may be superior to theophylline and aminophylline because it requires only one daily dose and has less effect on lower esophageal sphincter muscle.[170] Caffeine also has a higher therapeutic index value (toxic dose/therapeutic dose), but controlled studies have not confirmed that caffeine actually causes fewer adverse effects than aminophylline and theophylline.[169] Efficacy studies have shown caffeine to be equal to theophylline and aminophylline in the treatment of apnea and bradycardia.[175,176] One study indicated that

caffeine may be effective in treating apnea and bradycardia in patients unresponsive to theophylline.[169]

Investigations document that earlier extubation of infants can be achieved and post-extubation fatigue prevented with the use of methylxanthines.[170,171] Existing data concerning the use of caffeine in preventing postextubation diaphragmatic fatigue show that it is as effective as theophylline.[170]

Although methylxanthines (theophylline and aminophylline) have been used to treat acute bronchospasm, their efficacy for this purpose has been questioned. Investigations have shown that methylxanthines do not augment the efficacy of other agents (β_2-agonists, steroids) in patients with acute exacerbations of asthma.[177] Based on this evidence, aminophylline and theophylline should not be used for the initial treatment of asthma-like symptoms or bronchospasms in the neonate. In the case of the neonate in acute respiratory distress from a bronchospastic event, β_2-agonists may be preferred over methylxanthines.

Dosing and Monitoring

The appropriate dosing and monitoring of methylxanthine therapy are essential for efficacy and minimal toxicity. What is appropriate depends on the disease state being treated.

For the treatment of apnea and bradycardia and the prevention of diaphragmatic fatigue, aminophylline or theophylline therapy is usually initiated intravenously. Therapy is usually initiated (1) in anticipation of or after significant apnea and bradycardia have occurred, (2) before a premature infant is weaned from the ventilator, or (3) when the need to prevent or minimize diaphragmatic fatigue is anticipated.

A loading dose of 4–6.8 mg/kg of theophylline (5–8.5 mg/kg of aminophylline) is necessary to achieve a postloading dose concentration between 10 and 14 µg/ml.[167,170] The volume of theophylline distribution is highly

TABLE 10-3 ▲ Half-Life and Steady State of Methylxanthines in Neonates

Age Group	Half-Life (Hours)	Time to Steady State (Hours)
Theophylline/aminophylline		
Premature neonate	12–58	60–290
Term neonate	14	70
Infant	3.4	17
Child	1.2–10	20–30
Caffeine		
Premature neonate	33–144	165–720

Adapted from: Milsap RL, Hill MR, and Szefler SJ. 1992. Special pharmacokinetic considerations in children. In *Applied Pharmacokinetics: Principles of Therapeutic Drug Monitoring,* 3rd ed., Evans WE, Schentag JJ, and Jusko WJ, eds. Vancouver, Washington: Applied Therapeutics, 10-21–10-32.

variable and usually larger in the neonate (0.4–1 liters/kg) than the child (0.2–0.68 liters/kg), so the neonate requires larger loading doses for therapeutic concentrations.[20]

After a loading dose is administered, a maintenance dose of 3–7.5 mg/kg/day of theophylline (3.75–9.4 mg/kg/day aminophylline) divided into 2 or 3 doses should be instituted.[167–172] Unfortunately, there is no formula to determine at what age a neonate should receive twice daily or three times daily theophylline/aminophylline therapy. Because methylxanthine clearance is directly related to postconceptional and postnatal age, it would seem reasonable that younger patients should initially receive the lower end of the dosage range (3 mg/kg/day).[178] The dosing interval and the dose of methylxanthine should be determined by the therapeutic response of the neonate, the occurrence of adverse effects, and possibly the blood methylxanthine concentration.

Routine serum concentration determinations for theophylline and aminophylline should be performed during steady-state conditions and just before the next scheduled dose (trough). This will allow for a more useful interpretation of the concentration for dosage adjustment if needed. Steady-state conditions usually occur after a drug has been dosed for five half-lives (Table 10-3).[20] Concentrations should be obtained earlier than steady state if the patient exhibits signs and symptoms of toxicity or lack of efficacy.[179] Postloading concentrations obtained 30–60 minutes after a loading dose, along with clinical response, can help the clinician decide on the necessity of future loading doses.[167] It is inappropriate to wait until steady-state conditions are reached to monitor a theophylline concentration if the patient is exhibiting multiple episodes of apnea and bradycardia, suboptimal prevention of diaphragmatic fatigue, or symptoms of toxicity. At our institution, we monitor theophylline concentrations once weekly in stable patients so that dosing adjustments can be made for weight gain and maturing hepatic function.

Like theophylline and aminophylline, caffeine used in the treatment of apnea and bradycardia or prevention of diaphragmatic fatigue should be given initially in a loading dose. Caffeine is prepared as caffeine citrate, which is equivalent to one-half caffeine base for the same weight of citrate salt. The loading dose of caffeine citrate is 20 mg/kg (10 mg/kg caffeine base); the maintenance dose of 5–10 mg/kg/day caffeine citrate (2.5–5 mg/kg/day caffeine base) should be instituted 24 hours after the loading dose.[167–170,180]

Caffeine has a very long half-life in the premature neonate, and time to steady state may be as long as a month.[20] Samples for monitoring caffeine concentrations can be obtained as a trough during steady state. Concentrations should be monitored before discharge from the nursery even if the drug is not at steady state. As with theophylline, caffeine concentrations should be monitored before steady state if the patient is experiencing multiple episodes of apnea and bradycardia, suboptimal prevention of diaphragmatic fatigue, or adverse effects.[180] When theophylline, aminophylline, or caffeine is used for the prevention of diaphragmatic fatigue, the drug must be started at least 24 hours before the anticipated extubation.[170] A postdose concentration may be obtained to assure a therapeutic situation.

Currently, therapeutic theophylline concentrations for the treatment or prevention of apnea/bradycardia and diaphragmatic fatigue are 3–14 µg/ml based on various studies.[167,168,170,178,181] No added efficacy in the treatment of apnea/bradycardia has been observed with theophylline concentrations exceeding 14 µg/ml.[167] However, some clinicians note that theophylline concentrations of 20 µg/ml may be needed to eliminate or significantly reduce apnea/bradycardia.[181] Caffeine concentrations for the prevention or treatment of apnea/bradycardia are considered therapeutic in the range of 5–25 µg/ml.[180] Therapeutic effects of caffeine in the prevention of apnea/bradycardia and diaphragmatic fatigue have been noted at concentrations as low as 2.9 µg/ml, but the optimal therapeutic effect is not realized until a concentration of at least 10 µg/ml.[169]

Theophylline is converted to caffeine in the premature neonate's liver. Therefore, in patients receiving a methylxanthine in whom toxicity is observed and therapeutic theophylline concentrations exist, caffeine concentrations should be assessed simultaneously.[182] The methylxanthine concentration that may produce both adverse and therapeutic effects can vary among individual neonates. Clinical evaluation of the patient should always be considered the best evaluation tool for drug regimens.

Few data and much controversy exist on the subject of when methylxanthine therapy should be discontinued. Many studies have shown and many clinicians feel that when a neonate is no longer premature, he should no longer receive methylxanthine therapy for a "premature disease" such as apnea/bradycardia. Other clinicians prefer to monitor the neonate's progress through evaluation of pneumograms or data from apnea monitors. With this approach, a neonate who has not had a recorded apnea/bradycardia episode in two to three weeks should be considered a candidate for methylxanthine discontinuation.

The infant does not have to be weaned from caffeine, theophylline, and aminophylline, so the dose can be stopped when the clinician feels it is appropriate. Neonates may maintain therapeutic caffeine concentrations for two to three weeks, so it very important to observe them for apnea and bradycardia for at least a month after methylxanthine therapy is discontinued.

In the treatment of diaphragmatic fatigue, there are no clear-cut guidelines for discontinuing methylxanthine therapy. Some clinicians recommend discontinuing therapy three days after extubation and when clinically indicated.[183]

Adverse Effects

Various adverse effects have been reported with the use of methylxanthine therapy in neonates, including vomiting, tachyarrhythmias, seizures, tremor, agitation, gastroesophageal reflux, and electrolyte abnormalities. Progression of adverse effects is not always from less to more severe. Seizures or other serious adverse effects can be the initial presenting symptom of toxicity.

Toxicity does not always correlate with blood concentration. For example, neonates with theophylline concentrations of 30 µg/ml have been reported to exhibit only mild signs of toxicity.[184] Other neonates have manifested adverse effects with concentrations within the therapeutic range for the treatment of apnea/bradycardia (7–14 µg/ml).[167] Although increased concentrations of theophylline and caffeine have been shown to be efficacious, it would seem reasonable not to exceed therapeutic concentrations in the neonate and to

TABLE 10-4 ▲ Receptor Activity of Catecholamines

Drug	Receptors Stimulated	Effect
Dobutamine	β_1 β_2 (minimal) α_1 (minimal)	Increased heart rate and cardiac output
Dopamine	β_1, β_2, α_1 α_2 (minimal) Dopaminergic	Increased renal and mesenteric blood flow, increased heart rate, and increased blood pressure
Isoproterenol	β_1, β_2	Increased heart rate and cardiac output

Adapted from: Zaritsky A, and Chernow B. 1984. Use of catecholamines in pediatrics. *Journal of Pediatrics* 105(3): 341. Reprinted by permission.

closely monitor for adverse effects within the therapeutic range.

Various common conditions and drugs may affect theophylline and caffeine blood concentrations in the neonate. Birth asphyxia, erythromycin, and H_2 receptor antagonists can increase methylxanthine concentrations, necessitating a dosage reduction.[178,185] Drugs such as phenobarbital can increase theophylline requirements in neonates and infants.[186]

INOTROPIC AND VASOPRESSOR AGENTS

Mechanism of Action

Agents such as dopamine, dobutamine, and isoproterenol (catecholamines) can stimulate various types of receptors and exert many effects on different organ systems (Table 10-4).[187] Exogenous catecholamines can mimic the body's own endogenous substances or cause the release of endogenous catecholamines from nerve terminals. Although these agents are often considered in the treatment of shock, they can also be used as pharmacotherapeutic adjuncts to mechanical ventilation and as treatment for certain acute cardiopulmonary conditions of the neonate.[187–191]

Dopamine and dobutamine have been shown to exhibit nonlinear pharmacokinetics, making prediction of dose-response relationships difficult.[192,193] In addition, catecholamines do not exhibit the same pharmacodynamic effects in neonates as they do in adults and children. This is probably true because of adrenergic immaturity, down-regulation or decreased number of receptors, and inadequate amounts of endogenous catecholamines.[192] Thus, therapy with exogenous catecholamines in the neonate, although effective, may be associated with difficulties.

Uses, Comparisons, and Dosing

Dopamine at lower doses (2.5–10 µg/kg/minute) can increase renal blood flow and possibly heart rate.[190,191] Previous investigations have shown that dopamine given at doses of 5–10 µg/kg/minute can produce α_1-agonist effects such as increased mean arterial pressure (P$\overline{\text{aw}}$).[191] Another study found that doses >10 µg/kg/minute are usually needed to produce an increase in P$\overline{\text{aw}}$. The need for higher doses to produce P$\overline{\text{aw}}$ effects may be a result of the immature adrenergic system and decreased endogenous catecholamine stores in the neonate.[192]

Because dopamine does have a central vasodilation effect, adequate intravascular volume should be ensured before the initiation of therapy.[194] Dopamine has been used in patients with persistent pulmonary hypertension of the newborn (PPHN) with cardiac dysfunction or when systemic hypotension occurs with tolazoline therapy.[189,195] The use of dopamine in infants with PPHN to reverse right-to-left shunting by elevating systemic blood pressure cannot be recommended. The beneficial effects of dopamine are probably related to improvement in myocardial contractility and cardiac output.[196] Dopamine is more effective than dobutamine in increasing peripheral arterial pressure.[197]

Dobutamine is a β_1-agonist and has positive inotropic and chronotropic effects on the cardiac muscle. There is usually minimal increase in peripheral vascular resistance associated with the use of dobutamine in doses of 2–15 µg/kg/minute.[194] The therapeutic use of dobutamine is usually limited to cardiogenic or septic shock and may be used concurrently with dopamine in these situations.[187]

Isoproterenol is a potent β-adrenergic agonist that exerts positive chronotropic and inotropic effects. Because isoproterenol produces a greater chronotropic effect than dobutamine to achieve the same inotropic effect, dobutamine may be the preferred cardiotropic agent. Anecdotally, isoproterenol is said to produce a favorable transient decrease in pulmonary vascular resistance and pressure in patients with pulmonary hypertension.[192,194]

Adverse Effects

Catecholamines have short half-lives; therefore, adverse effects can be quickly corrected by discontinuing therapy.[198] Adverse effects that can occur with the use of dopamine include hypertension, tachycardia, and arrhythmia. Dopamine is an alkaline drug with a pH significantly different from skin and can therefore cause extreme pain and ischemic blanching when infiltrated. Diluted phentolamine (an α antagonist) has been used locally to treat dopamine infiltrations.[199]

Dobutamine can cause arrhythmias and intrapulmonary shunting. Although isoproterenol, like dobutamine and dopamine, can cause arrhythmias and tachycardia, its adverse effects are often more pronounced than those of other catecholamines.[194] Additionally, isoproterenol has been reported to aggravate ischemia and cause myocardial necrosis in adolescents.[200]

VASODILATING AGENTS

Mechanism of Action

Prostaglandins (PGE$_1$ and PGE$_2$) are primarily used to maintain patency of a patent ductus arteriosus (PDA) but occasionally have been used to treat PPHN. These agents produce both pulmonary and systemic vasodilation.[188]

Tolazoline is an α-adrenergic blocking agent exhibiting systemic and pulmonary vasodilator effects. It also has various other effects on the neonate, including cardiac and gastrointestinal stimulation as well as histaminelike stimulation of gastric secretion and peripheral vasodilation.[201]

A direct vasodilator, nitroprusside affects arterial and venous vascular beds equally. Although the cellular mechanisms of its therapeutic effects are not known, nitroprusside causes afterload and preload reduction.[202]

Uses and Comparisons

Because prostaglandins are not pulmonary "vasoselective," they offer no advantage over tolazoline. Tolazoline has never been compared to placebo in the treatment of infants with PPHN. Although the beneficial effects of tolazoline have been reported in case studies and numerous patients, these reports were based on nonrandomized, self-controlled design. All of the studies differed in outcome variables and causes of PPHN. The types of patients included in the tolazoline literature have been those with hyaline membrane disease, diaphragmatic hernia, persistent fetal circulation, meconium aspiration, and sepsis. When all of the literature concerning tolazoline is considered, an average 63 percent of the infants were judged to have a beneficial response with a wide variation in results (33–92 percent benefited).[195]

Benitz and Malachowski used nitroprusside to treat preterm and term infants with RDS and PPHN. They recommend that nitroprusside be used only when conventional therapy (mechanical ventilation, neuromuscular blockade, and sedation) fails.[202] Other pharmacotherapies may hold future promise in the treatment of PPHN: allopurinol, nifedipine, and magnesium sulfate.[196,203,204]

Dosing and Monitoring

Prostaglandin E_1 is given as a continuous infusion at doses of 0.05–0.1 µg/kg/minute. After therapeutic response is achieved, it should be reduced to the lowest effective dose. However, the required maintenance dose may be higher or lower than the initial dose and can range from 0.01 to 0.4 µg/kg/minute.[187]

Loading doses of tolazoline range from 1 to 2 mg/kg over one minute and have been followed by continuous infusions of 0.5–10 mg/kg/hour. Drummond and colleagues and Stevenson and associates have recommended the use of 1–2 mg/kg/hour of tolazoline based on effects on arterial blood gases and pulmonary artery pressure.[189,205] Tolazoline should be administered through branches of the superior vena cava to provide the highest possible concentration of the drug within the pulmonary arteries and to avoid left-to-right shunting through the patent foramen ovale.[198]

The dose of tolazoline should be reduced in patients with renal impairment. In fact, the drug probably should be used in patients with impending or existing renal compromise *only* if the benefits of therapy clearly outweigh the risks because accumulation of the drug can occur in these patients and adverse effects will increase.[195]

Nitroprusside infusions should be given initially at a rate of 0.25–0.5 µg/kg/minute and doubled every 15 to 20 minutes until the desired therapeutic response or a maximum dose of 6 µg/kg/minute is reached.[202]

When any of the preceding vasodilators are used in the neonate, continuous monitoring of central and peripheral arterial pressures and urinary output, and serial measurements of arterial blood gases are essential. Additional parameters need to be monitored based on the drug's adverse effect profile.

Adverse Effects

Prostaglandin E_1 has a short half-life; therefore, it could be reasoned that its adverse effects are short-lived with a reduction of dose or discontinuation of the drug. This may not be the case in the neonate with minimal cardiac reserve and an immature adrenergic system, and vigilant observation for adverse effects and prevention, if possible, is extremely important for safe and efficacious therapy.

Prostaglandin E_1 can cause apnea and respiratory depression as well as adverse cardiac effects such as hypotension, bradycardia, and arrhythmias. Diarrhea and inhibition of platelet aggregation can also occur. Reducing the rate of infusion after therapeutic effects are observed can attenuate the severity of PGE_1 adverse effects.[187]

Tolazoline has a long half-life (3–20 hours) in the neonate, indicating that it may not need to be given as a continuous infusion. In addition to pharmacokinetic data justifying single-dose regimens, a previous investigation has shown adverse effects to be more common in patients who received continuous infusion than in those who received single-dose tolazoline.[201]

Tolazoline-treated neonates exhibit various adverse effects resulting from the drug's varied mechanisms of action. Hypotension or hypertension can develop rapidly and profoundly; therefore, before initiating treatment, adequate blood volume should be ensured. Some clinicians recommend the concurrent use of dopamine. Edema and oliguria can result from the use of tolazoline. Pre-existing hemorrhage is a contraindication to tolazoline therapy because of the drug's ability to cause hematuria, gastrointestinal bleeding, and pulmonary hemorrhage.[198] Seizures have also been associated with the use of tolazoline.

Tolazoline's overall adverse effect rate approaches 50 percent. Part of the reason for this disturbing rate is that many investigators used higher doses of tolazoline (greater than 2 mg/kg/hour) without additional therapeutic benefit but with additional adverse effects.[195]

To avoid or lessen the hemodynamic adverse effects (hypotension and tachycardia) observed with the use of nitroprusside, low infusion rates (0.25 µg/kg/minute) should be used initially and increased slowly.[202] Nitroprusside infusion should also be decreased slowly to avoid rebound phenomenon (observed in adults). Cyanide and thiocyanate toxicity can develop with the use of nitroprusside in doses greater than 3 µg/kg/minute or longer than three days. Thiocyanide concentration should be monitored once daily after 72 hours of continuous infusion. Nitroprusside should be discontinued if this cyanide concentration is greater than 10–12 µg/ml.[206] This toxicity is more often observed in patients with renal impairment.[202]

NEUROMUSCULAR BLOCKING AGENTS AND SEDATIVES

Mechanism of Action

Neuromuscular blocking agents act at the neuromuscular junction. Two categories of neuromuscular blocking agents exist based on their interaction with the neuromuscular junction: (1) Nondepolarizing agents (curare, pancuronium, vecuronium, and atracurium) prevent neuromuscular transmission by preventing depolarization of the neuromuscular junction (they occupy acetylcholine-binding sites on postjunctional receptors). (2) Depolarizing agents such as the neuromuscular blocker succinylcholine inhibit neuromuscular transmission by acting as an agonist at the cholinergic receptor (this does not allow the neuromuscular junction to return to a resting state potential).[207] (The following discussion focuses on the nondepolarizing agents.)

Lorazepam, midazolam, and diazepam—benzodiazepines used for various conditions—are efficacious and safe adjuncts to mechanical ventilation.[208,209] Benzodiazepines are agonists of γ-aminobutyric acid (GABA), a neuroinhibitory transmitter, and are potent anxiolytics. These agents have no analgesic properties but do exert amnesic effects and have anticonvulsant properties.[209] Additionally, benzodiazepines may blunt the stress response through reducing circulating catecholamines, thus possibly preventing unfavorable hemodynamic changes such as increased blood pressure in the ventilated or agitated neonate.[210]

Uses and Comparisons

Skeletal muscle relaxants and sedation currently are used as adjuncts to mechanical ventilation. The use of neuromuscular blockade for the management of patients requiring mechanical ventilation remains controversial. Most studies of the use of skeletal muscle relaxants are uncontrolled and have different end points to evaluate efficacy. Investigations have found no difference in outcomes or positive changes in the numbers of pneumothoraces, level of PaO_2, or duration of oxygen therapy between neonates given neuromuscular blockade and those given placebo.[207]

Previously, neuromuscular blockade (paralysis) was used for infants who breathed out of phase with ventilators designed to permit airflow during mechanical inspiration. In the early 1970s, intermittent mandatory ventilation reduced the number of infants needing neuromuscular blockade.[211] Currently, many NICUs utilize paralysis to reduce barotrauma, prevent intraventricular hemorrhage, and decrease "fighting the ventilator" in some infants.[207] Other investigations have not found a beneficial effect associated with the use of neuromuscular blockade in mechanically ventilated neonates. Various results have been reported in patients with RDS and PPHN.

At present, neuromuscular blockade seems to have a variable effect on oxygenation of infants with RDS and PPHN.[207] Pancuronium therapy may help prevent IVH in selected neonates at risk.[212] For infants who breathe out of phase with the ventilator, neuromuscular blockade may be warranted.

Other nondepolarizing neuromuscular blocking agents (vecuronium and atracurium) have also been used in the neonatal population.[213–216] Vecuronium has a shorter duration of activity than pancuronium and is excreted largely in the bile. Hepatic failure may increase the half-life of vecuronium, but renal failure does not affect vecuronium clearance.[213] Atracurium undergoes Hofman degradation, a nonenzymatic elimination mechanism; atracurium's clearance is therefore not dependent on renal or hepatic elimination pathways.[214,215]

Both pancuronium and vecuronium induce minimal release of histamine, whereas atracurium can cause substantial release of histamine.[213,217] This difference is manifested in more cutaneous adverse effects and a slight decrease in blood pressure in atracurium-treated patients.[217]

Newer neuromuscular blockers, such as pipecuronium and mivacurium, may in the future prove useful in neonates.[218,219] Pipecuronium is an intermediate- to long-acting agent in infants, and it is devoid of histamine-related adverse effects.[218] Mivacurium is a short-acting agent that can be used routinely for infants undergoing nonemergency intubation and used as an infusion in procedures of longer duration. Its excretion is slightly prolonged in patients with renal failure.[219]

Neuromuscular blocking agents are not sedatives or pain medications. Appropriate sedation and pain control are an important part of the therapeutic management of neonates who require mechanical ventilation.

Sedation for procedures and sedation for mechanical ventilation have different objectives and probably should have different approaches pharmacotherapeutically. Neonates under-

going computerized tomography and magnetic resonance imaging often require short-term sedation. In the past, chloral hydrate has been used for this purpose.[220] Although chloral hydrate appears to be effective when used in a one- or two-dose regimen, repeated therapy can cause adverse effects. Chloral hydrate is metabolized to trichloroethanol and trichloroacetic acid.[221,222] Because of immature hepatic metabolism, these acids can accumulate, and cardiac toxicity can result from their accumulation.[222,223] After single doses of chloral hydrate, metabolites have been detected in the blood for longer than one week after administration.[223]

Benzodiazepines such as diazepam, lorazepam, and midazolam have been used successfully in the term and premature neonate as an adjunct to mechanical ventilation. As mentioned earlier, they have potent anxiolytic properties. Of the three benzodiazepines used in neonates, diazepam is the least desirable because of pharmacologically active metabolites.[209] Lorazepam and midazolam are shorter acting than diazepam. Lorazepam has no pharmacologically active metabolites, and midazolam's metabolites have little central nervous system activity.[210]

Midazolam and lorazepam have been shown to be effective in sedating older infants and children for short procedures. Repeated dosing has been used to sedate neonates, infants, and children requiring mechanical ventilation. These agents are probably preferable to chloral hydrate when repeated administration is needed in the neonate.

Dosing and Monitoring

Pancuronium, because of its longer half-life, is usually given by IV push, 0.06–0.09 mg/kg, every one to two hours as needed to maintain neuromuscular blockade. Repeated doses of pancuronium can prolong neuromuscular blockade for hours or days.[207]

Vecuronium, 150 μg/kg, has a duration of activity of 30–40 minutes and is frequently readministered if the IV push route is used. Continuous infusions of 1–2 μg/kg/minute have been used to maintain neuromuscular blockade in mechanically ventilated infants. When a continuous infusion of vecuronium is used, less drug is needed to maintain neuromuscular blockade than with IV push regimens. Because of its large volume of distribution, a loading dose of 150 μg/kg of vecuronium should be used immediately before institution of a continuous infusion.[213] Atracurium can also be given by continuous IV infusion in the neonate at 6 μg/kg/minute with a loading dose of 400 μg/kg.[214]

Chloral hydrate can be given at peroral doses of 25–50 mg/kg for sedation for procedures. Repeat doses of 25–50 mg/kg can be given if sufficient sedation is not achieved within 30–45 minutes. In any case, the total dose should not exceed 100 mg/kg, or 1 gm, in any patient. The vital signs and cardiac monitoring of the patient should be observed closely after the administration of chloral hydrate and probably up to 24 hours after the procedure.[220]

Midazolam or lorazepam doses of 0.05–0.1 mg/kg can be used intravenously for sedation or repeated every two to four hours for sedation in infants requiring mechanical ventilation.[208,224] Lorazepam can be administered orally, rectally, or intravenously. Midazolam can be administered orally, rectally, intravenously, or intranasally. Administration by the oral route may decrease the effectiveness of midazolam because of first-pass metabolism in the liver.[225]

Midazolam is given by continuous infusion in children and adults for seizures and sedation during mechanical ventilation. But because of the benzyl alcohol content of all parenteral benzodiazepines, this method of delivery is not appropriate for neonates.

Adverse Effects

The most commonly occurring adverse effects associated with the use of pancuronium in neonates include tachycardia, peripheral edema, and hypertension. Inadvertent extubation may occur in a neonate who is paralyzed; therefore, careful observation of the neonatal patient receiving neuromuscular blockade therapy is essential. Neuromuscular blockade obscures recognition of seizures, and some clinicians recommend concurrent phenobarbital therapy for patients receiving any neuromuscular blocking agent. As mentioned earlier, prolonged and profound muscular paralysis can result from pancuronium, so the agent should be withdrawn as soon as possible. Concurrent aminoglycoside therapy can also cause prolongation of pancuronium neuromuscular blockade.[207]

Vecuronium seems to cause few or no adverse cardiac effects and is not dependent on renal function for elimination. Therefore in premature neonates, the drug can be given without regard for decreased renal function.[213] Both vecuronium and atracurium have shorter half-lives than pancuronium, which is perhaps an advantage in the neonatal patient when prolonged neuromuscular blockade is not desired.[213,214] Atracurium is not dependent on liver or renal function for elimination and so may be an advantage for the neonatal patient. As discussed, atracurium in higher doses may cause some histamine release.[217]

Chloral hydrate can cause respiratory depression and severe gastrointestinal upset and vomiting because of its high osmolality. Additionally, its metabolites have extremely long half-lives and may cause cardiovascular adverse effects. Finally, the metabolites of chloral hydrate may have the ability to displace bilirubin from albumin-binding sites.[221–223]

Benzodiazepines can cause hypotension and respiratory depression in neonates. All sedatives should be weaned before anticipated extubation so as not to prolong mechanical ventilation. As discussed earlier, parenteral benzodiazepines contain benzyl alcohol. Therefore, any symptoms of fetal gasping syndrome, tachyarrhythmias, acidosis, and changes in respiratory pattern should be scrutinized carefully for the cause.

MISCELLANEOUS AGENTS

Cromolyn sodium is a mast cell–stabilizing agent that has been used for the treatment of asthma in adults and children. It is a prophylactic medication in that it cannot be used to control an acute exacerbation, but used only to prevent further asthma attacks. In adults and children, cromolyn sodium is an excellent respiratory anti-inflammatory drug and is particularly useful in patients with inflammatory lung disease associated with allergies.[226] Given its mechanism of action, cromolyn sodium might be expected to be efficacious in an infant with a disease such as BPD. There is, however, a paucity of data available concerning the use of cromolyn in the neonate.

Yamamoto and Kojima reported that pulmonary function tests did improve in a neonate given nebulized cromolyn sodium.[227] In a placebo-controlled, blinded, randomized investigation, Watterberg and Murphy failed to demonstrate any benefits of cromolyn sodium given prophylactically to a group of infants with RDS.[228] Abstracts have reported beneficial effects of cromolyn sodium in neonates.[229–232]

Nedocromil sodium is a newer anti-inflammatory agent similar to cromolyn sodium that seems to be effective in the treatment of asthma.[233] Nedocromil sodium is usually given at a dose of 2 inhalations four times daily. No systemic adverse effects have been reported with the use of cromolyn sodium or nedocromil sodium.[226,233] Both agents need initial studies (nedocromil) and additional studies (cromolyn) to assess the appropriateness of these therapies

in neonates and infants with early or long-established BPD.

Doxapram is an analeptic with peripheral and central respiratory stimulant properties.[234] In neonates with central or mixed apnea that is theophylline resistant, doxapram may be effective for short-term use.[235] Peliowski and Finer demonstrated that doxapram dramatically reduced the number of episodes of apnea in a neonatal patient, but the effect could not be observed beyond one week.[234]

Doxapram is usually given as an intravenous infusion. A loading dose of 5.5 mg/kg followed by a continuous infusion of 1 mg/kg/hour was initially recommended.[236] Newer data indicate that a dose of 0.2 mg/kg/hour is effective in neonates with theophylline-resistant idiopathic apnea of prematurity.[237] Although doxapram is effective when given perorally, it should not be given by this route because gastrointestinal bleeding, premature teeth buds, and possible necrotizing enterocolitis have been observed.[238] The intravenous form of doxapram contains benzyl alcohol; therefore, neonates receiving it should be monitored for signs of benzyl alcohol toxicity.[234]

SUMMARY

Providing pulmonary drug therapy to the premature neonate is difficult and challenging because of unique situations present in no other patient group. The pharmacokinetics of commonly used drugs in the pediatric and adult population have only recently become elucidated in the neonatal population. Lack of suitable neonatal dosage forms necessitates extemporaneous preparation of drugs. Until recently, drug delivery systems did not take into account the differences of patients who may weigh as little as 400 gm. Pharmacotherapeutic studies have widened our knowledge of efficacious drugs that can be used to treat the premature neonate, but the outcomes of these pharmacologic treatments are still often misunderstood. Although these therapeutic orphans have come far in obtaining equal consideration in efficacious, safe, pharmacotherapeutic therapies, there is still much to learn from our littlest patients before they will no longer be orphans.

ACKNOWLEDGMENT

Special thanks to Ms. Bonnie J. Oldham and Ms. Jackie L. Rosencrance for their secretarial support. The author thanks many in the Respiratory Care Department of Charleston Area Medical Center for their technical support.

DEDICATION

This chapter is dedicated to my late father, Paul H. Wandstrat.

REFERENCES

1. Shirkey H. 1968. Therapeutic orphans. *Journal of Pediatrics* 72(1): 119–120.

2. Gilman JT, et al. 1989. Rapid sequential phenobarbital treatment of neonatal seizures. *Pediatrics* 83(5): 674–678.

3. Welling PG. 1977. Influence of food and diet on gastrointestinal drug absorption. *Journal of Pharmacokinetics and Biopharmaceutics* 5(4): 291–334.

4. Besunder JB, Reed MD, and Blumer JL. 1988. Principles of drug biodisposition in the neonate: A critical evaluation of the pharmacokinetic-pharmacodynamic interface. *Clinical Pharmacokinetics* 14(4 part 1): 189–216.

5. Hyman PE, et al. 1983. Effects of external feeding on the maintenance of gastric acid secretion function. *Gastroenterology* 84(2): 341–345.

6. Keene MFL, and Hewer EE. 1929. Digestive enzymes of the human fetus. *Lancet* 1: 767–769.

7. Reed MD. 1989. Developmental pharmacology: Relationship to drug use. *Annals of Pharmacotherapy* 23(7–8 supplement): S21–S26.

8. Hillemeier AC, et al. 1981. Delayed gastric emptying in infants with gastroesophageal reflux. *Journal of Pediatrics* 98(2): 190–193.

9. Yu VYH. 1975. Effect of body position on gastric emptying in the neonate. *Archives of Disease in Childhood* 50(7): 500–504.

10. Cavell B. 1981. Gastric emptying in infants with congenital heart disease. *Acta Paediatrica Scandinavica* 70(4): 517–520.

11. Siegel M, et al. 1982. Gastric emptying in prematures of isocaloric feedings with differing osmolalities. *Pediatric Research* 16(2): 141–147.

12. Hillman LS, Martin LA, and Haddad JG. 1979. Absorption and maintenance dosage of 25-hydroxycholecalciferol (25-HCC) in premature infants. *Pediatric Research* 13(4 Abstract 449): 400.

13. Kostenbauder HB, et al. 1975. Bioavailability and single dose pharmacokinetics of intramuscular phenytoin. *Clinical Pharmacology and Therapeutics* 18(4): 449–456.

14. Ginsberg CM, McCracken GH, and Zweighaft TC. 1982. Serum penicillin concentrations after intramuscular administration of benzathine penicillin G in children. *Pediatrics* 69(4): 452–454.

15. Brachet-Liermain A, Goutieres F, and Aicardi J. 1975. Absorption of phenobarbital after the intramuscular administration of single doses in infants. *Journal of Pediatrics* 87(4): 624–626.

16. Tyrala EE, et al. 1977. Clinical pharmacology of hexachlorophene in newborn infants. *Journal of Pediatrics* 91(3): 481–486.

17. Armstrong RW, et al. 1969. Pentachlorophenol poisoning in a nursery for newborn infants. Part II: Epidemiologic and toxicologic studies. *Journal of Pediatrics* 75(2): 317–325.

18. Fisch RO, et al. 1963. Methemoglobinemia in a hospital nursery. *Journal of the American Medical Association* 185: 760–763.

19. Evans NJ, et al. 1985. Percutaneous administration of theophylline in the preterm infant. *Journal of Pediatrics* 107(2): 307–311.

20. Milsap RL, Hill MR, and Szefler SJ. 1992. Special pharmacokinetic considerations in children. In *Applied Pharmacokinetics: Principles of Therapeutic Drug Monitoring*, 3rd ed., Evans WE, Schentag JJ, and Jusko WJ, eds. Vancouver, Washington: Applied Therapeutics, 10-1–10-32.

21. Friis-Hansen B. 1961. Body water compartments in children: Changes during growth and related changes in body composition. *Pediatrics* 28: 169–181.

22. Friis-Hansen B. 1971. Body composition during growth. *Pediatrics* 47(1): 264–274.

23. Booker HE, and Darcey B. 1973. Serum concentrations of free diphenylhydantoin and their relationship to clinical intoxication. *Epilepsia* 14(2): 177–184.

24. Kurz H, Mauser-Ganshorn A, and Stickel HH. 1977. Differences in the binding of drugs to plasma proteins from newborn and adult man. *European Journal of Clinical Pharmacology* 11(6): 463–467.

25. Morselli PL, Franco-Morselli R, and Bossi L. 1980. Clinical pharmacokinetics in newborns and infants: Age related differences and therapeutic implications. *Clinical Pharmacokinetics* 5(6): 485–527.

26. Piafsky KM. 1980. Disease-induced changes in the plasma binding of basic drugs. *Clinical Pharmacokinetics* 5(3): 246–262.

27. Friedman Z, et al. 1978. Indomethacin disposition and indomethacin-induced platelet dysfunction in premature infants. *Journal of Clinical Pharmacology* 18(5-6): 272–279.

28. Brodersen R. 1974. Competitive binding of bilirubin and drugs to human serum albumin studied by enzymatic oxidation. *Journal of Clinical Investigation* 54(6): 1353–1364.

29. Roberts RJ. 1984. Pharmacologic principles in therapeutics in infants. In *Drug Therapy in Infants,* Roberts RJ, ed. Philadelphia: WB Saunders, 1–12.

30. Ritschel WA, ed. 1986. *Handbook of Basic Pharmacokinetics,* 3rd ed. Hamilton, Illinois: Drug Intelligence Publications, 155.

31. Dothey CI, et al. 1989. Maturational changes of theophylline pharmacokinetics in preterm infants. *Clinical Pharmacology and Therapeutics* 45(5): 461–468.

32. Juchau MR. 1980. Drug metabolism by the human fetus. *Clinical Pharmacokinetics* 5(4): 320–339.

33. Chiba K. 1980. Michaelis-Menten pharmacokinetics of diphenylhydantoin and application in the pediatric age patient. *Journal of Pediatrics* 96(3 part 1): 479–484.

34. Weinberger MM, and Ginchansky E. 1977. Dose-dependent kinetics of theophylline disposition in asthmatic children. *Journal of Pediatrics* 91(5): 820–824.

35. Whelton A. 1982. Antibiotic pharmacokinetics and clinical application in renal insufficiency. *Medical Clinics of North America* 66(1): 267–281.

36. Arant BS Jr. 1978. Developmental patterns of renal functional maturation compared in the human neonate. *Journal of Pediatrics* 92(5): 705–712.

37. Koren G, and James A. 1987. Vancomycin dosing in preterm infants: Prospective verification of new recommendations. *Journal of Pediatrics* 110(5): 797–798.

38. Wandstrat TL, and Phelps SJ. 1994. Vancomycin dosing in neonatal patients: The controversy continues. *Neonatal Network* 13(3): 33–39.

39. Nahata MC, et al. 1983. Tobramycin kinetics in newborn infants. *Journal of Pediatrics* 103(1): 136–138.

40. West JR, Smith HW, and Chasis H. 1948. Glomerular filtration rate, effective renal blood flow and maximal tubular excretory capacity in infancy. *Journal of Pediatrics* 32: 10–18.

41. Radde IC. 1985. Mechanisms of drug absorption and their development. In *Textbook of Pediatric Clinical Pharmacology,* MacLeod G, and Radde IC, eds. Philadelphia: PSG Publishing, 17–43.

42. Kaplan J, et al. 1974. Pharmacologic studies in neonates given large doses of ampicillin. *Journal of Pediatrics* 84(4): 571–577.

43. Nelson JD, Shelton S, and Kusmiesz H. 1975. Clinical pharmacology of ticarcillin in the newborn infant: Relation to age, gestational age, and weight. *Journal of Pediatrics* 87(3): 474–479.

44. Gilman JT, et al. 1989. Rapid sequential phenobarbital treatment of neonatal seizures. *Pediatrics* 83(5): 674–678.

45. Gal P, Ransom JL, and Weaver RL. 1990. Gentamicin in neonates: The need for loading doses. *Journal of Perinatology* 7(3): 254–257.

46. Gilman JT, and Gal P. 1986. Inadequacy of FDA dosing guidelines for theophylline use in neonates. *Drug Intelligence and Clinical Pharmacy* 20(6): 482–484.

47. Duckles SP, and Banners W. 1984. Changes in vascular smooth muscle reactivity during development. *Annual Review of Pharmacology and Toxicology* 24: 65–83.

48. Boerus LO. 1978. Drug-receptor interactions and biologic maturation. In *Clinical Pharmacology and Therapeutics,* Mirkin BL, ed. Chicago: Year Book Medical Publishers, 3–22.

49. Giacoia GP. 1990. The future of neonatal therapeutic drug monitoring. *Therapeutic Drug Monitoring* 12(4): 311–315.

50. Gal P. 1988. Therapeutic drug monitoring in neonates: Problems and issues. *Drug Intelligence and Clinical Pharmacy* 22(4): 317–323.

51. Wandstrat TL, and Kaplan B. 1995. Use of erythropoietin in premature neonates: Controversies and the future. *Annals of Pharmacotherapy* 29(2): 166–173.

52. Zukowsky K, et al. 1994. Pulmonary function testing in the critically ill neonate. Part III: Case studies. *Neonatal Network* 13(4): 31–35.

53. Ernst JA, et al. 1983. Osmolality of substances used in the intensive care nursery. *Pediatrics* 72(3): 347–352.

54. Brand JM, and Greer FR. 1990. Hypermagnesemia and intestinal perforation following antacid administration in a premature infant. *Pediatrics* 85(1): 121–124.

55. Atakent Y, et al. 1984. The adverse effects of high oral osmolar mixtures in neonates. *Clinical Pediatrics* 23(9): 487–491.

56. Manufacturer communication (letter). September 1, 1989. Lackey Kaven Roxane Laboratories, Inc.

57. White KC, and Harkavy KL. 1982. Hypertonic formula resulting from added oral medications. *American Journal of Diseases of Children* 136(10): 931–933.

58. Gershanik J, et al. 1982. The gasping syndrome and benzyl alcohol poisoning. *New England Journal of Medicine* 307(22): 1384–1388.

59. American Academy of Pediatrics Committee on Fetus and Newborn Committee on Drugs. 1983. Benzyl alcohol: Toxic agent in neonatal units. *Pediatrics* 72(3): 356–357.

60. Jardine DS, and Rogers K. 1989. Relationship of benzyl alcohol to kernicterus, intraventricular hemorrhage, and mortality in preterm infants. *Pediatrics* 83(2): 153–160.

61. Weissman DB, et al. 1990. Letter to the editor: Benzyl alcohol administration in neonates. *Anesthesia and Analgesia* 70(6): 673–674.

62. LeBel M, et al. 1988. Benzyl alcohol metabolism and elimination in neonates. *Developmental Pharmacology and Therapeutics* 11(6): 347–356.

63. Hindmarsh KW, et al. 1983. Urinary excretion of methylparaben and its metabolites in preterm infants. *Journal of Pharmaceutical Sciences* 72(9): 1039–1041.

64. Taketomo C, et al. 1994. *Pediatric Dosage Handbook 1993–1994,* 2nd ed. Hudson, Ohio: Lexi-Comp, 456.

65. Glasgow AM, et al. 1983. Hyperosmolality in small infants due to propylene glycol. *Pediatrics* 72(3): 353–355.

66. Pleasants RA. 1989. Intravenous delivery systems: Overview of systems and patient care implications. Glaxo Inc., 1–56.

67. Nahata MC. 1987. Effect of IV drug delivery systems on pharmacokinetic monitoring. *American Journal of Hospital Pharmacy* 44(11): 2538–2542.

68. Nahata MC. 1986. Delayed delivery of antibiotics by retrograde intravenous infusion. *American Journal of Hospital Pharmacy* 43(9): 2237–2239.

69. Seay RE, Edgren BE, and Schilling CG. 1991. Cost avoidance using syringe pumps to administer fat emulsion in a neonatal intensive-care unit. *American Journal of Hospital Pharmacy* 48(9): 1972–1974.

70. Leff RD, and Roberts RJ. 1988. Enteral drug administration practices: Report of a preliminary survey. *Pediatrics* 81(4): 549–551.

71. Estoup M. 1994. Approaches and limitations of medication delivery in patients with enteral feeding tubes. *Critical Care Nurse* 14(1): 68–72, 77–79.

72. Cameron D, Clay M, and Silverman M. 1990. Evaluation of nebulizers for use in neonatal ventilator circuits. *Critical Care Medicine* 18(8): 866–870.

73. Watterberg KL. 1991. Delivery of aerosolized medication to intubated babies. *Pediatric Pulmonology* 10(2): 136–141.

74. Kao LC, et al. 1984. Isoproterenol inhalation effects on airway resistance in chronic bronchopulmonary dysplasia. *Pediatrics* 73(4): 509–514.

75. Grigg J, et al. 1992. Delivery of therapeutic aerosols to intubated babies. *Archives of Disease in Childhood* 67(1 spec no): 25–30.

76. Silverman M. 1990. Aerosol therapy in the newborn. *Archives of Disease in Childhood* 65(8): 906–908.

77. Sly PD, and LeSouef PN. 1991. Inhaled therapy in pediatrics. *Journal of Paediatrics and Child Health* 27(1): 7–10.

78. Davis JM, Sinkin RA, and Aranda JV. 1990. Drug therapy for bronchopulmonary dysplasia. *Pediatric Pulmonology* 8(2): 117–125.

79. Cabal LA, Larrazabal C, and Ramanathan R. 1987. Effects of metaproterenol on pulmonary mechanics, oxygenation, and ventilation in infants with chronic lung disease. *Journal of Pediatrics* 110(1): 116–119.

80. Stefano JL, Bhutani VK, and Fox WW. 1991. A randomized placebo-controlled study to evaluate the effects of oral albuterol on pulmonary mechanics in ventilator-dependent infants at risk of developing BPD. *Pediatric Pulmonology* 10(3): 183–190.

81. Bruno DS, Parker DH, and Slaton G. 1989. Response of pulmonary mechanics to terbutaline in patients with bronchopulmonary dysplasia. *American Journal of the Medical Sciences* 297(3): 166–168.

82. Dipalma JR. 1985. Beta₂ agonists for acute asthma. *American Family Physician* 31(5): 184–187.

83. McFadden ER. 1985. Clinical use of β-adrenergic agonists. *Journal of Allergy and Clinical Immunology* 76(2 part 2): 352–356.

84. Rosan RC. 1975. Hyaline membrane disease and a related spectrum of neonatal pneumopathies. *Perspectives in Pediatric Pathology* 2: 15–60.

85. Lenney W, and Milner AD. 1978. At what age do bronchodilator drugs work? *Archives of Disease in Childhood* 53(7): 532–535.

86. Tepper RS. 1987. Airway reactivity in infants: A positive response to methacholine and metaproterenol. *Journal of Applied Physiology* 62(3): 1155–1159.

87. Gomez-Del Rio M, et al. 1986. Effect of a beta-agonist nebulization on lung function in neonates with increased pulmonary resistance. *Pediatric Pulmonology* 2(5): 287–291.

88. Motoyama EK, et al. 1987. Early onset of airway reactivity in premature infants with bronchopulmonary dysplasia. *American Review of Respiratory Disease* 136(1): 50–57.

89. Manufacturer data. 1993. Ventolin syrup. Package insert. Glaxo Inc.

90. Shim C, and Williams MH. 1980. Bronchial response to oral versus aerosol metaproterenol in asthma. *Annals of Internal Medicine* 93(3): 428–431.

91. Kaliner M. 1985. Mechanisms of glucocorticoid action in bronchial asthma. *Journal of Allergy and Clinical Immunology* 76(2 part 2): 321–329.

92. Kelly HW. 1991. Corticosteroids for acute severe asthma. *Drug Intelligence and Clinical Pharmacy Annals of Pharmacotherapy* 25(1): 72–79

93. Southgate WM. 1995. Aerosolized pharmacotherapy in the neonate. *Neonatal Network* 14(2): 29–36.

94. Lee H, Arnon S, and Silverman M. 1994. Bronchodilator aerosol administrated by metered dose inhaler and spacer in subacute neonatal respiratory distress syndrome. *Archives of Disease in Childhood* 70(3 spec no): F218–F222.

95. Wilkie RA, and Bryan MH. 1987. Effect of bronchodilators on airway resistance in ventilator-dependent neonates with chronic lung disease. *Journal of Pediatrics* 111(2): 278–282.

96. Kao LC, Durand DJ, and Nickerson BG. 1989. Effects of inhaled metaproterenol and atropine on the pulmonary mechanics of infants with bronchopulmonary dysplasia. *Pediatric Pulmonology* 6(2): 74–80.

97. Brundage KL. 1990. Bronchodilator response to ipratropium bromide in infants with bronchopulmonary dysplasia. *American Review of Respiratory Disease* 142(5): 1137–1142.

98. O'Callaghan C, Milner AD, and Swarbrick A. 1989. Paradoxical bronchoconstriction in wheezing infants after nebulized preservative free iso-osmolar ipratropium bromide. *British Medical Journal* 299(6713): 1433–1434.

99. Burg MB, Stoner L, and Cardinal J. 1973. Furosemide effect in isolated perfused tubules. *American Journal of Physiology* 225(1): 119–124.

100. Wahlig TM, Thompson TR, and Sinaiko AR. 1992. Drug use in the newborn. *Clinics in Perinatology* 19(1): 251–263.

101. Wells TG. 1990. The pharmacology and therapeutics of diuretics in the pediatric patient. *Pediatric Clinics of North America* 37(20): 463–504.

102. Rao M, et al. 1986. Antidiuretic hormone response in children with bronchopulmonary dysplasia during episodes of acute respiratory distress. *American Journal of Diseases of Children* 140(8): 825–828.

103. Oh W. 1991. Diuretic therapy. In *Neonatal Therapeutics*, Yeh TF, ed. St. Louis: Mosby-Year Book, 307–312.

104. Wells TG, et al. 1992. Pharmacokinetics and pharmacodynamics of bumetanide in neonates treated with extracorporeal membrane oxygenation. *Journal of Pediatrics* 121(6): 974–980.

105. Kao LC, Warburton D, and Sargent CW. 1983. Furosemide acutely decreases airway resistance in chronic bronchopulmonary dysplasia. *Journal of Pediatrics* 103(4): 624–629.

106. Giacoia GP, and Pineda R. 1991. Diuretics, hypochloremia, and outcome in bronchopulmonary dysplasia patients. *Developmental Pharmacology and Therapeutics* 16(4): 212–220.

107. Stefano JL, and Bhutani VK. 1990. Role of furosemide therapy after booster-packed erythrocyte transfusions in infants with bronchopulmonary dysplasia. *Journal of Pediatrics* 117(6): 965–970.

108. Kao LC, Warburton D, and Cheng M. 1984. Effect of oral diuretics on pulmonary mechanics in infants with chronic bronchopulmonary dysplasia: Results of a double-blind crossover sequential trial. *Pediatrics* 74(1): 37–44.

109. Albersheim SG, and Solimano AJ. 1989. Randomized, double-blind controlled trial of long-term diuretic therapy for bronchopulmonary dysplasia. *Journal of Pediatrics* 115(4): 615–620.

110. Rush MG, and Engelhardt B.1990. Double-blind, placebo-controlled trial of alternate-day furosemide therapy in infants with chronic bronchopulmonary dysplasia. *Journal of Pediatrics* 117(1 part 1): 112–118.

111. Cachero S, and Lofland G. 1990. Combination of metolazone and furosemide in the treatment of edema in the first month of life. *Child Nephrology and Urology* 10(3): 161–163.

112. Arnold WC. 1984. Efficacy of metolazone and furosemide in children with furosemide-resistant edema. *Pediatrics* 74(5): 872–875.

113. Peterson G, and Rumack B. 1980. Pharmacology of furosemide in the premature newborn infant. *Journal of Pediatrics* 97(1): 139–143.

114. Reed MD, Besunder JB, and Blumer JL. 1988. Neonatal clinical pharmacology: Principles and practice. In *Neonatal Respiratory Care,* Carlo WA, and Chatburn RL, eds. Chicago: Year Book Medical Publishers, 237–259.

115. Hufnagle KG, and Khan SN. 1982. Renal calcifications: A complication of long-term furosemide therapy in preterm infants. *Pediatrics* 70(1): 360–363.

116. Vileisis RA. 1990. Furosemide effect on mineral status of parenterally nourished premature neonates with chronic lung disease. *Pediatrics* 85(3): 316–322.

117. Cooperman LB, and Rubin IL. 1973. Toxicity of ethacrynic acid and furosemide. *American Heart Journal* 85(6): 831–834.

118. Tuzel IH. 1981. Comparison of adverse reactions to bumetanide and furosemide. *Journal of Clinical Pharmacology* 21(11–12 part 2): 615–619.

119. Walker PC, and Shankaran S. 1988. The bilirubin-displacing capacity of bumetanide in critically ill neonates. *Developmental Pharmacology and Therapeutics* 11(5): 265–272.

120. Shankaran S, and Poland R. 1977. The displacement of bilirubin from albumin by furosemide. *Journal of Pediatrics* 90(4): 642–646.

121. Ng PC. 1993. The effectiveness and side effects of dexamethasone in preterm infants with bronchopulmonary dysplasia. *Archives of Disease in Childhood* 68(3 spec no): 330–336.

122. Watts CL, and Bruce MC. 1992. Effect of dexamethasone therapy on fibronectin and albumin levels in lung secretions of infants with bronchopulmonary dysplasia. *Journal of Pediatrics* 121(4): 597–607.

123. NIH. 1994. Effects of corticosteroids for fetal maturation on perinatal outcomes. Consensus statement, February 28–March 2. 12(2): 1–24.

124. Ryan CA, and Finer NN. 1995. Antenatal corticosteroid therapy to prevent respiratory distress syndrome. *Journal of Pediatrics* 126(2): 317–319.

125. Kari MA, and Heinonen K. 1993. Dexamethasone treatment in preterm infants at risk for bronchopulmonary dysplasia. *Archives of Disease in Childhood* 68(5 spec no): 566–569.

126. Gladstone IM, and Ehrenkranz RA. 1989. Pulmonary function tests and fluid balance in neonates with chronic lung disease during dexamethasone treatment. *Pediatrics* 84(6): 1072–1076.

127. O'Shea TM, et al. 1993. Follow-up of preterm infants treated with dexamethasone for chronic lung disease. *American Journal of Diseases of Children* 147(6): 658–661.

128. Cummings JJ, and D'Eugenio DB. 1989. A controlled trial of dexamethasone in preterm infants at high risk for bronchopulmonary dysplasia. *New England Journal of Medicine* 320(23): 1505–1510.

129. Collaborative Dexamethasone Trial Group. 1991. Dexamethasone therapy in neonatal chronic lung disease: An international placebo-controlled trial. *Pediatrics* 88(3): 421–427.

130. Konig P, and Shatley M. 1992. Clinical observations of nebulized flunisolide in infants and young children with asthma and bronchopulmonary dysplasia. *Pediatric Pulmonology* 13(4): 209–214.

131. Yuksel B, and Greenough A. 1992. Randomized trial of inhaled steroids in preterm infants with respiratory symptoms at follow up. *Thorax* 47(11): 910–913.

132. LaForce WR, and Brudno DS. 1993. Controlled trial of beclomethasone dipropionate by nebulization in oxygen- and ventilator-dependent infants. *Journal of Pediatrics* 122(2): 285–288.

133. Yeh TF, and Torre JA. 1990. Early postnatal dexamethasone therapy in premature infants with severe respiratory distress syndrome: A double-blind, controlled study. *Journal of Pediatrics* 117(2): 273–282.

134. Cloutier MM. 1993. Nebulized steroid therapy in bronchopulmonary dysplasia. *Pediatric Pulmonology* 15(2): 111–116.

135. Ohlsson A, et al. 1992. Randomized controlled trial of dexamethasone treatment in very-low-birth-weight infants with ventilator-dependent chronic lung disease. *Acta Paediatrica* 81(10): 751–756.

136. Couser RJ, and Ferrara TB. 1992. Effectiveness of dexamethasone in preventing extubation failure in preterm infants at increased risk for airway edema. *Journal of Pediatrics* 121(4): 591–596.

137. Courtney SE, and Weber KR. 1992. Effects of dexamethasone on pulmonary function following extubation. *Journal of Perinatology* 12(3): 246–251.

138. Tellez DW, and Galvis AG. 1991. Dexamethasone in the prevention of postextubation stridor in children. *Journal of Pediatrics* 118(2): 287–290.

139. Knoppert DC, and Mackanjee HR. 1994. Current strategies in the management of bronchopulmonary dysplasia: The role of corticosteroids. *Neonatal Network* 13(3): 53–60.

140. Yoder MC, Chua R, and Tepper R. 1991. Effects of dexamethasone on pulmonary inflammation and pulmonary function of ventilator-dependent infants with bronchopulmonary dysplasia. *American Review of Respiratory Diseases* 143(5 part 1): 1044–1048.

141. Kazzi NJ, Brans YW, and Poland RL. 1990. Dexamethasone effects on the hospital course of infants with bronchopulmonary dysplasia who are dependent on artificial ventilation. *Pediatrics* 86(5): 722–727.

142. Mammel MC, et al. 1983. Controlled trial of dexamethasone therapy in infants with bronchopulmonary dysplasia. *Lancet* 1(8338): 1356–1358.

143. Avery GB, et al. 1985. Controlled trial of dexamethasone in respirator-dependent infants with bronchopulmonary dysplasia. *Pediatrics* 75(1): 106–111.

144. Mammel MC, et al. 1987. Short-term dexamethasone therapy for bronchopulmonary dysplasia: Acute effects and 1-year follow-up. *Developmental Pharmacology and Therapeutics* 10(1): 1–11.

145. Harkavy KL, et al. 1989. Dexamethasone therapy for chronic lung disease in ventilator- and oxygen-dependent infants: A controlled trial. *Journal of Pediatrics* 115(6): 979–983.

146. Cumming JJ, D'Eugenio DB, and Gross SJ. 1989. A controlled trial of dexamethasone in preterm infants at high risk for bronchopulmonary dysplasia. *New England Journal of Medicine* 320(23): 1505–1510.

147. Noble-Jamieson CM, Regev R, and Silverman M. 1989. Dexamethasone in neonatal chronic lung disease: Pulmonary effects and intracranial complications. *European Journal of Pediatrics* 148: 365–367.

148. Yeh TF, et al. 1990. Early postnatal dexamethasone therapy in premature infants with severe respiratory distress syndrome: A double-blind controlled study. *Journal of Pediatrics* 117(2 part 1): 273–282.

149. The Collaborative Dexamethasone Trial Group. 1991. Dexamethasone therapy in neonatal chronic lung disease: An international placebo-controlled trial. *Pediatrics* 88(3): 421–427.

150. Mammel MC, et al. 1987. Short-term dexamethasone therapy for bronchopulmonary dysplasia: Acute effects and 1-year follow-up. *Developmental Pharmacology and Therapeutics* 10(1): 1–11.

151. Ferrara TB, Couser RJ, and Hoekstra RE. 1990. Side effects and long-term follow-up of corticosteroid therapy in very low birthweight infants with bronchopulmonary dysplasia. *Journal of Perinatology* 10(2): 137–142.

152. Uemura Y, and Akiya S. 1981. Steroid induced retinopathy. In *Proceedings of the Conference on Retinopathy of Prematurity*. Columbus, Ohio: Ross Laboratories, 1:162–181.

153. Ramanathan R, Siassi B, and deLemos RA. 1995. Severe retinopathy of prematurity in extremely low birth weight infants after short-term dexamethasone therapy. *Journal of Perinatology* 15(3): 178–182.

154. Harkavy KL, Scanlon JW, and Chowdhry PK. 1989. Dexamethasone therapy for chronic lung disease in ventilator dependent infants: A controlled trial. *Journal of Pediatrics* 115(6): 979–983.

155. Kazzi NJ, Brans YW, and Poland RL. 1990. Dexamethasone effects on the hospital course of infants with bronchopulmonary dysplasia who are dependent on artificial ventilation. *Pediatrics* 86(5): 722–727.

156. Werher J, et al. 1992. Hypertrophic cardiomyopathy associated with dexamethasone therapy for bronchopulmonary dysplasia. *Journal of Pediatrics* 120(2 part 1): 286–289.

157. Vallejo G, et al. 1994. Ganciclovir treatment of steroid-associated cytomegalovirus disease in a congenitally infected neonate. *Pediatric Infectious Disease Journal* 13(3): 239–241.

158. Eisenfeld L, Rosenkrantz TS, and Block C. 1994. Effect of corticosteroids on the maturation of neutrophil motility in very low birthweight neonates. *American Journal of Perinatology* 11(2): 163–166.

159. Brownlee KG, et al. 1992. Catabolic effect of dexamethasone in the preterm baby. *Archives of Disease in Childhood* 67(1): 1–4.

160. O'Neil EA, Chwals WJ, and O'Shea M. 1992. Dexamethasone treatment during ventilator dependency: Possible life threatening gastrointestinal complications. *Archives of Disease in Childhood* 67(1 spec no): 10–11.

161. Fontana M, Massironi E, and Rossi A. 1993. Ranitidine pharmacokinetics in newborn infants. *Archives of Disease in Childhood* 68(5 spec no): 602–603.

162. Kelly EJ, Chatfield SL, and Brownlee KG. 1993. The effect of intravenous ranitidine on the intragastric pH of preterm infants receiving dexamethasone. *Archives of Disease in Childhood* 69(1 spec no): 37–39.

163. Agarwal AK, et al. 1990. Role of cimetidine in prevention and treatment of stress induced gastric bleeding in neonates. *Indian Pediatrics* 27(5): 465–469.

164. Vandenplas Y, and Sacre L. 1987. The use of cimetidine in newborns. *American Journal of Perinatology* 4(2): 131–133.

165. Ziemniak JA, Wynn RJ, and Aranda JV. 1984. The pharmacokinetics and metabolism of cimetidine in neonates. *Developmental Pharmacology and Therapeutics* 7(1): 30–38.

166. Strauss A, Brakin M, and Norris K. 1992. Adrenal responsiveness in very-low-birth weight infants treated with dexamethasone. *Developmental Pharmacology and Therapeutics* 19(2–3): 147–154.

167. Muttitt SC, Tierney AJ, and Finer NN. 1988. The dose response of theophylline in the treatment of apnea of prematurity. *Journal of Pediatrics* 112(1): 115–121.

168. Capers CC, Ward ES, and Murphy JE. 1992. Use of theophylline in neonates as an aid to ventilator weaning. *Therapeutic Drug Monitoring* 14(6): 471–474.

169. Davis JM, Spitzer AR, and Stefano JL. 1987. Use of caffeine in infants unresponsive to theophylline in apnea of prematurity. *Pediatric Pulmonology* 3(2): 90–93.

170. Sims ME, et al. 1989. Comparative evaluation of caffeine and theophylline for weaning premature infants from the ventilator. *American Journal of Perinatology* 6(1): 72–75.

171. Rooklin AR, and Moomjian AR. 1979. Theophylline therapy in bronchopulmonary dysplasia. *Journal of Pediatrics* 95(2): 882–885.

172. Davi MJ, et al. 1978. Physiologic changes induced by theophylline in the treatment of apnea in preterm infants. *Journal of Pediatrics* 92(1): 91–95.

173. Persson CG, et al. 1982. Tracheal relaxant and cardiostimulant actions of xanthines can be differentiated from diuretic and cns-stimulant effects. Role of adenosine antagonism? *Life Sciences* 31(24): 2673–2681.

174. Reese J, and Prentice G. 1994. Dose conversion from aminophylline to theophylline in preterm infants. *Archives of Disease in Childhood* 71(1): F51–F52.

175. Bairam A, et al. 1987. Theophylline versus caffeine: Comparative effects in treatment of idiopathic apnea in the preterm infant. *Journal of Pediatrics* 110(4): 636–639.

176. Fuglsang G, et al. 1989. The effect of caffeine compared with theophylline in the treatment of idiopathic apnea in premature infants. *Acta Paediatrica Scandinavica* 78(5): 786–788.

177. Strauss RE, Wertheim DL, and Bonagura VR. 1994. Aminophylline therapy does not improve outcome and increases adverse effects in children hospitalized with acute asthmatic exacerbations. *Pediatrics* 93(2): 205–210.

178. Gilman JR, Gal P, and Levine RS. 1986. Factors influencing theophylline disposition in 179 newborns. *Therapeutic Drug Monitoring* 8(1): 4–10.

179. Gal P, and Gilman JA. 1986. Concerns about the food and drug administration guidelines for neonatal theophylline dosing. *Therapeutic Drug Monitoring* 8(1): 1–3.

180. O'Donnell J. 1994. Theophylline misadventures. *Neonatal Network* 13(3 part 2): 19–28.

181. Gal P, and Wyble LE. 1992. Respiratory distress syndrome in the newborn. In *Pharmacotherapy: A Pathophysiologic Approach,* DiPiro JT, et al., eds. New York: Elsevier Science Publishing, 466–481.

182. Hendeles L, and Weinberger M. 1983. Theophylline: a "state of the art" review. *Pharmacotherapy* 3(1): 2–44.

183. Viscardi RM, et al. 1985. Efficacy of theophylline for prevention of post-extubation respiratory failure in very low birth weight infants. *Journal of Pediatrics* 107(3): 469–472.

184. Gal P, Roop C, and Robinson H. 1980. Theophylline-induced seizures in accidentally overdosed neonates. *Pediatrics* 65(3): 547–549.

185. Skinner MH. 1990. Adverse reactions and interactions with theophylline. *Drug Safety* 5(4): 275–285.

186. Yazdani M, et al. 1987. Phenobarbital increases the theophylline requirement of premature infants being treated for apnea. *American Journal of Diseases of Children* 141(1): 97–99.

187. Ward RM. 1994. The use of therapeutic drugs. In *Neonatology: Pathophysiology and Management of the Newborn,* 4th ed., Avery GB, Fletcher MA, and MacDonald MG, eds. Philadelphia: JB Lippincott, 1271–1299.

188. Kulik TJ, and Lock JE. 1984. Pulmonary vasodilator therapy in persistent pulmonary hypertension of the newborn. *Clinics in Perinatology* 11(3): 693–701.

189. Drummond WH, et al. 1981. The independent effects of hyperventilation, tolazoline, and dopamine on infants with persistent pulmonary hypertension. *Journal of Pediatrics* 98 (4): 603–611.

190. Girardin E, et al. 1989. Effect of low dose dopamine on hemodynamic and renal function in children. *Pediatric Research* 26(3): 200–203.

191. Klarr JM, et al. 1994. Randomized blind trial of dopamine versus dobutamine for the treatment of hypotension in preterm infants with respiratory distress syndrome. *Journal of Pediatrics* 125(10): 117–122.

192. Vivienne M, Miall-Allen VM, and Whitelaw AG. 1989. Response to dopamine and dobutamine in the preterm infant less than 30 weeks gestation. *Critical Care Medicine* 17(11): 1166–1169.

193. Banner W, et al. 1991. Nonlinear dobutamine pharmacokinetics in a pediatric population. *Critical Care Medicine* 19(7): 871–873.

194. Driscoll DJ. 1987. Use of inotropic and chronotropic agents in neonates. *Clinics in Perinatology* 14(4): 931–949.

195. Phillips JB. 1990. Treatment of PPHNS. In *Fetal and Neonatal Cardiology,* Long WA, Tooley WH, and McNamara DG, eds. Philadelphia: WB Saunders, 692–701.

196. Walsh-Sukys MC. 1993. Persistent pulmonary hypertension of the newborn—The black box revisited. *Clinics in Perinatology* 20(1): 127–143.

197. Greenough A, and Emery EF. 1993. Randomized trial comparing dopamine and dobutamine in preterm infants. *European Journal of Pediatrics* 152(11): 925–927.

198. Yeh TF, and Luken JA. 1988. Persistent pulmonary hypertension of the newborn. In *Neonatal Respiratory Care,* Carlo WA, and Chatburn RL, eds., Chicago: Year-Book Medical Publishing, 101–111.

199. Fiser DH, et al. 1988. Cardiovascular and renal effects of dopamine and dobutamine in healthy, conscious piglets. *Critical Care Medicine* 16(4): 340–345.

200. Matson JR, and Loughlin GM. 1978. Myocardial ischemia complicating the use of isoproterenol in asthmatic children. *Journal of Pediatrics* 92(5): 776–778.

201. McMillan DD, and Sauve RS. 1986. Bolus and continuous infusion of tolazoline in neonates with hypoxemia. *Developmental Pharmacology and Therapeutics* 9(3): 192–200.

202. Benitz WE, and Malachowski N. 1984. Use of sodium nitroprusside in neonates: Efficacy and safety. *Journal of Pediatrics* 106(1): 102–110.

203. Abu-Osba YK, et al. 1991. Treatment of severe persistent pulmonary hypertension of the newborn with magnesium sulphate. *Archives of Disease in Childhood* 67(1): 31–35.

204. Boda D, et al. 1984. Effect of allopurinol treatment in premature infants with idiopathic respiratory distress syndrome. *Developmental Pharmacology and Therapeutics* 7(6): 357–367.

205. Stevenson DK, et al. 1979. Refractory hypoxemia associated with neonatal pulmonary disease: The use and limitations of tolazoline. *Journal of Pediatrics* 95(4): 595–599.

206. Michocki R. 1995. Hypertensive emergencies. In *Applied Therapeutics,* 5th ed., Young LY, and Koda-Kimble MA, eds. Vancouver, Washington: Applied Therapeutics, 17–10.

207. Costarino AT, and Polin RA. 1987. Neuromuscular relaxants in the neonate. *Clinics in Perinatology* 14(4): 965–989.

208. Mohan OE, and Hershenson MB. 1988. Metabolic and hemodynamic effects of midazolam in critically ill infants. *Anesthesiology* 69(3): 750A.

209. Franck LS, and Gregory GA. 1993. Clinical evaluation and treatment of infant pain in the neonatal intensive care unit. In *Pain Relief in Infants, Children, and Adolescents,* Schechter NL, Berde CB, and Yaster M, eds. Baltimore: Williams & Wilkins, 519–535.

210. Krieman MJ, et al. 1992. Effects of adinazolam on plasma catecholamine, heart rate and blood pressure responses in stressed and non-stressed rats. *Neuropharmacology* 31(1): 33–38.

211. Kirby R, et al. 1972. Continuous flow ventilation as an alternative to assisted or controlled ventilation in infants. *Anesthesia and Analgesia* 51(6): 871–875.

212. Perlman JM, and Goodman S. 1985. Reduction in intraventricular hemorrhage by elimination of fluctuating cerebral blood-flow velocity in preterm infants with respiratory distress syndrome. *New England Journal of Medicine* 312(21): 1353–1357.

213. Eldadah MK, and Christopher JL. 1989. Vecuronium by continuous infusion for neuromuscular blockade in infants and children. *Critical Care Medicine* 17(10): 989–992.

214. Kalli I, and Meretoja OA. 1988. Infusion of atracurium in neonates, infants and children. *British Journal of Anaesthesia* 60(6): 651–654.

215. Goudsouzian NG. 1988. Atracurium infusion in infants. *Anesthesiology* 68(2): 267–269.

216. Fisher DM, and Miller RD. 1983. Neuromuscular effects of vecuronium (ORG NC45) in infants and children during N_2O, halothane anesthesia. *Anesthesiology* 58(6): 519–523.

217. Watkins J. 1986. Histamine release and atracurium. *British Journal of Anaesthesia* 58(supplement): 19–22.

218. Basta SJ. 1992. Clinical pharmacology of mivacurium chloride: A review. *Journal of Clinical Anesthesia* 4(2): 153–163.

219. Pittet JF, and Tassonyi E. 1990. Neuromuscular effect of pipecuronium bromide in infants and children during nitrous oxide-alfentanil anesthesia. *Anesthesiology* 72(3): 432–435.

220. Rumm PD, and Takao RT. 1990. Efficacy of sedation of children with chloral hydrate. *Southern Medical Journal* 83(9): 1040–1043.

221. Anyebuno MA, and Rosenfeld CR. 1991. Chloral hydrate toxicity in a term infant. *Developmental Pharmacology and Therapeutics* 17(1–2): 116–120.

222. Reimche LD, et al. 1989. Chloral hydrate sedation in neonates and infants—Clinical and pharmacologic considerations. *Developmental Pharmacology and Therapeutics* 12(2): 57–64.

223. Mayers DJ, and Hindmarsh W. 1991. Chloral hydrate disposition following single-dose administration to critically ill neonates and children. *Developmental Pharmacology and Therapeutics* 16(2): 71–77.

224. Gal P, and Mize R. 1990. Lorazepam dosing in neonates: Application of objective sedation scores. *Annals of Pharmacotherapy* 24(3): 326–327.

225. Tuel DC, and Weis FR. 1990. Oral midazolam for a mentally retarded patient. *Anesthesiology* 72(1): 216–217.

226. Thomson NC. 1992. Anti-inflammatory therapies. *British Medical Bulletin* 48(1): 205–220.

227. Yamamoto C, and Kojima T. 1992. Disodium cromoglycate in the treatment of bronchopulmonary dysplasia. *Acta Paediatrica Japonica* 34(6): 589–591.

228. Watterberg KL, and Murphy S. 1993. Failure of cromolyn sodium to reduce the incidence of bronchopulmonary dysplasia: A pilot study. *Pediatrics* 91(4): 803–806.

229. Shook LA. 1988. Improved lung resistance and compliance during cromolyn therapy in infants with bronchopulmonary dysplasia. *Pediatric Research* 24(4): 524A.

230. Stenmark KR. 1985. Recovery of platelet-activating factor and leukotrienes from infants with severe bronchopulmonary dysplasia: Clinical improvement with cromolyn treatment. *American Review of Respiratory Disease* 131(4): 236A.

231. Fisher J. 1992. Effect of cromolyn sodium on respiratory status of ventilated preterm infants. *Pediatric Research* 31(4 part 2): 307A.

232. DeGiulio PA. 1988. Effects of pretreatment with cromolyn and cold-induced airway reactivity in bronchopulmonary dysplasia. *Pediatric Research* 23(4): 503A.

233. Armenio L, et al. 1993. Double blind, placebo controlled study of nedocromil sodium in asthma. *Archives of Disease in Childhood* 68(2): 193–197.

234. Peliowski A, and Finer NN. 1990. A blinded, randomized, placebo-controlled trial to compare theophylline and doxapram for the treatment of apnea of prematurity. *Journal of Pediatrics* 116(4): 648–653.

235. Brion LR, et al. 1991. Low-dose doxapram for apnea unresponsive to aminophylline in very low birthweight infants. *Journal of Perinatology* 11(4): 359–364.

236. Jamali F, et al. 1988. Doxapram dosage regimen in apnea of prematurity based on pharmacokinetic data. *Developmental Pharmacology and Therapeutics* 11(5): 253–257.

237. Kumita H, et al. 1991. Low-dose doxapram therapy in premature infants and its CSF and serum concentrations. *Acta Paediatrica Scandinavica* 80(8–9): 786–791.

238. Tay-Uyboco J, et al. 1991. Clinical and physiologic responses to prolonged nasogastric administration of doxapram for apnea of prematurity. *Biology of the Neonate* 59(4): 190–200.

NOTES

11 Continuous Positive Airway Pressure for Neonates

Debra Bingham Jones, MS, RN,C
Diane Deveau, MS, RNC

There has been interest in the use of continuous positive airway pressure (CPAP) for treating respiratory distress in neonates since the late 1960s. In 1971, George Gregory, an anesthesiologist working in an NICU, and his team were the first to publish research on CPAP used for neonates with idiopathic respiratory distress syndrome.[1] His surprising success led to multiple studies examining the physiology and potential clinical application of CPAP during the 1970s and early 1980s.[1–9]

During this period, mechanical ventilation for neonates was also being developed and refined, and there were very few choices for management of neonatal respiratory distress. Currently, there are several options, including some that are new and very exciting. However, the use of nasal prong CPAP, even for the very ill or premature infant, remains a viable alternative to mechanical ventilation.

In most NICUs today, CPAP is used as one respiratory care option. Unfortunately, in some units, CPAP has earned a reputation for being cumbersome, time-consuming, and not effective enough to handle many cases of neonatal respiratory distress. There are contradictions among the studies designed to assess the clinical application, effectiveness, and physiologic consequences of CPAP. Comparisons can be very difficult because the amount of positive end-expiratory pressure (PEEP) used, the type of pressure-generating device, and the method of delivering CPAP vary greatly from study to study and from center to center.

Since 1974, Babies and Children's Hospital of the Columbia-Presbyterian Medical Center in New York City has used CPAP consistently and effectively as its primary mode of neonatal respiratory support. This chapter discusses the benefits of neonatal CPAP, the methodology used by Columbia-Presbyterian Medical Center, and strategies for enhancing the effectiveness of the therapy while minimizing patient complications.

REDUCING CHRONIC LUNG DISEASE

Chronic lung disease, originally defined as the need for supplemental oxygen at 28 days of life, is a prevalent and often debilitating complication of respiratory therapy in neonates. Respiratory care practices can have a significant impact on the number of cases and severity of the disease. In 1979, Wung and colleagues at Columbia-Presbyterian published a study describing the use of nasal prong CPAP instead of mechanical ventilation that decreased the incidence of bronchopulmonary dysplasia (BPD).[10]

A 1987 survey by Avery and coworkers revealed large differences in the percentage of chronic lung disease among infants in eight tertiary care centers. Columbia-Presbyterian Medical Center, one of the eight centers studied, had one of the best survival rates for low birth weight infants, yet it also had a significantly lower rate of chronic lung disease.[11] The major difference between this center and others was the consistent early application of nasal prong CPAP and the resulting decreased dependence on mechanical ventilation. This remains true today, because basic respiratory care practices have changed very little for the majority of neonates with respiratory distress born at or transferred to Columbia-Presbyterian.

PHYSIOLOGIC PRINCIPLES

The terms CPAP and PEEP are sometimes interchanged and confused. Continuous positive airway pressure is the system that allows positive end-expiratory pressure and a variable amount of oxygen to be continuously delivered to the airways of a spontaneously breathing patient. The amount of pressure is constant and is present during both the inspiratory and expiratory phases. During mechanical ventilation, PEEP is generated at the end of exhalation, between delivered breaths. General physiologic principles demonstrate the primary and secondary effects of PEEP and CPAP.

PRIMARY EFFECTS

Prevention of Atelectasis

Prevention of atelectasis is the primary benefit of neonatal CPAP because the most commonly encountered respiratory illnesses in the neonate include some degree of atelectasis resulting in respiratory distress. Continuous

positive airway pressure provides enough pressure to mechanically stabilize the air sacs, preventing collapse.

It is well documented that CPAP not only prevents alveolar collapse but actually recruits additional alveoli for gas exchange. *Prevention* of atelectasis is critical because it is much easier to maintain an expanded alveolus than to re-expand it.

Conservation of Surfactant

Surfactant production is low in the premature infant, and available surfactant can be quickly depleted, leading to alveolar collapse. When the alveoli collapse, surfactant is consumed at an even higher rate because of decreased surface area.[12] Continuous positive airway pressure acts to stabilize the alveolar wall mechanically, until production of surfactant is adequate. There is also some evidence that the use of CPAP in infants with respiratory distress syndrome (RDS) enhances surfactant release.[13]

Again, the early application of CPAP is critical to prevent or decrease the loss of existing surfactant. In addition, CPAP reduces the chance of damage to Type II pneumocytes that can be caused by high inspiratory pressures generated by mechanical ventilation.

Decreased Intrapulmonary Shunting

Physiologic shunting within the lung occurs when the web of blood vessels cannot exchange carbon dioxide and oxygen within the collapsed alveolus. If gas exchange does not occur over a widespread area, hypoxia and hypercarbia can result. With CPAP, right-to-left intrapulmonary shunting of blood decreases, which lessens ventilation-to-perfusion mismatch and results in improved gas exchange and increased arterial oxygen tension.

Increased Functional Residual Capacity

Functional residual capacity (FRC) is the air remaining in the lungs after exhalation. Gas exchange continues between breaths, with FRC functioning as an important reserve of air. In many infants with respiratory illnesses, FRC is greatly diminished, which decreases activity tolerance and increases the chance of hypoxia. Continuous positive airway pressure increases a neonate's ability to adjust to episodes of greater respiratory demands, such as nursing or medical procedures, feeding, or activity.[14]

Increased Compliance

When the functional residual capacity is improved, compliance is generally also improved. The alveoli are kept partially distended by CPAP and so are easier to expand during a neonate's breathing efforts. However, compliance can decrease if too much distending pressure is applied and the alveoli become overdistended.[15,16]

Increased Airway Diameter, Splinted Airway, and Diaphragm

By the mechanical action of its distending pressure, CPAP stabilizes and slightly distends the airways. Because of this increase in airway diameter, resistance is lowered during both inspiration and exhalation. Airway collapse is lessened or prevented, and premature babies exhibit a reduction in obstructive or mixed type apnea.[17–19]

Regularized Respiration

Neonates' breathing patterns become more regular on CPAP, probably because of the mechanical effects of the distending pressure which stabilize the chest wall and reduce thoracic distortion.[13,19] Premature infants are predisposed to chest wall distortion because of their flexible chest structure and lack of musculature. This makes them more prone to periods of irregular breathing and apnea.[19]

Decreased Tidal Volume, Respiratory Rate, Minute Ventilation

The majority of newborns on CPAP experiences a decrease in their respiratory rate and tidal volume; therefore, minute ventilation is decreased (minute ventilation = tidal volume × respiratory rate). In spite of the decrease in minute ventilation, the $PaCO_2$ remains stable or falls, demonstrating that alveolar ventilation is adequate. This phenomenon probably occurs from the recruitment of additional alveoli and reduction of dead space brought about by the CPAP.[20]

SECONDARY EFFECTS

Regional changes in cardiac, renal, and cerebral blood flow distribution due to PEEP have been documented. These changes, which are sometimes contradictory among the studies, are influenced by the infant's disease process, the CPAP delivery system, and the amount of pressure generated. There is no documentation that intestinal or hepatic blood flow is affected.[12]

Cardiac

Cardiac output is generally decreased with the introduction of PEEP, although clinically the effect may not be significant. The effect will be more pronounced with higher levels of PEEP that decrease venous return. Sturgeon and associates found no change in cardiac output in adults on CPAP.[21]

Neonates with hyaline membrane disease often demonstrate right-to-left shunting through the foramen ovale and left-to-right shunting through the ductus arteriosus.[13] This contributes significantly to the hypoxemia, pulmonary fluid retention, and morbidity seen in many of these newborns.

The effects of PEEP on cardiac function were studied in premature lambs, and some beneficial effects were found. The shunting through the foramen ovale was decreased, which improved oxygenation. Right ventricular output was increased without significant change in left ventricular output or pulmonary vascular resistance. Left-to-right ductal flow also decreased.[22] These consequences will have a positive effect on cardiac output and oxygenation.

Renal

There have been some studies on the renal effects of PEEP. Urinary output, glomerular filtration, and sodium and potassium excretion are decreased, and renal blood flow is either reduced or redistributed. The water- and sodium-retaining hormonal systems—antidiuretic hormone and aldosterone—are stimulated, and there is an antidiuretic effect.[23,24] These changes are reversible when PEEP is withdrawn.

Neurologic

Some studies suggest that intracranial pressure is increased with PEEP, especially when CPAP is delivered by a headbox.[12,25,26] One study found that the application of PEEP does not increase intracranial pressure. The pressure is dissipated through the venous systems between the pulmonary and cerebral circulations; the exact mechanism is unknown.[27]

Again, the amount of PEEP and the patient's lung compliance seem to play an important role in determining the degree of the effect. Higher levels of PEEP, coupled with less compliant lungs, are associated with higher intracranial pressures and decreased cerebral perfusion pressure. The clinical consequences of these effects in neonates are essentially unknown.

INDICATIONS FOR CPAP

There are three indications for the use of nasal prong CPAP: (1) respiratory distress of any origin (except congenital diaphragmatic hernia), (2) as a bridge when weaning from mechanical ventilation, and (3) apnea and bradycardia of the premature newborn.

TREATMENT FOR NEONATAL RESPIRATORY DISTRESS

Neonatal respiratory distress can present in a number of ways. Commonly observed signs and symptoms include grunting, retracting, flaring, tachypnea, decreased breath sounds, cyanosis, lethargy, and irritability. Further clinical evidence can be obtained by oximetry, transcutaneous monitoring, arterial blood gas analysis, and radiology. The etiology of respiratory distress includes a variety of pulmonary diseases, cardiac disease, neuromuscular disease, and sepsis. Nasal prong CPAP can be very effective in stabilizing the respiratory status while the underlying disease process is evaluated and treated. Common neonatal respiratory problems successfully treated with nasal prong CPAP alone include RDS, meconium aspiration syndrome, pulmonary edema, transient tachypnea of the newborn, and BPD.

Only in the case of unrepaired congenital diaphragmatic hernia should nasal prong CPAP be avoided. The risk in this situation involves distending pressure being delivered to the gastrointestinal tract that is abnormally lodged in the chest cavity. This would potentially increase the size of the gastrointestinal tract and decrease lung expansion even further.

The importance of early application of CPAP to prevent atelectasis and minimize the spiral of acute respiratory distress leading to respiratory failure cannot be overemphasized. Treatment with CPAP is most effective when applied promptly after respiratory distress is recognized. Early application of CPAP reduces the need for intermittent positive pressure ventilation and the duration of respiratory assistance—even in very low birth weight infants.[28–30] Recognition of respiratory distress often occurs shortly after delivery, and it can frequently be anticipated, as in the case of premature delivery or the presence of thick meconium.

At Columbia-Presbyterian, there is a small transitional nursery located in the labor and delivery area that is used for the purpose of immediate stabilization of the compromised neonate. Resuscitation is performed according to the American Heart Association/American Academy of Pediatrics Neonatal Resuscitation Program guidelines, and the neonate can be evaluated by nursery personnel with all of the necessary equipment. Infants are not electively intubated for prophylactic administration of surfactant. (At Columbia-Presbyterian, exogenous surfactant may be administered as a rescue protocol for extreme respiratory distress but is not used for prophylaxis.)

Because the staff anticipates the use of CPAP for most newborns admitted to this nursery, a CPAP unit is always set up, but it is left dry and securely covered to prevent contamination. In this way, CPAP can be applied to an infant only a few minutes old. Neonates who required bag and mask ventilation or even intubation for resuscitation subsequently may be placed on nasal prong CPAP.

As resuscitation efforts become effective, the rate of delivered breaths is slowed, and the neonate is encouraged to breathe spontaneously. The newborn is allowed several minutes to respond to this treatment before a decision is made to intubate. Of course, if there are symptoms of severe cardiopulmonary distress, the baby is immediately intubated and receives mechanical ventilation until the acute phase has resolved.

WEANING FROM MECHANICAL VENTILATION

At Columbia-Presbyterian, as well as other medical centers, the use of CPAP has facilitated weaning from mechanical ventilation. Engelke, Roloff, and Kuhns reported less atelectasis, lower respiratory rates, better arterial blood gases, and no reintubations.[28] Andreasson and colleagues, using a face mask system on very premature infants, reported improved oxygenation and decreased frequency of apnea.[31]

Other centers have not experienced this success.[32,33] This may be a result of differences in methods of delivering CPAP, staff comfort with a potentially labile infant on CPAP, or differences in criteria for extubation. In the case of an infant with RDS, it is clear that although

premature infants may no longer need mechanical breaths or inspiratory pressure, they may not be able to fully support the work of breathing and gas exchange on their own.

Mechanical ventilation can be harmful even at low settings when continued until the infant matures. Also, repeated extubation failures are detrimental to the patient's stability and leave him open to the risks of repeated episodes of atelectasis and reintubation. Extubation of the relatively stable infant can be considered sooner when oxygen and PEEP can be delivered via nasal prong CPAP.

TREATMENT FOR APNEA AND BRADYCARDIA

Apnea and bradycardia in the neonate can also be successfully treated with CPAP. There are three types of apnea in the neonate: central, obstructive, and mixed. The majority of neonatal apneas have an obstructive component. Obstructive apnea and mixed apnea are the most responsive to the application of CPAP because of the mechanical effects of chest wall stabilization and the splinting of the airways and diaphragm. Central apnea seems to show little or no response to CPAP.[14,18,19,34] Treatment with CPAP can frequently be used alone for apnea, or methylxanthines can be used as an adjunct, often at lower doses than would be needed without the use of CPAP.

ADMINISTRATION OF PRESSURE

Since the use of CPAP began, researchers have been seeking the "optimal" level of PEEP to relieve respiratory distress while causing the fewest complications. Low levels of PEEP (0–3 cm of pressure) generally do little lung damage and avoid the problem of overinflation but may not be high enough to overcome atelectasis.[35] Moderate levels of PEEP (4–7 cm) recruit alveoli to prevent atelectasis, but there is some risk of overinflation.[36]

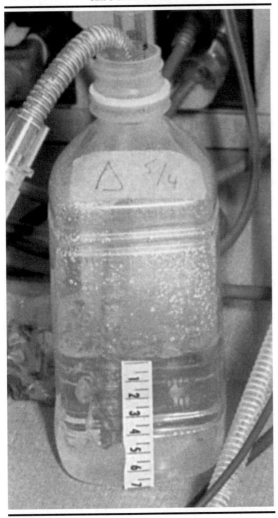

Most complications, such as decreased lung compliance, air leak, impaired venous return, and increased $PaCO_2$, occur at high levels of PEEP (8 cm or greater).[35,37-39] Many of the changes in the cardiopulmonary, renal, and cerebral circulations have been studied at the higher levels of PEEP, therefore, it is unclear if the same changes would occur at lower levels of PEEP.

The method of generating the positive pressure also varies, which causes some differences from institution to institution in ease of setup, cost, and technical difficulties. Most centers generate CPAP from an infant ventilator or an exhalation valve. There is a built-in manometer to read the pressure level, alarm limits can be set, the staff is familiar with manipulating the equipment, machines and tubing are already stocked, and the appearance is conventional.

Potential economic disadvantages, especially for a smaller hospital, include maintaining a supply of expensive equipment that might not otherwise be needed, and not being able to implement CPAP because the ventilator is needed by a sicker patient.

Clinically, any pressure-generating device can deliver excessive PEEP and cause pneumothorax or lung damage. A simple way of regulating pressure is to submerge the expiratory tubing under solution for the desired level of PEEP. At Columbia-Presbyterian, PEEP is delivered by leaving 7 cm of 0.25 percent acetic acid solution in its plastic container, then submerging the expiratory end of the CPAP tubing 5 cm into the solution to generate PEEP of +5 cm. The tubing is secured at the neck of the container by a 5 ml syringe with the cap and plunger removed (Figure 11-1).

This archaic looking method was chosen for cost, availability, and safety reasons. This system is inexpensive, readily available, easily replaced and maintained, and places no limit on the number of patients who can be on CPAP at any time. Leaving no more than 7 cm of solution in the container decreases the risk of delivering more than 7 cm of CPAP.

Manipulating the amount of gas flow can change the amount of pressure delivered to the neonate (pressure = flow × resistance). A minimal flow of 5 liters per minute is necessary to generate sufficient pressure and flush carbon dioxide from the system. A maximum flow of 10 liters per minute minimizes the risk of increased distending pressure to the lungs and excessive airflow into the abdomen via the esophagus. Flow is also a very important component of CPAP because the continuous flow of inspired gas does part of the work of breathing.[40]

The CPAP system can be assessed to be intact via manometer readings or by observing gentle bubbling in the solution bottle. *Note:* With nasal prong CPAP, manometer readings can fluctuate because the distending pressure is delivered to and measured at the nares instead of the trachea. Evaluating the neonate clinically instead of focusing on manometer fluctuations is the most useful indicator of how the neonate is tolerating CPAP.

With the solution bottle system, the amount of bubbling can fluctuate and even be intermittent if the neonate is clinically stable. Vigorous bubbling is unnecessary and generally indicates an excessive liter flow rate. If the liter flow is adequate, low manometer readings or lack of bubbling is caused by a leak within the system, nasal prongs that are too small and allow air to escape from the nares, or pressure escaping through the neonate's open mouth.

Although the effectiveness of PEEP and CPAP has been documented, clinically it is also very important to select the best delivery system. Discussions of the effectiveness of CPAP among NICUs can be confused by the different means available of administering the CPAP to the baby. Common methods include endotracheal tubes, nasopharyngeal prongs or tubes, face masks or hoods, and various types of nasal prongs.

ENDOTRACHEAL TUBE CPAP

Delivering CPAP by endotracheal tube ensures delivery of a specified amount of pressure directly to the lungs. If the infant should deteriorate, mechanical ventilation can begin immediately because the infant is already intubated. However, CPAP delivered by endotracheal tube has some serious drawbacks.

The endotracheal tube is longer and narrower than the neonate's trachea. Resistance is increased in tubes with longer lengths and smaller diameters.[41] The common analogy is one of breathing through a straw. The work of breathing becomes much harder, and fatigue leading to apnea or symptoms of respiratory distress are likely. It is always desirable to decrease the work of breathing in infants because respiratory muscle fatigue may contribute to respiratory failure.[42]

At Columbia-Presbyterian, when an infant has been mechanically ventilated, there is a trial of endotracheal CPAP for 15 minutes before extubation is attempted. This challenge is very stressful for some neonates, and it is quite common for the infant to have improved oxygenation and less distress when extubated and placed on nasal prong CPAP.

Some centers advocate manipulation of the amount of PEEP to improve oxygenation, and this can be easily achieved by endotracheal CPAP. However, because endotracheal CPAP is delivered directly to the lungs it leaves no way for the neonate to "pop off" excess pressure, whether delivered deliberately or inadvertently.

The risks of increased levels of PEEP were already described. Other drawbacks of endotracheal CPAP include laryngeal, tracheal, and vocal cord irritation or damage, increased risk of infection, need for sterile endotracheal suctioning technique, delay of feedings, and undetected endotracheal tube malposition.

NASOPHARYNGEAL CPAP

Nasopharyngeal CPAP involves one tube or a set of longer prongs inserted through the nares to rest in the pharynx. Although this method avoids the risks associated with endotracheal tubes, it shares the key problem of increased resistance. To facilitate passage and decrease trauma, these tubes are narrower than the airway. Also, they are long enough to reach the pharynx, and the neonate is forced to work

TABLE 11-1 ▲ Evaluation of Respiratory Status

Visual Observation (at rest and when awake)
Respiratory rate
Retractions (upper and lower chest)
Nasal flaring
Overall work of breathing
Comparison of upper and lower chest movement
    (synchronized, lag on inspiration, or "see-saw")

Auditory/Auscultation
Breath sounds
Grunting (inspiratory or expiratory)

Machine Based
Oximetry
Blood gas analysis
Radiography
Transcutaneous monitoring

harder to breathe through a long, narrow tube or tubes.

These tubes also create moderate to large amounts of secretions, which may be difficult and time-consuming to clear, but it is essential to keep the system patent and effective. Retropharyngeal abscess secondary to nasopharyngeal CPAP is rarely reported, but remains a potentially serious complication.[43]

FACE MASK CPAP

Face masks were once a common method of applying CPAP, and they are still used in a few centers. It can be very difficult to initiate and maintain a secure enough seal between the face and the mask to generate positive pressure and yet not damage the skin. There is a large amount of dead space in the mask, which can lead to carbon dioxide retention. The mouth and nose are relatively inaccessible, and suctioning can be difficult because PEEP will be lost. Gastric distention, especially at high flow rates, is also a problem.

NASAL PRONG CPAP

Nasal prongs are an easy and effective way to deliver CPAP. There are a few types of nasal prongs commercially available for neonates, and each NICU has developed strategies for keeping the prongs in place. Those systems that require constant readjustment, especially for the active infant, have earned CPAP a reputation for being hard to work with and not very useful. Careful selection of the type of prong used will decrease staff labor and increase CPAP effectiveness. The ideal prongs have the following characteristics:

- They are short, wide, and thin walled to allow for maximal airflow and decreased resistance.
- They are very soft and flexible to minimize trauma.
- They come in a variety of sizes to ensure a good fit for all neonates.
- They are easily and firmly secured, even on an active neonate, so therapy is continuous with minimal effort.
- They are designed to minimize the chance of tissue damage or irritation. Prongs set on a bridge rest off the face. Prongs that must be set firmly up the nose to generate sufficient pressure should be avoided because this can predispose to nasal septum breakdown.
- The tubing is lightweight and flexible, so that neonates can be positioned comfortably and the CPAP system adjusted to them instead of vice-versa.

Nasal prong CPAP has the lowest incidence of pneumothorax, comparable to the rate of spontaneous pneumothorax.[12] Another major advantage of nasal prong CPAP is the speed with which the system can be applied and removed. If the equipment is at hand, it only takes a few minutes. A professional staff member can be trained to quickly set up and apply CPAP with minimal risk to the infant, should he show signs of deterioration. The prongs are easy to remove for suctioning and are quickly replaced. The mouth is left free for feedings, pacifiers, or hygiene.

It is also easy to try a stable baby off CPAP. The prongs are simply removed from the nares and the baby observed for signs of increasing distress. Weaning a chronically ill child from CPAP can be done by an on/off schedule that takes only a few minutes to perform and can be cut short at any time if distress occurs.

Note: CPAP cannot be discontinued even briefly by shutting off the gas flow but leaving the prongs in place. Newborns are obligate nose breathers, so either the prongs must be removed from the nares, or a supply of fresh gas must be provided.

CARE OF THE INFANT ON NASAL PRONG CPAP

RESPIRATORY ASSESSMENT

A system-by-system evaluation of the neonate's response to CPAP should be done regularly to determine the effectiveness of the treatment and guide the care that is given. One of the key components of this evaluation is the response of the infant's respiratory system.

There are several methods to employ when evaluating an infant's respiratory response and the effectiveness of CPAP (Table 11-1). In a high-tech environment of machine-based assessments, it is important to take the time and make the effort to be skilled in low-tech physical assessment skills. Many decisions about the management of a neonate on CPAP are based on the physical examination rather than machine values. This is because an infant will make many physical adjustments in the method and rate of breathing in an effort to maintain homeostasis *before* technological tools indicate a change in respiratory status.

A change in the infant's oxygen saturation, blood gas values, and x-ray film are often late indications of the degree of respiratory distress. For example, after a visual assessment of the neonate's retractions, respiratory rate, and overall work of breathing, the size of prongs being used may be determined to be too small

because the infant is not breathing comfortably and air is leaking around the prongs. A decision to change the size of the prongs can be made before any deterioration is evidenced in the infant's oxygen saturation, blood gas values, and/or x-ray film.

Another example: During a trial off CPAP, the infant may become tachypneic and show an increase in the work of breathing by retracting and nasal flaring. The decision to replace the CPAP will depend more on the neonate's clinical response, even if the oxygen saturation level, blood gas values, and x-ray film remain unchanged. Just as a nurse does not wait for an infant to become hypothermic before initiating a neutral thermal environment, so a nurse must use physical assessment skills in her decision to resume CPAP before there are changes in the blood gas and x-ray.

The Silverman-Andersen Retraction Score is available to help quantitate the nurse's visual assessments of the neonate (Chapter 3).[44] The index can be particularly useful for the nurse who is learning to evaluate respiratory distress. These observations must be communicated in the written record and in discussions with colleagues.

The frequency of evaluating the infant's respiratory status depends on the severity of his condition. In most situations, an evaluation every two to three hours is adequate as long as continuous oxygen saturation monitoring is maintained. When evaluating respiratory status, make visual observations of the infant's breathing when at rest and compare these to the infant when awake or agitated. Visual observations are early indicators of how well the CPAP is working as well as the severity and progression of the respiratory disease. When breath sounds are auscultated, the CPAP prongs need to be removed from the infant's nares. When using the immersion technique for generating pressure, the bubbling can interfere with auscultation of breath sounds.

AIRWAY CARE

Humidity

The percentage of humidity being delivered in the CPAP system is an important component that is often overlooked. The preferred percentage of humidity needed is 90–100 percent. Most humidifiers have a button or knob to make the necessary adjustments in the amount of humidity being delivered.

The importance of providing adequate humidity in the system cannot be overemphasized. If the humidity of the gas being administered is not adequate, the infant's mucous membranes become extremely dry, making it difficult to suction the nasopharynx without causing irritation and bleeding in the area. If there is bleeding, scabs form that may block off part of the airway and cause pain and trauma to the infant whenever suctioning takes place. In addition, without adequate humidity, the infant's secretions will be thicker and more tenacious, making them more difficult to remove and leading to a decreased effectiveness of the CPAP system.

An airway blocked by edema, thick secretions, and scabs requires more frequent suctioning. The need for frequent suctioning leads to more trauma in the area and a vicious cycle has begun. All of these complications may be avoided if the percentage of humidity delivered remains above 90 percent. Adequate humidity in the CPAP system also improves pulmonary toilet for infants with meconium aspiration syndrome.

A clinical indicator of adequate humidity is the amount of "rain out" in the system. With 90–100 percent humidity, rain out in the CPAP tubing will require emptying approximately every two to three hours. If no rain out occurs,

then the percentage of humidity is lower than desired.

Temperature

Careful monitoring of the temperature of the delivered gas is important. In general, the temperature of the gas should be maintained close to the desired body temperature: 36.5°C (97.7°F). An in-line thermometer located outside the heat source of a radiant warmer or incubator will accurately measure the temperature of the gas being delivered to the infant.

Every three hours, the nurse should evaluate and document the temperature of the gas in order to make appropriate adjustments. If the gas being delivered is lower than body temperature, then the infant's secretions will be thicker and more difficult to suction. If the temperature is higher than 100°F, the gas can burn or damage the mucosa of the nasopharynx or lungs.

The administration of cold or hot gas can adversely affect the infant's body temperature. Body temperatures outside the neutral thermal range will have a negative impact on the infant's respiratory status by affecting oxygen consumption, blood vessel size, and oxygen saturation.

CARE OF THE NASAL SEPTUM

Meticulous attention to the nasal septum is an important aspect of nursing care for the infant on CPAP. Nasal septum breakdown is caused by the pressure of the nasal prongs on the nasal septum. Increased pressure on the nasal septum leads to decreased circulation in the area and pressure necrosis. The only way to prevent nasal septal breakdown is to prevent pressure on the septum. The use of creams or barriers to prevent breakdown has not been shown to be effective and may have adverse effects.

Five components are key in helping the nurse keep the prongs off the nasal septum: (1) the type and size of nasal prongs, (2) the hat used for anchoring and positioning the tubing and prongs, (3) proper positioning of the neonate and prongs, (4) use of lightweight tubing, and (5) use of a Velcro mustache. The effectiveness of these interventions needs to be routinely assessed and documented by the nurse.

Type and Size of Prongs

The type and size of prongs used has the greatest impact on the prevention of nasal septum breakdown. Choose prongs that are designed to work without applying pressure to the nasal septum. (At Columbia-Presbyterian, we use the nasal prongs manufactured by Hudson, RCI because these prongs were developed based on Dr. Wung's specifications.) Nasal prongs should fill the nostrils completely without force, and part of the prong should remain outside of the nose. In this way, the bridge of the prongs cannot possibly press into the septum, as shown in Figure 11-2.

Choosing large prongs with a snug fit will help keep the prongs in place, saving nursing time and decreasing the amount of nasal irritation. The size of prong needed will vary based on the manufacturer's recommendations, the infant's size, and the infant's physical features. For the newborn weighing <700 gm, the nostrils may need to be slightly dilated with a cotton swab lubricated in saline to allow a larger size prong to fit. Prongs that fit snugly are ideal for the very low birth weight infant because a snug fit will help hold the prongs off the nasal septum while decreasing airway resistance.

Hat

The hat works best if it is snug and stationary on the neonate's head. If the hat moves around, then the prongs will also move around. A length of 2-, 3-, and occasionally 4-inch stockinette seems to work best. (The hats that come with commercial prongs usually do not seem to fit well and easily slide off the infant's head.)

FIGURE 11-2 ▲ Correct size and positioning of prongs.

This 18-day-old, 35-week gestation infant remains on CPAP for retractions and tachypnea after extracorporeal membrane oxygenation for congenital diaphragmatic hernia.

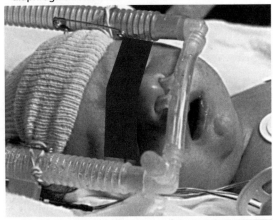

From: Jones DB, and Deveau D. 1991. Nasal prong CPAP: A proven method for the reduction of chronic lung disease. *Neonatal Network* 10(4): 7–15. Reprinted by permission.

The width of the stockinette is determined by the size of the neonate's head. Neonates who weigh <1,000 gm usually require 2-inch stockinette, and those who weigh >1,000 gm usually require 3-inch stockinette.

The length needed also varies; usually 11 inches will provide enough length to make a wide 2–3-inch rim and secure the hat at the crown (Figure 11-3). A 2–3-inch rim is made by folding the stockingnette twice; this is where the tubing is secured into place. A tie or rubber band at the crown of the head helps prevent the hat from slipping down.

After 24 to 36 hours, the hat will usually be stretched out and need to be replaced. As the hat loosens, the nurse will have more difficulty keeping the prongs in their proper position. Although a snug hat is important, it should not be so tight that it leaves ridges in the infant's skin. This would indicate that the hat is tight enough to possibly decrease perfusion to the area.

The proper position of the hat is resting along the lower part of the ears and across the

FIGURE 11-3 ▲ **A 13-day-old infant born at 27 weeks gestation and 588 gm on room air CPAP.**

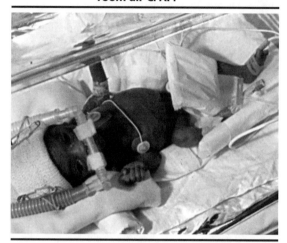

FIGURE 11-4 ▲ **A Velcro mustache and nasal suctioning (on room air CPAP).**

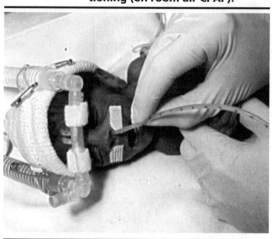

neonate's forehead. Make sure that the infant's earlobes are lying flat and are not folded. Clean behind the neonate's earlobes at least daily. If intravenous or arterial lines need to be placed in the infant's scalp while he is on CPAP, a hole may be cut in the hat to facilitate visualization of this area.

Tubing

Lightweight respiratory tubing should be used. In-line water collection bottles should be avoided because the additional weight added to the tubing can pull the prongs toward the nasal septum. The twist of the tubing in one direction or another affects the ease of keeping the prongs in the nostrils and whether the tubing rests on the infant's cheeks. The tubing needs to be adjusted so that it does not press into the infant's cheeks (Figures 11-2 and 11-3).

The tubing is anchored onto the hat by the use of Velcro or safety pins and rubber bands. Each nurse may determine the method that works best. (Figures 11-2 and 11-3 show the use of safety pins and rubber bands.) No matter which method is used, the primary consideration is that the tubing be held securely in place with enough room to make necessary fine

adjustments up and down. When using safety pins and rubber bands, point the safety pins toward the crown of the infant's head rather than the face, making sure the pins do not go through all thicknesses of the rim of the hat into the infant's scalp.

Mustache on the Philtrum

No matter how well the hat fits, how lightweight the tubing is, how the baby is positioned, or the size and type of prongs used, it is difficult in some infants to keep the prongs off the septum. On these occasions, a Velcro mustache placed over a piece of Tegaderm has been used effectively at Columbia-Presbyterian to maintain the prongs in proper position (Figure 11-4). Because of the moisture in the humidified gas and nasal and oral secretions, the Tegaderm and Velcro will loosen eventually, making it easy to replace.

ABDOMINAL DISTENTION

A neonate on nasal prong CPAP will have some gastric and intestinal distention or "CPAP belly" (Figure 11-5). It is unclear whether this is caused by the baby swallowing air, the amount of pressure in the system, decreased gut motility, or a combination of these. Research conducted by Jaile-Marti and colleagues has

FIGURE 11-5 ▲ A soft distended abdomen, "CPAP belly" (on 23 percent nasal prong CPAP).

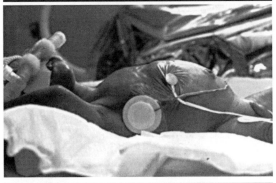

From: Jones DB, and Deveau D. 1991. Nasal prong CPAP: A proven method for the reduction of chronic lung disease. *Neonatal Network* 10(4): 7–15. Reprinted by permission.

FIGURE 11-6 ▲ Gentle aspiration of air from the stomach of a 13-day-old infant born at 27 weeks gestation and 588 gm, while on room air nasal prong CPAP.

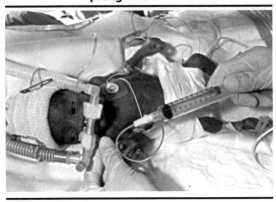

shown that CPAP belly is benign and can be differentiated from necrotizing enterocolitis.[45]

The clinical characteristics of a benign CPAP belly are a softly distended abdomen without skin discoloration and no instability of the vital signs. Bowel loops may be a sign of necrotizing enterocolitis or may just be from the CPAP; further investigation is warranted and careful monitoring is indicated.

To help reduce the amount of distention, the stomach should be gently aspirated every three to four hours using an orogastric tube and a syringe (Figure 11-6). After aspirating the stomach, remove the tube and document the amount of air obtained. Leaving the orogastric tube indwelling may lead to unwanted irritation and vagal stimulation without any clinical benefit and may even increase the amount of air the baby swallows.

If the neonate is on bolus gavage feedings, simply aspirate the stomach prior to feeding the infant. If a neonate is on continuous feedings and has some abdominal distention, the feeding is interrupted, and air and stomach contents are aspirated gently with a syringe. Any milk aspirated is then returned to the stomach, and the continuous feeding is restarted.

When a neonate is suffering from severe respiratory illness, there does not seem to be as much abdominal distention as there is when he starts to improve. The infant who is older and has been stable on CPAP for weeks also seems to have fewer problems with abdominal distention.

POSITIONING

The labile infant in severe respiratory distress will do better if he is positioned supine or on one side or another using a small neck roll and supportive nesting rolls and elevating the head of the bed approximately 30 degrees (Figure 11-3). Limiting the amount of handling and manipulation of the equipment and patient decrease the amount of stress on the infant.

Positioning an infant prone while on CPAP often requires more time and many adjustments, especially for less experienced nurses. The supine or side-lying position for a labile infant allows for better visualization of the infant's breathing and quicker access for suctioning. Once the neonate is more stable, which is often just a matter of days, alternating between supine, prone, and side-lying positions is recommended.

The stable infant on CPAP with abdominal distention will usually have less abdominal distention if placed prone. A pad under the infant's chest is a simple way to position the baby prone (Figure 11-7). Rolls or other creative devices can be employed to facilitate positioning. (Figure 11-8 provides an example of side-lying positioning.)

FEEDING

Decisions regarding whether or not to feed a neonate on CPAP are made based on the infant's respiratory and physiologic status and the type of CPAP used. If the CPAP is being delivered via an endotracheal tube, then feeding is done cautiously because of the risk of aspiration.

When a neonate is on nasal prong CPAP, tube feeding is done via an orogastric tube. The tube feedings may be done intermittently or maintained as a continuous feeding, depending on the condition of the infant.

Infants on nasal prong CPAP may nipple feed if they are clinically stable. An older, more stable infant who can tolerate short periods off CPAP may be nipple fed without the CPAP, but most infants need CPAP during their feeding if they need it other times.

SUCTIONING

An infant on nasal prong CPAP has an increase in secretions secondary to the humidified gas blowing into the nostrils and irritation in the area from the prongs. An infant on nasal prong CPAP will need to be suctioned at least every two to three hours. If the infant experiences repeated apnea and bradycardia or shows a gradual decline in oxygen saturation levels, one of the first considerations is to determine if there are secretions blocking the airway. Although controversial and not well studied, chest physiotherapy by percussion and/or vibration is done prior to suctioning in most infants at Columbia-Presbyterian's NICU. This is espe-

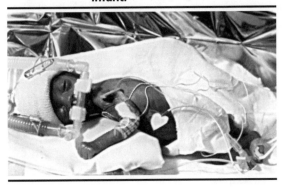

FIGURE 11-7 ▲ The use of a chest pad to facilitate prone positioning of a 13-day-old infant.

cially important if the infant's underlying disease is due to aspiration or the infant has a potential for atelectasis.

If the infant's nasopharynx is dry and difficult to suction, the use of a few drops of normal saline prior to suctioning can help lubricate the area and reduce the trauma of suctioning. As mentioned previously, if the nasal passages are dry or the secretions are extremely thick and tenacious, the percentage of humidity being delivered needs to be re-evaluated.

The size of suction catheter needed will depend on the size of the infant. If the catheter is too small, suctioning will not be effective, and the infant will have difficulty breathing. If the catheter is too large, it can cause trauma to

FIGURE 11-8 ▲ The use of rolls and a teddy bear to position a 13-day-old infant in the side-lying position while on nasal prong CPAP.

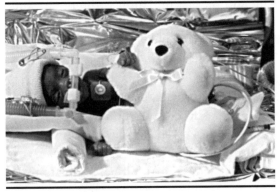

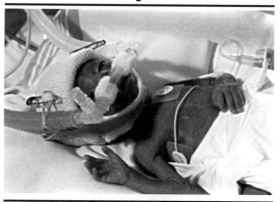

the area. Most infants can be suctioned effectively with a #8 French catheter (Figure 11-4).

MAINTENANCE OF THE EQUIPMENT

CHANGING THE EQUIPMENT

The CPAP equipment needs to be changed every two to three days. When changing the equipment of a labile or very low birth weight infant, it is often necessary for two people to work together. All of the new equipment needs to be connected and checked to be sure that it is functioning prior to the removal of the old system. An infant weighing <1,000 gm is often dependent on CPAP and may experience apnea and bradycardia immediately when taken off. The apnea and bradycardia will usually be resolved quickly when the CPAP is back on.

TROUBLESHOOTING AND OTHER CLINICAL ISSUES

Fluctuations in the amount of pressure being delivered in the system may simply be due to the opening and closing of the infant's mouth. For the majority of infants treated with CPAP, it is not necessary to continuously maintain exactly 5 cm H_2O pressure. However, if the infant is extremely labile, requires ≥40 percent oxygen, and/or is showing signs of deterioration, a chin strap can help keep the mouth

closed and maintain a more constant PEEP (Figure 11-9). The chin strap should be loose enough that the mouth can still open slightly, allowing for a "pop off" of excess pressure if needed. A baby who is stable enough to eat does not need a chin strap.

A sudden loss of all pressure can be noted by the lack of bubbling in the solution bottle, an alarm from the pressure monitor, an alarm from the ventilator, a drop in oxygen saturation, or apnea and bradycardia. The loss of pressure can be caused by a leak in the system such as disconnected tubing, dislocated prongs, or mechanical malfunction. A system check is warranted to see where the breakdown has occurred. If it is determined that the level of PEEP needs to be adjusted, it is advisable to remove the prongs from the infant's nares before making any changes and then test the system before replacing the prongs.

Frequent apnea and bradycardia occurring in the infant on CPAP require a re-examination of the equipment to look for any leaks in the system. The baby is checked for hyper- or hypoflexion of the neck that could lead to narrowing of the trachea. If no external mechanical problem can be identified, the neonate should be suctioned gently and quickly to check for blockage of the airway by secretions. The most common place to find the blockage is in the nasopharynx.

Excessive bubbling, an increase in pressure, or increased abdominal distention can be caused by setting the flow in the system too high. The range for all babies is between 5 and 10 liters/minute. If the flow is set too low, there can be carbon dioxide retention in the system. Most infants will require a flow of 7 liters/minute.

Although CPAP may be successfully used by an experienced staff on even very ill, labile infants, there are limitations. Refer to Table 11-2 for Columbia-Presbyterian's guidelines for

TABLE 11-2 ▲ **Indications for Mechanical Ventilation for Neonates at Columbia-
Presbyterian Medical Center**

1. Marked retractions on CPAP
2. Frequent, prolonged apnea on CPAP
3. PaO_2 <50 mmHg with FiO_2 80–100 percent
4. $PaCO_2$ >65 mmHg (after stabilization)
5. Cardiovascular collapse
6. Unrepaired congenital diaphragmatic hernia

neonatal intubation. Arterial blood gas determinations are an excellent way to assess the adequacy of ventilation and the acid-base status.
However, when the clinician reviews an arterial blood gas reading, she needs to evaluate the
entire clinical picture, not just the blood gas
values. For example, spontaneously breathing
infants requiring CPAP during the stabilization period should not be intubated because
the $PaCO_2$ is >65 mmHg. "Watchful waiting"
as the infant recovers from what occurred *in
utero* is the key to effective respiratory management in this situation and others. The cost-
benefit ratio of each decision that involves yet
another invasive procedure must be carefully
considered.

WEANING FROM CPAP

An infant on CPAP who no longer is showing signs of respiratory distress, does not have
apnea and bradycardia, and is not prone to
atelectasis can usually be successfully weaned
from CPAP. The postdelivery age when an
infant is ready to be weaned will vary greatly.
For example, a full-term infant with transient
tachypnea of the newborn may need the CPAP
for only a few hours, but an infant less than
1,000 gm may remain on room air CPAP for
8–10 weeks because of apnea, bradycardia, and
a high potential for atelectasis.

At Columbia-Presbyterian Medical Center,
weaning is done by taking the CPAP off to see
how the infant will breathe without this support. Usually after a few hours, the infant will

become tachypneic and need to go back on
CPAP. The infant usually is taken on and off
CPAP over several days until he can permanently tolerate being off. There is no set time
frame or protocol for how this is done because
every infant responds differently because of variations in size and disease process. As stated earlier, it is important to resume CPAP before
the oxygen saturation level drops and/or there
are changes visible on the x-ray; the visual and
physical exams of the infant dictate whether
the CPAP stays off or goes back on. Any infant
taken off CPAP who is not breathing comfortably and at a regular rate or has frequent
apnea and bradycardia is not ready to be weaned
from CPAP.[46]

SUMMARY

Continuous positive airway pressure is a safe,
effective, and relatively inexpensive way of providing respiratory support to infants in mild to
moderate respiratory distress. Early application
is especially beneficial to treat symptoms and
prevent further deterioration.

Although there are many methods to administer CPAP therapy, careful patient assessment
and attention to detail always remain important. The methods used at Babies and Children's
Hospital of the Columbia-Presbyterian Medical Center have been cited in this chapter as an
example of how nasal prong CPAP can be the
backbone of neonatal respiratory management
in an acute and semiacute nursery setting.

REFERENCES

1. Gregory GA, et al. 1971. Treatment of idiopathic respiratory distress syndrome with continuous positive airway
pressure. *New England Journal of Medicine* 284(24):
1333–1339.
2. Vidyasagar D, and Chernick V. 1971. Continuous positive transpulmonary pressure in hyaline membrane disease: A simple device. *Pediatrics* 48(2): 296–299.
3. Kattwinkel J, et al. 1973. A device for administration of
continuous positive airway pressure by the nasal route.
Pediatrics 52(1): 131–134.
4. Barrie H. 1972. Simple method of applying continuous
positive airway pressure in respiratory distress syndrome.
Lancet 1(7754): 776–777.

5. Harris TR. 1972. Continuous positive airway pressure applied by face mask. *Pediatric Research* 6: 410.

6. Caliumi-Pellegrini G, et al. 1974. Twin nasal cannula for administration of continuous positive airway pressure to newborn infants. *Archives of Disease in Childhood* 49(3): 228–230.

7. Vidyasagar D, Phildes RS, and Salem MR. 1974. Use of Amsterdam infant ventilator for continuous positive pressure breathing. *Critical Care Medicine* 2(2): 89–90.

8. Chernick V. 1973. Continuous distending pressure in hyaline membrane disease: Of devices, disadvantages, and a daring study. *Pediatrics* 52(1): 114–115.

9. Wung JT, et al. 1975. A new device for CPAP by nasal route. *Critical Care Medicine* 3(2): 76–78.

10. Wung JT, et al. 1979. Changing incidence of bronchopulmonary dysplasia. *Journal of Pediatrics* 95(5): 845–847.

11. Avery MA, et al. 1987. Is chronic lung disease in low birthweight infants preventable? A survey of eight centers. *Pediatrics* 79(1): 26–30.

12. Ahumada C. 1988. Continuous distending pressure. In *Assisted Ventilation of the Neonate,* 2nd ed., Goldsmith JP, and Karotkin EH, eds. Philadelphia: WB Saunders, 133–141.

13. Cotton RB. 1992. Pathophysiology of hyaline membrane disease (excluding surfactant). In *Fetal and Neonatal Physiology,* Polin RA, and Fox WW, eds. Philadelphia: WB Saunders, 892.

14. Martin RJ, et al. 1977. The effect of low continuous positive airway pressure on the reflex control of respiration in preterm infants. *Journal of Pediatrics* 90(6): 976–981.

15. Saunders RA, Milner AD, and Hopkin IE. 1976. The effects of continuous positive airway pressure on lung mechanics and lung volumes in the neonate. *Biology of the Neonate* 29(3–4): 178–186.

16. Field D, et al. 1985. Effects of positive end expiratory pressure during ventilation of the preterm infant. *Archives of Disease in Childhood* 60(9): 843–847.

17. Miller MJ, et al. 1990. Effects of nasal CPAP on supraglottic and total pulmonary resistance in preterm infants. *Journal of Applied Physiology* 68(1): 141–146.

18. Miller MJ, et al. 1985. Continuous positive airway pressure selectively reduces obstructive apnea in preterm infants. *Journal of Pediatrics* 106(1): 91–94.

19. Hagan R, et al. 1977. Neonatal chest wall afferents and regulation of respiration. *Journal of Applied Physiology* 42(3): 362–367.

20. Durand M, et al. 1983. Effect of continuous positive airway pressure on the ventilatory response to CO_2 in preterm infants. *Pediatrics* 71(4): 634–638.

21. Sturgeon CL Jr, et al. 1977. PEEP and CPAP: Cardiopulmonary effects during spontaneous ventilation. *Anesthesia and Analgesia* 56(5): 633–641.

22. Cotton RB, et al. 1980. Effect of positive-end-expiratory-pressure on right ventricular output in lambs with hyaline membrane disease. *Acta Paediatrica Scandinavica* 69(5): 603–606.

23. Annat G, et al. 1983. Effect of PEEP ventilation on renal function, plasma renin, aldosterone, neurophysins and urinary ADH and prostaglandins. *Anesthesiology* 58(2): 136–141.

24. Hall SV, et al. 1974. Renal hemodynamics and function with continuous positive pressure ventilation in dogs. *Anesthesiology* 41(5): 452–461.

25. Gabriele G, et al. 1977. Continuous airway pressure breathing with the head-box in the newborn lamb: Effects on regional blood flows. *Pediatrics* 59(6): 858–864.

26. Aidinis SJ, Lafferty J, and Shapiro HM. 1976. Intracranial responses to PEEP. *Anesthesiology* 45(3): 275–286.

27. Frost EAM. 1978. Effects of PEEP on intracranial pressure and brain compliance in brain-injured patients. *Journal of Neurosurgery* 47(2): 195–200.

28. Engelke SC, Roloff DW, and Kuhns LR. 1982. Postextubation nasal continuous positive airway pressure: A prospective controlled study. *American Journal of Diseases of Children* 136(4): 359–361.

29. Kamper J, et al. 1993. Early treatment with nasal continuous positive airway pressure in very-low-birth-weight infants. *Acta Paediatrica* 82(2): 193–197.

30. Bancalari E, and Sinclair JC. 1992. Mechanical ventilation. In *Effective Care of the Newborn,* Sinclair JC, and Bracken MB, eds. Oxford: Oxford University Press, 203.

31. Andreasson B, et al. 1988. Effects on respiration of CPAP immediately after extubation in the very preterm infant. *Pediatric Pulmonology* 4(4): 213–218.

32. Annibale DJ, et al. 1994. Randomized, controlled trial of nasopharyngeal continuous positive airway pressure in the extubation of very low birth weight infants. *Journal of Pediatrics* 124(3): 455–460.

33. Kim EH, and Boutwell WC. 1987. Successful direct extubation of very low birthweight infants from low intermittent mandatory ventilation rate. *Pediatrics* 80(3): 409–414.

34. Kattwinkel J, et al. 1975. Apnea of prematurity. *Journal of Pediatrics* 86(4): 588–592.

35. Bonta BW, et al. 1977. Determination of optimal continuous positive airway pressure for the treatment of IRDS by measurement of esophageal pressure. *Journal of Pediatrics* 91(3): 449–454.

36. Suter PM, Fairley B, and Isenberg MD. 1975. Optimum end-expiratory airway pressure in patients with acute pulmonary failure. *New England Journal of Medicine* 292(6): 284–289.

37. Hall RT, and Rhodes PG. 1975. Pneumothorax and pneumomediastinum in infants with idiopathic respiratory distress syndrome receiving continuous positive airway pressure. *Pediatrics* 55(4): 493–496.

38. Spitzer AR, Shaffer TH, and Fox WW. 1992. Assisted ventilation: Physiologic implications and complications. In *Fetal and Neonatal Physiology,* Polin RA, and Fox WW, eds. Philadelphia: WB Saunders, 902.

39. deLemos RA, et al. 1973. Continuous positive airway pressure as an adjunct to mechanical ventilation in the newborn with respiratory distress syndrome. *Anesthesia and Analgesia* 52(3): 328–332.

40. Katz JA, Draemer RW, and Gjerde GE. 1985. Inspiratory work and airway pressure with continuous positive airway pressure delivery systems. *Chest* 88(4): 519–526.

41. Wall MA. 1980. Infant endotracheal tube resistance: Effects of changing length, diameter, and gas density. *Critical Care Medicine* 8(1): 38–40.

42. Muller N, et al. 1979. Diaphragmatic muscle fatigue in the newborn. *Journal of Applied Physiology* 46(4): 688–695.

43. Jones SW, and King JM. 1993. Retropharyngeal abscess secondary to nasopharyngeal CPAP in a preterm neonate (letter). *Archives of Disease in Childhood* 68(5): 620.

44. Silverman WA, and Anderson DH. 1956. Evaluation of respiratory status. *Pediatrics* 17(1): 1–10.

45. Jaile-Marti J, et. al. 1992. Benign gaseous distention of bowel in premature infants treated with nasal prong continuous positive airway pressure: A study of contributing factors. *American Journal of Roentgenology* 158(1): 125–129.

46. Jones DB. 1995. *Infant Nasal Prong Continuous Positive Airway Pressure*. Videotape. Temecula, California: Hudson, RCI.

NOTES

12 Pulmonary Function Testing in the Critically Ill Neonate

James A. Cullen, RN
Susan S. Spinner, MSN, RN
Jay S. Greenspan, MD

The ability to assess pulmonary function in neonates is not new. It has been possible for years to measure respiratory pressure, airflow, and volume and to calculate pulmonary mechanics, energetics, and functional residual capacity (FRC). Because of difficulties in making these measurements, however, and the time required to interpret the data, these values have not been clinically useful.

Recent advances in computer-assisted technology as well as miniaturization of equipment now allow simple and rapid pulmonary function assessment of the critically ill neonate at the bedside. When these studies are performed carefully, the results are reproducible and accurate. In the future, these data will be even more readily available and may be utilized on-line to assess the infant's immediate status, much like vital signs or transcutaneous oxyhemoglobin saturation data are used now.

An understanding of the indications for, and information obtained from, pulmonary function profiles of critically ill neonates will be critical to nursing care in the future. These data have important implications for ventilatory management, assessment of interventions, and evaluation of new technologies.

The indications for and benefits of pulmonary function testing in the critically ill neonate vary with gestation, postnatal age, and clinical condition. A pulmonary function test in a neonate at risk for pulmonary disease can provide an assessment of the type and progression of a pulmonary abnormality, assess the response to therapeutic interventions, diagnose unsuspected pathology, and possibly suggest a prognosis.

Such testing needs to be performed routinely in infants at risk for respiratory disease, in those with acute changes in respiratory status, and in those being evaluated for new respiratory problems or therapeutic interventions. The general guidelines and goals of pulmonary function evaluation, as well as some of the information learned through routine testing and specific protocols are discussed in this chapter.

THE PULMONARY FUNCTION PROFILE

The pulmonary function profile represents all available pulmonary information obtainable on a particular infant. Because not all tests can be performed on an infant, this profile needs to be tailored for each patient. A basic

FIGURE 12-1 ▲ A schematic of a pneumotachograph, which attaches to a face mask or endotracheal tube to measure flow.

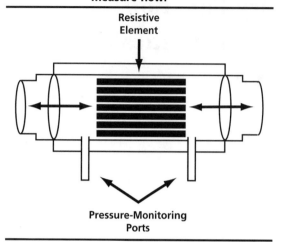

FIGURE 12-2 ▲ Normal tidal flow-volume relationship.

Note even flow on inspiration (lower portion of the loop) and expiration (upper portion) as gas is inhaled and exhaled through normal airways.

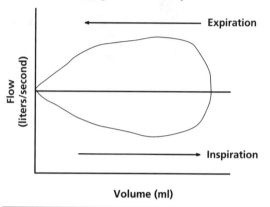

pulmonary function profile typically includes measurement of (1) pulmonary mechanics (compliance, resistance, time constant), (2) energetics (work of breathing), and (3) lung volume or FRC.

State-of-the-art equipment has made rapid evaluation at the bedside possible for even the sickest infants. These basic measurements therefore should be included along with an assessment of respiratory rate, oxyhemoglobin saturation, and physical examination as a pulmonary profile of any infant with lung disease. Although these tests generally provide accurate, reproducible results, their utility and safety depend on proper preparation, positioning, and monitoring before and during testing.

LUNG MECHANICS

Ventilation is the result of changes in pressure, flow, and volume over time. During spontaneous breathing, the contraction of the diaphragm and expansion of the rib cage drive inspiration. Mechanical ventilators drive inspiration using positive pressure to expand the chest. In both situations, expiration is passive.

To provide effective ventilation under either spontaneous or artificial conditions, respiratory effort must be sufficient to overcome the intrinsic properties of the lung that oppose air movement: the elastic and resistive components or the mechanics of the respiratory system. Surface tension, lung tissue, the chest wall and abdomen all contribute resistance to air movement. By monitoring the changes in pressure and flow in the respiratory system, these components can be quantified.

Pulmonary mechanics can be tested under two conditions: (1) during active, uninterrupted breathing (dynamic mechanics) and (2) during interrupted breathing, produced by briefly occluding the airway at one or more points in the cycle (static mechanics). The techniques discussed in this section refer to measuring dynamic mechanics, this being the most common technique in use currently.

Monitoring Flow

The most common direct method of monitoring flow is **pneumotachography**. A pneumotachograph consists of a tube containing an element that creates resistance to flow and pressure-monitoring ports on both sides of the resistive element (Figure 12-1). The resistive element can be a series of smaller tubes or a mesh screen. As air moves through the pneumotachograph during inspiration and expiration, a pressure difference that is proportional to the flow rate is created across the resistive element.

For intubated infants, a pneumotachograph is connected to the endotracheal or tracheostomy tube. For infants who are not on mechanical ventilation, it can be attached to a face mask. The pneumotachograph has standard connectors on both ends so the device can be connected to standard ventilation equipment such as an endotracheal tube, face mask, or ventilator circuit.

In a computerized pulmonary function testing system, the flow signal can be sampled many times a second and integrated with time to calculate tidal volume. The computer can then graphically display the relationship of flow and volume for a breath as a flow-volume loop (Figure 12-2). Flow-volume loops are useful in evaluating the infant for flow restrictions due to tracheobronchomalacia or bronchospasm.

Another technique for measuring flow is hot-wire **anemometry**. This technique is relatively new to neonatal respiratory care, but it has already been incorporated into the newest generation of mechanical ventilators to monitor tidal volume. Instead of a resistive element, as in pneumotachography, the anemometer contains a filament, or hot wire. The filament is maintained at a constant temperature regardless of the amount of flow moving across it. To maintain a constant temperature, voltage is supplied to the filament as gas flow changes. The change in voltage correlates with flow. As with pneumotachography, the flow signal is integrated with time to yield tidal volume.

Anemometers are less expensive than larger testing systems and can provide valuable real-time assessment data. Changes in tidal volume can be monitored with other parameters to detect changes in the infant's condition or to signal the need for interventions such as suctioning. Anemometers have less dead space than

pneumotachographs and can be used to monitor an infant for long periods without compromising ventilation.

Monitoring Pressure

Airway pressure monitoring, including peak inflating and end distending pressures as well as mean airway pressure, is an integral part of managing mechanical ventilation. For most ventilation schemes, the pressure sensor is placed at the airway opening and is displayed on the ventilator. To appropriately determine pulmonary mechanics, however, other pressure readings are needed.

In most cases, **transpulmonary pressure** is measured during pulmonary function testing. Transpulmonary pressure is the pressure across the lung, from the airway opening to the pleural space. Airway opening pressure is sampled at a port on the pneumotachograph connector closest to the patient.

Intrapleural pressure is not sampled directly, but can be safely and accurately estimated by monitoring esophageal pressure.[1] Specially designed balloons or water-filled catheters are made for this application. A catheter is passed into the esophagus until the tip is in the distal third. Pressure signals can be viewed on-line during testing.

A typical computer display is shown in Figure 12-3. Transpulmonary pressure, flow, and volume can be viewed on a single screen to monitor breathing during testing and to assess the quality of the pressure and flow signals before testing begins. Pressure can also be graphically displayed in relation to volume, plotted in a pressure-volume loop (Figure 12-4).

Sampling and Breath Analysis

Pressure and flow signals are sampled by a computer-driven testing system.[2] Sampling usually takes less than 60 seconds, depending on the infant's respiratory rate. Each breath is analyzed for artifact caused by air leaks or excessive patient movement. Breaths with significant

FIGURE 12-3 ▲ Typical scalar tracing showing pressure, flow, and volume for consecutive breaths.

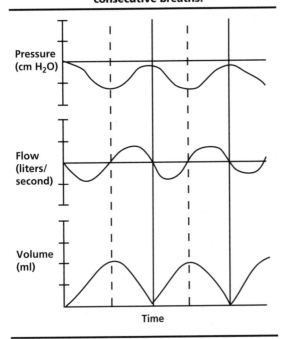

FIGURE 12-4 ▲ A typical pressure-volume loop for a single breath.

The points of zero flow, connected by the dashed line, depict pulmonary compliance. The area within the loop represents resistive work of breathing.

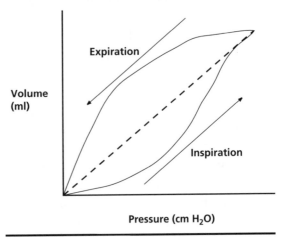

artifact are not included in the calculations. Each breath can be reviewed manually by the clinician, who can further check the quality of the breaths sampled. Once a satisfactory sample is obtained—usually ten breaths—the computer makes final calculations and generates an averaged data report.

As the pressure and flow signals are integrated with time and each other, a number of pulmonary function parameters can be quantified and calculated: tidal volume, respiratory rate, minute ventilation, inspiratory and expiratory times, peak inspiratory and expiratory flow, peak pressure changes, as well as mechanics and energetics.[3]

ENERGETICS

Compliance

This term describes the elastic properties of the lung. It is defined as the unit change in volume per unit change in pressure and expressed in ml/cm H_2O. When the change in

volume (tidal volume) is expressed in terms of the change in transpulmonary pressure, the resulting measurement is lung compliance. Surface tension, lung tissue, the chest wall, and the abdomen all contribute to compliance. If there is a large amount of interstitial fluid in the lungs, lung tissue becomes less compliant. This is true in both the acute and chronic phases of respiratory distress syndrome. The chest wall can adversely affect compliance when there is chest wall edema or if the infant is paralyzed. A distended abdomen displaces the diaphragm upward and resists movement during inspiration, decreasing compliance.

Respiratory system compliance includes the compliance of the chest wall. However, the difference between chest wall and lung compliance measurements in neonates is generally minimal because the neonatal chest wall is highly compliant and therefore does not have a significant effect on the elastic properties of the lung.[4]

Pulmonary compliance depends on lung volume. The lungs of a newborn premature infant with surfactant deficiency typically have a low

FIGURE 12-5 ▲ The change in compliance with different lung volumes.

Individual breaths have low compliance (flattening of the compliance curve) at low or high lung volumes.

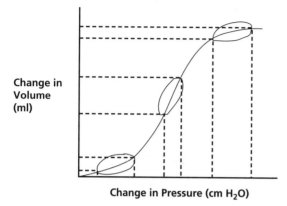

Adapted from: Harris TR, and Wood BR. 1996. Physiologic principles. In *Assisted Ventilation of the Neonate*, Goldsmith JP, and Karotkin EH, eds. Philadelphia: WB Saunders, 32. Reprinted by permission.

volume as a result of atelectasis.[5] The transpulmonary pressure required to inflate these lungs would be high in relation to the change in volume, yielding low compliance values. Conversely, an overdistended lung—such as occurs in a child with air trapping or one who is on excessively high ventilator pressures—will also have poor pulmonary compliance because the lungs are stretched to capacity and cannot easily accommodate additional volume.[6] Figure 12-5 illustrates this relationship of compliance and lung volume.

Pulmonary compliance is also related to the size of the infant's lungs. In this regard, larger lungs (an adult versus an infant, for instance) will move more volume per change in pressure than smaller lungs. To appropriately compare compliance values from an infant on different days, or between infants, therefore requires some means of normalizing for lung size. Dividing the measured pulmonary compliance by the infant's weight is the simplest method of normalization. Pulmonary compliance is then expressed as ml/cm H_2O/kg. Other means of

normalization are to divide the measured compliance by body length or to divide measured compliance by FRC. Normalization utilizing FRC is sometimes referred to as the "specific compliance."[7]

There is a difference between dynamic and static compliance. Compliance, as defined in this text, is the unit change in volume per unit change in pressure. Graphically it is represented as the slope of a line between any two points on a pressure volume curve (Figure 12-4). Dynamic compliance is obtained by measuring volume and pressure changes over the entire breath. Static compliance is measured by holding inflation at different points during inspiration for pressure and volume readings. The difference between the two is technique as well as the respiratory rate dependence of dynamic compliance. When the airway is occluded during testing under static conditions, airway and alveolar pressure have time to equilibrate throughout the lung. When dynamic mechanics are measured, the changes in volume and pressure are influenced by respiratory rate and airway resistance.[7–9] Lung segments that expand more slowly than others may result in lower dynamic compliance values. Dynamic compliance is therefore respiratory rate–dependent.[10]

Pulmonary Resistance

Airflow in the respiratory system is also subject to resistance, which is generated primarily by the airways, but to a lesser extent by the lung parenchyma and chest wall. Pulmonary resistance is typically measured by assessing transpulmonary pressure and dividing by flow. Airway resistance is affected by several factors, including the radius and length of the airway, the viscosity of gas in the airways, flow, and the driving pressure required to generate that flow.[6]

The relationship between these factors and resistance was first described by Poiseuille in the following formula:[11]

$$Flow = \frac{P \pi r^4}{8 h l}$$

in which P is driving pressure, r is the airway radius, h is viscosity, and l represents length. In this formula, the relationship between airway length, size, and resistance can be seen. Of critical importance is the exponential relationship between airway size and resistance. If airway size is reduced by half, airway resistance would not double, but would increase 16 times.

Resistance is proportional to airway length. If an infant has fewer airways—as can be seen in infants with pulmonary hypoplasia due to diaphragmatic hernia—airway resistance may be lower than in an infant with normal lungs.

Poiseuille's formula is used to describe resistance and flow under laminar conditions—that is, in the absence of turbulence. Airflow is closest to laminar in distal airways; some turbulence is present in the trachea and larger airways. Excessive turbulence can be generated when high flow rates are used to deliver air through an endotracheal tube. Resistance is increased in the pressure of turbulent flow.

Endotracheal tubes introduce new sources of resistance into the respiratory system. By necessity, these tubes are smaller than the infant's upper airway, and the smaller tube size dictates an increase in resistance.[12] To decrease the impact of tube length on resistance, endotracheal tubes are usually shortened by several centimeters once the infant is intubated.

For infants on mechanical ventilation, the additional resistance generated by the tube has little impact on ventilation. Intubated infants weaning from ventilation, however, may not be able to generate enough pressure and flow to overcome this additional resistance.

Respiratory Time Constant

Inspiration and expiration do not occur at constant rates. The rate at which tidal volume is inhaled or exhaled depends on both the elastic and resistive properties of the lungs. The

time constant, calculated by multiplying compliance and resistance, reflects these properties. A time constant is measured in seconds and reflects how long inspiration or expiration takes. By definition, one time constant reflects the amount of time needed to move 63 percent of the tidal volume. Three time constants are needed to move 95 percent of tidal volume because the time constant is exponential.

Knowledge of an infant's time constants can be useful in some cases of neonatal lung disease.[13] Infants with airway diseases such as tracheobronchomalacia generally have disproportionately high airway resistance compared to compliance. In these infants, the expiratory time constant will be long, reflecting the elevated resistance and the relatively good compliance. If such an infant is on a high ventilator rate, the expiratory time allowed by the ventilator may be less than is needed, as indicated by the time constant. When this occurs, the infant is at risk for air trapping.

Work of Breathing

The amount of work required to overcome the elastic and resistive forces of the lung is termed "the resistive work of breathing," which is one measure of pulmonary energetics. The work of breathing indicates how much energy is required to generate a breath, either by the infant breathing spontaneously or by the ventilator during assisted ventilation. When compliance is poor or resistance is high, the work of breathing will be high. Work is defined as force times distance and is normalized to weight.

LUNG VOLUME

Functional Residual Capacity

The pulmonary function profile is incomplete without an assessment of FRC—the volume of gas in communication with the airways. An important indicator of lung status that can be utilized alone to alter management strategies,

FIGURE 12-6 ▲ Pulmonary function testing circuit to determine functional residual capacity by the helium dilution technique.

The infant can be connected to the circuit from a ventilator or when breathing spontaneously. The drop in helium concentration following connection of the infant to the closed breathing circuit (gray line) is proportional to lung volume.

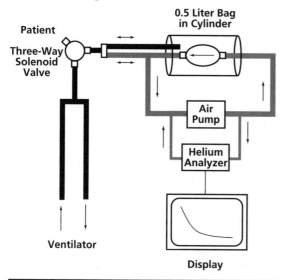

this measurement is particularly useful as a complement to other measures of pulmonary function. In this regard, compliance, resistance, and other measures of lung function can be markedly altered by changes in FRC. FRC can be assessed through several techniques.

The **helium dilution technique** is a simple method of determining FRC that can be performed on even the sickest infant.[5,14–17] This technique requires the infant's airway to be connected, at the end of a normal expiration, to a reservoir of known volume and helium concentration. The drop in helium concentration over 30 to 90 seconds is proportional to the lung volume at the time of connection, which can be easily calculated (Figure 12-6).

Several parameters could affect the accuracy of the measurement. Leaks around the face mask or endotracheal tube, oxygen consumption over the 30–90 seconds of equilibration, and prolonged lung time constants can all affect

measurements.[18] In addition, the calibration and inaccuracies of the helium analyzer can complicate measurements. Some critically ill infants do not tolerate changes in ventilation or oxygen concentration for prolonged periods of time, necessitating a rapid method of testing. Many of these issues have been addressed by the development of computerized equipment, and accurate FRC measurement is now possible at the bedside of even the most critically ill neonate.

The FRC can also be measured in newborns by a **nitrogen washout technique.**[19] For this method, the infant breathes 100 percent oxygen continuously, and the expired gas is sampled for nitrogen content. The integration of the nitrogen concentration curve of the exhaled gas can be utilized to determine the functional residual capacity.

Problems with this technique include the necessity of breathing 100 percent oxygen, inaccuracies when the infant is already breathing high oxygen concentrations, and difficulties with gas leaks. Like the helium dilution technique, computerization has permitted this method to be employed at the neonate's bedside.

OTHER MEASURES

Many other tests are available to determine pulmonary function. Some of these, such as plethysmography, and occlusion methods, can be substituted for some of the techniques previously discussed to produce similar measures of lung function.[20–25]

Other tests are available to expand the pulmonary function profile. Many are designed to test pulmonary drive, strength and endurance, distribution of ventilation, perfusion, pulmonary blood flow, and diffusion.[26–32] Still other tests can assess lung activity outside the range of normal tidal breathing (as in forced expiratory flows) or in unusual circumstances (as in bronchoprovocation tests).[33–42] Although many of these tests are very useful in certain circumstances, their utility in evaluating the acutely ill neonate is limited, and they are not discussed here.

TESTING INTERVALS

A complete pulmonary function profile includes not only measurements made at one point in time, but an entire series of measurements made over the infant's hospital course. As testing becomes easier to carry out accurately and less invasive, it will become more prevalent. Systems for on-line continuous pulmonary function evaluation, which may be the standard in the near future, are currently available. If such a system is not available in your institution, a baseline study performed soon after birth can guide the initial management strategy and be used in explaining the severity of the lung disease to the infant's parents.

A single test, however, cannot guide management for more than a few days—or even a few hours in some cases. Only repeated measurements allow the clinical team to assess each infant as an individual and to determine the appropriate type and level of respiratory support.

A baseline evaluation can be made as soon as the infant has been stabilized in the intensive care nursery. In some cases, testing may be needed while the infant is being stabilized, to aid in determining a diagnosis. For example, a term infant who presents with severe hypoxia can have one of several diagnoses, each with different degrees of pulmonary dysfunction.

Diagnoses to be ruled out for this infant may include congenital heart disease, pneumonia, or idiopathic persistent pulmonary hypertension of the newborn. For infants with pneumonia, the presence of interstitial lung disease may be reflected by lung compliance and elevated airway resistance. The FRC may also be reduced. These changes may not be seen if the infant has heart disease or pulmonary hypertension, which are not associated with parenchymal lung disease.

An infant with pulmonary hypertension may have a relatively normal pulmonary function profile or, in severe cases, may have a diminished FRC. In this scenario, a pulmonary function test adds significant assessment data and is useful in determining the diagnosis.

The absence of significant pulmonary function abnormalities on one study early in the infant's course does not exclude the possibility of severe lung disease. This is particularly true of premature infants with respiratory distress syndrome, whose pulmonary function deteriorates as atelectasis, caused by surfactant deficiency, progresses. These infants may require little respiratory support at birth but deteriorate within hours, requiring high levels of support. This progression stresses the value of serial testing, to assess the need for interventions such as surfactant replacement.

Once the infant has been stabilized, repeat testing can be scheduled. Initially, testing may be needed on a daily basis or more frequently to help assess the infant's response to treatment or the need for other interventions. Weekly testing while the infant remains on ventilation is helpful in monitoring recovery and can also be used to predict the infant's readiness for extubation. A final study prior to discharge can serve as a baseline for pulmonary follow-up.

NURSING IMPLICATIONS

The high-risk neonate presents special challenges in diagnosis, treatment, and follow-up. The ability to meet these challenges can be aided by an integrated clinical-physiologic approach utilizing state-of-the-art pulmonary function testing, coupled with appropriate therapeutic measures of respiratory management. Bedside pulmonary function testing is rapidly becoming an important tool in the armamentarium of the nurse caring for these infants. These data, which can be obtained and documented by the nurse at the bedside, can be integrated into every aspect of the nursing care plan. By utilizing this tool and understanding and analyzing the results, the nurse adds another dimension to her assessment skills, which influences appropriate intervention for the neonate.

Pulmonary function data can be utilized much like the arterial blood chemistry: to assess status, effect change, alter management, and guide prognosis. A complete understanding of the capabilities and limitations of such data will be important to all the infant's caretakers. Changes in infant mechanical ventilators and critical care beds may facilitate on-line pulmonary function data procurement.

PREPARING THE INFANT

The expertise of the intensive care nurse is invaluable in ensuring safe, accurate, and reproducible data. Although the tests are noninvasive and relatively simple to perform, manipulation of the infant is often required.

During pulmonary testing, the nurse assures good positioning, maintains a stable airway, and monitors for changes in the infant's status. To safely obtain accurate pulmonary function data, it is necessary to prepare the infant for testing in the following ways:

1. Attend to feeding needs:
- Schedule testing so that it won't conflict with the infant's feeding schedule.
- Delay testing until one hour after feeding.
- If gavage feedings are being used, aspirate stomach contents with a syringe, and remove the gastric tube before inserting the esophageal balloon. Remove naso/orogastric tubes to allow placement of the balloon catheter.

2. Quiet the infant:
- Consider sedation with chloral hydrate in older infants, particularly those with bronchopulmonary dysplasia (BPD). This will facilitate passage of the esophageal balloon and permit sampling of quiet breathing. Chloral hydrate causes transient decreases in respiration rate and tidal volume but otherwise does not have a significant effect on pulmonary function.
- If chloral hydrate is not used, hold an infant who is irritable during testing. This can be done without affecting test results as long as the infant can breathe freely.

3. Maintain proper head and neck position:
- Place the infant supine with the head in the midline and the neck in the neutral position. If the neck is flexed or hyperextended, the upper airway may be narrowed, creating artificially high airway resistance—even for intubated infants.
- In a nonintubated infant, avoid excessive compression of the face mask to the face—this will alter airway resistance measurements.
- Assess the effect of neck and head position by monitoring flow-volume loops on-line before testing begins. If significant airway obstruction is present, the flow-volume loop will show inspiratory or expiratory flow restriction.

4. Prepare the parents:
- Explain in detail the rationale for testing and the information that will be gained from it.
- Reassure parents that testing poses little risk to the infant and that he will be monitored closely throughout the procedure.
- Stress that testing does not interfere with the oxygen delivery or ventilatory support the infant is receiving.
- Reassure parents that sedation with chloral hydrate will not interfere with breathing and

will make the infant more comfortable during the test.

- If parents wish to be present, encourage one of them to hold the infant during testing. It is possible to measure pulmonary mechanics and lung volume while the infant is being held, as long as his head and neck are held in the optimal position.

USING THE DATA

Pulmonary function tests are an important assessment tool for the bedside nurse because they allow clinical observations about an infant's changing status to be further investigated. In addition, on-line pulmonary function analysis can facilitate improvement in hand ventilation and suctioning techniques.

The nurse can also use pulmonary function data to alter the infant's care plan and determine the necessity and timing for retesting. Nurses have used this tool as a potent teaching device: It allows parent teaching and discharge planning to be more precisely formulated. The data obtained from pulmonary function testing can thus be used to formulate the infant's care plan as early as the next shift and as far into the future as planning home care. Pulmonary function testing is also an important research tool that has largely gone untapped by nursing.

ROLE OF PULMONARY FUNCTION DATA

MANAGEMENT OF ACUTE LUNG DISEASE

The pulmonary function profile varies with the infant's diagnosis. Soon after birth, preterm infants present with low lung compliance and reduced FRC, while airway resistance is relatively normal.[43,44] Reductions in compliance and lung volume are related to both high alveolar surface tension and atelectasis.

When these infants are treated with surfactant, FRC and oxygenation improve within 2 hours of treatment, but a significant improvement in compliance may not be seen for 12 hours following surfactant administration.[5,45,46] Pulmonary function evaluation of the preterm infant may help to (1) determine the need for frequency of surfactant replacement therapy or other pulmonary interventions (such as high-frequency ventilation) and (2) define the pulmonary process and prognosis.[43,47]

During the first few weeks of life, pulmonary mechanics may worsen as new problems develop. Sequential testing of pulmonary mechanics in extremely low birth weight neonates shows a decrease in compliance and an increase in pulmonary resistance between one and two weeks of life.[44,48] These measurements return to week 1 values by four weeks of age. Although not universally observed in all preterm infants, this "worsening" during the second week probably has a multifactorial etiology. Pulmonary problems at this time can result from sepsis and pneumonia, a patent ductus arteriosus, or the early stages of chronic lung disease and inflammation.

In ventilator-dependent, low birth weight neonates at two weeks of age, airway reactivity and bronchospasm may represent a new problem, and airway management can be a challenge. Pulmonary function analysis can again be utilized to diagnose bronchospasm and to evaluate the effectiveness of interventions (such as a bronchodilator) (Figure 12-7).[33,34]

Tracheobronchomalacia can be diagnosed by examining flow-volume loops for evidence of airway collapse on expiration. Infants with airway collapse will have very high expiratory resistance values and prolonged time constants. By monitoring flow-volume loops on-line while adjusting positive end-expiratory pressure (PEEP) levels, the nurse can minimize expiratory collapse.

Finally, testing may be useful in optimizing treatment in infants on pulmonary support.

(A) Pretreatment, with flow limitation evident on the expiratory limb, which is consistent with elevated expiratory resistance. Following treatment (B), a modest increase in tidal volume and improvement in expiratory flow can be seen.

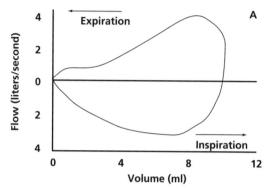

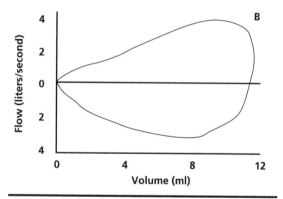

Mechanical support needs to be fine-tuned on a regular basis to diminish the work of breathing and barotrauma and to improve lung healing.

Pulmonary function values improve slowly over weeks in premature infants recovering from respiratory distress syndrome. Airway reactivity may present a significant management challenge; pulmonary function testing can be used to assess the infant's response to changes in ventilator settings or to bronchodilator administration. Pulmonary mechanics can remain abnormal even after the infant has been weaned from mechanical ventilation and oxygen.

Like that of a preterm infant, the pulmonary function profile of a term infant with respira-tory compromise also differs with the diagnosis. Infants with congenital diaphragmatic hernia may present with reduced compliance and FRC resulting from a combination of lung hypoplasia and compression by displaced abdominal viscera. Airway resistance in these patients may be low because of the decreased number of airways in the affected lung regions.

Infants with meconium aspiration syndrome will also have reduced lung compliance and FRC. Airway resistance may be high in these infants because of the presence of debris in the airways.

Abnormal pulmonary function values may indicate the need for other forms of therapy for these infants, such as extracorporeal membrane oxygenation (ECMO). In particular, knowledge of low FRC, which may predict impending respiratory failure, may facilitate timely initiation of treatment or transfer to a tertiary center for the appropriate treatment.

For infants on ECMO, pulmonary function testing has been used to monitor lung recovery and to assess readiness to wean from ECMO back to conventional ventilation. The role of pulmonary analysis in predicting lethal lung hypoplasia and the response to newer modalities (such as nitric oxide and liquid ventilation therapies) is currently being evaluated.

MANAGEMENT OF CHRONIC LUNG DISEASE

Although much has been learned about bronchopulmonary dysplasia during the 25 years since its initial description, chronic lung disease remains a significant complication of prematurity. Substantial advances in understanding its pathophysiology and pathogenesis are reflected in new therapeutic interventions.

Much current research is directed toward the role of prevention. New approaches for accelerating lung maturation with combined maternal steroid therapy, surfactant replacement therapy, high-frequency ventilation, antioxidant administration, and other pharmacologic strategies to minimize lung injury are being explored. Other technologies such as perfluorochemical liquid ventilation, and perhaps inhaled nitric oxide therapy, may be added to the clinical regimen for some infants with severe neonatal respiratory failure.

Less information is available on mechanisms that can hasten lung healing. Ongoing studies of inflammatory products, growth factors, and cytokines may lead to new therapies that will favorably influence the fibroproliferative phase of the disease.

While advances in neonatal care have given infants weighing less than 750 gm a better than 60 percent chance of survival, the incidence of BPD has increased at the same time.[49] In the extremely immature neonate, the initial respiratory disease progresses to BPD in as many as 55 percent of infants.[49,50] The medical and social impact of BPD continues to remain a significant problem, not only in infancy, but through the first year of life. These infants create a large emotional and financial burden for their parents, caregivers, and society with their prolonged initial hospitalization, home care, increased need for rehospitalization, and associated problems.

Preparation for Discharge

One approach to controlling costs, managing care, and minimizing the need for intense, prolonged treatment is to determine a plan of care well before discharge. As with any nursing problem, successful discharge planning begins at the time of admission. There is a need to have objective data to define pulmonary morbidity, evaluate potential therapies and interventions, and integrate the infant's pulmonary status into the discharge plan. Even though an infant may be breathing room air for several weeks, significant pulmonary morbidity may still exist.

Pulmonary function testing at discharge can assess for the presence of residual parenchymal dysfunction, airway reactivity, and increased work of breathing. Such abnormalities can be unrecognized in the unstressed infant at the time of discharge but can be exacerbated by intercurrent illness or additional stressors at home (such as a smoky environment and cold or less-humidified air).

An understanding of such susceptibility promotes more effective anticipatory guidance and may suggest prophylactic therapy. It is not unusual, for instance, to suggest on a discharge evaluation that a bronchodilator be available for infants who seem to respond well to this therapy. In addition, the infant's nutritional status may be related to the work of breathing, and caloric requirement estimates can be correlated with pulmonary function analysis.

Once a discharge pulmonary function test is obtained, a teaching plan can be developed, and parents can learn how to handle this aspect of their infant's care at home. In addition, the pulmonary needs can be fully ascertained, social services can be integrated, and home care can be coordinated in a timely fashion.

Rehospitalization

BPD severity ranges widely. The most severe form, occurring in 0.5 to 19 percent of all very low birth weight infants, is seen in those who require oxygen and/or ventilator treatment for more than three months.[51] Their morbidity is higher than that of infants with chronic lung disease who do not require such treatment.

To reduce costs, many institutions transfer infants to a rehabilitation hospital soon after they are weaned from the ventilator. Bachrach and colleagues document savings of $60,000 per patient transferred to a rehabilitation hospital.[52]

With the aid of pulmonary function testing, early diagnosis of lung injury and prediction of the severity and chronicity of the infant's disease will enhance goal setting for these infants and help reduce hospitalization and facilitate early transfer to a rehabilitative facility. Such a program would result in markedly decreased lengths of stay and reduced hospital costs, without an increase in morbidity or mortality. The focus could then shift from acute care needs to training for home care and technological support for home oxygen therapy, thereby facilitating effective and efficient discharge planning.

SUMMARY

Respiratory insufficiency is a primary or secondary diagnosis in more than 80 percent of the infants admitted to intensive care. These high-risk neonates present special challenges in diagnosis, treatment, and follow-up. It is difficult to accurately determine the nature of an infant's respiratory dysfunction on the basis of physical examination and arterial blood gases alone. In addition, response to therapies varies dramatically among infants who are considered to have similar disease processes.

A more detailed analysis of the pathophysiology of the pulmonary disease is essential if appropriate therapies are to be instituted. Pulmonary function testing, with its ability to describe and quantify neonatal lung disease, offers such an analysis. Although the basic tools of history and physical assessment will remain the mainstay of infant evaluation, these new tests will facilitate a more physiologic approach, which should result in less morbidity, mortality, and cost.

REFERENCES

1. Beardsmore CS, et al. 1980. Improved esophageal balloon technique for use in infants. *Journal of Applied Physiology* 49(4): 735–742.

2. Bhutani VK, et al. 1988. Evaluation of neonatal pulmonary mechanics and energetics: A two factor least mean square analysis. *Pediatric Pulmonology* 4(3): 150–158.

3. Bancalari E. 1986. Pulmonary function testing and other diagnostic laboratory procedures. In *Neonatal Pulmonary Care,* Thibeault DW, and Gregory GA, eds. Norwalk, Connecticut: Appleton & Lange, 49–73.

4. Comroe JH Jr, et al. 1962. *The Lung: Clinical Physiology and Pulmonary Function Tests.* Chicago: Year Book Medical Publishers.

5. Goldsmith LS, et al. 1991. Immediate improvement in lung volume after exogenous surfactant: Alveolar recruitment versus increased distention. *Journal of Pediatrics* 119(3): 424–428.

6. Fisher JB, et al. 1988. Identifying lung overdistention during mechanical ventilation using volume-pressure loops. *Pediatric Pulmonology* 5(1): 10–14.

7. Polgar G. 1986. Mechanical properties of lung and chest wall. In *Neonatal Pulmonary Care,* Thibeault DW, and Gregory GA, eds. Norwalk, Connecticut: Appleton & Lange, 195–233.

8. Guslits BG, et al. 1987. Comparison of methods of measurement of compliance of the respiratory system in children. *American Review of Respiratory Disease* 136(3): 727–729.

9. Migdal M, et al. 1987. Compliance of the total respiratory system in healthy preterm and full-term newborns. *Pediatric Pulmonology* 3(4): 214–218.

10. Wanner A, et al. 1974. Relationship between frequency dependence of lung compliance and distribution of ventilation. *Journal of Clinical Investigation* 54(5): 1200–1213.

11. West JB. 1995. Mechanics of breathing. In *Respiratory Physiology.* Baltimore: Williams & Wilkins, 103–105.

12. LeSouef PN, England SJ, and Bryan AC. 1984. Total resistance of the respiratory system in preterm infants with and without an endotracheal tube. *Journal of Pediatrics* 104(1): 108–111.

13. Mammel MC, et al. 1989. Determining optimum inspiratory time during intermittent positive pressure ventilation in surfactant-depleted cats. *Pediatric Research* 7(4): 223–229.

14. Fox WW. 1988. Measurement of functional residual capacity in infants using the helium dilution method. In *Neonatal Pulmonary Function Testing: Physiological, Technical, and Clinical Considerations,* Bhutani VK, Shaffer TH, and Vidyasagar D, eds. Ithaca, New York: Perinatology Press, 81–90.

15. Antunes MJ. 1992. Decreased functional residual capacity predates requirement for ECMO and lung opacification during ECMO. *Pediatric Research* 31(4 part 2): 192A.

16. Antunes MJ. 1995. Prognosis with preoperative pulmonary function and lung volume assessment in infants with congenital diaphragmatic hernia. *Pediatrics* 96(6): 1117–1122.

17. Antunes MJ, et al. 1994. Continued pulmonary recovery observed after discontinuing extracorporeal membrane oxygenation. *Pediatric Pulmonology* 17(3): 143–148.

18. Fox WW, et al. 1979. Effects of endotracheal tube leaks on functional residual capacity determination in intubated neonates. *Pediatric Research* 13(1): 60–64.

19. Gerhardt T, et al. 1985. A simple method for measuring functional residual capacity by N_2 washout in small animals and newborn infants. *Pediatric Research* 19(11): 1165–1169.

20. Auld PAM, et al. 1963. Measurement of thoracic gas volume in the newborn infant. *Journal of Clinical Investigation* 42(4): 476–483.

21. Avery ME, et al. 1963. Impedance pneumograph and magnetometer methods for monitoring tidal volume. *Journal of Applied Physiology* 18(5): 895–903.

22. Beardsmore CS, et al. 1989. Measurement of lung volumes during active and quiet sleep in infants. *Pediatric Pulmonology* 7(2): 71–77.

23. Beardsmore CS, Stocks J, and Silverman M. 1982. Problems in measurement of thoracic gas volume in infancy. *Journal of Applied Physiology: Respiratory, Environmental and Exercise Physiology* 52(4): 995–999.

24. Duffty P, et al. 1981. Respiratory induction plethysmography (Respitrace): An evaluation of its use in the infant. *American Review of Respiratory Disease* 123(5): 542–546.

25. Grunstein MM, et al. 1987. Expiratory volume clamping: A new method to assess respiratory mechanics in sedated infants. *Journal of Applied Physiology* 62(5): 2107–2114.

26. Greenspan JS, et al. 1992. Increased respiratory drive and limited adaptation to loaded breathing in bronchopulmonary dysplasia. *Pediatric Research* 32(3): 356–359.

27. Motoyama EK, et al. 1987. Early onset of airway reactivity in premature infants with bronchopulmonary dysplasia. *American Review of Respiratory Disease* 136(1): 50–57.

28. Motoyama EK. 1977. Pulmonary mechanics during early postnatal years. Part II. *Pediatric Research* 11(3): 220–223.

29. Bose CL, et al. 1986. Measurement of cardiopulmonary function in ventilated neonates with respiratory distress syndrome using rebreathing methodology. *Pediatric Research* 20(4): 316–320.

30. Duara S, et al. 1991. Metabolic and respiratory effects of flow-resistive loading in preterm infants. *Journal of Applied Physiology* 70(2): 895–899.

31. Duara S, et al. 1985. Preterm infants: Ventilation and P_{100} changes in CO_2 and inspiratory resistive loading. *Journal of Applied Physiology* 58(6): 1982–1987.

32. Sly PD, Lanteri C, and Bates J. 1990. Effect of thermodynamics of an infant plethysmograph on the measurement of thoracic gas volume. *Pediatric Pulmonology* 8(3): 203–208.

33. Greenspan JS, DeGiulio PA, and Bhutani VK. 1989. Airway reactivity as determined by a cold air challenge in infants with bronchopulmonary dysplasia. *Journal of Pediatrics* 114(3): 452–454.

34. Greenspan JS, Wolfson MR, and Shaffer TH. 1991. Airway responsiveness to low inspired gas temperature in preterm neonates. *Journal of Pediatrics* 118(3): 443–445.

35. Morgan WJ. 1988. Evaluation of forced expiratory flow in infants. In *Neonatal Pulmonary Function Testing: Physiological, Technical, and Clinical Considerations*, Bhutani VK, Shaffer TH, and Vidyasagar D, eds. Ithaca, New York: Perinatology Press, 107–123.

36. Prendiville A, Green S, and Silverman M. 1987. Paradoxical response to nebulized salbutamol in wheezy infants, assessed by partial expiratory flow-volume curves. *Thorax* 42(2): 86–91.

37. Stefano JL, et al. 1986. Inductive plethysmography—a facilitated postural calibration technique for rapid and accurate tidal volume determination in low birth weight premature newborns. *American Review of Respiratory Disease* 134(5): 1020–1024.

38. Taussig LM, et al. 1982. Determinants of forced expiratory flows in newborn infants. *Journal of Applied Physiology* 53(5): 1220–1227.

39. Taussig LM. 1977. Maximal expiratory flow at functional residual capacity: A test of lung function for young children. *American Review of Respiratory Disease* 116(6): 1031–1038.

40. Tepper R, and Reister T. 1993. Forced expiratory flows and lung volumes in normal infants. *Pediatric Pulmonology* 15(6): 357–361.

41. Tepper RS, et al. 1986. Expiratory flow limitation in infants with bronchopulmonary dysplasia. *Journal of Pediatrics* 109(6): 1040–1046.

42. Tepper RS, et al. 1986. Physiologic growth and development of the lung during the first year of life. *American Review of Respiratory Disease* 134(3): 513–519.

43. Goldman SL, et al. 1983. Early prediction of chronic lung disease by pulmonary function testing. *Journal of Pediatrics* 102(4): 613–617.

44. Greenspan JS, Abbasi S, and Bhutani VK. 1988. Sequential changes in pulmonary mechanics in the very low birth weight (≤1,000 grams) infant. *Journal of Pediatrics* 113(4): 732–737.

45. Couser RJ, et al. 1990. Effects of exogenous surfactant therapy on dynamic compliance during mechanical breathing in preterm infants with hyaline membrane disease. *Journal of Pediatrics* 116(1): 119–124.

46. Davis JM, et al. 1988. Changes in pulmonary mechanics after the administration of surfactant to infants with respiratory distress syndrome. *New England Journal of Medicine* 319(8): 476–479.

47. Gerhardt T, et al. 1987. Serial determination of pulmonary function in infants with chronic lung disease. *Journal of Pediatrics* 110(3): 448–456.

48. Abbasi S, and Bhutani VK. 1990. Pulmonary mechanics and energetics of normal, non-ventilated low birthweight infants. *Pediatric Pulmonology* 8(2): 89–95.

49. Collaborative European Multicenter Study Group. 1988. Surfactant replacement therapy for severe neonatal respiratory distress syndrome: An international randomized clinical trial. *Pediatrics* 82(5): 683–690.

50. Abbasi S, et al. 1993. Long-term pulmonary consequences of respiratory distress syndrome in preterm infants treated with exogenous surfactant. *Journal of Pediatrics* 122(3):446–452.

51. Avery ME, et al. 1987. Is chronic lung disease in low birth weight infants preventable? A survey of eight centers. *Pediatrics* 79(1): 26–30.

52. Bachrach SJ, et al. 1993. Early transfer to a rehabilitation hospital for infants with chronic bronchopulmonary dysplasia. *Clinical Pediatrics* 32(9): 535–541.

13 High-Frequency Ventilation: The Current Challenge to Neonatal Nursing

Tracy Karp, RNC, MS, NNP

Over the past 30 years, conventional mechanical ventilators (CMV) have been used with increasing success to treat infants suffering a variety of cardiorespiratory diseases.[1,2] The addition of surfactant therapy has further increased survival rates and lessened morbidity.[3] Although death occurs in fewer and fewer patients, complications such as bronchopulmonary dysplasia (BPD) and pulmonary air leak syndrome may occur in some survivors.[1,2,4–6] Bronchopulmonary dysplasia continues to occur in 6–30 percent of infants weighing <1,500 gm, with rates up to 70 or 80 percent in infants weighing <1,000 gm.[5,7,8] These complications may be secondary to trauma to the lungs from excessive tidal volumes, high levels of inspired oxygen, and elevated levels of positive pressure ventilation.[9–12]

A method of ventilation more effective than traditional time-cycled, pressure-limited ventilation, one that uses smaller tidal volumes and possibly less peak inspiratory pressure to sustain infants, might decrease the mortality and morbidity from respiratory failure.[13] High-frequency ventilation (HFV) may be such a method.

During the last 17 years, HFV has become an increasingly popular method of providing respiratory support to infants with severe lung disease.[14–17] Use of HFV has expanded from experimental therapy in a few nurseries to a common means of respiratory support in more than 300 nurseries.[14,18]

Currently, five HFV devices are approved by the U.S. Food and Drug Administration (FDA) for use in children.[14] High-frequency ventilation has influenced neonatal nursing care from the beginning of its usage and continues to do so.[19–23] This chapter presents a broad overview of HFV and the nursing management and care of infants receiving this therapy.

INTRODUCTION

High-frequency ventilation is a type of mechanical ventilation that provides at least four times the normal neonatal respiratory rate and a tidal volume close to or less than anatomical dead space (ADS).[24] The respiratory frequencies (breaths or cycles) generally range from 240 breaths per minute or 4 Hertz (Hz) to 3,000 breaths per minute or 50 Hz.[25,26] The normal upper limit of spontaneous neonatal respirations is usually less than 60 breaths per minute.[2]

With HFV, respiratory gas flow and support of oxygenation and ventilation may be provided by various systems, including jet impulse, flow interruption, and bias flow oscillations by piston or diaphragm drivers.[14,15,26–28]

This chapter focuses mainly on HFV provided by either high-frequency jet ventilation (HFJV) devices or high-frequency oscillatory ventilation (HFOV) devices. An example of an HFJV device is the Life-Pulse high frequency jet ventilator (Bunnell, Inc., Salt Lake City, Utah). This is a microprocessor-controlled, positive pressure-limited, time-cycled HFV device. Examples of HFOV devices include Sensormedics 3100 ventilator (SensorMedics, Inc., Yorba Linda, California) and the Infant Star High Frequency Ventilator (Infrasonics, Inc., San Diego, California). The SensorMedics is a piston-driven, time-cycled, pressure-limited device; the Infrasonics is a high-frequency flow interrupter device that provides an oscillatory type wave pattern using a Venturi device. It is important to note that the release of new devices and modification of existing devices are constantly occurring. The description of mentioned devices does not indicate an endorsement of such devices.

HISTORICAL PERSPECTIVE

Though HFV is a relatively recent technique in the treatment of infants and adults with respiratory failure, the idea is not new. In 1915, Henderson, Chillingworth, and Whitney noted that panting dogs maintained adequate gas exchange with tidal volumes less than ADS.[29] Brisco, Foster, and Comroe noted in 1954 that alveolar ventilation could be maintained with small tidal volumes.[30] In 1959, John H. Emerson, a pioneer in respiratory devices, built and patented an apparatus for vibrating the patient's airway. Although it was never used on patients,

this was the first true high-frequency oscillation (HFO) device.[31]

During the 1970s, interest in high-frequency ventilation increased. In 1972, Lunkenheimer and associates reported the ability to ventilate dogs with the use of HFO delivered by a loudspeaker unit.[32] Klain and Smith, in 1977, and Sjostrand, in 1980, successfully used HFJV to support adults during bronchoscopy or airway surgery.[33,34]

During the early 1980s, reports of HFV use in neonatal patients began to appear. Most of these early cases were either attempts to rescue infants failing conventional ventilation or short-term experiments.[35,36] In 1981, Marchak and associates reported the first successful short-term treatment of respiratory distress syndrome (RDS) with HFV using an oscillatory system.[37] Two years later, Pokora and coworkers described the successful short-term treatment of neonates with intractable respiratory failure and progressive pulmonary air leaks using HFJV.[38]

By 1984, Harris and Christensen had treated 22 infants with pulmonary interstitial emphysema (PIE) who were unresponsive to conventional therapy. Sixteen of these infants had a favorable response to HFJV, requiring less ventilatory support; 11 infants survived.[39] At about the same time, HFOV was shown to be successful in treating premature baboons with PIE.[40]

Also in 1984, Carlo and associates showed the ability of HFJV to ventilate infants with respiratory distress syndrome using less airway pressure than CMV.[41] This supported the earlier high-frequency oscillation work of Frantz, Werthammer, and Stark.[42] Thus in the early 1980s, there was preliminary evidence showing that HFV was potentially effective in improving the survival of infants with severe RDS, pulmonary air leak, and intractable respiratory failure.

During the 1980s, HFV was also used to treat persistent pulmonary hypertension of the newborn (PPHN). Pauly and associates, in 1987, used HFJV to treat nine infants with PPHN who were failing CMV. Four responded. From their limited experience, they concluded that if the infant showed no improvement after three hours on HFV, alternative forms of support, such as extracorporeal membrane oxygenation (ECMO), should be considered.[43] However, Carlo and colleagues, in 1989, were not able to show improvement in a group of patients with PPHN who were treated with a different HFJV device.[44]

In 1988, Kohelet and associates reported their ability to rescue infants with PPHN using HFOV. Of 41 infants rescued, 83 percent survived.[45] Also using HFOV, Carter and coworkers were able to rescue about 46 percent of the patients with PPHN (and other diseases) referred to their nursery for ECMO therapy. They found that of all patient groups, those with meconium aspiration syndrome (MAS) or pulmonary hypoplasia were least likely to respond to HFOV.[46] During the mid- to late 1980s, studies continued to validate the efficacy of HFV in a variety of disease states with a variety of devices.

In 1986, Gonzalez and colleagues found decreased gas flow through pneumothoraces in neonates receiving HFJV (Life-Pulse, Bunnell, Inc.) versus CMV. They found that gas flow rates out of chest tubes decreased from 227 ± 96 ml/minute during CMV to 104 ± 59 ml/minute on HFJV.[47]

Also in 1986, Clark and associates reported successful rescue of infants with PIE and air leak using HFOV.[48] In 1987, Mammel and colleagues reported improved survival rates in their seven-year experience with HFJV rescue for intractable pulmonary air leaks and very severe respiratory failure.[49]

In 1989, two significant papers were published. The first was a report of the large NIH-sponsored randomized comparison trial of HFOV versus CMV as the primary treatment for infants with RDS. More than 670 infants were enrolled and treated with either the "local" CMV device or a piston-driven, fixed I:E ratio HFOV device. The results showed no improvement in survival and no reduction in air leaks or BPD. There was, however, a small but significant increase in Grade III and IV intraventricular hemorrhage (IVH) in the study group.[50] These findings led to much controversy concerning the study design and interpretation of the results.[12,51]

Spitzer, Butler, and Fox, also in 1989, reported their experience with 176 patients rescued by HFJV. Fifty-four percent of the infants survived, and ventilation and oxygenation were improved with HFJV.[52]

During the 1990s, more randomized clinical studies using HFV to treat infants with RDS, PIE, and other air leaks were reported. In 1990, Carlo and associates reported a small, randomized trial of early HFJV use in infants with RDS. They were not able to show an improvement in survival or a decrease in the development of BPD. There was no increase in IVH rate.[53]

In 1992, Clark and colleagues reported a small, randomized trial using HFOV in infants with RDS. They treated three groups: one with CMV, one with CMV and HFOV, and one with HFOV alone. They reported no difference in survival but a decrease in BPD among the group treated only with HFOV. There was no statistically significant increase in the incidence of IVH.[54]

In these studies, there was not widespread use of surfactant preparations. By the mid-1990s, reports of the use of HFV with surfactant for infants with RDS began to appear. In 1995, Patel and Klein reported a rescue study of 114 patients with birth weights <1,000 gm treated with HFOV or CMV after surfactant therapy. This retrospective review focused mainly on safety issues, IVH, and outcome status. Although investigators felt the HFO-treated patients were sicker than the CMV-treated patients, they found no differences between the two groups in rates of IVH, pneumothorax, BPD, survival, or outcome.[55]

More recently, in 1996 Gerstmann and colleagues reported the results of a multicenter, randomized, controlled trial of the efficacy of HFOV after surfactant therapy among infants <35 weeks gestational age. The HFOV was started within the first few hours of life. The HFOV group had similar mortality but less chronic lung disease and reduced hospital costs than infants receiving both CMV and surfactant.[56] Also in 1996, Wiswell and associates reported on the use of HFJV for early treatment of RDS in infants <33 weeks gestational age. In their study there was no difference in pulmonary outcomes or hospital cost when compared to those treated with CMV. Infants ventilated with HFJV with the strategy used in this study, were more likely to have a poor outcome (death, grade IV IVH, or cystic periventricular leukomalacia).[57]

In examining the treatment of air leaks, Keszler and associates, in 1991, reported on 144 infants who were randomized to CMV or HFJV for treatment of PIE. The HFJV group had a better response than the CMV group and improved survival, but there were no differences between the groups in the incidence of BPD or IVH.[58]

In 1993, the HiFO Study Group, a multicenter research consortium, reported a randomized trial investigating the effect of HFOV on the development of air leak syndrome. They found fewer new air leaks in the HFOV group than in controls and no differences in BPD. Intraventricular hemorrhage rates were much

lower than those found in the NIH sponsored HIFI Study Group, but there were methodological differences.[50,59]

Another type of high-frequency (flow interrupter) respirator, the Volumetric Diffusive Respirator (VDR-1) (Percussionaire Corp., Sands Point, Indiana) has been used to treat neonates.[60,61] Bodenstein and colleagues treated 79 infants using a rescue protocol; 60 percent survived.[60]

In 1993, Pardou and coworkers used the VDR-1 with a low mean airway pressure (Pa̅w) strategy to treat infants with RDS in a randomized, controlled trial. They found no differences in mortality or morbidity between the VDR-1 and the CMV groups. They concluded that, though the machine was safe, it offered no advantage over CMV with the strategy used.[62]

High-frequency ventilation has also been used to support infants undergoing various surgical procedures. For example, HFJV has been used during and after surgery for congenital tracheal stenosis, tracheoesophageal fistula, and cardiac and abdominal defect repairs.[63,64] Davis and associates reported in 1994 that HFJV provided better gas exchange at lower Pa̅w when compared to CMV in a group of nine infants undergoing Blalock-Taussig shunt placement.[65] Postoperative cardiac function was improved with HFJV in a small group of patients after they underwent the Fontan procedure.[66]

The patients who have sparked the most interest are those with congenital diaphragmatic hernia. Early reports on the use of HFV in these patients were not encouraging. Although there was some clinical improvement, survival was poor.[67-69] More recently, improved outcome has been reported, especially with HFOV.[70,71] Regardless of the device used, treatment of infants with congenital diaphragmatic hernia remains challenging.

The efficacy of HFV treatment of infants with meconium aspiration syndrome has been described. In 1983, Mammel and associates first reported a comparison of HFJV (Instrument Device Corporation, Pittsburgh, Pennsylvania) and CMV in an adult cat model. They found, at comparable $P\overline{aw}$, higher pulmonary vascular resistance, pulmonary artery pressure, and alveolar-arterial oxygen differences when the animals were on HFJV rather than CMV.[72] In 1985, Trindale and coworkers compared HFJV (Bunnell device) to CMV in a meconium aspiration piglet model. They found that HFJV required a peak inspiratory pressure (PIP) 50 percent lower than that of CMV to keep the PCO_2 equal.[73]

Keszler and associates studied combined jet ventilation in a MAS puppy model. In their study, combined HFJV/CMV (sighs) provided the best oxygenation and ventilation at less $P\overline{aw}$ and PIP than CMV alone.[74] Finally, in a piglet model, Wiswell and coworkers studied the effect of surfactant added to HFJV therapy. They found no benefit to the added surfactant therapy.[75]

More recently, use of HFV in infants with meconium aspiration syndrome and respiratory failure has been viewed in terms of predicting the need for or avoidance of ECMO. By using HFJV, Baumgart and colleagues avoided ECMO in 38 percent of patients with MAS. They also noted that, in general, patients responded within one to six hours.[76] Carter's group avoided the use of ECMO in 50 percent of infants with MAS by using HFOV.[46] Varnholt and associates, in 1992, used HFOV to rescue 46 percent of infants referred for ECMO. Of their HFOV infants, 50 percent suffered air leak (either continued or new).[77]

Also in terms of avoiding ECMO, Clark, Yoder, and Sell reported in 1994, a randomized crossover trial comparing HFOV and CMV. Although there was no ultimate difference in outcome or ECMO usage because of crossover, HFOV was able to rescue 63 percent of those failing CMV, and CMV was able to rescue 23 percent of the patients. These investigators concluded that HFOV was a safe and effective device to avoid ECMO therapy.[78]

As part of Clark, Yoder, and Sell's study and a larger retrospective review, Paranka and colleagues reported on predictors of HFOV failure. They found that the presence of congenital diaphragmatic hernia, lung hypoplasia, and an arterial-to-alveolar oxygen ratio of ≤ 0.05 at initiation or 0.08 after six hours of HFOV predicted the need for ECMO or death.[79]

High-frequency ventilation has also been used in conjunction with other specialized therapies. Davis and associates, in 1992, reported on the use of rescue treatment with a combination of HFJV and surfactant to avoid ECMO in infants with severe respiratory failure. Of the 28 patients, 25 survived.[80]

The use of nitric oxide and HFV is increasing. In 1994, Lynch and colleagues reported the combined use of HFJV and nitric oxide.[81] By 1995, Wilford and coworkers reported on a delivery system for nitric oxide and HFOV.[82] Although these reports shared anecdotal experiences of safety and efficiency, these systems require much adaptation, monitoring, and vigilance to ensure consistent, safe nitric oxide delivery.

By 1997, there was a large body of information supporting the use of certain types of HFV therapy as rescue treatment. The success of the therapy seems to be affected by patient population, device, strategy, timing of use, and the clinical environment. Also, limited human data to support the use of early HFV therapy in infants with RDS are beginning to accumulate. However, the current clinical human trials still do not yet support the primary use of these devices for the widespread initial treatment of infants with RDS.

Research on HFV is continuing on a large scale. Both experimental design and large experiential studies continue to gather data. Until further work is completed, most HFV usage will be limited to early rescue applications. Nursing has an obligation to generate a part of this body of knowledge.

A PHYSIOLOGIC FRAMEWORK

Despite being studied for decades, HFV is a phenomenon still being described and explored. A review of basic theory and physiology that may explain how HFV supports respiratory gas exchange will provide a basic framework for understanding. Two excellent reviews are available in the literature.[83,84]

CONVENTIONAL MECHANICAL VENTILATION

The CMV device supports gas exchange by mimicking many normal physiologic processes. Fresh gas is delivered to the lungs as bulk flow in tidal volumes much greater (>6–8 ml/kg) than anatomic dead space. During inspiration, positive pressure is used to force bulk gas flow through the larger airways. Gas moves through the smaller airways and to the alveolar region mostly by passive diffusion.[10] Varying amounts of positive end-expiratory pressure (PEEP) are used to prevent airway and alveolar collapse.[2]

Oxygenation during CMV depends mostly on the amount of ambient oxygen (FiO_2) and mean airway pressure ($\overline{Paw}$) used to deliver the gas.[85,86] The ventilatory parameters that comprise the mean airway pressure are the PEEP, PIP, inspiratory time, and rate.[87] The effect of $\overline{Paw}$ on oxygenation may be related to enhanced alveolar recruitment and stabilization, creating an optimal lung volume.[14,88] High mean airway pressure may be detrimental to oxygenation if it leads to excessive lung volumes or reduction in pulmonary blood flow or cardiac output.

FIGURE 13-1 ▲ **CO_2 elimination equation.**

CO_2 Elimination:

- CMV: $\dot{V}CO_2 = V_T \times f$
- HFV: $\dot{V}CO_2 = (V_T)^a \times f^b$
  $a = 1.5\text{–}2.2$
  $b = 0.5\text{–}1$

F = frequency, V_T = Tidal volume
$\dot{V}CO_2$ = volume of CO_2 per unit of time

Adapted from: Clark R. 1994. High frequency ventilation. *Journal of Pediatrics* 124(5): 661–670; and Fredberg JJ. 1989. Summary: Pulmonary mechanics during high frequency ventilation. *Acta Anesthesiology Scandinavica* (90 supplement): 170–171. Reprinted by permission.

Carbon dioxide elimination during CMV is dependent upon alveolar ventilation, which is the product of tidal volume (minus dead space) and respiratory frequency.[88] Ventilation can be enhanced by increasing either tidal volume or frequency. However, ventilation can be hampered by excessive tidal volume or $\overline{Paw}$, as both can lead to alveolar distention, or by respiratory rates that do not allow sufficient exhalation time.[89,90]

Exhalation during CMV is a passive event occurring by the natural recoil of the chest. The time necessary to deflate (or inflate) the lung is known as the time constant. It takes three to five time constants for the lung to empty to its functional residual capacity. The time constant is the product of airway resistance and lung compliance.[88] If the time allowed for exhalation is shorter than the time constant, gas trapping will occur and lead to alveolar distention and impaired carbon dioxide elimination.[90,91]

HIGH-FREQUENCY VENTILATION

During HFV, respiratory gas exchange can be explained by a combination of traditional gas exchange concepts described previously, and unique concepts (described later) related to HFV.[14,16,17,27,83] Oxygenation during HFV appears to depend on $\overline{Paw}$ and ambient FiO_2,

FIGURE 13-2 ▲ **Pendelluft.** Representation of interregional gas mixing caused by different time constants in two lung units. The fast (1) time constant unit can be seen to be filling at end expiration. The slow (2) time constant unit fills at the end of inspiration. Tracheal flow is zero at this time, and this effect thus augments alveolar tidal volume.

$t_1 < t_2$

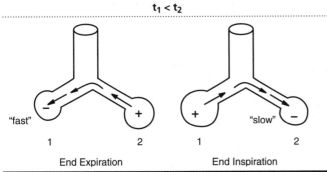

From: Wetzel RC, and Gioia FR. 1987. High frequency ventilation. *Pediatric Clinics of North America* 34(1): 20. Reprinted by permission.

as with CMV.[92] The key is having optimal lung volumes for the disease state being treated.[12] Lung volumes vary less during HFV than CMV, possibly because of the small size of each breath.[17] The P$\overline{aw}$ used to support the lung volume may be higher or lower than that required during CMV, depending upon the device and where the pressure is measured.[16,41,93,94]

High-frequency ventilation can effectively eliminate carbon dioxide.[17,21,95–98] Tidal volume and respiratory frequency influence the rate of carbon dioxide elimination.[14,99] (This relationship is illustrated in Figure 13-1.) Although there are differences in devices, tidal volume, though very small, has the greatest impact on carbon dioxide elimination. The delivery of the tidal volume and how it changes can be device specific.

As with CMV, for all HFV devices, tidal volume delivery is sensitive to lung compliance and resistance. For HFJV devices (such as Life-Pulse, Bunnell, Inc.), tidal volume change is generally related to amplitude or *delta p* (PIP – PEEP) as long as the inspiratory time does not vary. For HFO devices, tidal volume can vary based

on amplitude, power, and percentage of inspiratory time.[17] Thus, changes in frequency alone can affect tidal volume. Though the relationships are complex and changing, there are probably optimal frequencies for each type of device and disease state.[12,95,97,100,101]

Another important factor affecting carbon dioxide elimination is gas trapping in the lung. Reducing the risk of gas trapping requires that there be sufficient time for exhalation and that lung overinflation be avoided.[91] All HFV devices can cause gas trapping if used inappropriately. Avoiding lung overinflation, using the shortest inspiratory time possible, ensuring sufficient exhalation time, and eliminating obstructions will reduce the risk of gas trapping.[16,90,91,96,102]

GAS EXCHANGE MECHANISMS

We know that gas exchange can occur during HFV, even when tidal volume approaches or is less than anatomic dead space.[83,84,103] Numerous physiologic mechanisms are responsible, the most important being convection and diffusion.

Convection

During HFV, high kinetic/potential energy breaths are given. Although the individual volumes of each breath may be less than anatomic dead space, gas movement can still occur in a bulk fashion.[83] Direct aeration of proximal airways and central alveolar units can occur because of short transit times from the main airways.[10,83] These alveolar units may provide a significant portion of the total gas exchange because of local hyperventilation.[103] That is, the PCO_2 in these central units may be much lower than in the surrounding or more peripheral alveolar units.

FIGURE 13-3 ▲ The quicker the puff, the sharper the spike. Forward movement of gas in the center and backward movement of gas at the walls.

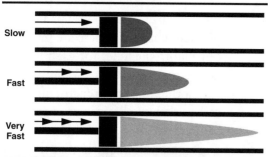

From: Harris TR, and Wood BR. 1996. Physiologic principles. In *Assisted Ventilation of the Neonate*, 3rd ed., Goldsmith JP, and Karotkin EH, eds. Philadelphia: WB Saunders, 21–68. (Modified from: Henderson Y, Chillingworth FP, and Whitney JL. 1915. The respiratory dead space. *Journal of Physiology* 38[1]: 5). Reprinted by permission.

Convective mixing and recirculation of gas can occur between neighboring respiratory units during the whole respiratory cycle.[104] This interregional mixing or "pendelluft" is due to the different time constants of the respiratory units. This results in out-of-phase gas movements and facilitates convective exchange (Figure 13-2).

Convective flow streaming is another means of gas transport. Henderson, Chillingworth, and Whitney showed that the more energy or speed generating a puff of smoke, the greater the forward movement of the center of the puff (Figure 13-3).[29] A parabolic-shaped puff or breath is formed from the development of asymmetric velocity profiles. During exhalation, there are blunt flow profiles in the opposite direction, but the elongated center portion does not return to the starting point.[105] At the end of a breath, there is a small net forward movement (Figure 13-4). During HFV (especially jet ventilation), gas tends to flow down the center or inner core of the tube (or airway) and out along the outer walls (Figure 13-5).[105,106]

Diffusion

Diffusion describes gas exchange by random (brownian) movement. This exchange occurs

FIGURE 13-4 ▲ Asymmetric velocity profiles.

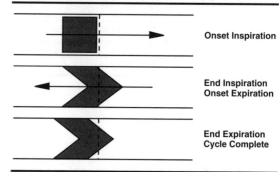

From: Wetzel RC, and Gioia FR. 1987. High frequency ventilation. *Pediatric Clinics of North America* 34(1): 22. Reprinted by permission.

in any part of the lung where there is a gradient, not only in the terminal respiratory units.

Taylor Dispersion

In 1954, Taylor described the augmented movement and radial diffusion of gas in situations of parabolic gas flow (HFV breath) (Figure 13-6).[107] This augmented diffusion can occur wherever gas meets, including situations such as the coaxial flow in the larger airways and convective streaming farther out in the lung.

During HFV, this diffusion process is facilitated by the increased surface area between two gases because of increased viscous drag.[108] Actual gas exchange may be hampered by Taylor dispersion because of the diffusion of carbon

FIGURE 13-5 ▲ Helical pattern of convective streaming during HFJV.

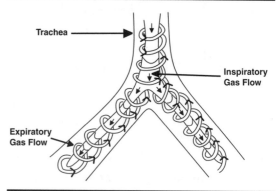

Adapted by Solon JF, from: Rausch K via Ellis R, unpublished data, Milpitas, California. Reprinted by permission.

FIGURE 13-6 ▲ Taylor dispersion. The inspiratory gas front is parabolic, and this provides a greatly increased area over which radial molecular diffusion can occur, as represented by the arrows.

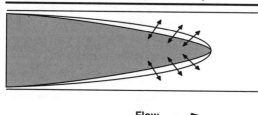

Flow ⟶

From: Wetzel RC, and Gioia FR. 1987. High frequency ventilation. *Pediatric Clinics of North America* 34(1): 21. Reprinted by permission.

FIGURE 13-7 ▲ A representation of which mechanisms of gas transport predominate in given lung regions.

1 Convection
2 Taylor Type
3 Velocity Profiles
4 Interregional (Pendelluft)
5 Molecular Diffusion

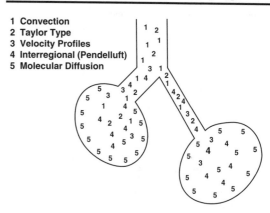

From: Wetzel RC, and Gioia FR. 1987. High frequency ventilation. *Pediatric Clinics of North America* 34(1): 23. Reprinted by permission.

dioxide from the expiring gas into the fresh gas. The high-energy HFV cycles probably result in the delivery of more total fresh gas to the respiratory units before significant contamination can occur. This preserves the diffusion gradient needed to move carbon dioxide out of the blood.[109]

Various aspects of direct ventilation and convective and diffusive mechanisms of gas transport are probably responsible for the majority of gas exchange during HFV. These mechanisms are not restricted to any one anatomic area. Convective forces are probably more dominant in areas where bulk flow occurs, and diffusion forces in areas where it stops. There must also be areas of overlap and simultaneous operation (Figure 13-7).

Traditional concepts, such as bulk flow, need to be modified in regard to HFV, but they still have validity in many situations. Tidal volumes greater than ADS have been measured during HFJV, but these include entrained gases without increased pressure.[10] Entrainment refers to the ability to provide, without extra driving pressure, additional respiratory gases during a breath or cycle.[10,88] This can occur in HFV, but usually not in CMV. The mechanism resulting in entrainment is unclear.

Bulk gas flow may also occur as a result of an accumulation of breaths, rather than as an iso-

lated event during a single breath.[83] More research is necessary before this phenomenon is fully described and understood. In order to have generalizable results, investigators must further attempt to standardize the process of and procedure for providing HFV. Unfortunately, this remains unlikely given the continuing trends in HFV research and manufacturing.

CLINICAL DEVICES: STRATEGIES AND INDICATIONS

Anecdotal and experimental evidence has accumulated to support the use of HFV therapy in various disease states and clinical situations (these are presented in Table 13-1). When considering the indications for high-frequency ventilation, it is most important to individualize them to each NICU. The type of device, experience with the device, and alternate therapies must all be considered.

HFV therapy must be used early enough to improve outcome and decrease complications, rather than as a last resort. Yet the timing of use should not be so early as to expose the infant to unnecessary risks and complications. Whenever possible, HFV use should be

TABLE 13-1 ▲ **Clinical Indications for Use of High-Frequency Ventilation**

Severe respiratory failure

Extraventilatory air leak syndromes

Failing CMV

Persistent pulmonary hypertension

Before and after other therapies

ECMO

Cardiac surgery

Congenital diaphragmatic hernia surgery

Airway surgery

Adapted from: Karp T. 1993. High frequency ventilation: Life in the fast lane? Presented at Neonatal Nurses National Conference, Nottingham, England, September 25; and Clark RH. 1994. High-frequency ventilation. *Journal of Pediatrics* 124(5): 661–670. Reprinted by permission.

in the context of a research study. This builds up the knowledge and experience base. Finally, considering the current data, HFV should not be used in situations where CMV has a track record of success.

GENERAL CONCEPTS

High-frequency ventilation is provided to the patient by specialized devices. The general classification and comparisons of these devices are based on the method of HFV employed and operating characteristics. The high-frequency devices in current clinical use deliver gas during inspiration under positive pressure. Negative pressure devices are under laboratory investigation.[110]

Some general operating characteristics of HFJV and HFOV devices are listed in Table 13-2. An understanding of key concepts will be useful in managing the patient on HFV:

- Frequency (or rate) refers to the breaths or cycles the machine can deliver.
- The waveform refers to the "shape" of the breath delivered. Waveform may influence how gas travels in and out of the lung.
- Exhalation refers to how the gas gets out of the lung. Passive exhalation relies on the natural recoil of the chest (as in CMV). Active exhalation refers to actual pulling or assist-

ing the gas out of the chest by generating a type of "negative" pressure or pull during exhalation.

- The inspiratory-to-expiratory (I:E) ratio refers to the time allotted to inspiration as compared to expiration for each breath. It is affected by rate. When the time for inspiration is the same as that for expiration, the I:E ratio is 1:1. For most devices, especially those with passive exhalation, more time is needed for expiration than inspiration.
- Tidal volume (in Table 13-2) refers to the size of the breath in relation to anatomic dead space. The amount of pressure used, gas flow, endotracheal tube size (or change in size), and the time allowed for inspiration all contribute to determining tidal volume. In general, the more pressure, gas flow, time allowed for inspiration, and the larger endotracheal tube, the larger the delivered tidal volume.

High-frequency ventilation may be provided as a single therapy or in combination with traditional mechanical ventilation. The device may be a stand-alone machine (SensorMedics 3100), a stand-alone machine that works in tandem with a conventional ventilator (Life-Pulse high frequency jet ventilator), or a machine that combines both capabilities (Infant Star High Frequency Ventilator). Device configurations are constantly being changed by manufacturers, so the user must be up to date on their recommendations.

MONITORING ISSUES

Currently, most neonatal ventilation is provided by positive pressure. The caregiver monitors the pressure signal produced by various pressure transducers with results displayed either on the ventilator or on an attached monitor. The pressure readings during CMV are most often sampled at the patient connector and measured by a transducer located in the ventilator.

TABLE 13-2 ▲ General Operating Characteristics of HFJV and HFOV Devices

Characteristic	HFJV	HFOV
Frequency in cycles per minute (Hz/minute)	150–660 (2.5–12)	300–3000 (5–50)
Inspiratory waveform	Triangular/spike	Sine wave
Exhalation	Passive	Active
Tidal volume (usually)	<CMV >Anatomic dead space	<CMV < or >anatomic dead space

The pressure values displayed usually represent the pressure transmitted through the endotracheal tube to the lung.[14] As the ventilator rate increases, the endotracheal tube acts as a resistor, decreasing the amplitude of the signal. Thus, at high rates, the pressure in the lung can be less than that measured at the endotracheal tube connector. The exception is when gas trapping occurs, in which case the pressure in the lung may be higher than that on the monitor display. The key to preventing this problem is to ensure expiratory time sufficient to avoid gas trapping and a buildup of pressure.

With HFOV devices, the attenuation of the pressure signal can be significant, especially when a 1:2 I:E ratio is used.[94] In other words, the pressure (amplitude) signal sampled by the device at the patient connector may be much higher than the actual pressure (amplitude) in the lung.[14,111–113]

With an HFJV device, such as the Bunnell Life-Pulse, the pressure signal is sampled at the end of the triple-lumen endotracheal tube. The transducer is located in the patient box, close to the patient connector, rather than back in the ventilator. This arrangement allows for measurement of an undampened signal. The pressure values displayed on the ventilator reflect those in the trachea.[16]

GENERAL PATIENT MANAGEMENT PRINCIPLES

General guiding principles for management of the patient on HFV depend on disease state and device. One must (1) provide enough mean airway pressure to (2) stabilize optimal lung volumes while (3) avoiding gas trapping and cardiac impairment.[14,113,114]

Optimal lung volumes depend upon the disease state. In general, there should be no significant atelectasis, no extraventilatory air, no hyperinflation, and good ventilation-to-perfusion matching. At optimal lung volume, there will be appropriate oxygenation and ventilation and the least risk of lung injury.

The mean airway pressure required to achieve optimal lung volume will depend upon the disease state and device. It may be high or low, depending upon what you want to accomplish. The optimal $\overline{Paw}$ will provide the optimal lung volume with the fewest adverse side effects.[115] The challenge is the difficulty of monitoring lung volume (see Chapter 12). The most frequent tool is the chest x-ray, along with the physical examination, vital signs, and blood gas analysis.[16,116] In addition, frequent echocardiography may be a tool for the evaluation of venous return and associated decrease in cardiac output during HFV.[114,117]

Although there are device-specific issues, most concepts can be employed with either type of device. A key to successful treatment with high-frequency ventilation is maintaining lung volumes.[12] Some treatments and procedures, such as suctioning, which require disconnecting the infant from the ventilator circuit, will result in some degree of lung deflation. Lung volume can be restored with either a sustained inflation (sigh) or a gradual increase in $\overline{Paw}$ on the HFV device until oxygenation or chest x-ray improves.[17] Caution must be used with both sustained inflations and increased $\overline{Paw}$ because they can impede venous return, decrease cardiac output, and damage the airways.[114,117,118]

FIGURE 13-8 ▲ Patient box.

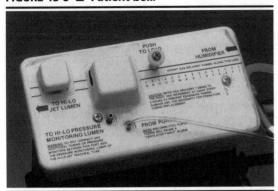

FIGURE 13-9 ▲ Triple lumen ET tube.

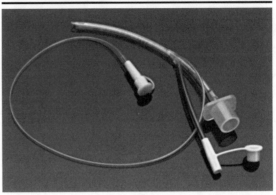

Surfactant and HFV may be synergistic in their effects.[119,120] Surfactant can be used before and during HFV therapy.[55,119] It is usually administered with the infant off HFV because reflux of surfactant into the endotracheal tube can occur, as can tube obstruction, especially when small amplitudes are employed. Surfactant usage must be considered when various HFV research and clinical strategies are compared. More research in this area is required.

The clinical strategies focus on pulmonary management, but other patient needs must not be forgotten. The key to successful HFV is stable and effective hemodynamics. Frequently, intravascular volume and inotropic support are needed—especially when high $\overline{Paw}$ is required to resolve atelectasis. Additional attention to nutrition, pain control, and parent needs is essential to provide a holistic approach to the care of the patient.[116]

HIGH-FREQUENCY JET VENTILATION[14–16,21,115]

A method of providing HFJV is by the use of the Life-Pulse high frequency jet ventilator. This device is a microprocessor-controlled, positive pressure-limited, time-cycled, high-frequency ventilator. The jet pulses are delivered from a valve box located close to the patient (Figure 13-8). The size of these jet pulses (tidal volume) is controlled by the jet PIP and length of inspiration. Inspiration time is generally held at 20 milliseconds. Therefore, tidal volume is not affected by rate changes unless inspiratory time is specifically changed. This valve box also contains the airway pressure–monitoring transducer.

The valve box is connected to the patient by two methods. One method is via a special triple-lumen endotracheal tube (Hi-Lo Jet endotracheal tube; Mallinckrodt, Inc., St. Louis, Missouri) (Figure 13-9). This Hi-Lo endotracheal tube has the jet injector site near the end of the tube within its main barrel. Just proximal to this site is the pressure-monitoring lumen. The main barrel of this tube allows for exhalation, delivery of CMV gas, and suctioning. The lumen of the Hi-Lo tube is 0.5 mm larger than the corresponding conventional ET tube.

Another method of connection to the patient is a specialized triple-lumen endotracheal tube adapter, the "jet nozzle" (Figure 13-10).[121] This new adapter allows care providers the choice of using either the Hi-Lo or a conventional endotracheal tube.[122] The adapter is useful in situations in which one wishes to avoid reintubation or when Hi-Lo tubes do not fit because of very small patient size. The use of the adapter alters the pressure measurement and jet delivery site to the top of the endotracheal tube.

FIGURE 13-10 ▲ Jet nozzle ET tube adapter.

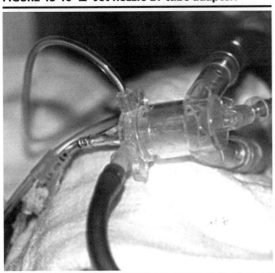

The Life-Pulse ventilator provides HFV in tandem with a CMV device. The CMV device provides the PEEP and background CMV breaths (sighs) as needed. The gas flow to create the jet impulses is governed by a microprocessor-controlled pressure regulator that adjusts to meet the operating conditions. This gas flow, or servopressure, changes in response to lung volume, respiratory compliance, or airway resistance. In the absence of an air leak in the system, rising servopressure usually indicates improved compliance. A drop may indicate increased airway resistance, decreased compliance, or tension pneumothorax.[123]

The key concepts for HFJV usage are as follows:

- Oxygenation is related to P$\overline{aw}$, carbon dioxide removal, and tidal volume.
- Generally, HFJV allows use of a lower P$\overline{aw}$ and PIP as compared to CMV.
- The HFJV (Life-Pulse, Bunnell, Inc.) requires use of a background CMV device to provide PEEP. The CMV device also sustains inflations (sighs) when recruitment of an atelectatic lung is needed.

- It can utilize "elevated or high" P$\overline{aw}$ strategy to support oxygenation and optimal lung volumes.
- It requires a specific type of endotracheal adapter or tube.

Clinical Strategies

When dealing with an infant with restrictive lung disease and air leak syndromes such as PIE and pneumothorax, the goal in using HFJV is to use less PIP and P$\overline{aw}$ to allow the air leaks to heal. It is suggested to start with a PIP 10–20 percent less than that used for CMV. The P$\overline{aw}$ should be the same or less by 1–2 cm H_2O to support oxygenation. The PEEP can be the same or greater by one. The HFJV rate is usually started at 420 breaths per minute.

As the infant is placed on HFJV, the CMV is weaned to a rate of 5 and, if possible, an HFJV PIP less than that used for CMV. For patients with air leak injury, lower tandem CMV rates (down to 0) or only continuous positive airway pressure (CPAP) can be used when oxygenation is adequate. This approach is used to avoid further air leak injury. The CPAP levels must be high enough to stabilize open alveoli, but not excessive so as to prevent healing. The risk of delayed air leak healing from the CPAP level needed to support oxygenation must be balanced against the trauma of the CMV rate (large tidal volume breaths).

Atelectatic disorders, such as RDS, require a somewhat different strategy. The PIP may be slightly reduced or the same as the CMV setting. The PEEP setting will be 1–3 cm H_2O higher than the CMV setting. The HFJV rate will be 420 breaths per minute.

Again, the infant is weaned from background CMV support, but if oxygenation falls, the CMV PIP may need to be slightly higher than the HFJV PIP. This is to help recruit atelectatic air spaces. The CMV support, usually PIP, is reduced as rapidly as lung volume stabilization allows; then the HFJV PIP is reduced as tolerated. However, to prevent atelectasis PEEP may need to remain elevated as PIP is decreased.

Obstructive disorders, such as MAS, can be treated by HFJV. The device is used to support gas exchange and facilitate debris removal. Until stabilized, the patient may require high HFJV and background settings. Often, once the infant's lung volume is restored, he can be effectively ventilated (or hyperventilated) with HFJV at a lower PIP.

One must constantly assess the patient for gas trapping. Sufficient expiratory time is essential to avoid significant gas trapping. Expiratory time can be gained by lowering the HFJV rate (to as low as the 240–360 breaths per minute range).[115] This is indicated by an increasing I:E ratio.

Weaning from HFJV has not been systematically studied. In general, the therapy is used during the acute phase of the disease. Most infants are weaned by 7 to 14 days.[21] The air leaks, if present, should be resolved for 1 to 2 days before weaning. Methods of weaning vary, but they usually involve decreasing the tidal volume (PIP) to a maintenance level and reducing the HFJV rate to 250–350 breaths per minute. Support from CMV is increased with emphasis on using small (4–6 ml/kg) tidal volume breaths.

HIGH-FREQUENCY OSCILLATING VENTILATORS[14,15,17]

The majority of HFOV in the U.S. is provided by two devices:

1. The SensorMedics 3100 ventilator is a time-cycled, pressure-limited device that uses a piston-driven diaphragm to move bias gas flow. The resulting oscillations of gas are delivered to the patient in a push-pull fashion via a rigid tube connected to a traditional endotracheal tube.

The size of the oscillations, known as amplitude, are controlled by the driving pressure (or stroke volume) of the piston. Inspiratory time is a percentage of the breath cycle. It is adjustable and usually set at 33 percent to provide an I:E ratio of 1:2. This is to reduce the risk of gas trapping. Frequency is adjustable from 300 to 1,500 cycles per minute (5–25 Hz). It is usually set between 600 and 900 cycles per minute (10–15 Hz).

Tidal volumes are usually less than anatomic dead space and adjusted by changing the amplitude of the cycle. An adequate amplitude will provide a tidal volume that will cause minimal chest vibrations. However, tidal volume is also highly dependent upon inspiratory time. Because inspiratory time is a percentage of the time cycle, it will change when the frequency is altered. Reducing the frequency will increase the inspiratory time and therefore the tidal volume. Conversely, increasing frequency will decrease inspiratory time and tidal volume.

Mean airway pressure is provided by PEEP. The PEEP is controlled by continuous fresh gas (bias flow) and the resistance of a low-pass filter. PEEP is usually adjusted by manipulations of this low-pass filter.

2. The Infant Star Ventilator with HFO module is a high-frequency flow interrupter device that provides oscillatory wave patterns using a Venturi device. Although it is a "hybrid" type of device, it acts similarly to the piston-driven oscillator.

Inspiratory time is fixed at 18 milliseconds, so its I:E ratio is variable. At the usual operating frequency of 900 breaths per minute (15 Hz), the I:E ratio is 1:2.7. Low-rate tandem ventilation (sighs) is often provided.[55]

The basic concepts for HFOV usage are as follows:

- Oxygenation is dependent upon P$\overline{\text{aw}}$, and ventilation is dependent on tidal volume.

- The HFOV allows for the use of higher mean airway pressure compared to CMV.
- It allows for ventilation with very small (less than ADS) tidal volumes.
- It requires stabilization of lung volumes. Adjusting support as lung volumes change is critical to success.
- It requires close monitoring of cardiac output, which may be reduced as the lung volume stabilizes.
- It uses a standard endotracheal tube.

Clinical Strategies

The approach to treating homogeneous processes such as RDS or diffuse atelectasis is one of increasing the Paw to open and stabilize the lung volume. The Paw is increased by 1–2 cm H_2O over CMV. If oxygenation is poor, the Paw is further increased in 1–2 cm H_2O steps. The Paw needed to stabilize the lung volume may be as high as 25–30 cm H_2O. However, significant changes in lung volume can occur with small changes in Paw. The ventilatory rate is set at 600–900 breaths per minute (10–15 Hz) with an I:E ratio of 1:3 or 1:1, depending upon the device. The amplitude of the oscillations (tidal volume) is adjusted to move the chest.

For nonhomogeneous lung disease such as meconium aspiration or pneumonia, one tries to use a Paw 1–2 cm H_2O less than CMV. The rate, I:E ratio, and amplitude are the same as for homogeneous disease. Because the HFOV oscillations are very small, their effectiveness may be reduced when the airways are full of secretions or meconium.

The approach to air leak syndrome depends on the severity and the predominant underlying pathology. If the lung volumes are low, a modified high lung volume strategy may be used. Rapid weaning is necessary once lung volumes are stabilized. If the air leak is severe, with gas trapping, then a lower lung volume strategy is employed. Risk for gas trapping

increases when the airways are contaminated with debris. Airway collapse may occur if Paw is too low.

Weaning, as with HFJV, has not been well studied. Amplitudes are decreased to minimal levels. Some patients have been directly extubated, but most are returned to low CMV settings.[119]

COMPLICATIONS

Although HFV appears to be efficacious in treating pulmonary air leak and respiratory failure, several serious complications have been reported. Most complications are similar to those seen with CMV and include air leaks, bronchopulmonary dysplasia, and intraventricular hemorrhage. Rates, incidences, and severity vary according to the type of device and the ventilation strategy used.[14,17,49,50] A key factor in the complications seen appears to be the learning curve of the care providers.

Complications can be either "chronic" (such as BPD and IVH) or acute (such as air leak syndromes, impaired cardiac output, or airway damage). Various complications have been attributed to certain machines and ventilation strategies, but few causal relationships have been identified and generalizations are limited. The same ventilator used with different clinical strategies can produce different rates of complications or injury.[12,60,61,118]

AIR LEAKS

Air leaks, including pneumothorax, pneumopericardium, pneumoperitoneum, pneumomediastinum, and pulmonary interstitial emphysema, have been reported in infants being treated with HFV.[14,15,109] Pneumopericardium was reported in 13 percent of infants treated with HFJV in a study done in 1987.[49] Mammel and Boros later speculated that this pneumopericardium rate might have been in part secondary to the suctioning practice used at that time. A more recent study has not found pneumopericardium to be a problem.[15]

The etiology of the air leaks is multifactorial. Two factors that may be of greater importance with HFV than CMV include lung overdistention caused by high P̄aw and inadvertent gas trapping.[14,15,91] The gas trapping may be due to insufficient expiratory time, airway collapse, or inadvertent PEEP.[124] In 1993, it was suggested that the incidence of new air leaks can be reduced by using HFOV with an appropriate strategy and closely monitoring infants with RDS.[58]

BRONCHOPULMONARY DYSPLASIA

BPD occurs in many patients treated with HFV, especially those treated after a prolonged course of CMV. Most studies show no difference in BPD rates between groups of infants treated with HFV and CMV.[50,58] One small study by Clark and associates did show a reduction of BPD in the group treated only with HFV.[54] Again, there may be some developing evidence that early use of HFV may reduce BPD.[56,119] No published data suggest that HFV alters the course of respiratory failure in severe, established BPD.

INTRAVENTRICULAR HEMORRHAGE

This is a multifactorial complication that has been reported at varying rates in infants treated with HFV. Infants with severe IVH were excluded from the early experimental trials. However, there was no increased incidence of IVH in the survivors of rescue therapy.

In 1989, the HIFI study showed a significant increase in severe IVH in the HFOV-treated infants as compared to the CMV infants (26 versus 18 percent). There was also an increase in the incidence of periventricular leukomalacia (12 versus 7 percent).[50] A review of this study focused on how differences among strategies, devices, and centers influenced results.[51] There was speculation that increased impair-

ment of venous return might have resulted in the increase in IVH. This increase was not found in Japan by Ogawa and coworkers, who reported a small, randomized study with IVH rates of 15 percent in HFV-treated subjects and 13 percent for CMV subjects.[125]

In a more recent study involving HFO, there was no significant difference in the incidence of IVH between groups treated with HFO and CMV. But because of methodology issues, the authors concluded that the "association between HFOV and IVH remains open."[59] In the HFJV study of PIE, there was no significant difference in IVH rates between CMV and HFJV groups, but there was a trend toward a lower incidence in the HFJV group.[58] This is countered by the more recent experience of Wiswell and associates who had an increased incidence of IVH with HFJV usage.[57]

CARDIAC IMPAIRMENT/HYPOTENSION

High-frequency ventilation can cause impaired hemodynamics.[114,126] This complication is most commonly seen when lung overdistention occurs; therefore, using strategies that avoid lung overdistention will avoid significant cardiac impairment.[116,127]

Hypotension occurs in many infants treated with HFV, and this may be related to primary pathology, cardiac impairment, or hyperventilation. Therapy is focused on avoiding or correcting the underlying cause and providing supportive care such as volume infusion and inotropic support. If no improvement occurs and the cardiac impairment remains severe, the ventilatory strategy or even the device may have to be changed.

AIRWAY DAMAGE

Airway damage can occur in any infant treated with mechanical ventilation.[118,128–130] Airway damage spans a wide spectrum, but most attention has been focused on necrotizing tracheobronchitis, a condition of acute inflammation, extensive hemorrhage, tissue necrosis, erosion of tracheal epithelium, increased thick secretions, and mucus plugging.[118,128–130] Necrotic debris can slough off the trachea and, together with the thick secretions, lead to total or partial airway obstruction. This may require emergency intervention such as bronchoscopy to remove airway debris.[130,131]

The cause of necrotizing tracheobronchitis is most likely multifactorial.[15] Lack of proper humidification of respiratory gases is considered an important etiologic factor.[128,129] Early models of HFV systems, especially HFJV, provided humidification of respiratory gases by a variety of methods, both singly and in combination. Current models provide extensive humidity, to the point of "rain out" in some cases.

Direct trauma has also been suggested as a factor for the etiology of necrotizing tracheobronchitis.[118] This trauma may be due to a strategy of high Pāw being provided in an uninterrupted pattern or to direct shear forces.[132] Therapy is aimed at early recognition and minimizing trauma and airway intervention. Bronchoscopy may be necessary for diagnosis and to clear the airway.

The incidence of necrotizing tracheobronchitis seems to have decreased, but it may occur on either a microscopic or clinical level in 2–4 percent of patients on HFV.[133] A 1995 report by Nicklaus suggested that follow-up for airway injury should continue even after discharge. Manifestation of the injury (webs and scars) may not become symptomatic until years after therapy.[134]

Mucostasis has also been reported in some patients on HFV.[17] This usually occurs in infants with some pre-existing lung injury and may be facilitated by either the small tidal volumes employed or direct pressure. If plugging becomes severe, the infant may have to be removed from HFV. However, for other infants,

it appears that HFV—especially HFJV—facilitates secretion removal.

Reactive airway disease may also be part of the airway damage spectrum.[21] Characterized by severe bronchospasm, this process probably results from irritation of the airways during ventilation—especially in the presence of infection.

MECHANICAL PROBLEMS

As with all devices, mechanical failures or problems can occur. The ventilators used for HFV have evolved from crude devices to sophisticated, highly technical machines with many built-in safeguards. Proper connection of pressure-monitoring devices as well as an accurate understanding of alarm states are imperative if application of high airway pressure to the patient is to be avoided.

Use of HFV may expose the patient to certain undefined risks such as silicone debris from the ventilator circuit.[135] Proper patient positioning is necessary to avoid risk of water intoxication from either the humidifier or breathing circuits. However, prolonged placement in any one position may lead to skin breakdown, especially in the occipital area.[136]

As with all methods of mechanical ventilation, HFV has adverse side effects and complications. These complications must be closely monitored and reported as use of these devices increases. Careful analysis of benefits versus risks is required prior to widespread usage of any treatment modality.

NURSING CARE

Nursing care of infants during HFV therapy is based on the nursing process and general standards of neonatal nursing and has evolved over the last 15 years.[137] Initially, care was based on brief experiences with a limited number of patients.[19,20,138–140] Now, care is based on larger and larger numbers of patient contacts for longer time periods.[21–23,141–144]

TABLE 13-3 ▲ Assessment of Chest Vibrations

Lack of or decreased chest wall motion can be caused by:
    Plugged, dislodged, or malpositioned ET tube
    Massive pneumothorax
    Machine failure or gas leak
    Not enough PIP or amplitude
    Gas trapping
Excessive chest wall motion can be caused by:
    Excessive PIP or amplitude
    Improved compliance
    Machine failure

Most patients receiving HFV are critically ill, though there is now increased use of HFV in less acutely ill infants. Many patients treated with HFV are subjects in one or more research studies and may receive other highly technical treatments such as ECMO or experimental therapies such as nitric oxide. The clinical course is often one of worsening lung disease reflected by deteriorating blood gas values and chest x-ray films. Frequently, extensive air leak syndrome has developed or worsened. These complex patients require the adaptation, revision, and evaluation of various aspects of nursing practice to integrate HFV technology into bedside care.

ASSESSMENT

Assessment of patients on HFV is frequent and extensive, consisting mainly of inspection, auscultation, and palpation. Although the basic nursing methods for gathering data remain unchanged, the interpretation of the information is affected by HFV technology. Assessment is also influenced by underlying disease state and drug usage.

Respiratory System

Assessment of the respiratory system is dramatically affected by HFV. The high breath rates and small tidal volume of each cycle cause significant chest vibration. The amount of chest movement is directly related to the size or amplitude of the cycle and makes counting total respiratory rates impractical.

During normal ventilator operation, the vibrations are continuous, except when some type of sustained inflation is given. During HFJV, the chest vibrations will be interrupted when the CMV PIP or the infant's spontaneous breaths exceed the HFJV PIP. These pauses are very short and have no obvious adverse effect on most infants.

It is important to constantly monitor the amount of vibration because it appears to be related to tidal volume delivery. As HFOV amplitude or HFJV PIP is reduced, the amplitude of the vibrations decreases. Lack of vibration is usually due to too small a tidal volume or airway obstruction and may precede an acute deterioration (Table 13-3). The status of chest vibration is assessed formally every 30 minutes and informally whenever the patient is observed.

Spontaneous respirations can occur provided the infant is not hypocapnic or receiving paralytic agents. These breaths are best assessed by inspection for retractions and other signs of distress. Spontaneous aeration is usually not heard until marked improvement in pulmonary compliance occurs.

The breath sounds created by HFV have a loud "jack hammer rumbling" quality with a high-pitched tone. Different than traditional breath sounds, these provide much information, especially when monitored over time. Decreased tone of these sounds may indicate poor ventilation or pneumothorax. Higher-pitched tones, especially those of musical quality, seem to indicate mucus secretions, plugs, or bronchospasm. Decreasing or absent breath sounds may indicate airway obstruction, especially when accompanied by very small amplitude cycles.

The patient should be assessed frequently for the presence of air leaks. Changes in the air leak rate or occurrence of new leaks will alter therapeutic plans. Constant vigilance for new air leaks, especially pneumopericardium, is vital.

Although it is unclear if pneumopericardium is more frequent with HFV than CMV, it does occur. In situations of acute deterioration, especially with cardiovascular compromise, pneumopericardium must be considered.

Assessment of tracheal secretions is very important during HFV. Changes in tracheal secretion consistency and color may be the first warning signs of developing necrotizing tracheobronchitis or nosocomial pneumonia.

Cardiovascular System

Most infants requiring HFV therapy have concomitant cardiovascular compromise. This may be secondary to the underlying disease state, therapeutic maneuvers, or lung overinflation. Pulmonary hypertension and poor left ventricular output are the most common alterations seen. The high lung volumes and/or high mean airway pressures required to support these infants may hamper venous return and impair cardiac output. Accumulation of extraventilatory air may also hamper venous return and subsequent cardiac output. Cardiovascular assessment utilizes auscultation, inspection, and palpation as well as other information such as urine output and acid-base status.

Physical assessment of the cardiovascular system is hampered by the inability to hear heart sounds during HFV operation. Murmurs usually cannot be heard unless they are very loud, and pulse rate cannot be counted unless the ventilator is on standby or disconnected. Evaluation for murmurs may require a temporary pause in HFV therapy. Ability to locate the point of maximal impulse (PMI) is greatly limited by the chest vibration, except in infants with an extremely active precordium. The PMI is usually seen in the subxiphoid area. Assessment of peripheral pulses is hampered by the total body vibration. The more peripheral pulses (radial and posterior tibial) are less affected than the central pulses (femoral and brachial) because of the distance from the vibrating thorax.

During HFV operation, electrocardiogram and vascular pressure waveforms can show movement artifact. The degree of artifact appears to depend upon the vigor of the body movement, pulmonary compliance, and transducer sensitivity. The central venous pressure waveform is the most affected, with intrathoracic pressure fluctuations readily visible. Despite motion artifact, the pressure value seems valid and useful.

Other Systems

Assessment of the gastrointestinal tract is influenced by the body vibrations and noise produced during HFV. Gross assessment can be performed, but fine assessments, such as bowel sound and liver evaluation, can be difficult. Abdominal distention and tenderness can still be determined, and stooling is not impaired. Tolerance of feedings can be monitored as with CMV.

The genitourinary system is not affected by HFV. The use of paralytic and sedative agents in these infants will necessitate frequent evaluation for urinary retention.

Assessment for alterations in skin integrity should be done frequently. In Primary Children's Medical Center's (PCMC) experience, the body vibration does not seem to increase the incidence of skin breakdown. In fact, the movement may help reduce impairment in those infants who are paralyzed.

Assessment of the neurologic status depends more upon the severity of the underlying disease state, any specific complications, and pharmacotherapy than it does on HFV therapy. Some infants are obtunded; others are active and alert. With adequate ventilation and oxygenation, infants do not appear distressed while on HFV. Behavioral signs of distress are interpreted in their usual context. Developmental states and signs can also be assessed. Seizure activity can be observed. Fontanel, tone, and basic reflexes can be assessed within limitations of patient status.

Equipment and Monitoring Needs

Because patients receiving HFV are generally critically ill, constant assessment of vital signs and blood gas values is necessary. The noise and vibration produced by HFV precludes many normal assessment activities: Heart sounds cannot be heard, so continuous heart rate monitoring is vital. At PCMC, the nurses find it useful to employ a monitor that can determine the heart rate from both the QRS complex and the arterial waveform. Chest movement artifact may alter EKG waveform, depending on electrode placement.

Continuous blood gas monitoring is required as with any critically ill child. Carbon dioxide monitoring is mandatory because HFV may alter the blood levels significantly in a very short period of time. Oxygen saturation and PO_2 monitors (internal or transcutaneous) can be used to assess the patient's oxygenation status. Bedside pulmonary mechanics monitoring is increasing.

For patient safety, the nurse must be familiar with the HFV monitoring device displays and alarms. As new ventilators or new models of previously used devices are introduced, the bedside nurse must be kept up to date with new operating and troubleshooting procedures. Failure to do so may put the patient at increased risk for harm. Physiologic and patient parameters to monitor include but are not limited to:

- Arterial blood gases
- Oxygen saturation
- Transcutaneous CO_2 and O_2
- Central venous pressure
- Heart rate
- Respiratory rate
- Blood pressure
- Temperature
- Pulmonary function tests
- Specific ventilator parameters

Nursing Diagnosis and Goals

Nursing diagnoses are derived from the information obtained during the patient assessment. General diagnoses such as altered respiratory gas exchange are adapted to reflect HFV usage.

One example is the diagnosis of "potential for airway obstruction." Although airway obstruction can occur with any form of mechanical ventilation, the use of HFV may increase the potential for mucostasis or necrotizing tracheobronchitis. The use of very small tidal volumes, especially with HFOV, may limit the ability of the ventilator to clear small amounts of secretions from the endotracheal tube. Also suctioning is limited in the early stages of therapy for many disease states because suctioning may reduce lung volumes. All these factors increase the potential for airway obstruction. If airway obstruction is severe, the infant may need to have HFV amplitude increased or background rate adjusted (if applicable) or be returned to CMV.

Patient care goals are derived from the nursing diagnosis. Nursing care can be focused by the use of adapted nursing diagnoses that reflect the influence of new technology. Both short- and long-term goals are developed, including goals to provide a supportive, developmentally sound, and safe environment that facilitates recovery. Goals may direct the gathering and interpreting of data, so interventions can be timely and complications avoided.

Interventions

Nursing care interventions are individualized according to acuity and patient need. Many general nursing interventions are similar to those for infants requiring CMV (see Chapter 7).

Certain interventions are the result of the HFV technology and are device dependent. For infants receiving HFJV therapy, the first nursing activity is assistance with the placement of the special triple-lumen jet endotracheal tube. This procedure can place

TABLE 13-4 ▲ **Selected Nursing Interventions**[21,23,143]

Intervention	HFJV	HFOV
Endotracheal suctioning	• Can perform with HFJV on or off. When HFJV off, procedure is similar to that with CMV. When HFJV is on, normal saline irrigant is instilled down the green "jet" tube. • Place suction catheter down main tube with continuous suction applied. • Avoid manual bagging. • Adjust HFJV or CMV setting to facilitate recovery.	• Perform with HFOV off. • Avoid procedure as much as possible to limit disconnection from HFOV. Actual procedure similar to CMV. • Avoid hand bagging. • Increase $\overline{Paw}$ if needed to facilitate recovery.
Positioning	• Patient can be placed in all positions. Limited by short, but flexible, length of "jet" tubing to patient box. • Patient box sits next to head. • Patient can be moved while connected to HFJV. • Patient can be held by parents to facilitate bonding.	• Generally no position changes during first 48 hours requiring disconnection of HFOV. • Changes while on HFOV limited by rigid tubing that delivers bias flow. Head to toe movement on either a horizontal or vertical axis can be employed. • Patient can be held by parents. • Infant must always remain elevated above the rigid tubing to prevent aspiration of condensed water from circuit humidity. • Side cuts may be placed in sidewalls of radiant warmer to facilitate positioning.

additional stress on an already compromised patient. Taping the jet tube in place correctly is of greater significance than with conventional tubes. The green jet line is placed facing anterior (the lower lip). This puts the bevel of the jet tube in a left oblique position, which seems to facilitate ventilation. The intubation procedure often necessitates a chest radiograph to document placement. This will not be necessary for patients using the "jet nozzle" adapter.

For HFOV, no change in the endotracheal tube is required to initiate therapy; however, a change to a different sized tube can dramatically affect the tidal volume delivered for any given amplitude. The use of HFV can require modification of both suctioning and positioning procedures.[23,136,144–146] Table 13-4 discusses these selected nursing interventions.

Patient response to ventilator changes on HFV is somewhat unpredictable. As previously discussed, oxygenation is related to mean airway pressure and normal lung volumes, and ventilation is related to tidal volume (or amplitude/*delta*

p). Frequent blood gas analysis is required during the initiation of therapy, weaning after normal lung volumes are established, and periods of instability. Chest films may also be taken as often as every four to six hours during these periods. Currently, chest films are the most common means of evaluating lung volumes.

Alteration in ventilator settings usually takes many factors into consideration. A team approach with frequent consultation is needed. Because much of the care for these infants is based on anecdote and experience, tremendous flexibility in treatment plans is necessary.

PLAN EVALUATION AND REVISION

Evaluation of nursing care occurs frequently because of the complexity of these patients. The process is ongoing, providing feedback into the various steps of the nursing process. Most of the evaluation activities occur on an informal level at the bedside among the staff nurse, primary care provider, attending physician, and family.

Evaluation must also occur on a formal level. Various mechanisms utilized to accomplish this can include but are not limited to (1) formal nursing care rounds, (2) patient care conferences, and (3) quality assessment meetings. In these conferences and meetings, parents and medical, social service, clergy, and nursing staff, as well as other family members and support people (where appropriate), review the case or pertinent issues. The information and decisions from these conferences are then integrated into the daily nursing care plan.

The steps of the nursing process require that the information obtained, goals established, interventions performed, and evaluations conducted be analyzed to provide the basis for revision of the care plan. Revision is required frequently because of the limited ability to predict responses to HFV and occurs as the patient's condition progresses or deteriorates.

Because most infants on HFV now survive, the degree of residual chronic lung disease will be a prime factor in the planning of future care. If the chronic lung disease is severe or air leaks persist, prolonged HFV may be required. If improvement does not occur, then planning must be made for either the use of alternate technology (such as ECMO) or care of the infant and family during the terminal portion of hospitalization. Usually, death is due to progressive respiratory failure. The terminal period may be prolonged by the ability of HFV to support ventilation in infants with very diseased lungs.

PARENT CARE

The nursing process is applied not only to the infant undergoing HFV but also to the parent(s). The emotional stress of parents is very great when an infant is sick at birth. The prospect of placing their baby on HFV may increase that stress. Not only are these infants generally extremely ill, but they are receiving a nonstandard, and at times experimental, therapy to which their responses can be unpredictable. This may create additional stress for the parent. High-frequency ventilation technology is offered often in hopes of rescuing the child who has not responded to CMV and surfactant. Yet for some extremely ill infants, such as those with pulmonary hypoplasia, this may only delay death.

The HFV technology and the parent's level of stress require additional nursing care for family education and support. Parents are encouraged to participate in care as much as is feasible. This is especially true with long-term use of HFV. Infants on HFV can be held, though provisions need to be made for the additional equipment and special positioning requirements. For the infant who is terminally ill, ongoing assessment of the infant and family and frequent, open communication with the family can help to ensure appropriate support during this difficult period. The families of all patients undergoing HFV therapy should be provided social service support.

ADMINISTRATIVE AND PROFESSIONAL ISSUES

The introduction of HFV technology affects the management of the intensive care unit especially in the areas of personnel and capital costs. Staffing requirements are increased in order to provide adequate patient coverage. Nursing hours per patient day increase as the acuity of the patient population increases. Additional education time is often required to orient the staff to HFV technology. This is especially true in units that use the technology only on an infrequent basis. Especially with infrequent usage or new usage, HFV technology may increase job stress.

Capital costs and bedside physical space requirements may increase. Additional ventilators and related equipment, such as blenders and carts, must be purchased. Costs per ventilator can be in the $20,000 range. Debate about how many and which type of machines need to be purchased frequently occurs.

The HFV technology can also be a revenue source, depending upon the reimbursement mechanism for the patient. Patient referral population may increase, but this is less an issue now as more and more units have HFV devices. Debate about when to transfer a patient failing HFV technology to a unit that has ECMO or nitric oxide capabilities may occur.

High-frequency technology can also be a marketing tool for both patient and staff recruitment. And, although HFV provides an additional means to save infants who were going to die, there may be a social and emotional cost. Certain infants who eventually will die are supported for longer periods than is possible with CMV. Ethical issues regarding appropriate patient selection and resource utilization further increase the stress inherent in the care of critically ill infants.

Another source of stress is the use of a machine that can be unpredictable in terms of patient response and action—especially to those with limited experience. There is always some degree of mistrust for anything new or different. The bedside nurse must be prepared to return the infant to CMV at a moment's notice. Improvements in machine reliability and device refinements have greatly reduced, but not eliminated, this source of stress. Additional stress on nursing and other personnel can be caused by more documentation, education, patient assignment changes, and additional staffing resource requirements. Even the care environment is affected by HFV. In general, noise level in many nurseries is significantly increased.

There are also many positive influences brought about by the introduction and utilization of HFV technology. Outcome for many infants appears to be improved. Nursing has been given an opportunity to broaden its theoretical basis for care. New concepts of physiology are learned and old ones evaluated. New methods of responding to crises are now available, and the nurse plays an integral collaborative role in the therapy.

Unit-based research has been influenced and affected by HFV technology. Nursing participation has occurred in many of the research projects. Involvement in medical research seems to have fostered interest in nursing research. Experience with the introduction of HFV technology can also help pave the way for the introduction of other technologies such as ECMO and nitric oxide therapy. The involvement in rescue therapy, early therapy, research, education, and the evolution of nursing practice seems to have made a positive impact on job satisfaction.

SUMMARY

High-frequency ventilation is now a more than 16-year-old "new" technology. It has been shown to be useful for rescue ventilation with infants suffering severe respiratory failure and possibly useful as an early therapeutic device for infants not responding to CMV.

As with many technologies, HFV has had a considerable influence on our nursing care. It has required evaluation, adaptation, and increased collaboration of our patient care and unit management practices. Our nursing care approach continues to evolve. This evolution is hampered by a continued lack of nursing research to support many of our assertions. For this, nurses take responsibility and are even more committed to validate our care through nursing research.

So where does this leave us? There are many questions about the future:

- Will HFV devices become the "standard" ventilators used on all infants?
- How will the devices themselves change?
- What ventilation strategy will we use and when?
- Can HFV therapy prevent lung injury and BPD?

- What will be the "real" effect of HFV on IVH?[147]
- What will be the effect of HFV in combination with other therapies such as surfactant replacement therapy, synchronized intermittent mandatory ventilation, nitric oxide, ECMO, or liquid ventilation?
- What is the role of HFV during patient transport?[148]
- What about use in older patients?
- How will nursing care evolve in response to HFV?
- Where do families fit in?

Our current and future challenge is to answer these and other questions in a collaborative, multidisciplinary fashion based on research and enhanced by our art of caring.

REFERENCES

1. Hodson WA, and Truog WE. 1994. Principles of management of respiratory problems. 1994. In *Neonatology: Pathophysiology and Management of the Newborn*, 4th ed., Avery GB, Fletcher MA, and MacDonald MG, eds. Philadelphia: JB Lippincott, 478–503.

2. Carlo WA, Martin RJ, and Fanaroff AV. 1992. Assisted ventilation and complications of respiratory distress. In *Neonatal-Perinatal Medicine: Diseases of the Fetus and Infant*, 5th ed., Fanaroff AA, and Martin RJ, eds. St. Louis: Mosby-Year Book, 820–834.

3. Long W, ed. 1993. *Clinics in Perinatology: Surfactant Replacement Therapy*. Philadelphia: WB Saunders, 696–831.

4. Northway WH, Rosen RC, and Porter DY. 1967. Pulmonary disease following respirator therapy of hyaline membrane disease. *New England Journal of Medicine* 276(7): 357–368.

5. Avery ME, et al. 1987. Is chronic lung disease in low birth weight infants preventable? A survey of eight centers. *Pediatrics* 79(1): 26–30.

6. Mandansky DL, et al. 1979. Pneumothorax and other forms of pulmonary air leak in newborns. *American Review of Respiratory Disease* 120(4): 729–737.

7. Holtzman RB, and Frank L, eds. 1992. *Clinics in Perinatology: Bronchopulmonary Dysplasia*. Philadelphia: WB Saunders, 485–695.

8. Abman SH, and Groothius JR. 1994. Pathophysiology and treatment of bronchopulmonary dysplasia: Current issues. *Pediatric Clinics of North America* 41(2): 277–315.

9. National Institute of Health, Division of Lung Disease, National Heart, Lung, and Blood Institute. 1979. Workshop on bronchopulmonary dysplasia. *Journal of Pediatrics* 95(5 part 2): 815–819.

10. Bancalari E, and Goldberg RN. 1987. High-frequency ventilation in the neonate. *Clinics in Perinatology* 14(3): 581–597.

11. Parker JC, Hernandez LA, and Peevy KJ. 1993. Mechanisms of ventilator induced lung injury. *Critical Care Medicine* 21(1): 131–143.

12. Gerstmann DR, deLemos RA, and Clark RH. 1991. High frequency ventilation: Issues of strategy. *Clinics in Perinatology* 18(3): 563–580.

13. Truog WE, and Jackson JC. 1992. Alternative modes of ventilation in the prevention and treatment of bronchopulmonary dysplasia. *Clinics in Perinatology* 19(3): 621–648.

14. Clark R. 1994. High-frequency ventilation. *Journal of Pediatrics* 5(1): 661–670.

15. Mammel M, and Boros S. 1996. High frequency ventilation. In *Assisted Ventilation of the Neonate: Principles of Mechanical Ventilation*, 3rd ed., Goldsmith JP, and Karotkin EH, eds. Philadelphia: WB Saunders, 199–214.

16. Harris TR, and Bunnell JB. 1993. High-frequency jet ventilation in clinical neonatology. In *Neonatology for the Clinician*, Pomerance JJ, and Richardson CJ, eds. Norwalk, Connecticut: Appleton & Lange, 311–323.

17. Clark RH, and Null DM. 1993. High-frequency oscillatory ventilation. In *Neonatology for the Clinician*, Pomerance JJ, and Richardson CJ, eds. Norwalk, Connecticut: Appleton & Lange, 289–309.

18. Myrer ML. 1992. New trends in neonatal mechanical ventilation. *Critical Care Nursing Clinics of North America* 4(3): 507–513.

19. Karp TB, et al. 1986. High frequency jet ventilation: A neonatal nursing perspective. *Neonatal Network* 4(5): 42–50.

20. Inwood S, Finley GA, and Fitzhardinge PM. 1986. High-frequency oscillation: A new mode of ventilation for the neonate. *Neonatal Network* 4(5): 53–58.

21. Karp T. 1991. High-frequency jet ventilation. In *Acute Respiratory Care of the Newborn*, Nugent J, ed. Petaluma California: NICU INK, 147–170.

22. Haney C, and Allingham TM. 1992. Nursing care of the neonate receiving high frequency jet ventilation. *Journal of Obstetric, Gynecologic, and Neonatal Nursing* 21(3): 187–195.

23. Avila K, Mazza LV, and Morgan-Trujillo L. 1994. High-frequency oscillatory ventilation: A nursing approach to bedside care. *Neonatal Network* 13(5): 23–30.

24. Slutsky AS, et al. 1981. High frequency ventilation: A promising new approach to mechanical ventilation. *Medical Instrumentation* 15(2): 229–233.

25. Bunnell B. 1990. High frequency ventilation of infants. In *Current Perinatology*, vol. 2, Rathi M, ed. New York: Springer-Verlag, 173–201.

26. Randel R. 1993. High frequency ventilation. Presented at the ninth annual meeting of the National Association of Neonatal Nurses, Orlando, Florida.

27. Wetzel RC, and Gioia FR. 1987. High frequency ventilation. *Pediatric Clinics of North America* 34(1): 15–38.

28. 1983. Special conference report: High frequency ventilation for immature infants. *Pediatrics* 71(2): 280–287.

29. Henderson Y, Chillingworth FP, and Whitney JL. 1915. The respiratory dead space. *American Journal of Physiology* 38(1): 1–19.

30. Brisco WR, Foster RE, and Comroe J Jr. 1954. Alveolar ventilation at very low tidal volumes. *Pediatric Research* 7(7): 27–30.

31. Emerson JH. 1959. Apparatus for vibrating portions of a patient's airway. U.S. patent no. 2,918,917.

32. Lunkenheimer PP, et al. 1972. Application of transtracheal pressure oscillations as a modification of "diffusion" respiration. *British Journal of Anaesthesia* 44(6): 627–631.

33. Klain M, and Smith RB. 1977. High frequency percutaneous transtracheal jet ventilation. *Critical Care Medicine* 5(6): 280–287.

34. Sjostrand U. 1980. High frequency positive pressure ventilation (HFPPV), a review. *Critical Care Medicine* 8(6): 345–364.

35. Butler WJ, et al. 1980. Ventilation by high frequency oscillation in humans. *Anesthesia and Analgesia* 59(8): 577–584.

36. Carlon GC, et al. 1981. Clinical experience with high frequency jet ventilation. *Critical Care Medicine* 9(1): 1–6.

37. Marchak BE, et al. 1981. Treatment of RDS by high-frequency oscillatory ventilation: A preliminary report. *Journal of Pediatrics* 99(2): 287–292.

38. Pokora T, et al. 1983. Neonatal high frequency jet ventilation. *Pediatrics* 72(1): 27–32.

39. Harris TR, and Christensen RD. 1984. High frequency jet ventilation of pulmonary interstitial emphysema. *Pediatric Research* 18(4): 326A.

40. Ackerman NB Jr, et al. 1984. Pulmonary interstitial emphysema in the premature baboon with hyaline membrane disease. *Critical Care Medicine* 12(6): 512–516.

41. Carlo WA, et al. 1984. Decrease in airway pressure during high-frequency jet ventilation in infants with respiratory distress syndrome. *Journal of Pediatrics* 104(1): 101–107.

42. Frantz I, Werthammer J, and Stark A. 1983. High frequency ventilation in premature infants with lung disease: Adequate gas exchange at low tracheal pressure. *Pediatrics* 71(4): 483–488.

43. Pauly TH, et al. 1987. Predictability of success of high-frequency jet ventilation in infants with persistent pulmonary hypertension. Ross Special Conference in Neonatology: Two Great Debates (program syllabus), 172A.

44. Carlo WA, et al. 1989. High frequency jet ventilation in neonatal pulmonary hypertension. *American Journal of Diseases of Children* 143(2): 233–238.

45. Kohelet D, et al. 1988. High frequency oscillation in the rescue of infants with persistent pulmonary hypertension. *Critical Care Medicine* 16(5): 510–516.

46. Carter J, et al. 1990. High frequency oscillatory ventilation and extracorporeal membrane oxygenation for the treatment of acute neonatal respiratory failure. *Pediatrics* 85(1): 159–164.

47. Gonzalez F, et al. 1986. Decreased gas flow through pneumothoraces in neonates receiving high-frequency jet ventilation versus conventional ventilation. *Journal of Pediatrics* 110(3): 464–466.

48. Clark RH, et al. 1986. Pulmonary interstitial emphysema treated by high frequency oscillatory ventilation. *Critical Care Medicine* 14(11): 926–930.

49. Mammel MC, et al. 1987. High frequency jet ventilation: The Children's Hospital of St. Paul experience and viewpoint. Ross Special Conference in Neonatology: Two Great Debates (program syllabus), 181–182.

50. High-Frequency Oscillatory Ventilation Study Group. 1989. High-frequency oscillatory ventilation compared with conventional mechanical ventilation in the treatment of respiratory failure in premature infants. *New England Journal of Medicine* 320(2): 88–93.

51. Bryan AC, and Froese AB. 1991. Reflections on the HIFI trial. *Pediatrics* 87(4): 565–567.

52. Spitzer AR, Butler S, and Fox WW. 1989. Ventilatory response to combined high frequency jet ventilation and conventional mechanical ventilation for rescue treatment of severe lung disease. *Pediatric Pulmonology* 7(4): 244–250.

53. Carlo WA, et al. 1990. Early randomized intervention with high frequency ventilation in respiratory distress syndrome. *Journal of Pediatrics* 117(5): 765–770.

54. Clark RH, et al. 1992. Prospective randomized comparison of high frequency oscillatory and conventional ventilation in respiratory distress syndrome. *Pediatrics* 89(1): 5–12.

55. Patel CA, and Klein JM. 1995. Outcome of infants with birth weights less than 1,000 g with respiratory distress syndrome treated with high-frequency ventilation and surfactant replacement therapy. *Archives of Pediatric and Adolescent Medicine* 149(3): 317–321.

56. Gerstmann DR, et al. 1996. The Provo multicenter early high-frequency oscillatory ventilation trial: Improved pulmonary and clinical outcome in respiratory distress syndrome. *Pediatrics* 98(6 part 6): 1044–1057.

57. Wiswell TE, et al. 1996. High-frequency jet ventilation in the early management of respiratory distress syndrome is associated with a greater risk for adverse outcomes. *Pediatrics* 98(6 part 1) 1035–1043.

58. Keszler M, et al. 1991. Multi-center controlled trial comparing high-frequency jet ventilation and conventional mechanical ventilation in newborn infants with pulmonary interstitial emphysema. *Journal of Pediatrics* 119(1): 85–93.

59. HiFO Study Group. 1993. Randomized study of high-frequency oscillatory ventilation in infants with severe respiratory distress syndrome. *Journal of Pediatrics* 122(4): 609–619.

60. Bodenstein CJ, et al. 1987. VDR-1 programmable high-frequency ventilation in severe neonatal respiratory failure. Ross Special Conference in Neonatology: Two Great Debates (program syllabus), 181–182.

61. Gaylord MS, Quissell BJ, and Lair ME. 1987. High frequency ventilation in the treatment of infants weighing less than 1,500 grams with pulmonary interstitial emphysema: A pilot study. *Pediatrics* 79(6): 915–921.

62. Pardou A, et al. 1993. High frequency ventilation and conventional mechanical ventilation in newborn babies with respiratory distress syndrome: A prospective, randomized trial. *Intensive Care Medicine* 19(7): 406–410.

63. Schur MS, et al. 1988. High-frequency jet ventilation in the management of congenital tracheal stenosis. *Anesthesiology* 68(6): 952–955.

64. Donn SM, et al. 1990. Use of high-frequency jet ventilation in the management of congenital tracheoesophageal fistula associated with respiratory distress syndrome. *Journal of Pediatric Surgery* 25(12): 1219–1221.

65. Davis DA, et al. 1994. High-frequency jet versus conventional ventilation in infants undergoing Blalock-Taussig shunts. *Annals of Thoracic Surgery* 57(4): 846–849.

66. Meliones JN, et al. 1991. High-frequency jet ventilation improves cardiac function after the Fontan procedure. *Circulation* 84(5 supplement): 364–368.

67. Harris TR, et al. 1984. High frequency jet ventilation treatment of neonates with congenital left diaphragmatic hernia. *Clinical Research* 32(2): 123A.

68. Bohn D, Tamura M, and Bryan C. 1984. Respiratory failure in congenital diaphragmatic hernia: Ventilation by high frequency oscillation. *Pediatric Research* 18(4): 387A.

69. Boros SJ, et al. 1985. Neonatal high frequency ventilation: A four year experience. *Pediatrics* 75(4): 657–663.

70. Stoddard R, et al. 1993. Treatment of congenital diaphragmatic hernia (CDH) with high frequency oscillatory ventilation (HFOV). *Pediatric Pulmonology* 15(6): 367.

71. Miguet D, et al. 1994. Preoperative stabilization using high frequency oscillatory ventilation in the management of congenital diaphragmatic hernia. *Critical Care Medicine* 22(9): S77–S82.

72. Mammel MC, et al. 1983. Comparison of high-frequency jet ventilation and conventional mechanical ventilation in a meconium aspiration model. *Journal of Pediatrics* 103(4): 630–634.

73. Trindale O, et al. 1985. Conventional versus high frequency jet ventilation in a piglet model of meconium aspiration: Comparison of pulmonary and hemodynamic effects. *Journal of Pediatrics* 107(1): 115–120.

74. Keszler M, et al. 1986. Combined high frequency jet ventilation in a meconium aspiration model. *Critical Care Medicine* 14(1): 34–37.

75. Wiswell T, et al. 1994. Surfactant therapy and high frequency jet ventilation in management of a piglet model of meconium aspiration syndrome. *Pediatric Research* 36(4): 494–500.

76. Baumgart S, et al. 1992. Diagnosis-related criteria in consideration of extracorporeal membrane oxygenation in neonates previously treated with high frequency jet ventilation. *Pediatrics* 89(3): 491–494.

77. Varnholt V, et al. 1992. High frequency oscillatory ventilation and extracorporeal membrane oxygenation in severe persistent pulmonary hypertension of the newborn. *European Journal of Pediatrics* 151(10): 769–774.

78. Clark RH, Yoder BA, and Sell MS. 1994. Prospective, randomized comparison of high frequency oscillation and conventional ventilation in candidates for extracorporeal membrane oxygenation. *Journal of Pediatrics* 124(3): 447–454.

79. Paranka MS, et al. 1995. Predictors of failure of high frequency oscillatory ventilation in term infants with severe respiratory failure. *Pediatrics* 95(3): 400–404.

80. Davis J, et al. 1992. High frequency jet ventilation and surfactant treatment of newborns with severe respiratory failure. *Pediatric Pulmonology* 13(1): 108–112.

81. Lynch JM, et al. 1994. Nitric oxide delivery with high frequency jet ventilation. Eleventh Annual Conference on High-Frequency Ventilation of Infants, Snowbird, Utah (abstract and presentation).

82. Wilford L, et al. 1995. Delivery of nitric oxide via a high frequency oscillatory ventilator. Twelfth Annual Conference on High-Frequency Ventilation of Infants, Snowbird, Utah (abstract and presentation).

83. Chang HK. 1984. Mechanisms of gas transport during high frequency ventilation. *Journal of Applied Physiology* 56(3): 553–563.

84. Drazen J, Kamm RD, and Slutsky AS. 1984. High frequency ventilation. *Physiological Review* 64(2): 505–543.

85. Boros SJ. 1979. Variation in inspiratory:expiratory ratio and airway pressure wave form during mechanical ventilation: The significance of mean airway pressure. *Journal of Pediatrics* 94(1): 114–117.

86. Ciszek TA, et al. 1981. Mean airway pressure—significance during mechanical ventilation in neonates. *Journal of Pediatrics* 99(1): 121–126.

87. Jacob J, et al. 1980. The contribution of PDA in the neonate with severe RDS. *Journal of Pediatrics* 96(1): 79–87.

88. Carlo WA, and Martin RJ. 1986. Principles of neonatal assisted ventilation. *Pediatric Clinics of North America* 33(2): 221–237.

89. Cartwright DW, Willis MM, and Gregory GA. 1984. Functional residual capacity and lung mechanics at different levels of mechanical ventilation. *Critical Care Medicine* 12(5): 422–427.

90. Frantz I, and Close RH. 1985. Elevated lung volumes and alveolar pressure during jet ventilation of rabbits. *American Review of Respiratory Disease* 131(1): 134–138.

91. Bancalari A, et al. 1987. Gas trapping with high frequency ventilation: Jet versus oscillatory ventilation. *Journal of Pediatrics* 110(4): 617–622.

92. Chan V, and Greenough A. 1993. Determinants of oxygenation during high frequency oscillation. *European Journal of Pediatrics* 152(4): 350–353.

93. Carlo WA, Chatburn RL, and Martin RJ. 1987. Randomized trial of high-frequency jet ventilation versus conventional ventilation in respiratory distress syndrome. *Journal of Pediatrics* 110(2): 275–282.

94. Gerstmann DR, et al. 1990. Proximal, tracheal and alveolar pressures during high frequency oscillatory ventilation in normal rabbit model. *Pediatric Research* 28(4): 367–373.

95. Korventranta H, et al. 1987. Carbon dioxide elimination during high frequency jet ventilation. *Journal of Pediatrics* 111(1): 107–113.

96. Johnston J, et al. 1987. Exhalation time effects on arterial and venous blood oxygen content and arterial PCO_2 during high frequency jet ventilation of surfactant depleted cats. *Pediatric Pulmonology* 3(1): 19–23.

97. Smith DW, Frankel LR, and Ariagno RL. 1987. Influences of ventilator rate and inspiratory time (T_I) on tidal volume (V_T), rate of CO_2 elimination (V_ECO_2) and lung (LV) using the Bunnell Life-Pulse high frequency ventilator. *Pediatric Pulmonology* 3(10): 377A.

98. Slutsky AS, Drazen J, and Kamm RD. 1985. Alveolar ventilation at high frequencies using tidal volumes smaller than anatomical dead space. *Lung Biology in Health and Disease* 25(2): 137–176.

99. Fredberg JJ. 1989. Pulmonary mechanics during high frequency ventilation. *Acta Anaesthesiologica Scandinavica* 90(supplement): 170–171.

100. Chan V, Greenough A, and Milner AD. 1993. The effect of frequency and mean airway pressure on the volume delivery during high frequency oscillation. *Pediatric Pulmonology* 15(3): 183–186.

101. Bohn DJ, et al. 1980. Ventilation by high frequency oscillation. *Journal of Applied Physiology* 48(4): 710–716.

102. Weisberger SA, et al. 1986. Effects of varying inspiratory and expiratory times during high frequency jet ventilation. *Journal of Pediatrics* 108(4): 596–600.

103. Permutt S, Mitzner W, and Weinmonn G. 1985. Model of gas transport during high-frequency ventilation. *Journal of Applied Physiology* 58(6): 1956–1970.

104. Allen JL, et al. 1985. Alveolar pressure magnitude and a synchrony during high-frequency oscillation of excised rabbit lungs. *American Review of Respiratory Disease* 132(2): 343–349.

105. Haselton FR, and Scherer PW. 1980. Bronchial bifurcation of respiratory mass transport. *Science* 208(4): 69–71.

106. Scherer PW, and Haselton FR. 1982. Convective exchange in oscillatory flow through bronchial-tree models. *Journal of Applied Physiology* 53(4): 1023–1033.

107. Taylor GI. 1954. Dispersion of matter in turbulent flow through a pipe. *Proceedings of the Royal Society of London* 223(1155): 446–468.

108. Jaegar MJ, Kursweg UH, and Banner MJ. 1984. Transport of gases in high frequency ventilation. *Critical Care Medicine* 12(9): 708–710.

109. Bunnell B. 1987. *Life-Pulse High Frequency Ventilator Operator's Manual,* revision 9. Salt Lake City, Utah: Bunnell, Inc.

110. Eyal FG, et al. 1986. Comparison of high-frequency negative-pressure oscillation with conventional mechanical ventilation in normal and saline lavaged cats. *Critical Care Medicine* 14(8): 724–729.

111. Perez Fontan JJ, Heldt GP, and Gregory GA. 1986. Mean airway pressure and mean alveolar pressure during high frequency jet ventilation in rabbits. *Journal of Applied Physiology* 61(2): 456–463.

112. Smith DW, Frankel LR, and Ariagno RL. 1988. Dissociation of mean airway pressure and lung volume during high frequency oscillatory ventilation. *Critical Care Medicine* 16(5): 531–535.

113. Venegas JG, and Fredberg JJ. 1994. Understanding the pressure cost of ventilation: Why does high-frequency ventilation work? *Critical Care Medicine* 22(9): S49–S57.

114. Acherman RJ, et al. 1994. Cardiovascular effects of high frequency (HFOV) with optimal lung volume strategy in term infants with adult respiratory distress syndrome (ARDS). Eleventh Annual Conference on High-Frequency Ventilation of Infants, Snowbird, Utah (abstract and presentation).

115. Richards E, and Bunnell B. 1995. Fundamentals of patient management during high frequency jet ventilation. *Neonatal Intensive Care* 8(3): 22–27.

116. Bollinger E, et al. 1996. Nursing care. In *Assisted Ventilation of the Neonate,* 3rd ed., Goldsmith JP, and Karotkin EH, eds. Philadelphia: WB Saunders,125–149.

117. Minton S, et al. 1995. Echocardiography as an important clinical tool for patient care management during HFOV. Twelfth Annual Conference on High-Frequency Ventilation of Infants, Snowbird, Utah (abstract and presentation).

118. Wiswell TE, et al. 1988. Tracheal and bronchial injury in high-frequency oscillatory ventilation and high-frequency flow interruption compared with conventional positive-pressure ventilation. *Pediatrics* 112(2): 249–256.

119. Gertsmann D, et al. 1995. Early high frequency oscillatory ventilation in VLBW neonates: A multicenter retrospective analysis. Twelfth Annual Conference on High-Frequency Ventilation of Infants, Snowbird, Utah (abstract and presentation).

120. Froese AB, et al. 1993. Optimizing alveolar expansion prolongs the effectiveness of exogenous surfactant therapy in adult rabbits. *American Review of Respiratory Disease* 148(3): 569–577.

121. Wood B, Adams A, and Richardson P. 1995. Double port endotracheal tube adapter for high frequency jet ventilation. Twelfth Annual Conference on High-Frequency Ventilation of Infants, Snowbird, Utah (abstract and presentation).

122. Richardson P. 1995. Personal communication concerning the double port E-T adapter.

123. Bunnell B. 1995. Personal communication concerning servo-pressure.

124. Pramanik A, Romero M, and Wissing D. 1987. Inadvertent positive end expiratory pressure (PEEP): A complication of high frequency jet ventilation. *Pediatric Pulmonology* 3(10): 376A.

125. Ogawa Y, et al. 1993. A multicenter randomized trial of high frequency oscillatory ventilation as compared with conventional mechanical ventilation in preterm infants with respiratory failure. *Early Human Development* 32(1): 1–10.

126. Traverse JH, et al. 1988. Impairment of hemodynamics with increasing mean airway pressure during high frequency oscillatory ventilation. *Pediatric Research* 49(1): 21–28.

127. Kinsella JP, et al. 1991. High-frequency oscillatory ventilation versus intermittent mandatory ventilation: Early hemodynamic effects in the premature baboon with hyaline membrane disease. *Pediatric Research* 29(2): 160–166.

128. Ophoven JP, et al. 1984. Tracheobronchial histopathology associated with high frequency jet ventilation. *Critical Care Medicine* 12(9): 829–832.

129. Kirpalani H, et al. 1985. Diagnosis and therapy of necrotizing tracheobronchitis in ventilated neonates. *Critical Care Medicine* 13(10): 792–797.

130. Harris TR, Gooch WM, and Wilson JF. 1984. Necrotizing tracheobronchitis associated with high frequency jet ventilation. *Clinical Research* 32(2): 132A.

131. Pietsch JB, et al. 1985. Necrotizing tracheobronchitis: A new indication for emergency bronchoscopy in the neonate. *Journal of Pediatric Surgery* 20(4): 391–393.

132. Wiswell TE, et al. 1990. Different high frequency strategies: Effect on the propagation of tracheobronchial histopathologic changes. *Pediatrics* 85(1): 70–78.

133. Mammel MC, and Boros SJ. 1987. Airway damage and mechanical ventilation: A review and commentary. *Pediatric Pulmonology* 3(6): 443–447.

134. Nicklaus P. 1995. Airway complications of jet ventilation in neonates. *Annals of Otology, Rhinology, and Laryngology* 104(3): 24–29.

135. Minton S, et al. 1987. Silicone particulate debris in the Life-Pulse high frequency jet ventilator. *Pediatric Pulmonology* 3(10): 375A.

136. Schmidt J, et al. 1995. Skin breakdown with high frequency oscillatory ventilation. Twelfth Annual Conference on High-Frequency Ventilation of Infants, Snowbird, Utah (abstract and presentation).

137. NANN. 1993. *Standards of Care for Neonatal Nursing Practice.* Petaluma, California: National Association of Neonatal Nurses.

138. Warren TE, and Howell C. 1983. High-frequency jet ventilation: A nursing perspective. *Heart and Lung* 12(4): 432–437.

139. Griffin JP, and Carlon GC. 1984. Pulmonary aspects of critical care and rehabilitation. *Heart and Lung* 13(3): 250–254.

140. Loder BJ, Guy Y, and Carlon GC. 1984. Critical care nurse and high-frequency ventilation. *Critical Care Medicine* 12(9): 798–799.

141. Gordin P. 1989. High frequency jet ventilation for severe respiratory failure. *Pediatric Nursing* 15(6): 625–629.

142. White C, Richardson C, and Raibstein L. 1990. High-frequency ventilation and extracorporeal membrane oxygenation. *Clinical Issues in Critical Care Nursing* 1(2): 427–444.

143. Inwood S. 1991. High frequency oscillation. In *Acute Respiratory Care of the Neonate,* Nugent J, ed. Petaluma, California: NICU INK, 171–184.

144. Utah Valley Regional Medical Center. 1992. Care of infants of high frequency ventilation. *NBICU Policy and Procedure Manual.* Provo, Utah.

145. Olson DL, et al. 1986. Policies and procedures: High frequency jet ventilation: Endotracheal suction procedure. *Neonatal Network* 4(5): 66–68.

146. Guntupalli K, Sladen A, and Klain M. 1984. High-frequency jet ventilation and tracheobronchial suctioning. *Critical Care Medicine* 12(9): 791–792.

147. Clark RH, et al. 1996. Intraventricular hemorrhage and high-frequency ventilation: A meta-analysis of prospective clinical trials. *Pediatrics* 98(6 part 1): 1058–1061.

148. Stanley M. 1996. Clinical outcome of high frequency jet ventilation in transport. Thirteenth Annual Conference on High-Frequency Ventilation of Infants, Snowbird, Utah (abstract and presentation).

NOTES

14 Extracorporeal Membrane Oxygenation in the Newborn

Jan Nugent, RNC, MSN, MD
Gerry Matranga, RNC, MN, NNP

Recent advances in technology have challenged clinicians to consider alternative therapies for the 5–10 percent of infants with severe pulmonary dysfunction who respond poorly to maximal conventional ventilatory, medical, and surgical treatment.[1] The past decade has witnessed intense research in the field of high-frequency ventilation and extracorporeal membrane oxygenation (ECMO).[2] In the clinical arena, these new techniques have found application in the care of neonatal respiratory distress.

After current standard therapy has been exhausted, ECMO can provide life-saving cardiopulmonary support in some neonates with predictably fatal pulmonary failure. Nurses caring for these infants need a basic understanding of the principles of ECMO perfusion as well as excellent physical assessment and psychosocial skills. The nurse's ability to provide this sophisticated level of care will have direct and significant impact on the outcome of this mode of therapy.

CONVENTIONAL VENTILATOR THERAPY

Despite significant advances in the care of infants with severe pulmonary dysfunction, respiratory failure remains the most frequent cause of neonatal death. Failure of conventional ventilator therapy accounts for an estimated 15,000 neonatal deaths annually.[3] Contributing respiratory pathology includes respiratory distress syndrome; meconium aspiration syndrome; persistent pulmonary hypertension of the newborn (PPHN), which may occur as a primary entity or as a secondary complication of respiratory failure; and pulmonary hypoplasia associated with congenital diaphragmatic hernia.

Conventional ventilator therapy includes use of 100 percent oxygen, positive pressures, and rapid ventilator rates via a pressure-limited, time-cycled, continuous flow mechanical ventilator. Frequent adjuncts to this therapy are use of inotropic agents (dopamine, dobutamine) to augment systemic circulation, pulmonary vasodilators (tolazoline, prostaglandin E_1) to reduce pulmonary vascular resistance, and sodium bicarbonate to induce alkalosis and dilate pulmonary vasculature.[4–7] Additions to conventional therapy such as exogenous surfactant and nitric oxide have improved the outcome of standard therapy.[8–10]

Unfortunately, the aggressive management required to treat severe pulmonary parenchymal dysfunction and PPHN can contribute significantly to acute parenchymal damage. This can lead to therapeutic failure and death or chronic respiratory disease. An estimated 10 percent of infants who survive the acute stages of their disease may be chronically crippled by bronchopulmonary dysplasia from barotrauma and oxygen toxicity.[11]

A HISTORICAL PERSPECTIVE

"The process of prolonged extracorporeal circulation (cardiopulmonary bypass) achieved by extrathoracic vascular cannulation," ECMO, provides cardiorespiratory support for infants in reversible, profound respiratory or cardiac failure.[11]

Rashkind and associates were the first to report use of neonatal extracorporeal oxygenation via femoral arteriovenous shunt through a bulb oxygenator in 1965.[12] Initial work with a membrane oxygenator was reported by other investigators during the late 1960s and early 1970s.[13–15] There were no survivors reported in these early trials, but the work of these clinicians established the feasibility of ECMO as a treatment modality and demonstrated the need for further refinements in apparatus and technique.

The chief problems the early investigators encountered were fairly daunting. The heart-lung machine required a large blood reservoir, which necessitated complete suppression of coagulation and a large priming volume. The oxygenator, which functioned by direct exposure of blood to oxygen, damaged blood cells and proteins if operated for more than a few hours. The blood pump hemolyzed red cells and caused significant leukopenia. Vascular access was a problem: Umbilical vessels or vessels in the leg were used to gain access to the infant's circulation, but these proved too small to provide extracorporeal flow sufficient for adequate respiratory support.

The final concern was that of coagulation control because extracorporeal therapy required

that the patient be heparinized until coagulation ceased. This practice was safe for only a limited period of time because of the real potential of producing life-threatening hemorrhage when extended over a period of days. No simple laboratory procedure for instantaneous evaluation of clotting time existed. This made accurate titration of systemic anticoagulants impossible.[16]

Medical researchers, lured by the prospect of developing a clinical revolution in cardiopulmonary support, began extensive clinical trials supported by grants from the National Institutes of Health. Kolobow and coworkers began work on the roller pump and membrane lung in 1969, demonstrated the superior blood compatibility of silicone in a membrane lung in 1974, and published data on long-term survivability of lambs perfused up to ten days in 1976.[17–19]

Concurrent clinical work on the technique of extracorporeal circulation via extrathoracic vascular access was begun by Bartlett and coworkers in 1971. They managed their first newborn patient in 1973 and to date have performed more than 100 neonatal ECMO procedures. Of these infants, 45 were reported in the literature in 1982—with a 55 percent survival rate.[20] The years of painstaking research had led to dramatic improvements in machinery and patient management.

Since that time, the survival rate has improved because of extensive experience with the technique, case selection, and earlier intervention. Bartlett and associates determined that ECMO was safe (the risks of the treatment itself were less than the risks of the disease) and effective in trials that included 55 moribund patients treated in three centers over a nine-year period. Of the 40 infants with birth weights of more than 2 kg, 28 (70 percent) survived. Of the 15 infants with birth weights of less than 2 kg, 3 (20 percent) survived.[20–22]

Encouraged by the reported overall survival rate of 56 percent, groups in several major medical centers began to evaluate the use of ECMO in neonates.[3,23] During this phase of clinical research, ECMO was used when all other therapy had failed and the infant was considered moribund. The moribund condition was quantified by objective criteria predictive of high mortality (more than 80 percent), chief of which were the newborn pulmonary insufficiency index and the alveolar-arterial gradient (Table 14-1).[24–26]

Prompted by the successful outcome of this phase of research, Bartlett and associates designed and conducted a prospective, controlled, randomized study. From October 1982 until April 1984, a group of 12 infants with birth weights >2 kg who met 80 percent mortality risk criteria entered the study. One patient was randomly assigned to conventional therapy and died. The 11 patients randomly assigned to ECMO survived.[22]

This study used the "randomized play-the-winner" technique, which assigns an infant to treatment based on the outcome of each previous patient in the study—that is, if one treatment is more successful, more patients are randomly assigned to it. This randomly assigned pattern was to continue until ten patients had been treated with ECMO or ten control patients died.[22] The researchers utilized this methodology to address the scientific/ethical issue of withholding an unproven but potentially lifesaving treatment. Thus some patients were saved from exposure to an inferior treatment. The research of this phase documented that survival is better with ECMO (90 percent) than with conventional ventilation.[22] These results, the small study size, and the statistical method used generated significant controversy.[27,28]

This controversy compelled O'Rourke and associates to design a prospective clinical trial

TABLE 14-1 ▲ Criteria Predictive of Potential Mortality

1. Newborn Pulmonary Insufficiency Index (NPII)
The NPII score is a single-number cumulation of oxygen requirement, acidosis, and time. This score assesses the severity of an infant's respiratory distress in the first day of life. It is calculated by plotting the newborn's FiO_2 and pH on a graph over the first 24 hours of life. The NPII graph has 10 percent FiO_2 increments and one-tenth pH increments on the vertical axis and hourly time increments on the horizontal axis. The score is determined by the number of boxes outlined between the FiO_2 and pH lines when the plotted FiO_2 is greater than the plotted pH on the graph.[38,68] In the past, the NPII was used effectively as a measure of high mortality risk (greater than 80 percent). Since the advent of induced alkalosis as a treatment for PPHN, the NPII has not been applicable.[22,68,69]

2. Alveolar-arterial gradient >620 mmHg for 12 hours
Alveolar-arterial oxygen difference ($AaDO_2$) is a measure of alveolar efficiency in transporting oxygen to pulmonary capillaries. Use of this criterion assumes that the baby is ventilated with 1.0 FiO_2 and that the $PACO_2 = PaCO_2$. The following calculation is used:
$$AaDO_2 = (FiO_2)\ (713) - PaO_2 - PaCO_2$$
The numerical value 713 assumes an atmospheric pressure of 760 mmHg minus vapor pressure (47 mmHg); PaO_2 and $PaCO_2$ are measured by assaying arterial blood gases. Retrospective reviews demonstrate that an $AaDO_2$ >620 for 12 consecutive hours correlates with greater than 80 percent mortality.[25,26,68]

3. Acute deterioration despite optimal therapy: either a PaO_2 <40 mmHg or a pH ≤7.15 for two hours

4. Lack of response to treatment of PPHN. (Two of the following indications for three hours): PaO_2 <55 mmHg; pH <7.4; hypotension

5. Severe barotrauma, with four of the following indications:
    Interstitial emphysema
    Pneumothorax
    Pneumopericardium
    Pneumoperitoneum
    Subcutaneous emphysema
    Persistent air leak for 24 hours
    Mean airway pressure of ≥15 cm H_2O

6. Congenital diaphragmatic hernia with respiratory failure:[22,38,71]
PaO_2 <80 mmHg on FiO_2 >0.8/24 hours after surgery
$PaCO_2$ >40 mmHg (2 hours after surgery) with ventilation index (mean airway pressure × respiratory rate) >1,000 [71]

7. The oxidation index
The oxidation index can be utilized to predict mortality and the incidence of bronchopulmonary dysplasia. The oxygenation index is calculated by dividing the product of the FiO_2 (times 100) and the mean airway pressure by the postductal PaO_2:
$$\frac{Mean\ Airway\ Pressure \times FiO_2 \times 100}{Postductal\ PaO_2}$$
Retrospective data demonstrate that an oxidation index ≥40 correlates with a predicted mortality risk of 80–90 percent; an index ≥25–40 correlates with a 50–60 percent mortality.[11]

Adapted from: Nugent J. 1986. Extracorporeal membrane oxygenation in the neonate. *Neonatal Network* 4(5): 29. Reprinted by permission.

comparing ECMO with conventional mechanical ventilation (CMV). To limit the number of infants assigned to what might ultimately be a less effective therapy, they used an adaptive design with both a randomized and nonrandomized phase. If the therapies were proven to be of equal efficiency, all patients would have been randomized. The mortality rates did differ significantly, and the assignment of patients to CMV was halted after the tenth patient. Enrolled in the study were 39 newborns (weight >3 kg, 39–40 weeks gestation) with severe PPHN and respiratory failure who met 85 percent mortality criteria. The overall survival of ECMO-treated infants was 99 percent (28 of 29), compared with 60 percent (6 of 10) in the CMV group.[29]

To date, the ECMO registry (published by ELSO, Extracorporeal Life Support Organization), which includes data from institutions in the U.S. and abroad, lists more than 11,000 infants treated with ECMO since 1975 and documents an overall survival rate of 80 percent. These statistics include all the early cases at participating medical institutions.[30] Bartlett and colleagues, in a published summary of their group's first 100 cases, validate an overall survival rate of 72 percent.[31] In infants weighing more than 2 kg, the survival rate is 83 percent.[11] In experienced hands, this treatment modality has proven to be an effective life-support system for the very critically ill infant who is greater than 34 weeks gestation.

Bartlett and colleagues completed in 1989 a study that addressed the use of ECMO earlier in the course of the disease, at a time of lower predicted mortality. Neonates who met criteria for 50 percent predicted mortality using an oxygen index (OI) >25 were randomized to either ECMO or CMV. Those in the CMV group either improved or were offered late ECMO after meeting 80 percent predicted mortality. The study evaluated differences in length of hospital stay, length of mechanical ventilation, cost, and patient morbidity among groups receiving early ECMO, late ECMO, and CMV. Preliminary results suggest that the group with the least morbidity went on ECMO early (15 of 20 normal survivors versus 6 of 11 normal survivors in the late ECMO group and 1 of 5 normal survivors in the CMV group that did not receive ECMO). There was no statistical difference in cost.[32]

CRITERIA FOR USE OF ECMO

Extracorporeal membrane oxygenation is an extreme life-support procedure with significant inherent risks. Presently, neonates are considered candidates only if their risk of mortality is estimated at 80 percent or more, despite the use of 100 percent oxygen, high-pressure ventilation, and vasoactive drug therapy.

The ECMO procedure acts as a temporary heart-lung substitute. A neonate's pulmonary or cardiac pathology must be acute and reversible within the one-to-two-week period that it is feasible for ECMO to safely support the infant.[33] Neonatal disorders that may fit this criteria are respiratory distress syndrome, meconium aspiration syndrome, PPHN, congenital diaphragmatic hernia with respiratory failure, pneumonia, and selected cardiac anomalies.

Utilizing ECMO as a mode of therapy places the neonate at risk of life-threatening and serious physiologic and mechanical complications. Selection criteria must identify infants destined to die using conventional care while excluding the hypoxic neonate who would survive without ECMO.

To detect high-risk patients and exclude those with poor prognoses, the patient selection process must have a high degree of predictability and specificity. To achieve this specificity, each neonatal ECMO center must determine its own mortality indicators and criteria.[11]

Final selection is based on objective criteria predictive of greater than 80 percent mortality (see Table 14-1). Currently, the most frequently used criteria are oxygenation index and the alveolar-arterial oxygen gradient ($AaDO_2$).[30] In certain situations, the use of $AaDO_2$ results in either false negative or false positive results. The potential for this error lies in the $AaDO_2$ equation: The arterial carbon dioxide pressure ($PaCO_2$) and the arterial oxygen pressure (PaO_2) are weighted equally; hence it is the sum of these values, and not the individual numbers, that is important. If the sum is high and the resultant $AaDO_2$ is less than 620, the patient does not qualify; if the sum is low and the $AaDO_2$ is greater than 620, the patient does qualify. Infants with a high $PaCO_2$ and low PaO_2 may not qualify (sum is high), or infants with an artificially low $PaCO_2$ may qualify despite acceptable PaO_2 levels (sum is low). Further research is required to enhance specificity. At present, criteria based specifically on PaO_2 may decrease the false negative and false positive results.[33]

In the early stages of the development of such an invasive and inherently risky technique as ECMO, it was appropriate to begin with patients who had failed conventional therapy and were moribund. As more patients survive and the efficacy of this treatment modality is validated, the selection criteria have undergone and will continue to undergo a natural metamorphosis toward earlier intervention.

Contraindications to ECMO include the following:

1. Cyanotic congenital heart disease (uncorrectable anomalies)
2. Irreversible pulmonary damage
3. Any nonreversible condition incompatible with normal quality of life (such as bilateral pulmonary hypoplasia, certain chromosomal abnormalities, or severe neurologic damage)
4. Intracranial hemorrhage (>Grade I)
5. A birth weight <2 kg
6. Gestational age of <35 weeks

Before ECMO is initiated, each candidate has a pediatric cardiology evaluation and cranial ultrasound. An electroencephalogram may be indicated to rule out irreversible neurologic impairment.

In the infant with congenital heart disease (which can mimic PPHN), the treatment of choice would be palliative surgery. An exception would be the infant who, because of cardiovascular crisis, requires stabilization and life support prior to or after cardiac surgery.[34–36] The use of ECMO prior to surgery can potentially improve patient survival and/or eliminate the need for emergency palliative procedures in favor of complete intracardiac repair.[35]

Extracorporeal membrane oxygenation is not usually indicated in neonates who have received more than ten days of mechanical ventilation. Use of this criteria excludes infants with significant iatrogenic lung damage.[37]

An abnormal electroencephalogram, although not in itself a contraindication, will help the pediatric neurologist determine if the infant has irreversible neurologic damage. An electroencephalogram is of particular importance if neurologic assessment is hindered by chemical paralysis.

Intracranial hemorrhage (>Grade I) is a contraindication because the systemic heparinization of ECMO patients significantly increases the risk of extension of the hemorrhage.[37,38] Infants with Grade I intraventricular hemorrhage should be followed with a daily cranial ultrasound and ECMO discontinued in the event of an enlarging hemorrhage.[37]

A birth weight of less than 2 kg or a gestational age of less than 35 weeks is considered a contraindication because the incidence of intracranial hemorrhage occurring during ECMO in this group is significant.

FIGURE 14-1 ▲ Anteroposterior chest film demonstrates correct placement of (1) venous cannula (left arrow) in the right atrium via the right internal jugular vein and (2) the arterial cannula (right arrow) in the aortic arch via the right common carotid artery.

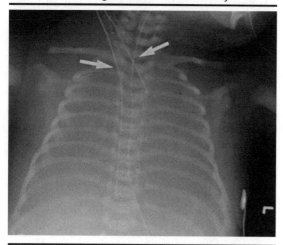

From: Nugent J. 1986. Extracorporeal membrane oxygenation in the neonate. *Neonatal Network* 4(5): 30. Reprinted by permission.

Consequently, the survival rate of these infants is discouragingly low.[22,31]

ROUTES OF PERFUSION

In the ECMO circuit, blood is drained from the venous system and diverted outside the body, where oxygen is added and carbon dioxide removed by the membrane oxygenator. The oxygenated blood is then returned to the patient. This support achieves adequate gas exchange and permits ventilator settings to be reduced to low parameters, minimizing barotrauma and oxygen toxicity. The two most common methods of perfusing infants on ECMO are venoarterial (VA) bypass and venovenous (VV) bypass.

VENOARTERIAL BYPASS

The VA route—presently the most common method of bypass—drains blood from the right side of the heart through a catheter placed in the right atrium via the right internal jugular vein. Oxygenated blood is returned through

the right common carotid artery into the ascending aorta (Figure 14-1).[38] The carotid artery is the arterial vessel of choice because it is the largest vessel able to provide adequate blood flow to the aortic arch. If the patient demonstrates cardiac failure, venoarterial bypass will be used.

The venoarterial route provides support for the heart and lungs by (1) decompressing the right ventricle and the pulmonary circulation, which decreases pulmonary artery pressure, pulmonary capillary filtration pressure, and right heart pressures, and (2) supporting the pumping action of the heart and systemic circulation mechanically, via the roller head pump.[38]

There are several technical advantages to this route: The lungs can be lavaged and suctioned without hazarding hypoxia, positive pressure ventilation can be reduced to minimal parameters, and stabilization and total respiratory support can be achieved in less time and at lower pump flow rates than with the venovenous route.[38,39]

There are two major risks inherent in venoarterial bypass: Emboli (air or particulate) could be infused directly into the arterial circulation, and the ligation of the carotid artery may inversely affect cerebral perfusion.[38]

VENOVENOUS BYPASS

The VV route has been used successfully to support neonates in respiratory failure.[39,40] The initial venovenous procedure necessitated two operative sites for cannulation: the internal jugular vein for blood drainage and the femoral vein for return of oxygenated blood. Technically, this form of venovenous bypass was more difficult to manage because two surgical incisions and dissections were needed and stabilization required more time. These patients were at risk for groin wound infections and serious venous insufficiency in the leg with the femoral vein ligation.[40] Despite these concerns, the research documenting the efficacy of venovenous bypass contributed to the development of a double-lumen, single venovenous catheter.

As early as 1985, studies were published documenting the efficacy of a venovenous double-lumen single catheter for bypass.[41] Recent publications have continued to document the effectiveness of this technique and support the use of this route of bypass.[42,43] This form of venovenous bypass involves cannulating the right atrium via the internal jugular vein with a double-lumen catheter (Figure 14-2). The venous blood is drained from the right atrium via the drainage lumen, circulated through a membrane oxygenator, and returned to the right atrium via the inflow lumen.

This route is advantageous because it does not require cannulation and ligation of the common carotid artery. Preload and afterload of the heart remain unchanged, the right atrium and ventricle are not decompressed, and hence there is no change in cardiac output or pulmonary artery pressure. Oxygenated blood returns to the right side of the heart and lungs, minimizing the danger of arterial embolization. Perfusing the pulmonary artery system with oxygenated blood theoretically should increase pulmonary arteriolar dilation and reduce right ventricular afterload.[43] There are disadvantages to the venovenous route: More time is required to stabilize the patient; inotropic support must be continued; ventilator settings must be weaned more slowly than with VA ECMO.

Because venovenous bypass does not provide direct circulatory support, this form of bypass has been limited to patients whose cardiac function is adequate to circulate oxygenated blood from the right atrium to the systemic circulation. Hence, evidence of left- or right-sided cardiac dysfunction via echocardiogram or clinical physiologic parameters (persistent metabolic acidosis, hypotension, or anuria despite maxi-

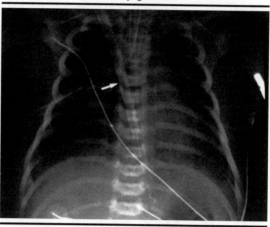

FIGURE 14-2 ▲ **Anteroposterior chest film** demonstrating correct placement of VVDL catheter in right atrium via internal jugular vein.

mal inotropic support) has been a relative contraindication to VV ECMO.[42]

However, studies comparing infants with severe lung disease treated with ECMO or conventional therapy found no significant differences in cardiac performance and concluded that cardiac failure is not a primary cause of clinical deterioration.[44] Additionally, echocardiographic measurements of infants on venovenous bypass demonstrate normalization and no deterioration of cardiac performance, establishing that ventricular dysfunction can be improved with VV bypass.[45] Further research is required to determine the specific degree of ventricular dysfunction that would limit the use of venovenous double-lumen (VVDL) bypass and dictate the need for venoarterial bypass. At the present time, approximately 16 percent of patients on VVDL bypass are converted to the venoarterial route because of inadequate support.[30]

The physical limitation of venovenous double-lumen ECMO is internal jugular vessel size. The double-lumen catheter used is a #14 French. Neonates weighing <2,500 gm frequently cannot be cannulated successfully. Displacement of the mediastinum in patients with

FIGURE 14-3 ▲ Components of the ECMO circuit: (a) PVC tubing with stopcocks, (b) silicone rubber bladder with infusion sites, (c) bladder box assembly, (d) roller pump, (e & f) membrane oxygenator and gas sources, (g & h) heat exchanger and water bath, (j) ACT machine, and (k) heparin infusion.

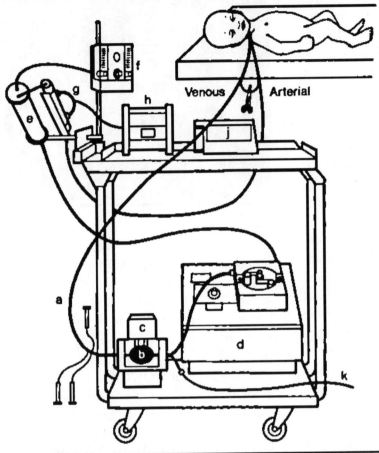

From: Nugent J. 1986. Extracorporeal membrane oxygenation in the neonate. *Neonatal Network* 4(5): 31. Reprinted by permission.

14-3). A detailed description of the development of the ECMO circuit is available in the literature.[46]

The cannulas are for removing deoxygenated venous blood and returning oxygenated blood to the infant's arterial circulation. ECMO bypass flow and the ability to deliver oxygen are limited by the volume of venous drainage blood. This volume is limited by the size and position of the venous drainage catheter. The venous catheter must be capable of delivering the total cardiac output (120–150 ml/kg/minute) and should be positioned to drain blood from the superior and inferior vena cava.[11]

The internal diameter of the cannulas has the greatest impact on resistance to flow. Because the ECMO system must be capable of providing total heart-lung support, cannulas of the largest possible internal diameter are inserted. This assures adequate venous drainage to support the required bypass flow rates. Argyle chest tubes ranging in size from 8 to 16 French have been the most widely used because they are thin walled and offer low resistance to flow.[46] However, specifically designed ECMO cannulae (Biomedicus, Elecath, Kendall) are available and demonstrate flow characteristics superior to the Argyle chest tubes.[47]

After the patient has received local anesthesia and morphine, the surgeon carefully isolates and dissects the right internal jugular vein and

a diaphragmatic hernia, tension pneumothorax, or prominent first rib may also prevent atraumatic introduction of the cannula.[42]

THE ECMO CIRCUIT

Components of the ECMO circuit include cannulas; a system of polyvinylchloride (PVC) tubing with Luer-Lok connectors, stopcocks, a silicone rubber bladder with infusion sites; bladder box assembly; roller pump; membrane oxygenator; and heat exchanger. An activated clotting time machine completes the system (Figure carotid artery. Both vessels are dissected regardless of route of perfusion. When the venovenous route is used, the carotid artery should also be dissected, thereby facilitating rapid conversion to the venoarterial route if needed. Extensive manipulation of the vessels can produce vasospasm. This prohibits cannulation with an adequate sized catheter. Application of topical papaverine will promote venodilation for accommodation of the venous catheter.[42]

The patient is systemically heparinized just before the cannulas are introduced. Before administering a heparin loading dose of 50–100 units/kg, the nurse assesses all invasive sites for adequate hemostasis.[42] Once the patient's activated clotting time has reached 250 seconds and prior to introduction of the internal jugular vein catheter, succinylcholine or pancuronium bromide (Pavulon) is given to prevent respiratory movement and air embolism.

To initiate venoarterial bypass, the carotid artery and the internal jugular vein are ligated distally preceding the introduction of the cannulas. Perfusion of the brain is maintained by collateral circulation through the external carotid artery, the circle of Willis, and the ophthalmic artery.[48]

The arterial cannula is advanced so that the catheter tip reaches just to the aortic arch. The venous cannula is positioned so that the tip lies in the right atrium with the side holes draining the right atrium and the superior vena cava.[49] The cannulas are flushed with a retrograde blood flow from the right atrium and aortic arch, sutured to the skin of the upper neck, and connected to the ECMO circuit tubing. The position of the cannulas is immediately determined by chest x-ray examination.

To initiate venovenous double-lumen catheter bypass, the distal portion of the internal jugular vein is ligated. A venotomy is created in the proximal jugular vein, and a lubricated double-lumen catheter is inserted and advanced to the right atrium.

The catheter is placed so the tip is in the right atrium and the most proximal venous drainage hole is within the superior vena cava. The arterial "angled Y" portion of the catheter should be oriented anteriorly on the infant's head. This will direct oxygenated blood from the arterial lumen of the catheter toward the tricuspid valve. The "angled Y" of the catheter is sutured to the skin behind the ear to prevent catheter rotation.[42] Correct catheter placement is assessed via chest radiograph and/or echocardiography.

The PVC tubing with its system of connectors, ports with stopcocks, and silicone bladder provides for circulation of blood from the infant through the components of the circuit as well as for removal of blood and administration of fluids, medications, and blood products. This system has a volume of approximately 350–400 ml.

Prior to cannulation, the circuit is primed: It is flushed with carbon dioxide, which aids in the removal of microbubbles by making them more soluble, and filled with a crystalloid solution. Albumin, 25 percent, is added to precondition and coat the circuit surface area, minimizing fibrinogen adherence and platelet destruction. This solution is displaced with citrated packed red blood cells to which calcium and heparin have been added. The pH of the blood is corrected with THAM, and 25 percent albumin is added to equalize oncotic pressure. It is essential to determine that the electrolytes, blood gases, and acid-base balance of the prime solution are physiologic prior to instituting bypass. Platelets are added to the prime solution once bypass is begun and the activated clotting time is within the desired range.

The system of ports with stopcocks on the PVC tubing and the infusion sites on the bladder provide access to the circuit. Each of the ports is designed for a singular purpose. The port closest to the patient is used to remove blood samples; the second, third, and fourth ports are for administering blood products, medications, and alimentation solutions. The number and position of stopcocks will vary with each institution's protocol.

Because fluid can stagnate in the bladder, infusing heparin, alimentation solutions, and medications through the ports is preferable to using the infusion sites on the bladder. These sites are suitable for administering blood products and, in emergencies, for removing air. To avoid contamination, sampling sites should be used for blood withdrawal only and infusion sites for infusion only.

Because all ECMO patients are heparinized, institutional protocols may recommend that all intravenous infusion sites be discontinued prior to cannulation. This reduces the possibility of bleeding from puncture sites. All medications, fluids, and blood products except platelets are given through the venous side of the ECMO circuit. The only exceptions are fluids infused via the umbilical catheters or peripheral arterial lines. When medications are given via syringe, care is taken to aspirate each syringe gently for air bubbles because there is no in-line air filter.

The same precautions and guidelines for safe administration of medications and blood directly into patients are used when medications and blood are infused into the ECMO circuit. Platelets are infused on the arterial side of the circuit between the membrane oxygenator and the heat exchanger. This prevents inadvertent filtration of platelets by the membrane oxygenator.

The bladder box assembly is a fail-safe alarm system. The collapsible silicone bladder distends with returning venous blood. If the flow into the ECMO circuit is not adequate, the bladder will collapse, causing a servoswitch to

sound an audible alarm and stop the roller pump. Upon re-expansion of the bladder, the servoswitch re-engages the pump, and normal pump operation continues.[38] This servoregulation feature prevents the pump flow rate from exceeding venous return.

Transducer-based technology that allows for servoregulation of extracorporeal flow, independent of bladder volume, is now available (Polystan). Transducers placed in-line in the circuit monitor premembrane (venous) and postmembrane (arterial) pressures. This advance in servoregulation technique allows for early detection of flow problems and timely intervention.

A decrease in premembrane pressure signals decreased venous return prior to the collapse of the silicone bladder. Causes of decreased and inadequate venous return are hypovolemia, kinked venous catheter, incorrect position of the venous catheter in the right atrium, inadequate catheter diameter, and pneumothorax. Adequate venous return is critical to achieving pump flows needed for cardiopulmonary support. Persistent decreased venous return promotes a hemodynamically unstable patient. Hence, the cause for decreased return must be recognized and corrected immediately. A rise in postmembrane pressure could indicate kinking of the arterial catheter, accidental clamping of the catheter, a clot in the membrane oxygenator or heat exchanger, or impending oxygenator failure.

The ECMO blood pump is a double-roller device that compresses and displaces the blood in the PVC tubing that is positioned in the pump raceway. The action of the pump pushes fluid forward, creating suction within the venous catheter. The pumping action will assist left ventricular function in an infant on venoarterial bypass. The pump is electrically powered and can be hand cranked or attached to a battery power source if a power failure occurs.

A digital display indicating the circuit flow in cubic centimeters per minute appears on the face of the pump.

The membrane oxygenator or lung (Sci-Med/Kolobow) is a solid, silicone, polymer membrane envelope with a plastic space screen. This is spirally wound around a spool and encased in a silicone rubber sleeve.[38] In the lung, oxygen is added, and carbon dioxide and water vapor are removed. Membrane oxygenators are the oxygenators of choice. They have the advantages of eliminating the blood/gas interface effects (damaging plasma proteins, lipoproteins, red cells), assuring constant blood volume, and providing ease of operation.[50]

A heat exchanger is located downstream from the oxygenator and provides warming of the blood, which is kept normothermic.[38] Heat loss from the blood occurs during ECMO from the cooling effect of ventilating gases inside the oxygenator and circuit exposure to ambient air temperature. It has been our experience that the infant also requires heat from a radiant heat source to maintain normal body temperature during the ECMO procedure.

A bubble detector (Polystan, Cobe, Shiley) can be placed distal (patient side) to the heat exchanger. It can detect air bubbles as small as 600 microns. If a bubble is detected, the roller head pump is immediately shut off and flow to the patient ceases.

Fiberoptic technology that provides continuous monitoring of arterial and venous blood gases is now available. These monitoring devices (Cardiovascular Devices, Inc.), which are integral parts of the arterial and venous sides of the PVC circuit, provide digital readouts of arterial pH, PaO_2, PCO_2, base excess/bicarbonate (BE/HCO_3^-) and venous pH, PvO_2, $PvCO_2$, and saturation. The arterial monitoring allows for assessment of membrane oxygenator function. Venous monitoring assists in assessing the adequacy of extracorporeal perfusion and the efficiency of the extracorporeal circulation in meeting the infant's metabolic needs.

An activated clotting time machine and an infusion pump are used intermittently to monitor the patient's activated clotting time and continuously infuse a heparin solution into the ECMO circuit. Once the loading dose of heparin is given at the time of cannulation, the activated clotting time is maintained at 180–250 seconds. Low-dose heparin of approximately 30–60 units/kg/hour is continuously infused into the circuit.

Heparin activity is monitored by whole blood activated clotting time. It is essential to use whole blood activated clotting time, rather than plasma partial thromboplastin time, because of the interactions between platelets, white cells, and heparin.[50] Activated clotting time is checked every 30–60 minutes, and the heparin infusion is titrated to keep the time within the desired range.

To control the amount of heparin administered, none is added to any other medications or fluids. An exception may be fluids infusing through umbilical catheters or peripheral arterial lines. Factors that influence heparin requirements are thrombocytopenia and abnormal coagulation studies.[38]

PHYSIOLOGY OF EXTRACORPOREAL CIRCULATION

Physiologic function during prolonged cardiopulmonary bypass differs considerably from normal physiology. The normal functions of blood flow, gas exchange, blood surface interface interactions, and reticuloendothelial functions are replaced in various degrees by the extracorporeal device.[50]

Venoarterial bypass drains blood from the right ventricle and returns oxygenated blood to the aortic arch. These flow dynamics significantly reduce preload and increase afterload. After initiation of venoarterial bypass, left

TABLE 14-2 ▲ ECMO Complications

Physiologic	Rationale and Treatment
Electrolyte/glucose/fluid imbalance	Sodium requirements decrease to 1–2 mEq/kg/day. Potassium requirements increase to 4 mEq/kg/day secondary to the action of aldosterone. Calcium replacement may be required if citrate is a component of prime blood anticoagulant. Hyperglycemia may occur if citrate-phosphate-dextrose anticoagulated blood is used: Reduce dextrose concentration of maintenance and heparin infusions. Maintain total fluid intake 100–150 ml/kg/day. Fluid intake should balance output; furosemide may be required if positive fluid balance occurs.[49]
Central nervous system deterioration: cerebral edema, intracranial hemorrhage, seizures	This significant complication of ECMO can be related to pre-ECMO hypoxia, acidosis, hypercapnea, or to vessel ligation. The drug of choice for seizures is phenobarbital. Serial EEGs and cranial ultrasounds may be required.
Generalized edema	Extracellular space is enlarged by distribution of crystalloid solution from the prime fluid, action of aldosterone and antidiuretic hormone, or tissue injury from hypoxia or sepsis. Furosemide or hemofiltration may be indicated if edema causes brain or lung dysfunction. Restrict fluid (80 ml/kg/day) until diuresis is established.
Renal failure	Acute tubular necrosis results from pre-ECMO hypotension and hypoxia. Monitor output and indicators of renal failure: blood urea nitrogen (BUN), creatinine. Increase renal perfusion by increasing pump flow and use of dopamine (5 µg/kg/minute). Hemodialysis may be added to the circuit if necessary.
Bleeding/thrombocytopenia	This is the most frequent cause of death. This is most common in infants requiring surgery or chest tubes. Large foreign surface of ECMO circuit lowers platelet function and count. Minimize with good control of ACT (180–200 seconds) and judicious use of platelets and fresh frozen plasma. All surgical procedures must be done with electrocautery. Amicar (30 mg/kg/hour) decreases intracranial and extracranial hemorrhage.[71]
Decreased venous return and/or hypovolemia	Infant must have adequate circulating volume to obtain adequate flow rates. Manifested by collapsing silicone bladder triggering bladder box alarm, decrease in extracorporeal flow rate, arterial pressure, and arterial pulse amplitude. Blood sampling, wound drainage, or peripheral vessel dilation may account for hypovolemia. Check for pneumothorax, partial venous catheter occlusion or malposition, which may decrease venous drainage and return. Replace volume with packed cells, fresh frozen plasma. Treat pneumothorax with chest tube placement. Raise level of bed to enhance gravity drainage of venous blood.
Hypertension	This is caused by hypervolemia due to overinfusion of blood products, which causes a larger percentage of blood to flow through malfunctioning lungs. Hypertension can also be caused by renal ischemia and excretion of renin/angiotension. Hypertension, secondary to hypervolemia, is manifested by widening pulse amplitude and decreasing systemic oxygenation at a fixed extracorporeal flow rate. Treat overinfusion by removing blood from the circuit. Renal hypertension may dictate use of captopril or labetalol.
Patent ductus arteriosus	Left-to-right shunting may occur, causing increased blood flow to the lungs, necessitating high pump flows without expected increase in PaO$_2$. Ligation may be indicated because weaning from ECMO will not be successful.
Cardiac stun	Transient loss (1–3 days) of ventricular contractility. Manifested by hypotension, marked decrease in aortic pulse pressure, poor peripheral perfusion, and decrease in PaO$_2$. Possibly due to mismatch between afterload and ventricular contractility during ECMO. Adjust pump flow to provide circulatory support, maintain inotropic therapy.[72]
Mechanical	**Rationale and Treatment**
Tubing rupture, air in circuit, oxygenator malfunction	Increase ventilator to pre-ECMO parameters. Take patient off bypass. Repair circuit, aspirate air, replace oxygenator. Be prepared to resuscitate infant.
Power failure	Always plug pump into hospital's emergency power supply. Hand crank until emergency power is available.
Decannulation	Apply firm pressure. Come off bypass; increase ventilator parameters. Repair vessel; replace blood volume. Be prepared to resuscitate infant.

Adapted from: Nugent J. 1986. Extracorporeal membrane oxygenation in the neonate. *Neonatal Network* 4(5): 33. Reprinted by permission.

ventricular performance decreases. The changes in preload and afterload probably cause an increase in workload on the left ventricle. This decrease in left ventricular function is transient and resolves in 48–72 hours.[45]

During ECMO, the venous catheter only partially drains the venous return from the right atrium. Hence, total systemic blood flow is the sum of residual left ventricular output and the ECMO pump flow rate. Calculations from a flow partition model demonstrate that in venoarterial bypass, blood flow from the arterial catheter in the aortic arch is preferentially directed to the upper body.

Coronary artery and abdominal blood flows are derived predominantly from the left ventricle. Oxygen delivery to the heart is therefore more closely related to the pulmonary status and pulmonary venous saturation than to the ECMO pump arterial oxygen content. These findings have implications when ECMO is instituted for postoperative management of compromised cardiac performance and may also contribute to the etiology of the cardiac stun syndrome (Table 14-2) seen in some infants following initiation of ECMO.[51]

In VVDL bypass, blood is drained from the right atrium and oxygenated blood is returned to the right atrium. Hence, systemic perfusion is dependent on the infant's native cardiac output. Preload and afterload of the heart are unchanged, and there is no selective distribution of systemic blood flow. Theoretically, because the coronary arteries are perfused by blood from the left ventricle, the increased oxygen content of the blood coming from the ECMO circuit via the left ventricle should improve the oxygen delivery to the coronary arteries if the infant is hemodynamically stable.[45,52]

VA bypass is instituted by draining venous blood by siphon into the extracorporeal circuit; a like amount of arterialized blood is returned to arterial circulation. As bypass flow is gradu-

ally increased, flow through the pulmonary artery decreases at a faster rate than bypass flow, reducing total flow in the systemic circulation. Peripheral and pulmonary hypotension may occur.

In venovenous double-lumen bypass, total systemic flow dynamics are not changed (there is no alteration in preload or afterload). However, peripheral hypotension does also occur with this route of perfusion. Though the exact mechanisms causing hypotension are not well understood, reduction in blood viscosity and the release of vasoactive substances may contribute to this phenomenon.[50] Blood volume replacement is required for correction of hypotension, optimal tissue perfusion, and prevention of metabolic acidosis.

It has also been demonstrated that hypotension after initiation of ECMO by either route is associated with decreased ionized calcium levels. The citrate in the prime blood may bind with ionized calcium, causing functional hypocalcemia and depressed cardiac performance.[52] Calcium should be added to the prime, normalizing ionized calcium in the circuit. Additionally, the infant's serum calcium levels should be monitored closely and corrected when indicated.

In VVDL perfusion, hypotension may also be due to removal of inotropic drugs when the catheter drains the right atrium. An extension tube may be attached to the arterial side of the double-lumen catheter, allowing additional infusion of inotropes during the initiation of bypass. As the patient's blood pressure stabilizes, he may be weaned from this infusion and the extension tube capped off.[42]

Extracorporeal membrane oxygenation via the venoarterial route is nonpulsatile, meaning that pulse contour decreases as venoarterial flow rate increases, and systemic perfusion is dependent on circuit flow and cardiac output. The precise nature of the physiologic effects of nonpulsatile flow during extracorporeal circulation has been the subject of controversy. Experts agree, however, that the kidney interprets the nonpulsatile flow as inadequate, resulting in renin and aldosterone production and antidiuresis.[50]

Venovenous bypass perfusion is pulsatile. The pulse contour does not change or dampen, and the systemic perfusion depends only on the infant's native cardiac output.[53]

The total flow to the patient during ECMO is a function of blood volume and the diameter of the venous catheter. An increase in blood volume at a stable ECMO flow will increase pulmonary-artery-to-left-atrial flow, decreasing the relative percentage of cardiopulmonary bypass. Conversely, a reduction in patient blood volume can inadvertently increase extracorporeal flow and decrease pulmonary-artery-to-left-atrial flow.

Total patient flow is the sum of extracorporeal flow plus pulmonary blood flow. Adequate flow in ECMO bypass is reached when oxygen delivery and tissue perfusion result in normoxia, normal pH, normal venous oxygen saturation (SvO_2), and normal organ function. Normal cardiac output in an infant is 120–150 ml/kg/minute. Total gas exchange and support are usually achieved at this flow rate.

Gas exchange is accomplished via the membrane lung. The lung consists of two compartments divided by a semipermeable membrane: Ventilating gas is on one side; blood is on the other. As the blood flows past the membrane, oxygen diffuses into the blood because of a pressure gradient between the 100 percent oxygen in the ventilating gas and the low oxygen pressure in mixed venous blood. The chemical binding of oxygen to hemoglobin proceeds very rapidly.

The limiting factor in oxygenation of flowing blood is the rate of oxygen diffusion through plasma. Therefore, the thickness of the blood film between the gas exchange membranes becomes the rate-limiting factor in oxygen transfer.

Simultaneously, carbon dioxide diffuses from the blood compartment, responding to a pressure gradient between the venous carbon dioxide pressure and the ventilating gas. The rate of carbon dioxide transfer is greater than that of oxygen; hence, a carbon dioxide–enriched mixture is usually necessary for ventilating the oxygenator. This prevents inadvertent hypocapnia, respiratory alkalosis, and cessation of the infant's spontaneous respirations.

The carbon dioxide pressure is controlled by gas flow through the membrane oxygenator. To remove excess carbon dioxide, the sweep flow (the total liter flow of oxygen, carbon dioxide, and compressed air to the oxygenator) may be increased. The manufacturer's recommended limit for sweep flow should not be exceeded. If the pressure on the gas side of the membrane exceeds that on the blood side, gas embolization could occur.

Oxygen transfer capacity of a membrane oxygenator is related to the rate of blood flow through the membrane and the degree of oxyhemoglobin desaturation of the blood entering the oxygenator. The flow rate at which venous blood leaves the oxygenator at 95 percent saturation is referred to as "rated flow."

As blood flow through the membrane oxygenator is increased, a point is reached when the thickness of the blood film limits the rate that oxygen can diffuse into the blood. At this point, the outflow blood exits at less than 95 percent saturation. The rated flow for a membrane oxygenator is that at which this limitation is reached.

The rated oxygen delivery is the amount of oxygen that can be taken up by the blood at the rated flow. Oxygen delivery is related to the flow and to the amount of unsaturated hemoglobin presented to the oxygenator per minute. Oxygen delivery depends entirely on flow; decreasing flow decreases delivery.[50]

In selecting an oxygenator, one should be sure that the "rated flow" is greater than cardiac output—that is, the infant's oxygen requirement should not exceed the oxygenating performance of the membrane lung. The Sci-Med 0.4 m^2 membrane lung has a rated flow of 40 ml/minute/m^2 with a recommended blood flow rate of 350 ml/minute; the 0.8 m^2 size has a rated flow of 60 ml/minute/m^2 with a recommended blood flow rate of 1,400 ml/minute. Either can be used effectively in the neonate, whose usual maximal flow rate requirement is 120–150 ml/kg/minute.

There are often factors that control systemic oxygenation during ECMO. Total oxygen delivery to tissues is equal to extracorporeal oxygen plus pulmonary oxygen. Increasing extracorporeal flow and decreasing patient lung flow will increase the infant's PaO_2. Decreasing extracorporeal flow and increasing patient lung flow will decrease the infant's PaO_2 as long as the infant's lung function is not adequate.

In VVDL bypass, higher pump flows and a larger membrane oxygenator (0.6 m^2 or 0.8 m^2) may be required to compensate for the problem of pump recirculation. Pump recirculation refers to drainage of oxygenated blood from the right atrium and return of that blood to the ECMO circuit. Consequently, less oxygenated blood is available for the infant's circulation because a portion of oxygenated circulating blood volume goes into the drainage cannula.

Recirculation can range from 5 to 29 percent of blood flow; hence, higher flows may be required to maintain oxygenation. Typical blood flow for optimal gas exchange in venovenous bypass is 100–120 ml/kg/minute versus 80–100 ml/kg/minute in venoarterial bypass.[42]

Because of recirculation, VV bypass does not result in as great a degree of oxygenation as does VA bypass. Oxygen tensions of 50–60 torr and oxygen saturations of 85–90 percent are accepted.[42] Increasing flow in VV bypass may increase recirculation and decrease patient oxygenation.

In situations where the patient is hypoxic and no additional recirculation is desired, an increase in extracorporeal flow is not indicated. Oxygenation may be improved by optimizing the infant's cardiac output and hemoglobin. Cardiac output may be improved by increasing venous return to the heart. This can be accomplished by reducing positive inspiratory pressure (PIP) and positive end-expiratory pressure (PEEP), thereby decreasing mean airway pressure and allowing increased venous return.[42]

A less than optimal hematocrit (less than 45 percent in venoarterial, 55 percent in venovenous) will decrease oxygenation. Rapid or overinfusion of blood products decreases oxygenation because a larger percentage of blood flow is shifted to the pulmonary-artery-to-left-atrial flow, decreasing the relative percentage of cardiopulmonary bypass. Care must be taken to recognize and avoid this problem.[38]

During ECMO, at least 80 percent of the cardiac output is exposed to a large artificial surface each minute. All blood cellular components and protein molecules come into contact with a foreign surface hourly. Flow patterns in the circuit include areas of stagnation and turbulence.[38] All these factors stimulate both the protein and the platelet arms of the clotting system.

Within seconds of blood exposure to a foreign surface, a molecular layer of protein adheres to the surface. One of these proteins is fibrinogen, which is converted into fibrin, and subsequent clot formation occurs within a few minutes. Other protein clotting factors are absorbed to some extent by foreign surface exposure, resulting in a decrease of clotting factors at the initiation of bypass. Concurrently,

TABLE 14-3 ▲ Circuit Emergency Procedures

Circuit Emergencies	
Air embolism (arterial)	Power failure
Tubing rupture	Gas source failure
Oxygenator malfunction	
Decannulation	
Pump failure	
↓	
Come off bypass	

Circuit Emergency Procedures	
Nurse	*ECMO specialist*
Ventilation	Clamp catheters
Anticoagulation	Open bridge
Chemical resuscitation	Remove gas source
Replace blood loss	Repair circuit

the liver and spleen increase synthesis of fibrinogen and other clotting factors, returning their serum concentrations to prebypass levels within a period of hours.[50]

Pre-exposure of the circuit's inner surface to albumin appears to minimize fibrin surface adherence and platelet destruction.[38] In the presence of heparin, fibrinogen is not converted to fibrin, and clotting does not occur.

Platelets show the greatest effect of exposure to a foreign surface, as evidenced by continuous platelet aggregate formation and decreasing platelet count and function. The concentration of platelets drops abruptly with onset of extracorporeal circulation and continues to fall as long as bypass continues. The thrombocytopenia is due in part to platelets adhering directly to the foreign surface but to a greater extent to platelets adhering to each other and to white cells, forming platelet aggregates of 2–200 micron units, which are infused into the patient. These aggregates are picked up by the liver, spleen, and to a lesser extent by the lung, where they are bound or phagocytized. Platelet aggregate formation is not detrimental to microcirculation, as is evidenced by lack of microembolic tissue damage even in prolonged bypass (16 days).[38,50]

Because a large number of platelet aggregates is generated continuously, it can be estimated that all circulating platelets are incorporated into aggregates every few hours. These platelets disaggregate and recirculate. The platelet count plateaus at 30,000–60,000/mm^3 when a balance between aggregation, regeneration from bone marrow, disaggregation, and recirculation is achieved.[38] This chronic thrombocytopenia requires frequent platelet transfusions.

Platelet transfusions are necessary when the platelet level drops below 100,000/mm^3. If the patient is experiencing abnormal amounts of bleeding, the platelet count is maintained at >100,000/mm^3, and the activated clotting time is restricted to 180–200 seconds. Platelet transfusions do increase heparin consumption, and to compensate, the heparin infusion may need to be increased. Transfusion of a whole unit of adult platelets (rather than platelet concentrate) may be preferable because platelets are very sensitive to contact and temperature.[11]

After cessation of extracorporeal circulation, clotting factors and platelets return to normal or above normal levels.[50] However, thrombocytopenia can occur up to four days after the cessation of ECMO. Platelet counts must be monitored during this critical period. Infants at highest risk for prolonged thrombocytopenia are those with meconium aspiration syndrome or sepsis and those whose ECMO course was marked by mechanical complications (tubing rupture, oxygenator malfunction, see Table 14-3).[54,55]

Physiologic changes occur as a result of systemic heparinization. Several of the steps between activation of the surface factor (Factor XII) and fibrin formation are inhibited by heparin.[50] This action results in prolonged clotting times. Heparin has an almost immediate onset of action following intravenous administration. It is inactivated by the liver and excreted by the kidney. Clotting times return to normal within two to six hours after the drug is discontinued.

The effects of prolonged extracorporeal circulation on blood cell survival and function demonstrate that hemolysis is negligible and the survival of red blood cells is not altered by continuous exposure to the ECMO circuit. All the various types of white cells decrease in concentration because of the combined effects of dilution and aggregation.

Studies of phagocytosis and bacterial killing of circulating leukocytes during extracorporeal circulation demonstrate significantly decreased phagocytic activity in the circulating white cells. It is postulated that these effects are due to the mechanical or chemical effects of the ECMO circuit on blood. It is thought that the phagocytes may become saturated with platelet aggregates, which reduce their ability to further phagocytize bacteria. White cell concentration rebounds after cessation of ECMO.[50]

Fluid and electrolyte changes occur frequently during extracorporeal circulation. Sodium retention, expanded extracellular fluid, and decreased total body potassium are characteristic changes. These conditions are thought to be attributable to (1) third spacing of albumin, the source of which is the circuit priming fluid; (2) the action of aldosterone, which causes sodium retention, expansion of extracellular fluid, and kaliuresis; and (3) fluid and electrolyte shifts from the intravascular to the extravascular space caused by hypoxic ischemic injury or sepsis.[56]

The goal of fluid management is to promote diuresis while maintaining adequate circulatory volume.[56] Potassium replacement is required, and excessive extracellular fluid can be removed via use of furosemide or continuous hemofiltration.[32] Calcium and magnesium levels can remain low throughout the ECMO run; correction is achieved with moderate supplementation via parenteral fluids.[50]

CARE OF THE INFANT UNDERGOING ECMO

Cannulation and the initiation of bypass usually occur in the NICU under local anesthesia and with operating room staff in attendance. This avoids the formidable risks inherent in moving a critically ill newborn to and from the operating room with bypass in progress. The operating room team provides an ECMO surgical case cart, an electrocautery unit, and a fiberoptic headlight. While the team is readying the surgical equipment, the ECMO specialist assembles and primes the circuit.

It is essential that the infant have an indwelling arterial line for arterial sampling as well as for continuous blood pressure monitoring. The site of choice is the umbilical artery; if this is not feasible, a postductal site such as the left radial artery will be utilized. A peripheral venous line may also be inserted in an extremity or in a scalp vein for infusion of parenteral fluids and medications during the surgical procedure. All necessary lines are kept to a minimum and are inserted prior to heparinization.

During the surgical procedure, the NICU nursing personnel constantly monitor the infant's cardiopulmonary status and administer the necessary medications. Blood products and emergency drugs are drawn up and are available. Initiation of bypass frequently causes hypotension, which is generally corrected with volume replacement. Care must be taken not to dislodge the infant's endotracheal tube and arterial or venous lines during the procedure.

Following cannulation, bypass is gradually instituted until approximately 80 percent of the infant's cardiac output is diverted through the ECMO circuit. This usually requires flow rates of 80–120 ml/kg/minute (Figure 14-4). At maximum flow, hypoxia, hypercarbia, and acidosis will be reversed. The infant will become normotensive, and vasoactive drugs and muscle

FIGURE 14-4 ▲ Example of an arterial pressure waveform and bypass flow rates. On venoarterial bypass, conduction and contraction continue even though little blood is flowing through the heart. The EKG pattern will remain normal. The normal peaked pattern of the arterial pressure waveform will flatten as bypass flow increases. Total bypass (70–80 percent of cardiac output) is reached when the arterial pressure tracing flattens and no peaked contours are evident during positive pressure inflation.

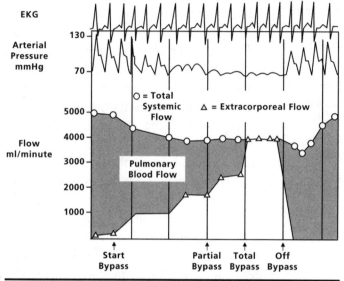

From: Chapman R, Toomasian J, and Bartlett R. 1988. *Extracorporeal Membrane Oxygenation Technical Specialist Manual,* 9th ed. Ann Arbor: University of Michigan, 8. Reprinted by permission.

sion. A decrease in SvO_2 indicates tissue hypoxia. The best end-point indicator for venovenous bypass is the PaO_2 or oxyhemoglobin saturation measured by pulse oximetry.[42] Continuous monitoring of venous and arterial oxyhemoglobin saturation via fiberoptic technology allows for optimal management of bypass flow.

Total blood flow to the infant on bypass is the sum of extracorporeal flow and pulmonary blood flow. Total oxygen delivery is the combination of extracorporeal oxygen delivery and pulmonary oxygen delivery. The resultant systemic arterial blood gases reflect the sum of these relative oxygen contents.

Oxygen delivery is maximized by maintaining the hematocrit at 45–55 percent. Blood products are also given to correct hypovolemia, excessive bleeding, and thrombocytopenia. Maintenance and alimentation fluids are administered at 80–120 ml/kg/day. The usual sodium requirement is 1–2 mEq/kg/day, with a potassium requirement of 4 mEq/kg/day. Gastric feedings may be initiated if bowel function is normal.

Significant insensible water loss can occur secondary to the radiant warmer and the membrane lung. Daily weights are the best indicator of fluid balance. A weight gain will occur the first 24–48 hours, followed by diuresis and weight loss. Antibiotics are ordered routinely, as well as frequent blood cultures and chest films.

The infant should receive endotracheal suctioning based on individual assessment and need. Hourly recording of vital signs, intake and output, neurologic checks, and arterial blood gases are mandatory. Oozing at the cannulation site may require frequent dressing changes. The amount of blood loss must be quantified and replaced.

relaxants may be discontinued. During venovenous bypass, an infusion of dopamine at 3–5 µg/kg/minute may be indicated because the infant is totally dependent on native cardiac output for blood pressure.[42]

Ventilator parameters are reduced to minimal settings to "rest" the lungs. Venovenous bypass may require higher resting parameters. The extracorporeal flow is adjusted to maintain systemic arterial PaO_2 at 60–80 torr in venoarterial and 50 torr in venovenous, $PaCO_2$ at 35–45 torr, pH at 7.35–7.45, SvO_2 at more than 70 percent; and arterial saturation at more than 90 percent in VA, 85–90 percent in VV bypass.

In the infant on venoarterial bypass, SvO_2 is considered an excellent indicator of adequate flow because it is a measure of tissue perfu-

The infant's position should be changed every one to two hours. Catheter dislodgement is a fatal complication; caution must be taken at all times to avoid inadvertent decannulation. The ECMO specialist should assist the nurse in all position changes.

Because of the thin-walled polyurethane construction of the venovenous double-lumen catheter, cannula kinking is a major problem. The infant's head and neck frequently remain immobilized in order to prevent kinking. Occupational therapists can help develop individualized nursing care plans addressing this immobility concern.

Wedges and blanket rolls can be useful when repositioning the infant. To provide greater stability to the catheter, place a protective "sleeve," fashioned from a large-diameter endotracheal tube, around the catheter proximal to the "angled Y."

COMPLICATIONS

Complications associated with ECMO are both physiologic and mechanical. Mechanical problems frequently create emergency situations that require immediate recognition and resolution. Tables 14-2 and 14-3 outline these complications with their rationale and corrective actions.

Mechanical complications occur in 27 percent of ECMO patients. The most common one is incorrect catheter placement (36 percent); the next most frequent is oxygenator failure (24 percent). Technical complications affect survival: One or more technical complications has resulted in 80 percent survival compared to 84 percent with no complications.[57]

Data collected from members of ELSO document that physiologic complications occur in approximately 63 percent of ECMO candidates. Neurologic complications (seizures, cerebral infarction) predominate (24 percent). Hemorrhagic complications (bleeding, hemolysis)

account for 21 percent, cardiopulmonary complications (cardiac arrest, pulmonary hypertension, pneumothorax, arrhythmias) for 17 percent, renal complications (creatinine >1.5 mg percent, use of dialysis/hemofiltration) for 14 percent, and metabolic complications (electrolyte imbalances, pH derangement) for 8 percent.[57]

Overall, 37 percent of ECMO patients have had no medical complications. Survival among these infants was significantly better than among those in whom one or more medical complications was present (95 versus 76 percent).[57]

A comparison of the complication rates of infants treated prior to 1984 to those of infants treated between 1984 and 1989 indicated that the annual rate of technical and medical complications has decreased. This reflects decreasing morbidity despite the rapidly expanding numbers of infants treated and new ECMO centers.[57]

When researchers compared complication data from venovenous ECMO to that from venoarterial ECMO, they found the incidence of neurologic complications was greater in the venoarterial group than in the venovenous double-lumen group, as was the incidence of symptomatic patent ductus arteriosus. Hemorrhage and mechanical complications were similar. Catheter kinking was limited to use of the double-lumen catheter. The increased rate of complications in the VA group reflects the fact that patients treated with venoarterial bypass are more unstable at the outset of ECMO.[51]

THE ECMO TEAM

The complex and challenging care of infants on ECMO requires a highly trained and skilled team of professionals that includes a physician, perfusionist, neonatal intensive care nurse, and ECMO specialist. The most important factor in maintaining ECMO for days or weeks is the team. Maintaining the procedure without mistakes requires constant, diligent concentration.

TABLE 14-4 ▲ Nursing Responsibilities and Interventions for ECMO

Prior to Cannulation

Responsibility	Intervention
Obtain and document baseline physiologic data	Record weight, length, head circumference.
	Draw blood samples for complete blood count (CBC), electrolytes, calcium, glucose, BUN, creatinine, PT/PTT, platelets, arterial blood gases.
	Record vital signs: heart rate, respiratory rate, systolic, diastolic, mean blood pressure, temperature.
Assure adequate supply of blood products for replacement	Draw type-and-cross match samples for two units of packed red cells, fresh frozen plasma.
	Keep one unit of packed cells and fresh frozen plasma always available in the blood bank.
Maintain prescribed pulmonary support	Maintain ventilator parameters.
	Administer muscle relaxants if indicated.
Assemble and prepare equipment	Prepare infusion pumps to maintain arterial lines and infusion of parenteral fluids and medications into the ECMO circuit.
	Place the infant on a radiant warmer with the head positioned at the foot of the bed to provide thermoregulation and access for cannulation.
	Attach infant to physiologic monitoring devices to monitor heart rate, intra-arterial blood pressure, transcutaneous oxygen, and other parameters.
	Insert urinary catheter and nasogastric tube; place to gravity drainage.
	Remove intravenous lines just prior to heparinization (optional).
	Prepare loading dose of heparin (50–100 units/kg).
	Prepare heparin solution for continuous infusion (100 units/ml/D$_5$W).
	Prepare paralyzing drug (pancuronium bromide, 0.1 mg/kg, or succinylcholine, 1–4 mg/kg).
	Assist in insertion of arterial line (umbilical or peripheral).
	Administer prophylactic antibiotics.

During Cannulation

Monitor cardiopulmonary status during procedure	Monitor heart rate and intra-arterial blood pressure continuously.
	Obtain blood gases after paralysis and during cannulation, as indicated by the infant's response to the procedure.
Be prepared to administer cardiopulmonary support	Have medications and blood products available to correct hypovolemia, bradycardia, acidosis, cardiac arrest.
Administer medications	Give loading dose of heparin systemically when vessels are dissected free and are ready to be cannulated.
	Give paralyzing drug systemically just prior to cannulation of internal jugular vein if infant has not been previously paralyzed.
Reduce ventilator parameters to minimal settings	Once adequate bypass is achieved, reduce PIP to 16–20 cm H$_2$O, PEEP to 4 cm H$_2$O, ventilator rate to 10–20 breaths per minute, and FiO$_2$ to 21–30%. Venovenous bypass patients may require greater respiratory support.

(continued on page 361)

Providing this mode of care is not feasible for many hospitals because of the expense and commitment involved in training personnel. The training of an ECMO specialist alone requires a minimum of 50–80 hours of class and laboratory work.

Both a nurse and an ECMO specialist are assigned to care for the ECMO patient each shift. The nurse is responsible for ongoing assessment, hemodynamic monitoring, data collection, administration of fluids and medications, and pulmonary care. The ECMO

TABLE 14-4 ▲ **Nursing Responsibilities and Interventions for ECMO** (continued)

During ECMO Run

Responsibility	Intervention
Monitor and document physiologic parameters	Record hourly: heart rate, blood pressure (systolic, diastolic, mean), respirations, temperature, transcutaneous PO_2, CO_2, oxygen saturation, activated clotting time (ACT), ECMO flow.
	Measure hourly accurate intake and output of all body fluids (urine, gastric contents, blood); measure every four hours: urine pH, protein, glucose, specific gravity; hematest all stools.
	Assess hourly: color, breath sounds, heart tones, murmurs, cardiac rhythm, arterial pressure waveform (Figure 14-4), peripheral perfusion.
	Perform hourly: neurologic check, including fontanel tension, pupil size and reaction, level of consciousness, reflexes, tone, and movement of extremities.
	Record ventilator parameters hourly.
	Assess weight and head circumference daily.
Monitor and document biochemical parameters	Draw arterial blood gases from umbilical or peripheral line as indicated.
	All other blood specimens are drawn from the ECMO circuit by the ECMO specialist: electrolytes, calcium, platelets, Chemstrip, hematocrit every four to eight hours, CBC, PT/PTT, BUN, creatinine, total and direct bilirubin, plasma hemoglobin, fibrinogen, fibrin split products, and blood culture as indicated.
Administer medications	Remove air bubbles and double-check dosages before infusion.
	Administer no medications IM or by venipuncture.
	Place all medications and fluids into the venous side of the ECMO circuit.
	Prepare and administer the arterial line (umbilical or peripheral) infusion.
	Administer parenteral alimentation.
Provide pulmonary support	Perform endotracheal suctioning based on individual assessment and need.
	Maintain patent airway; be alert to extubation or plugging.
	Obtain daily chest films and tracheal aspirate cultures as indicated.
	Maintain ventilator parameters.
Prevent bleeding	Avoid all of the following: rectal probes, injections, venipunctures, heelsticks, cuff blood pressures, chest tube stripping, restraints, chest percussion.
	Avoid invasive procedures: Do not change nasogastric tube, urinary catheters, or endotracheal tube unless absolutely necessary; use premeasured endotracheal tube suction technique.
	Observe for blood in the urine, stools, endotracheal or nasogastric tubes.
Maintain excellent infection control	Change all fluids and tubing daily.
	Change dressings daily and PRN.
	Clean urinary catheter site daily.
	Maintain strict aseptic and hand washing techniques.
	Use universal barrier precautions.
Provide physical care	Keep skin dry, clean, and free from pressure points.
	Give mouth care PRN.
	Provide range of motion as indicated.
	Turn side to side every one to two hours.
Provide pain management, sedation, stress reduction	Minimize noise level.
	Cluster patient care to maximize sleep period.
	Administer analgesia: fentanyl 9–18 µg/kg/hour (increased dosage due to fentanyl binding to membrane oxygenator).
	Manage iatrogenic physical dependency by following a dose reduction regime (reduce dose 10% every 4 hours)[73]
Be alert to complications and emergencies	See Tables 14-2 and 14-3.

Adapted from: Nugent J. 1986. Extracorporeal membrane oxygenation in the neonate. *Neonatal Network* 4(5): 34–35. Reprinted by permission.

TABLE 14-5 ▲ ECMO Specialist Responsibilities and Interventions

Responsibility	Intervention
Maintain and monitor ECMO circuit	Check circuit carefully for air, clots, tightness of connectors, stopcocks.
	Check bladder box alarm function.
	Monitor pump arterial and venous blood gases each shift to assess oxygenator function. Pump arterial PO_2 less than 100 mmHg, CO_2 retention, or leaking membrane indicates oxygenator failure.
Assess infant	Check cannula placement and stability.
	Assess breath sounds, neurologic status.
	Observe volume of fluid and blood drainage.
	Monitor vital signs and lab values.
Maintain prescribed parameters: pH 7.35–7.45 PaO_2 60–80 mmHg (VA) PaO_2 50 mmHg (VV) $PaCO_2$ 35–45 mmHg $\overline{Paw}$ 45–55 mmHg Hct 45–55% Platelets 70–100,000/mm³ SvO_2 >70% SaO_2 >90% (VA) SaO_2 >85% (VV) ACT 180–250 seconds	Maintain infant's systemic arterial blood gases by adjusting sweep gas and pump flow.
	Maintain mean arterial blood pressure, hematocrit, and adequate platelet count by infusion of appropriate blood products.
	Assess ACT hourly or PRN; titrate heparin infusion to maintain parameters.
Assist nurse in care	Draw *all* blood samples from circuit except systemic arterial blood gases.
	Coordinate recording of intake and output with nurse.
	Assist in all position changes.
	Administer and monitor all medications, blood products, and fluids placed into the pump circuit.
Be prepared to deal with pump emergencies	See Tables 14-2 and 14-3.

Adapted from: Nugent J. 1986. Extracorporeal membrane oxygenation in the neonate. *Neonatal Network* 4(5): 36. Reprinted by permission.

specialist is responsible for checking and monitoring the circuit, adjusting gas and pump flow, maintaining heparinization, administering appropriate blood products, drawing blood specimens, and documenting data.

The nurse practice acts in many states will not allow the nurse to delegate administration of medications and blood products to non-licensed personnel; hence this responsibility rests with the nurse if the ECMO specialist is not a registered nurse. Tables 14-4 and 14-5 outline nursing and ECMO specialist responsibilities and interventions.

WEANING AND DECANNULATION

Signs of improvement and indicators suggesting that the infant is ready to be weaned from ECMO consist of improvement of lung fields as seen on chest films, clinical findings of weight loss, improved aeration via chest auscultation, rising oxygen pressure (PaO_2 and SaO_2), and improved lung compliance. When the infant is initially on bypass, the lungs on x-ray examination appear opaque with variable volume loss; as pulmonary function improves, the lung fields begin to clear. Improvement shown on chest x-ray films usually lags behind clinical improvement.[58]

Weight loss, which results in a return to baseline, demonstrates a loss of excess extracellular fluid and often heralds improvement in pulmonary function. As the primary pathology resolves and pulmonary function improves, oxygenation in the fraction of the cardiac output traversing the lungs improves. This is indicated by a rise in the systemic PaO_2.

End-tidal carbon dioxide tension ($PetCO_2$) monitoring is useful for following improvement in lung function. After cannulation and prior to improvement in lung functioning, $PetCO_2$ will be lower than $PaCO_2$ because of impaired gas exchange. As pulmonary function improves, $PetCO_2$ values increase and are equal to $PaCO_2$.

Research has demonstrated that changes in lung compliance can be a sensitive indicator of a neonate's lung improvement while on ECMO. Lotze, Short, and Taylor demonstrated that lung compliance measurements can be used to monitor clinical course and improvement as well as to predict the patient's successful removal from bypass.[59]

Employment of sensitive measures of lung function, such as lung compliance, can be very useful in the weaning process and could potentially shorten total time on bypass. This is particularly important when the infant's condition warrants immediate cessation of bypass but arterial blood gas measurements are marginal, as when there is excessive bleeding. Continued clinical research in this area is needed.

Once improvement in pulmonary gas exchange has been ascertained, weaning the infant by decreasing the flow rate in small (10–20 ml) increments is begun. Decreasing the flow rate diverts less blood into the extracorporeal circuit and increases blood flow to the infant's lungs. The flow is decreased in this manner, usually over a period of days, until extracorporeal support is no longer needed to maintain adequate gas exchange at low ventilator settings. Weaning from venovenous bypass can be accomplished by decreasing the FiO_2 of the sweep gas and/or reducing pump flow.

When the flow rate is decreased to 50 ml/kg/minute, a state of "idling" is achieved. The infant will remain at this lowest possible flow rate for four to eight hours. Heparinization must be maintained for as long as the catheters are in place. During the idling period, the heparin infusion may need to be switched to the patient to maintain appropriate activated clotting time levels. If the infant's condition deteriorates, extracorporeal flow is increased, and support of the infant is resumed.

If improvement of lung function remains stable at low ventilator settings during idling, a test period with the infant off ECMO is attempted. The cannulas are clamped, and the circuit is slowly recirculated via the bridge to prevent stagnation. If it has not already been done during idling, the heparin infusion is now switched to the patient. The gas flow into the oxygenator is discontinued, the heat exchanger temperature is decreased, and all infusions into the ECMO circuit are discontinued and switched to the patient.[38]

Decannulation can proceed if blood gas values remain satisfactory (SaO_2 >90 percent on <50 percent FiO_2, $PetCO_2$ of 40 mmHg). The same preparation and equipment needed for cannulation are made available. Under local anesthesia, cannulas are removed and vessels ligated or repaired.

Until recently, the artery and vein have not been repaired because of significant post-ECMO risk of thrombus formation and embolization at the cannulation site.[60] However, studies indicate that carotid reconstruction can be performed safely with no significant morbidity or mortality in select ECMO patients.[61–63] Long-term follow-up of patients undergoing carotid repair will be needed to determine the efficacy of this procedure.

Succinylcholine or pancuronium bromide is given to the infant before decannulation to prevent air embolization. The ventilator settings are increased to compensate for loss of the infant's own ability to ventilate because of drug-induced paralysis.

After decannulation, the infant is weaned as tolerated from mechanical ventilation. Heparin reversal is usually not warranted because heparin is metabolized in a few hours. Once the infant's activated clotting time is within normal limits, routine NICU care can resume. Transfusions to correct anemia are frequently required during the first 24 hours after ECMO. Platelet counts should be followed closely because thrombocytopenia may persist for up to four days following decannulation.[54]

PARENTAL SUPPORT

Support of the family of the infant undergoing ECMO presents some unique challenges. Parents are usually in crisis: Their infant has been critically ill since birth, and they are aware that his chances for survival are poor. Parents are informed that the ECMO procedure itself is a method of last resort with no guarantee of positive outcome. The technical environment is overwhelming. It is not unusual to find the parent grieving and in a state of withdrawal.

Support should be given by listening, communicating, educating, and providing parent-infant and parent-parent support. Parents need continuous communication of concise, accurate information about their child's condition and the required procedures. They should be allowed access to their infant, and the staff should be empathetic and as reassuring as the situation will allow.

Parent-to-parent support utilizing parents whose infant has experienced ECMO is efficacious and a positive experience for all involved families. Parent support groups on local and national levels have been established to educate and assist ECMO parents. As proficiency with ECMO technology improves, the ECMO candidate has an increasingly better chance for survival, and every effort must be made to encourage parental involvement and bonding.

FOLLOW-UP AND OUTCOME

The survival rate for infants treated with ECMO is steadily improving, and in centers that provide this therapy, it is a feasible life-saving measure for neonates who might otherwise die. To date, overall survival of infants treated with ECMO is 80 percent. Survival of ECMO-treated infants with various pathologies is as follows: meconium aspiration, 94 percent; RDS, 84 percent; congenital diaphragmatic hernia, 58 percent; sepsis/pneumonia, 77 percent; and PPHN, 82 percent.[30]

Annual survival rates for infants supported with ECMO increased from 56 percent in 1981 to 86 percent in 1987 and have remained statistically unchanged. Survival rates for infants with all entry diagnoses have improved except for those with congenital diaphragmatic hernia. Even with the rapidly expanding numbers of infants treated and new ECMO centers, it is encouraging to see sustained excellent survival.[57]

Critical scrutiny of survivors is essential to properly assess the value and safety of the technique. Neonatal ECMO survivors are followed closely for possible complications caused by hypoxia and acidosis occurring both before and during the procedure. Survivors are systematically and periodically evaluated for the following parameters: growth and development, cardiorespiratory development, cerebrovascular status, and neurologic and psychological functioning. Early intervention and remediation are made possible if disabilities are identified.

In early follow-up studies, physical growth and development as well as cardiorespiratory development were reported as normal. All infants showed evidence of adequate cerebral blood flow to both hemispheres, despite the necessity of carotid artery ligation.[16,48] Ligation of the right carotid artery and internal jugular vein was not associated with a consistent lateralizing lesion.[64] Neurologic competence appropriate for age was reported in 83 percent of survivors in one study and 75 percent in another.[16,48]

Two recent long-term studies evaluating neonatal ECMO survivors have shown them to do at least as well neurologically and developmentally as comparable patients treated without ECMO.[65,66] A truly legitimate cohort of newborns who could compare with ECMO survivors does not exist because this group should have 80 percent mortality. Lacking this comparison group, one can only compare outcome in the ECMO-supported group with survivors of neonatal respiratory failure and PPHN treated with conventional therapy. Infants with respiratory failure and PPHN demonstrate impairment rates from 0 to 32 percent, with 18.6 percent having sustained neurologic and/or cognitive impairment.[65]

Schumacher and colleagues assessed the developmental outcome of 92 infants treated with ECMO from 1981 to 1987 and reported a handicap rate of 20 percent. Abnormal neurodevelopmental outcome was significantly associated with cerebral infarction and chronic lung disease. A disproportionate number of children in the oldest age group was handicapped. Eliminating these children from the study lowered the handicap rate to 16 percent, demonstrating that morbidity improves with experience.[65]

Differentiation between pre-existing deficits and those secondary to ECMO manipulation can be difficult. The functional normalcy of the majority of the survivors is encouraging and demonstrates that ECMO support can be accomplished safely and that subsequent normal development is possible.

With increasing experience, mortality rates have decreased, and it should be expected that morbidity will also decrease. Improvement in pre-ECMO management, selection criteria, and ECMO management should contribute to lower morbidity. However, enthusiasm for this procedure must be tempered by careful consideration of the inherent morbidity and mortality risks.

Centers using ECMO must be actively involved in ECMO research if further refinements in technique and reduction of morbidity and mortality are to be forthcoming. Researchers are seeking ways to eliminate the need for heparinization.[32,43] This would allow application of the technique to low birth weight infants by decreasing the risk of intracranial hemorrhage.

Research has substantiated the advantage of initiating ECMO support early in the neonate's disease rather than using it as a last resort.[31] Researchers reason that medical costs could be reduced and cardiorespiratory and neurologic outcome improved if intervention were not deferred until 80 percent or greater mortality was predicted.[16] With the advent of venovenous double-lumen bypass and avoidance of carotid ligation, it may be anticipated that entry criteria for ECMO support will be liberalized. Infants will be treated earlier in the course of respiratory failure, the need for total support will lessen, and morbidity and mortality will improve.[43]

As the number of ECMO centers escalates, it becomes mandatory to analyze morbidity data as they relate to quality of survival. Enthusiasm for this technique has promoted concern that ECMO centers are being established without a thorough understanding of the complexity, hazards, and uncertainties of this therapy. The American Academy of Pediatrics' Committee on Fetus and Newborn has published recommendations for ECMO centers that describe the rationale for establishing the need for a center as well as required institutional criteria.[67] Regionalization of ECMO centers is recommended to accommodate patient bed needs and provide a milieu of safe and effective ECMO care.[64]

REFERENCES

1. Chatburn R. 1984. High frequency ventilation: A report on a state of the art symposium. *Respiratory Care* 29: 839.

2. Bancalari E, and Goldberg RN. 1987. High-frequency ventilation in the neonate. *Clinics in Perinatology* 14(3): 581–597.

3. Krummel T, et al. 1982. Extracorporeal membrane oxygenation in neonatal pulmonary failure. *Pediatric Annals* 11(11): 905–908.

4. Drummond W, et al. 1981. The independent effects of hyperventilation, tolazoline and dopamine on infants with persistent pulmonary hypertension. *Journal of Pediatrics* 98(4): 603–611.

5. Ormagabal M, Kirkpatrick B, and Muellar D. 1980. Alteration of A-aDO$_2$ in response to tolazoline as a predictor of outcome in neonates with persistent pulmonary hypertension. *Pediatric Respiration* 14: 607.

6. Levin DL. 1980. Effects of inhibition of prostaglandin synthesis on fetal development, oxygenation, and the fetal circulation. *Seminars in Perinatology* 4(1): 35–44.

7. Lyrener RK, et al. 1985. Alkalosis attenuates hypoxic pulmonary vasoconstriction in neonatal lambs. *Pediatric Research* 19(12): 1268–1271.

8. Gluck L, and Nugent J. 1991. Surfactant replacement. In *Acute Respiratory Care of the Neonate,* Nugent J, ed. Petaluma, California: NICU INK, 185–196.

9. Kinsella J, et al. 1992. Low-dose inhalational nitric oxide in persistent pulmonary hypertension of the newborn. *Lancet* 340(8823): 819–820.

10. Kinsella J, et al. 1993. Clinical response to prolonged treatment of persistent pulmonary hypertension of the newborn with low doses of inhaled nitric oxide. *Journal of Pediatrics* 123(1): 103–108.

11. Ordiz R, Cillary R, and Bartlett R. 1987. Extracorporeal membrane oxygenation in pediatric respiratory failure. *Pediatric Clinics of North America* 34(1): 39–46.

12. Rashkind W, et al. 1965. Evaluation of a disposable plastic low flow volume pumpless oxygenator as a lung substitute. *Journal of Pediatrics* 66(1): 94–102.

13. Dorson W, et al. 1969. A perfusion system for infants. *Transactions—American Society for Artificial Internal Organs* 15: 155–157.

14. White J, et al. 1971. Prolonged respiratory support in newborn infants with a membrane oxygenator. *Surgery* 70(2): 288–296.

15. Pyle R, et al. 1975. Clinical use of membrane oxygenation. *Archives of Surgery* 110: 966–970.

16. Bartlett R. 1984. Extracorporeal oxygenation in neonates. *Hospital Practice* 19(4): 139–151.

17. Kolobow T, Zapol W, and Pierce J. 1969. High survival and minimal blood damage in lambs exposed to long term (1 week) veno-venous pumping with a polyurethane chamber roller pump with and without a membrane blood oxygenator. *Transactions—American Society for Artificial Internal Organs* 15: 172–173.

18. Kolobow T, et al. 1974. Superior blood compatibility of silicone rubber free of silica filler in the membrane lung. *Transactions—American Society for Artificial Internal Organs* 20: 269A–276A.

19. Kolobow T, Stool E, and Pierce J. 1976. Longterm perfusion with the membrane lung in lambs. In *Artificial Lungs for Acute Respiratory Failure: Theory and Practice,* Zapol WM, and Qvist J, eds. New York: Academic Press, 234–242.

20. Bartlett R, et al. 1982. Extracorporeal membrane oxygenation for newborn respiratory failure: Forty-five cases. *Surgery* 92(2): 425–433.

21. Bartlett RH, et al. 1976. Extracorporeal membrane oxygenation (ECMO) cardiopulmonary support in infancy. *Transactions—American Society for Artificial Internal Organs* 22: 80–93.

22. Bartlett R, et al. 1985. Extracorporeal circulation in neonatal respiratory failure: A prospective randomized study. *Pediatrics* 76(4): 479–487.

23. Hardesty R, et al. 1981. Extracorporeal membrane oxygenation: Successful treatment of persistent fetal circulation following repair of congenital diaphragmatic hernia. *Journal of Thoracic and Cardiovascular Surgery* 81(4): 556–569.

24. Wetmore N, et al. 1979. Defining indications for artificial organ support in respiratory failure. *Transactions—American Society for Artificial Internal Organs* 25: 459–461.

25. Kirkpatrick B, et al. 1983. Use of extracorporeal membrane oxygenation for respiratory failure in term infants. *Pediatrics* 72(6): 872–876.

26. Rapherty R, and Downes J. 1973. Congenital diaphragmatic hernia: Prediction of survival. *Journal of Pediatric Surgery* 8(5): 815–818.

27. Paneth N, and Wallenstein S. 1985. Extracorporeal membrane oxygenation and the play the winner rule. *Pediatrics* 76(4): 622–623.

28. Ware J, and Epstein M. 1985. Extracorporeal circulation in respiratory failure: A prospective randomized study. *Pediatrics* 76(5): 849–851.

29. O'Rourke P, et al. 1989. Extracorporeal membrane oxygenation and conventional medical therapy in neonates with persistent pulmonary hypertension of the newborn: A prospective randomized study. *Pediatrics* 84(6): 957–963.

30. Neonatal ECMO Registry 1996. Report of the Extracorporeal Life Support Organization, July. Unpublished data.

31. Bartlett R, et al. 1986. Extracorporeal membrane oxygenation (ECMO) in neonatal respiratory failure. *Annals of Surgery* 204(3): 236–245.

32. Bartlett R, et al. 1989. Prospective randomized study of cost effectiveness of neonatal ECMO. Ann Arbor, Michigan: ELSO chapter meeting, October.

33. Marsh D, Wilkerson S, and Cook L. 1988. Extracorporeal membrane oxygenation selection criteria: Partial pressure of arterial oxygenation versus alveolar-arterial oxygen gradient. *Pediatrics* 82(2): 162–166.

34. Klein M, et al. 1990. Extracorporeal membrane oxygenation for the circulatory support of children after repair of congenital heart disease. *Journal of Thoracic and Cardiovascular Surgery* 100(4): 498–505.

35. Hunkeler NM, et al. 1992. Extracorporeal life support in cyanotic congenital heart disease before cardiovascular operation. *American Journal of Cardiology* 69(8): 790–793.

36. von Alleman D, and Ryckman FC. 1991. Cardiac arrest in the ECMO candidate. *Journal of Pediatric Surgery* 26(2): 143–146.

37. O'Rourke PP. 1993. ECMO: Current status. *Neonatal Respiratory Diseases* 3(3): 1–11.

38. Chapman R, Toomasian J, and Bartlett R. 1988. *Extracorporeal Membrane Oxygenation Technical Specialist Manual.* Ann Arbor: University of Michigan Press.

39. Klein MD, et al. 1985. Venovenous perfusion in ECMO for newborn respiratory insufficiency: A Clinical comparison with venoarterial perfusion. *Annals of Surgery* 201(4): 520–526.

40. Andrews A, et al. 1983. Venovenous extracorporeal membrane oxygenation in neonates with respiratory failure. *Journal of Pediatric Surgery* 18(4): 339–346.

41. Zwischenberger JB, et al. 1985. Total respiratory support with single cannula venovenous ECMO: Double lumen continuous flow versus single lumen tidal flow. *Transactions—American Society for Artificial Internal Organs* 31: 610–615.

42. Anderson HL, et al. 1989. Venovenous extracorporeal life support in neonates using a double lumen catheter. *Transactions—American Society for Artificial Internal Organs* 35(3): 650–653.

43. Cornish JD, et al. 1993. Extracorporeal membrane oxygenation service at Egleston: Two year's experience. *Journal of the Medical Association of Georgia* 82: 471–475.

44. Karr SS, Martin GR, and Short BL. 1991. Cardiac performance in infants referred for extracorporeal membrane oxygenation. *Journal of Pediatrics* 118(3): 437–442.

45. Strieper MJ, et al. 1993. Effects of venovenous extracorporeal membrane oxygenation on cardiac performance as determined by echocardiographic measurements. *Journal of Pediatrics* 122(6): 950–955.

46. Bartlett RH, and Gazzaniga AB. 1978. Extracorporeal circulation for cardiopulmonary failure. *Current Problems in Surgery* 15(5): 1–96.

47. Rivera K, et al. 1990. Maximum flow rates for arterial cannulae used in neonatal ECMO (abstract). Sixth Annual Children's Hospital—National Medical Center—ECMO Symposium, February.

48. Krummel T, et al. 1984. The early evaluation of survivors after extracorporeal membrane oxygenation for neonatal pulmonary failure. *Journal of Pediatric Surgery* 19(5): 585–589.

49. German J, et al. 1980. Technical aspects in the management of the meconium aspiration syndrome with extracorporeal circulation. *Journal of Pediatric Surgery* 15(4): 378–383.

50. Bartlett R, and Gazzaniga A. 1980. Physiology and pathophysiology of extracorporeal membrane circulation. In *Techniques in Extracorporeal Circulation,* Ionescu M, ed. Boston: Butterworths, 1–43.

51. Anderson HL, et al. 1993. Multicenter comparison of conventional venoarterial access versus venovenous double-lumen catheter access in newborn infants undergoing extracorporeal membrane oxygenation. *Journal of Pediatric Surgery* 28(4): 530–535.

52. Kinsella JP, Gerstmann DR, and Rosenberg AA. 1992. The effect of extracorporeal membrane oxygenation on coronary perfusion and regional blood flow distribution. *Pediatric Research* 31(1): 80–83.

53. Meliones JN, et al. 1991. Hemodynamic instability after the initiation of extracorporeal membrane oxygenation: Role of ionized calcium. *Critical Care Medicine* 19(10): 1247–1251.

54. Anderson H, et al. 1986. Thrombocytopenia in neonates after extracorporeal membrane oxygenation. *Transactions—American Society for Artificial Internal Organs* 32: 534–537.

55. Anderson KD. 1993. Extracorporeal membrane oxygenation. As cited in Ashcraft KW, and Holder TM. *Pediatric Surgery,* 2nd ed. Philadelphia: WB Saunders, 967.

56. Heiss K, et al. 1987. Renal insufficiency and volume overload in neonatal ECMO managed by continuous ultrafiltration. *Transactions—American Society for Artificial Internal Organs* 33: 557–560.

57. Stolar CJH, Snedecor SM, and Bartlett RH. 1991. Extracorporeal membrane oxygenation and neonatal respiratory failure: Experience from the Extracorporeal Life Support Organization. *Journal of Pediatric Surgery* 26(5): 563–571.

58. Taylor G, Short B, and Driesmar P. 1986. Extracorporeal membrane oxygenation: Radiologic appearance of the neonatal chest. *American Journal of Roentgenology* 146: 1257–1259.

59. Lotze A, Short B, and Taylor G. 1987. Lung compliance as a measure of lung function in newborns with respiratory failure requiring extracorporeal membrane oxygenation. *Critical Care Medicine* 15(3): 226–229.

60. Anderson HL, et al. 1991. Venovenous extracorporeal membrane oxygenation in neonates using the double lumen catheter: Summary of 62 cases (abstract). Seventh Annual Children's Hospital—National Medical Center—ECMO Symposium, February.

61. Spector ML, et al. 1991. Carotid artery reconstruction in the neonate: Discharge data and eighteen month follow-up (abstract). Seventh Annual Children's Hospital—National Medical Center—ECMO Symposium, February.

62. Moulton SL, et al. 1991. Carotid artery reconstruction following neonatal extracorporeal membrane oxygenation. *Journal of Pediatric Surgery* 26(7): 794–799.

63. Riggs P, et al. 1991. Repair following ECMO: Colorflow doppler studies (abstract). Seventh Annual Children's Hospital—National Medical Center—ECMO Symposium, February.

64. Glass P, Miller M, and Short B. 1989. Morbidity for survivors of extracorporeal membrane oxygenation: Neurodevelopmental outcome at 1 year of age. *Pediatrics* 83(1): 72–78.

65. Schumacher MD, et al. 1991. Follow-up of infants treated with extracorporeal membrane oxygenation for newborn respiratory failure. *Pediatrics* 87(4): 451–457.

66. Hofkosh D, et al. 1991. Ten years of extracorporeal membrane oxygenation: Neurodevelopmental outcome. *Pediatrics* 87(4): 549–555.

67. American Academy of Pediatrics Committee on Fetus and Newborn. 1990. Recommendations on extracorporeal membrane oxygenation. *Pediatrics* 85(4): 618–619.

68. Andrews A, Bartlett R, and Roloff D. 1982. Mortality risk graphs for neonates with respiratory distress (abstract). *Pediatric Respiration* 16: 275A.

69. Beck R, Anderson KD, and Pearson GD. 1986. Criteria for extracorporeal membrane oxygenation in a population of infants with persistent pulmonary hypertension of the newborn. *Journal of Pediatric Surgery* 21(4): 297–302.

70. Wilson JM, et al. 1993. Amicar decreased the incidence of intracranial hemorrhage and other hemorrhagic complications of ECMO. *Journal of Pediatric Surgery* 28(4): 536–640.

71. Bohn D, et al. 1987. Ventilatory predictors of pulmonary hypoplasia in congenital diaphragmatic hernia, confirmed by morphologic assessment. *Journal of Pediatrics* 111(3): 423–431.

72. Martin G. 1993. Cardiac changes during prolonged extracorporeal membrane oxygenation. In *Extracorporeal Life Support*, Arenemen R, and Cornish D, eds. Boston: Blackwell Scientific Publications, 136.

73. Caron E, and Maguire DP. 1990. Current management of pain, sedation and narcotic physical dependency of the infant on ECMO. *Journal of Perinatal and Neonatal Nursing* 4(1): 63–74.

NOTES

15 The Role of Inhaled Nitric Oxide in Persistent Pulmonary Hypertension of the Newborn

John P. Kinsella, MD
Steven H. Abman, MD

Although persistent pulmonary hypertension of the newborn (PPHN) may occur as a discrete pathophysiologic disturbance (idiopathic PPHN), it more commonly complicates the course of various neonatal cardiopulmonary diseases, such as meconium aspiration syndrome, Group B streptococcal sepsis, and congenital diaphragmatic hernia.[1,2] Despite the diversity of clinical conditions accompanying PPHN, marked pulmonary hypertension and altered pulmonary vasoreactivity are its central pathophysiologic features. High pulmonary vascular resistance (PVR) results in right-to-left shunting of blood across the patent ductus arteriosus and foramen ovale, often causing critical hypoxemia.

Current therapy to reduce pulmonary hypertension includes mechanical hyperventilation, alkalosis, hyperoxia, and vasodilator drug therapy.[3] Attempts at reducing PVR with hyperventilation and hyperoxia may cause severe lung injury, contributing to further morbidity and mortality of PPHN. In addition, pulmonary vasodilator drug therapy is often unsuccessful because of concomitant systemic hypotension and an inability to achieve or sustain pulmonary vasodilation.[3] Indeed, effective treatment of PPHN has suffered from the lack of an agent that can effect *selective* and *sustained* pulmonary vasodilation.

Breakthroughs in vascular biology have provided exciting insights into such an agent. In response to physiologic and pharmacologic stimuli, the human vascular endothelium produces a short-acting substance—endothelium-derived relaxing factor (EDRF)—that diffuses to the vascular smooth muscle and causes vasodilation.[4,5] This factor has been identified as nitric oxide (NO), which has subsequently been shown to play important roles in both the physiologic control of vascular tone and the pathophysiology of many disease states.[6]

Recent reports suggest a potential clinical role for inhaled nitric oxide gas in the treatment of infants with severe PPHN. This chapter discusses the complex problem of PPHN, reviews the background investigations that led to the use of inhaled nitric oxide in infants with PPHN, and discusses the clinical studies of inhaled nitric oxide in the treatment of PPHN.

CLINICAL PRESENTATION

The newborn with PPHN often shows signs of respiratory distress, including tachypnea, retractions, and nasal flaring. Differential cyanosis may result from right-to-left shunting of blood across the patent ductus arteriosus, causing the delivery of desaturated blood to the lower body. However, this phenomenon is rarely apparent clinically if cardiac output is adequate.

Preductal (right arm) and postductal (lower extremity) oxygen saturation measurements will provide information about the presence of right-to-left shunting of blood across the ductus arteriosus. In infants with PPHN, postductal oxygen saturation levels will often be lower than preductal levels. For those infants in whom the extrapulmonary shunting occurs predominantly at the level of the foramen ovale, however, the preductal and postductal arterial saturation levels will be equal. Both infants with severe PPHN and those with severe parenchymal lung disease may present with low arterial partial pressure of oxygen in arterial blood (PaO$_2$) in high inspired oxygen.

The presence of a cardiac murmur should alert the clinician to the possibility of congenital heart disease; however, tricuspid regurgitation is often associated with PPHN and can produce a heart murmur. In patients with PPHN, tricuspid regurgitation is caused by increased right ventricular pressure due to high pulmonary vascular resistance. The murmur of tricuspid regurgitation often sounds like that of a ventricular septal defect: harsh and at the mid-left sternal border. In infants with PPHN, the second heart sound is often single and of increased intensity.

Initial laboratory tests should include evaluation for sepsis, polycythemia, hypoglycemia, and hypocalcemia. The chest radiograph is essential in determining the presence of parenchymal lung disease, heart size, relative pulmonary blood flow, and adequacy of lung inflation by mechanical ventilation. Although PPHN should be considered when the severity of hypoxemia is out of proportion to the

degree of pulmonary disease by chest radiograph, many conditions characterized by severe lung disease are also complicated by PPHN.

Although the previously described findings are helpful in the initial assessment of the cyanotic newborn, PPHN often cannot be reliably diagnosed clinically. However, structural heart disease can be ruled out and the contribution of pulmonary hypertension to systemic hypoxemia can be accurately measured with echocardiography. Two-dimensional echocardiography alone is often sufficient to diagnose many cyanotic heart lesions.

Two lesions that share clinical characteristics with PPHN may be difficult to diagnose. Total anomalous pulmonary venous return may be difficult to diagnose by echocardiography alone, and coarctation of the aorta may not be well defined when the ductus arteriosus is widely patent.

In most patients with PPHN, there are "windows" on the pulmonary vascular bed that can be used for noninvasive determination of relative systemic-pulmonary vascular resistances.[7] Pulsed-doppler and color-doppler studies are important tools in the diagnosis of PPHN. Doppler studies can be used to describe the direction of shunting at the patent ductus arteriosus and the foramen ovale. *Right-to-left or bidirectional shunting at the ductal and/or atrial level in a structurally normal heart defines PPHN.* Pulsed-doppler and continuous wave–doppler studies can be used to measure the peak velocity of the tricuspid insufficiency jet. This measurement can be used to reliably estimate the peak pulmonary artery pressure by employing the modified Bernoulli equation:

4 (peak velocity tricuspid regurgitation jet)^2 + central venous pressure

The actual value is not as important as the relationship of the pulmonary artery pressure to simultaneously measured systemic arterial pressure.

MANAGEMENT

Descriptions of PPHN management have commonly focused on the subset of patients with idiopathic PPHN. They have pulmonary hypertension of variable severity *without* concomitant lung disease. However, PPHN frequently occurs with the more common causes of neonatal respiratory distress, including disorders characterized by moderate to severe lung disease (such as meconium aspiration and bacterial pneumonia). Therefore, the therapeutic approach to PPHN requires meticulous attention to all aspects of the cardiopulmonary perturbations (pulmonary hypertension, decreased cardiac performance, and parenchymal lung disease) that characterize this syndrome.

Because of the diverse nature of diseases associated with PPHN, no single therapeutic approach will be effective in all patients. In general, the management goals for the infant with PPHN are as follows:

1. Reduce pulmonary vascular resistance.
2. Optimize lung inflation and treat any underlying pulmonary disease.
3. Sustain cardiac performance and systemic hemodynamic stability.

Systemic hypotension should be promptly treated, initially with volume infusion of a colloid solution (such as 5 percent albumin, Plasmanate, or fresh frozen plasma) in 10 ml/kg increments. Fresh frozen plasma is the solution of choice if there is evidence of a coagulopathy—prolonged prothrombin time, thrombocytopenia, clinical signs of bleeding diathesis. Although adequate systemic blood flow and substrate delivery should be determined by end-organ responses (such as urine flow rate or metabolic acidemia), these variables are time dependent, and rapid assessments of volume status are essential in the acute management of this disorder.

Initial fluid resuscitation should be based on clinical observations of skin perfusion, heart rate, and blood pressure. A mean arterial pressure <35–40 mmHg in the term newborn with PPHN should be considered severe hypotension.[8] A heart rate >160 beats per minute and a capillary refill time that exceeds 2 seconds suggest intravascular volume depletion. Volume resuscitation should be used with caution when systemic hypotension is related to poor cardiac performance, particularly when the heart is enlarged on a chest radiograph.

If volume resuscitation alone is ineffective in maintaining adequate blood pressure and systemic perfusion, cardiotonic agents (dobutamine and/or dopamine) should be administered (beginning at 5 µg/kg/minute and increasing to 20 µg/kg/minute). The chronotropic effects of isoproterenol may be helpful in improving systemic blood flow, but this agent also reduces systemic afterload and can worsen ventilation-to-perfusion matching in infants with parenchymal lung disease.

In infants with idiopathic PPHN (without significant lung disease), pulmonary management should be directed at minimizing overzealous mechanical ventilation and avoiding lung overinflation. Applying inappropriately high airway pressure to the normally compliant lung can lead to air leak (for example, pneumothorax) and adverse cardiopulmonary interactions (decreased cardiac output from reduced venous return and cardiac filling).

If adequate oxygenation (PaO_2 >80 torr) cannot be obtained with moderate ventilator settings (peak inspiratory pressure <35 cm H_2O), then consideration should be given to a trial of respiratory alkalosis. Some patients will respond to alkalosis (pH 7.50–7.55) with marked improvement in oxygenation, but if significant improvement is not promptly demonstrated, hyperventilation should be discontinued. Respiratory alkalosis can often be achieved with high-frequency ventilator devices, which may minimize peak distending pressures delivered to the lung.

FIGURE 15-1 ▲ **Schematic of the synthesis and action of endogenous nitric oxide.**

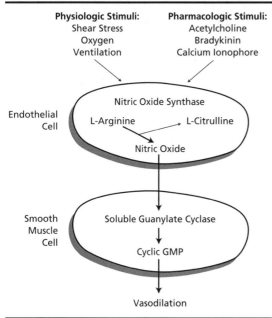

In the infant with severe lung disease and PPHN, treatment of the underlying lung disease is essential (and sometimes sufficient) to resolve the accompanying pulmonary hypertension. Because of the diverse nature of diseases complicating PPHN, there is no single approach to mechanical ventilation in this syndrome. Ventilator adjustments must be made with attention to radiographic changes of the accompanying lung disease and hemodynamic status (including intravascular volume, systemic perfusion, and cardiac performance).

Mechanical ventilation in infants with PPHN should be initiated with conventional intermittent mandatory ventilation. However, there is increasing interest in the potential role of high-frequency ventilation in managing these infants. In management of the patient with significant pulmonary parenchymal disease complicating PPHN, high-frequency oscillatory ventilation is an important adjunct. High-frequency oscillation allows more effective alveolar recruitment in diseases refractory to conventional ventilator therapy.

The efficacy of inhaled nitric oxide is probably improved when adequate lung inflation is achieved; alveolar recruitment with conventional mechanical ventilation is frequently ineffective. Indeed, one of the more common causes of suboptimal response to inhaled nitric oxide is the presence of severe parenchymal lung disease.

Current treatment to reduce pulmonary hypertension includes mechanical hyperventilation to cause respiratory alkalosis, vasodilator drug therapy, and metabolic alkalosis induced with sodium bicarbonate or THAM (tris-hydroxymethyl aminomethane). The latter is useful when ventilation is not adequate to allow the removal of carbon dioxide generated with bicarbonate therapy. Pulmonary vasodilator drug therapy (with such agents as tolazoline or sodium nitroprusside) is often unsuccessful because of concomitant systemic hypotension, adverse effects (such as gastrointestinal bleeding), or a failure of the drug to achieve or sustain pulmonary vasodilation.

Vasodilator drug therapy to decrease pulmonary vascular resistance in infants with PPHN has been limited by the lack of a truly selective pulmonary vasodilator drug. However, recent developments in vascular biology have elucidated the role of nitric oxide in transitional pulmonary vasoregulation and have set the stage for the first clinical trials of this pulmonary-specific inhalational vasodilator.

INHALED NITRIC OXIDE

When administered by inhalation, nitric oxide diffuses to vascular smooth muscle, stimulating cyclic-guanosine monophosphate (GMP) production and causing vasodilation (Figure 15-1). Its selectivity for the pulmonary circulation is due to the rapid and avid binding of nitric oxide by hemoglobin, decreasing its availability to the systemic circulation.[5] Although marked right-to-left shunting is the major cause of hypoxemia in infants with

FIGURE 15-2 ▲ **Low-dose nitric oxide causes marked increases in pulmonary blood flow in the newborn lamb.**

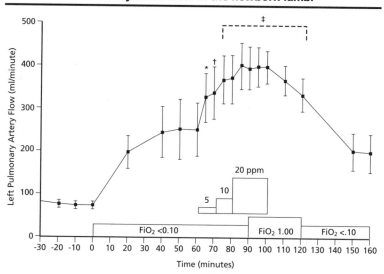

* $P <.05$, † $P <.01$, ‡ $P <.001$ compared with previous study period.

From: Kinsella JP, et al. 1992. Hemodynamic effects of exogenous nitric oxide in ovine transitional pulmonary circulation. *American Journal of Physiology* 263(3 part 2): H875–H880. Reprinted by permission.

PPHN, some newborns also have altered ventilation-to-perfusion matching due to parenchymal lung disease (for example, meconium aspiration). In addition to lowering PVR, inhaled NO further improves oxygenation by dilating those pulmonary arteries associated with the best ventilated lung units, thereby enhancing ventilation-to-perfusion matching.

Recent laboratory and clinical observations provided the rationale for using inhaled nitric oxide in the treatment of PPHN. Inhaled NO selectively reduced pulmonary vascular resistance in mature animals with pulmonary hypertension and caused selective pulmonary vasodilation in human adults with primary pulmonary hypertension during brief exposure.[9,10]

In the perinatal lung, endogenous nitric oxide formation modulates fetal PVR, contributes to the normal fall in PVR at birth, and maintains low PVR postnatally.[11–13]

ANIMAL STUDIES

The effects of exogenous nitric oxide on the transitional pulmonary circulation of newborn animals were first reported in 1992. The NO doses used in this study were based on the chronic ambient levels considered safe for adults by U.S. regulatory agencies. Studies were performed in near-term lambs using inhaled NO at doses of 5, 10, and 20 parts per million (ppm).[14]

Inhaled nitric oxide caused a dose-dependent increase in pulmonary blood flow in mechanically ventilated newborn lambs (Figure 15-2). This study demonstrated that low-dose inhaled NO causes potent, selective, and sustained pulmonary vasodilation in the newborn lamb. Inhaled NO at 20 ppm did not decrease coronary arterial or cerebral blood flow in this model.[15]

Other studies have subsequently confirmed these observations. Roberts and coworkers studied the effects of inhaled NO on pulmonary hemodynamics in mechanically ventilated, newborn lambs. They found that inhaled nitric oxide reverses hypoxic pulmonary vasoconstriction and that maximum vasodilation occurs at doses of ≥80 ppm. They also found that the vasodilation caused by inhaled NO during hypoxia is not attenuated by respiratory acidosis.[16]

Berger and associates investigated the effects of inhaled nitric oxide on pulmonary vasodilation in piglets with Group B streptococcal sepsis. They found that inhaled NO at 150 ppm for 30 minutes causes marked pulmonary vasodilation but is associated with significant increases in methemoglobin concentrations.[17]

FIGURE 15-3 ▲ Low-dose inhaled nitric oxide improves oxygenation in neonates with severe PPHN.

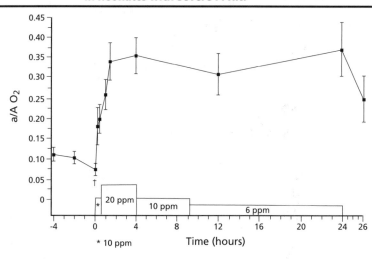

From: Kinsella JP, et al. 1992. Low-dose inhalational nitric oxide in persistent pulmonary hypertension of the newborn. *Lancet* 340(8823): 819–820. Reprinted by permission.

HUMAN STUDIES

Recent studies have demonstrated that inhaled nitric oxide causes marked improvement in oxygenation in many human newborns with PPHN. Roberts and colleagues reported that brief (30 minutes) NO inhalation at 80 ppm improves oxygenation in patients with PPHN; however, this response was sustained in only one patient after the nitric oxide was discontinued.[22]

Kinsella and associates also demonstrated rapid improvement in oxygenation in newborns with severe PPHN, using doses of nitric oxide at 20 ppm for four hours, then decreasing the dose to 6 ppm for the duration of treatment. This low-dose strategy resulted in sustained improvement in oxygenation (Figure 15-3).[23]

Corroborating studies in other animal models support the observations that inhaled NO causes potent, selective, and sustained pulmonary vasodilation at low doses (≤20 ppm).[18–21]

In a subsequent study, this low-dose strategy was used in an additional nine patients with severe PPHN, including two with congenital diaphragmatic hernia (Figure 15-4). In this study, eight patients had resolution of the underlying PPHN, and one patient with overwhelming sepsis showed an initial improvement in oxygenation but subsequently required treatment with extracorporeal membrane oxygenation for hemodynamic support.[24]

The efficacy of low-dose nitric oxide (≤20 ppm) in causing acute improvement in oxygenation in patients with severe PPHN has been corroborated in a 1994 study by Finer and associates. In a careful dose-response study, these investigators measured the improvement in oxygenation associated with NO doses ranging from 5 to 80 ppm. They found that the acute improvement in oxygenation in patients with PPHN was similar at all doses studied.[25]

Inhaled nitric oxide causes *sustained* improvement in oxygenation in patients with severe PPHN when clinical management includes meticulous attention to the nature of the underlying lung disease. In patients with severe PPHN and parenchymal lung disease or pulmonary hypoplasia (for example, congenital diaphragmatic hernia), optimal management may include high-frequency oscillation to recruit and maintain lung volume, thus promoting effective delivery of the inhalational vasodilator nitric oxide. Moreover, loss of apparent responsiveness to NO may occur because of deterioration in cardiac performance and progressive atelectasis (decreasing effective delivery of this inhalational agent to its site of action in terminal lung units).[26]

Not all neonates with hypoxemic respiratory failure have severe pulmonary hypertension. Pulmonary parenchymal disease can cause critical hypoxemia, and pulmonary vasodilator therapy would not be expected to be an effective therapy in this setting.

POTENTIAL TOXICITIES

Inhalational nitric oxide therapy remains investigational; but when it is approved for use in patients with PPHN, this treatment, because of its lack of systemic vascular effects, may replace other vasodilator therapies. Preliminary reports of inhalational NO therapy in patients with PPHN are encouraging, but many questions remain to be answered before its routine application can be accepted.

Although the clinical studies described were designed to investigate the hemodynamic effects of inhaled nitric oxide at "nontoxic" concentrations, concerns remain regarding potential toxicities, including methemoglobinemia and lung injury due to nitrogen dioxide, peroxynitrite, and hydroxyl radical formation.[27] Of particular concern are the potential effects of nitric oxide on inhibition of DNA synthesis and deamination of DNA.[28,29] The safe and effective application of inhalational NO therapy to neonates with severe cardiopulmonary failure must also take into account decreased antioxidant host defenses in the immature lung, the potential risk of surfactant inactivation, and down-regulation of endogenous nitric oxide synthesis.[30,31]

Moreover, the effects of inhaled nitric oxide may not be limited to the pulmonary vascu-

FIGURE 15-4 ▲ Effects of low-dose inhaled nitric oxide and high-frequency oscillatory ventilation in a patient with congenital diaphragmatic hernia.

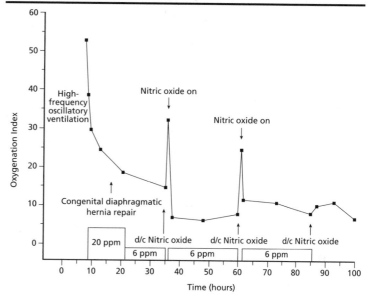

Brief discontinuation of nitric oxide caused marked worsening in oxygenation until 72 hours of therapy.

From: Kinsella JP, et al. 1993. Clinical responses to prolonged treatment of persistent pulmonary hypertension of the newborn with low doses of inhaled nitric oxide. *Journal of Pediatrics* 123(1): 106. Reprinted by permission.

lature. Preliminary evidence suggests that NO at high doses may modify the inflammatory response of alveolar macrophages, and circulating nitric oxide adducts could have adverse extrapulmonary effects.[32,33]

Another potentially important effect of nitric oxide inhalation at high doses is prolongation in bleeding time.[34] Endogenous NO inhibits platelet adhesion to the vascular endothelium, and this effect may be related to the formation of stable *S*-nitroso-proteins.[35,36] However, in a small study of premature infants treated with inhaled nitric oxide, no change in bleeding time occurred.[37]

As with most therapeutic agents, the complications associated with nitric oxide are likely dose dependent, and this agent should be used in the lowest effective dose. Controlled clinical trials are ongoing and provide the settings to clarify the potential toxicities of this new therapy.

DELIVERY AND MONITORING

Centers actively studying the role of inhaled NO in the treatment of PPHN have devised delivery systems that take advantage of the continuous flow nature of conventional neonatal ventilators. In one delivery system, nitric oxide from a relatively low concentration source tank (450 ppm) is blended with the gas within the afferent limb of the conventional ventilator. When conventional pressure-limited, continuous flow neonatal ventilators are used, the delivered nitric oxide dose depends on the flow rates of the NO gas and the ventilator circuit gas. Adequate control of dosing can be achieved using a low-flow meter attached to the nitric oxide tank if ventilator circuit bias gas flow is not changed.

The delivered nitric oxide dose is less predictable when ventilators with variable flow rates are used, and this system is inappropriate for volume-cycled ventilators that do not incorporate a continuous bias gas flow. A delivery system employing a two-stage gas blender technique has also been described.[38]

Monitoring delivered nitric oxide concentrations is essential because of the potential for toxicity at high doses. It is also important to measure nitrogen dioxide concentrations. Nitrogen dioxide is generated from NO in the presence of oxygen, and inspired nitrogen dioxide can cause pulmonary injury at relatively low concentrations.

The standard monitoring method for nitric oxide and nitrogen dioxide is chemiluminescence. However, electrochemical sensors for nitric oxide and nitrogen dioxide are less expensive than chemiluminescence analyzers, and these sensors may be reliable measurement devices.[39] Accurate calibration of both types of monitors is vital for correct gas concentration analysis. Delivered concentrations of these gases are routinely sampled at a side port on the endotracheal tube adapter. Both intermittent and continuous sampling methods have been employed. With either approach, care must be taken to correct for changes in ventilator pressure settings caused by aspiration of gas by the nitric oxide measurement device.

Marked deterioration in oxygenation can occur if NO is inadvertently withdrawn early in the course of severe PPHN (as might occur with routine suctioning). Modifications in suctioning methods may include avoidance of "bagging" during suctioning, or adding nitric oxide to the bag system during suctioning. Ambient concentrations of both nitric oxide and nitrogen dioxide are routinely monitored, and consideration should be given to scavenging ventilator exhaust gases if ambient concentrations increase above baseline levels.

SUMMARY

Occasionally PPHN presents as severe pulmonary hypertension without concomitant lung disease. Most cases of PPHN, however, are associated with pulmonary parenchymal diseases (such as meconium aspiration, pneumonia, and surfactant deficiency) and cardiac dysfunction. Therefore, the therapeutic approach to PPHN requires attention to the cardiac and pulmonary vascular components of this syndrome as well as the accompanying lung disease.

Inhalational nitric oxide therapy could prove to be an essential adjunct in the management of infants with PPHN. Such therapy, however, must be tailored to the underlying diseases, with appropriate modifications in response to cardiopulmonary changes over the course of the illness.

REFERENCES

1. Gersony WM, Duc GV, and Sinclair JD. 1969. "PFC" syndrome (persistence of the fetal circulation). *Circulation* 40(supplement 3): 87A.

2. Levin DL, et al. 1976. Persistent pulmonary hypertension of the newborn infant. *Journal of Pediatrics* 89(4): 626–630.

3. Drummond WH, et al. 1981. The independent effects of hyperventilation, tolazoline, and dopamine on infants with persistent pulmonary hypertension. *Journal of Pediatrics* 98(4): 603–611.

4. Ignarro LJ, et al. 1987. Endothelium-derived relaxing factor produced and released from artery and vein is nitric oxide. *Proceedings of the National Academy of Sciences of the United States of America* 84(24): 9265–9269.

5. Palmer RMJ, Ferrrige AG, and Moncada SA. 1987. Nitric oxide release accounts for the biological activity of endothelium-derived relaxing factor. *Nature* 327(6122): 524–526.

6. Moncada S, Palmer RMJ, and Higgs EA. 1991. Nitric oxide: Physiology, pathophysiology, and pharmacology. *Pharmacological Reviews* 43(2): 109–142.

7. Kinsella JP, et al. 1992. Cardiac performance in extracorporeal membrane oxygenation candidates: Echocardiographic predictors for extracorporeal membrane oxygenation. *Journal of Pediatric Surgery* 27(1): 44–47.

8. Kitterman JA, Phibbs RH, and Tooley WH. 1969. Aortic blood pressure in normal newborn infants during the first 12 hours of life. *Pediatrics* 44(6): 959–968.

9. Frostell C, et al. 1991. Inhaled nitric oxide: A selective pulmonary vasodilator reversing hypoxic pulmonary vasoconstriction. *Circulation* 83(6): 2038–2047. (Published erratum appears in *Circulation* 1991. 84[5]: 2212.)

10. Pepke-Zaba J, et al. 1991. Inhaled nitric oxide as a cause of selective pulmonary vasodilation in pulmonary hypertension. *Lancet* 338(8776): 1173–1174.

11. Abman SH, et al. 1990. Role of endothelium-derived relaxing factor during transition of pulmonary circulation at birth. *American Journal of Physiology* 259(6 part 2): H1921–H1927.

12. Davidson D, and Eldemerdash A. 1990. Endothelium-derived relaxing factor: Presence in pulmonary and systemic arteries of the newborn guinea pig. *Pediatric Research* 27(2): 128–132.

13. Fineman JR, Heymann MA, and Soifer SJ. 1991. N omega-nitro-L-arginine attenuates endothelium-dependent vasodilation in lambs. *American Journal of Physiology* 260(4 part 2): H1299–H1306.

14. Kinsella JP, et al. 1992. Hemodynamic effects of exogenous nitric oxide in ovine transitional pulmonary circulation. *American Journal of Physiology* 263(3 part 2): H875–H880.

15. Rosenberg AA, Kinsella JP, and Abman SH. 1995. Cerebral hemodynamics and distribution of left ventricular output during inhalation of nitric oxide. *Critical Care Medicine* 23(8): 1391–1397.

16. Roberts JD, et al. 1993. Inhaled nitric oxide reverses pulmonary vasoconstriction in the hypoxic and acidotic newborn lamb. *Circulation Research* 72(2): 246–254.

17. Berger JI, et al. 1993. Effect of inhaled nitric oxide during Group B streptococcal sepsis in piglets. *American Review of Respiratory Disease* 147(5): 1080–1086.

18. Zayek M, et al. 1993. Effect of nitric oxide on the survival rate and incidence of lung injury in newborn lambs with persistent pulmonary hypertension. *Journal of Pediatrics* 123(6): 947–952.

19. Zayek M, Cleveland D, and Morin FC. 1993. Treatment of persistent pulmonary hypertension in the newborn lamb by inhaled nitric oxide. *Journal of Pediatrics* 122(5 part 1): 743–750.

20. Etches PC, et al. 1994. Nitric oxide reverses acute hypoxic pulmonary hypertension in the newborn piglet. *Pediatric Research* 35(1): 15–19.

21. Nelin LD, et al. 1994. The effect of inhaled nitric oxide on the pulmonary circulation of the neonatal pig. *Pediatric Research* 35(1): 20–24.

22. Roberts JD, et al. 1992. Inhaled nitric oxide in persistent pulmonary hypertension of the newborn. *Lancet* 340(8823): 818–819.

23. Kinsella JP, et al. 1992. Low-dose inhalational nitric oxide in persistent pulmonary hypertension of the newborn. *Lancet* 340(8823): 819–820.

24. Kinsella JP, et al. 1993. Clinical responses to prolonged treatment of persistent pulmonary hypertension of the newborn with low doses of inhaled nitric oxide. *Journal of Pediatrics* 123(1): 103–108.

25. Finer NN, et al. 1994. Inhaled nitric oxide in infants referred for extracorporeal membrane oxygenation: Dose response. *Journal of Pediatrics* 124(2): 302–308.

26. Kinsella JP, and Abman SH. 1995. Recent developments in the pathophysiology and treatment of persistent pulmonary hypertension of the newborn. *Journal of Pediatrics* 126(6): 853–864.

27. Beckman JS, et al. 1990. Apparent hydroxyl radical production by peroxynitrite: Implications for endothelial injury from nitric oxide and superoxide. *Proceedings of the National Academy of Sciences of the United States of America* 87(4): 1620–1624.

28. Lepoivre M, et al. 1991. Inactivation of ribonucleotide reductase by nitric oxide. *Biochemical and Biophysical Research Communications* 179(1): 442–448.

29. Wink DA, et al. 1991. DNA deaminating ability and genotoxicity of nitric oxide and its progenitors. *Science* 254(5034): 1001–1003.

30. Haddad IY, et al. 1993. Mechanisms of peroxynitrite-induced injury to pulmonary surfactants. *American Journal of Physiology* 265(6 part 1): L555–L564.

31. Bult H, et al. 1991. Chronic exposure to exogenous nitric oxide may suppress its endogenous release and efficacy. *Journal of Cardiovascular Pharmacology* 17: S79–S82.

32. Turbow R, et al. 1994. Inflammatory responses and suppressed macrophage function following inhaled nitric oxide. *Pediatric Research* 35: 356A.

33. Stamler JS, et al. 1992. S-nitrosylation of proteins with nitric oxide: Synthesis and characterization of biologically active compounds. *Proceedings of the National Academy of Sciences of the United States of America* 89(1): 444–448.

34. Hogman M, et al. 1993. Bleeding time prolongation and NO inhalation. *Lancet* 341(8861): 1664–1665.

35. Radomski MW, Palmer RMJ, and Moncada S. 1987. Endogenous nitric oxide inhibits platelet adhesion to vascular endothelium. *Lancet* 2(8567): 1057–1058.

36. Simon DI, et al. 1993. Antiplatelet properties of protein S-nitrosothiols derived from nitric oxide and endothelium-derived relaxing factor. *Arteriosclerosis and Thrombosis* 13(6): 791–799.

37. Ahluwalia J, et al. 1994. Nitric oxide improves oxygenation in neonates with respiratory distress syndrome and pulmonary hypertension. *Pediatric Research* 36: 3A.

38. Wessel DL, et al. 1994. Delivery and monitoring of inhaled nitric oxide in patients with pulmonary hypertension. *Critical Care Medicine* 22(6): 930–938.

39. Mercier J, et al. 1993. Device to monitor concentration of inhaled nitric oxide. *Lancet* 342(8868): 431–432.

NOTES

16 Liquid Ventilation

Jay S. Greenspan, MD

Normal *in utero* pulmonary development depends on periodic breathing and an appropriate balance between production and exhalation of fetal lung fluid.[1,2] A successful transition to extrauterine life requires adequate pulmonary structural maturity to facilitate gas exchange as well as the presence of surfactant to lower surface tension in the pulmonary air spaces.[3]

Some or all of these processes may be insufficient in the prematurely delivered infant, or they may be disturbed by an abnormal perinatal course. A successful transition to extrauterine life without pulmonary-related morbidity and mortality in these infants may be difficult, even with optimal management.

In spite of the advances in respiratory therapy of infants over the past several decades, morbidity and mortality from lung disease remain a major problem in neonatal care. To address this problem, investigators have begun to explore liquid ventilation as an alternative approach to gas breathing. Though this technique may initially seem unusual, it is based on several basic physiologic principles and more than two decades of extensive animal research.

BACKGROUND

The impetus to pursue the clinical application of liquid ventilation in neonates has evolved from two arenas of research and development. Liquid ventilation has been studied as a means of accomplishing the following:

1. Reducing the high surface tension in terminal air spaces of the injured or premature lung. When filled with liquid, even the surfactant sufficient lung demonstrates increased compliance.[3-5]

Although current therapies utilizing exogenous surfactant replacement therapy have reduced morbidity and mortality for some groups of infants by reducing alveolar surface tension, the success of this therapy may be limited by unequal pulmonary distribution. Liquid ventilation would uniformly diminish surface tension and diminish pulmonary inflation pressures, thereby reducing the barotrauma necessary to achieve adequate gas exchange. Furthermore, liquid ventilation distends the immature pulmonary parenchyma, compensating in part for structural limitations and large distances between vascular channels and air spaces.[6-8]

TABLE 16-1 ▲ Physical Properties of Perfluorochemicals Used in Liquid Breathing

		Perfluorochemicals				
	Water	FC-77	RM-101	FC-75	Perfluorodecalin	Perflubron
Boiling point (°C)	100	97	101	102	140	143
Density at 25°C (gm/ml)	1	1.78	1.77	1.78	1.95	1.93
Viscosity at 25°C (centistokes)	1	0.8	0.82	0.82	2.9	1.1
Vapor pressure at 37°C (torr)	47	85	64	63	14	11
Surface tension at 25°C (dynes/cm)	72	15	15	15	19	18
Oxygen solubility at 25°C (ml gas/100 ml liquid)	3	50	52	52	49	53
Carbon dioxide solubility at 25°C (ml gas/100 ml liquid)	57	198	160	160	140	210

2. Removing pulmonary debris. A saline lavage technique was first utilized to treat pneumonitis induced by poisonous gas inhalation in animals more than 70 years ago.[9] Aspiration is a frequent complication of many neonatal pulmonary pathologic processes (such as pneumonia, meconium and amniotic fluid aspiration, and respiratory distress syndrome). Removal of this debris with liquid ventilation could provide an alternative to the standard techniques of suctioning and chest physiotherapy.

Many liquids will diminish surface tension and remove debris in the injured lung, but breathable fluids must also be able to dissolve adequate volumes of respiratory gases and be nontoxic, minimally absorbed, and easily excreted. Saline solubility for oxygen is only 3 ml/100 ml fluid at one atmosphere, or about 5 percent of that needed by the infant.[10] Much of the research during the 1960s and 1970s was directed at finding a safe, capable fluid and delivery system for liquid breathing.

During the 1980s, researchers refined liquid breathing techniques and utilized liquid ventilation as a physiologic tool to explore the unknowns of the prematurely delivered infant. The most recent work in the 1990s has determined the feasibility of liquid ventilation in the human and fine-tuned the technology to facilitate the initial large-scale clinical trials.

APPROPRIATE LIQUIDS FOR VENTILATION

Many liquids with high gas solubility, such as the synthetic and natural oils, are too viscous or toxic to serve as a respiratory medium. Perfluorochemicals are inert liquids derived by replacing all the carbon-bound hydrogen atoms on organic compounds with fluorine. Several techniques are available for the production of perfluorochemicals from compounds such as benzene.[11]

Oxygen is about 20 times more soluble in perfluorochemicals than in water, and carbon dioxide solubility varies with the specific chemical, but is generally high.[12] In addition to demonstrating excellent respiratory gas solubility, these liquids are insoluble in lipids or water; evaporate rapidly in room air; are odorless, colorless, and biologically inert; and have low surface tension properties. Initial experimentation by Clark and Gollan demonstrated the feasibility of small animals breathing perfluorochemicals during normobaric immersion.[10]

Some of the physical properties of perfluorochemicals that have been utilized in liquid breathing are listed in Table 16-1. In animal trials, these liquids have been used for periods as long as 16 days with no apparent ill effects. At the present time, there do not appear to be any physiologic limitations to the duration of exposure of mammals to perfluorochemicals in liquid breathing. The long-term toxicity, particularly in humans, however, remains unknown.

Following liquid ventilation, some animal species have shown a transient, mild deterioration in pulmonary mechanics after return to gas breathing. This is probably due to residual perfluorochemicals in the otherwise healthy lung.[11–19]

Histologic evaluation of prematurely delivered animals ventilated with perfluorochemicals and recovered to air respiration demonstrates decreased hyaline membrane formation, reduced injury to airway epithelium and distal air spaces, and clearance of alveolar debris.[15,17,20–22] Lung ultrastructure appears to remain intact following liquid breathing in healthy animals.

In long-term evaluations, no changes were found in the lungs of dogs on either light or electron microscopy examinations (except for a slight increase in alveolar macrophages), and adult monkeys have had normal pulmonary function as long as three years after treatment.[11,18,19]

Systemically, perfluorochemicals appear to be eliminated almost entirely through the lungs, with small amounts excreted through the skin. Little perfluorochemical is absorbed by the pulmonary circulation during therapy, although small amounts may remain stored in fat cells for years after liquid breathing.[11,23] The perfluorochemicals, however, appear to be biologically inert and do not undergo transformation or metabolism, which makes toxicity unlikely. Elimination of perfluorochemicals stored in fat cells appears to depend on subsequent re-entry into the circulation, with ultimate excretion occurring through the lungs and skin.

Much work has been done on the safety and efficacy of a 20 percent perfluorochemical emulsion to be utilized as an artificial blood substitute.[24] In this technique, much more perfluorochemical would be available for tissue absorption, thereby dramatically increasing potential toxicity. Yet this mode of administration appears to be safe. Although these studies suggest that there would be minimal or no long-term toxicity after perfluorochemical liquid ventilation, future investigation is necessary, particularly when considering the ventilation of human neonates.

The poor solubility of perfluorochemicals for substances other than gases affects clinical applications. All substrates for growth are insoluble, and hence these fluids are bacteriostatic. Unlike saline, perfluorochemicals do not wash out or alter the natural surfactant present at the gas-liquid interface.[11,25] Although the solubility characteristics of perfluorochemicals may limit effective debridement, when they were utilized in an animal model of human meconium aspiration, they effectively removed particulate matter and improved pulmonary function.[26] Biologically active agents such as vasoactive drugs, antibiotics, and artificial surfactants will not dissolve in perfluorochemical liquids, but these agents can be effectively pushed into the distal air spaces by the liquid when injected on inspiration.[27–29]

In addition to ventilator applications, perfluorochemicals possess qualities that make them applicable to radiologic procedures.[30] Low acoustic attenuation makes these liquids well suited for ultrasound technology; detailed images of the liquid-filled organ can be obtained with standard ultrasound technology. Perfluorochemicals are also radiopaque, resulting in a whitened lung on standard radiograph.

The presence of fluorine and/or bromine in perfluorochemicals makes them suitable adjuncts for magnetic resonance imaging. Lungs filled with perfluorochemicals by lavage, injection, or aerosol spray can be imaged in fine detail. In addition, because the amount of dissolved oxygen alters the spin-lattice relaxation time (T1) image of the nuclear magnetic resonance signal, magnetic resonance can be utilized to help determine both lung function and ventilation-to-perfusion matching.

LIQUID VENTILATION TECHNIQUES

Although the previously listed attributes tend to make perfluorochemicals an acceptable respiratory medium for gas exchange, these liquids also have high density, viscosity, and diffusion coefficients, which dramatically affect breathing strategy. In particular, the higher viscosity and markedly increased resistance to flow increases the work of breathing during spontaneous ventilation.[31–33]

The effect of resistance, along with a prolonged diffusion coefficient, necessitates an increased inspiratory time. Because expiratory flow rates are reduced markedly in the liquid-filled lung as compared to the gas-filled lung, expiratory time is also substantially greater than that seen during gas breathing.

Liquid breathing, therefore, is a process in which respiratory rate is slower, inspiratory and expiratory times are more prolonged, and an exchange period or "dwell" time is required for adequate gas exchange to occur.[33,34] Even with optimal ventilation schemes, the large work of breathing required to breathe perfluorochemicals results in fatigue during spontaneous ventilation.

Mechanical ventilators capable of ventilating liquids have been designed to compensate for these difficulties (Figure 16-1). These devices control ventilation through time cycling and pressure and/or are volume limiting—in short, they perform much like a conventional mechanical gas ventilator. These ventilators can also efficiently recirculate the fluid in a manner very similar to that used in current extracorporeal membrane oxygenation (ECMO) technology.

Unlike most forms of gas ventilation, liquid ventilation requires both an active inspiration and expiration to diminish the work of breathing and achieve adequate timing ratios. Animal studies indicate improved oxygenation with

controlled arterial carbon dioxide tension and acidosis with the use of these ventilators as compared to spontaneous liquid ventilation.[31–34]

Appropriate ventilator schemes have been designed and extensively evaluated. Investigators have demonstrated that several animal species can undergo liquid ventilation with various oxygenated perfluorochemicals, successfully recover to gas breathing, and survive without long-term compromise.[7,8,11,15,17,25,26,33,34] The clinical advantage of liquid ventilation over gas ventilation was demonstrated in a preterm lamb model, and liquid ventilation trials in severely ill human neonates showed the feasibility and potential of this modality in humans.[35,36]

When ventilated, perfluorochemicals are evenly distributed throughout the lung at low inflation pressures. Oxygenation of compromised or premature animals can generally be facilitated by placing them on liquid ventilation. Arterial oxygen tensions can be controlled by altering the oxygen content of the liquid or the functional residual capacity. Arterial carbon dioxide tensions and lung volume are regulated by altering inspiratory:expiratory timing ratios or driving pressure and flow rates.[33,34]

Healthy adult animals may experience some increase in alveolar-arterial oxygen gradient while on liquid ventilation. Minimal gains in surface tension reduction, ventilation-to-perfusion matching, and alveolar recruitment are outweighed by the increases in dead space.[18–20,37] Early ventilation trials in adult animals also demonstrated a small but significant production of metabolic acidosis.[38] This has been attributed to cardiovascular adjustments and increases in pulmonary vascular resistance due to compression of the vessels, which can be overcome by appropriate intravascular volume expansion.

If the animal has pulmonary compromise prior to liquid ventilation, the positive impact on surface tension, ventilation-to-perfusion

FIGURE 16-1 ▲ Technique for administration of perfluorochemicals via total liquid ventilation.

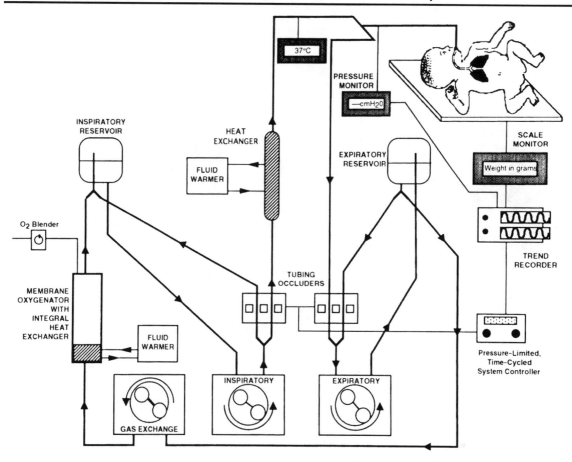

Active inspiration and expiration is generated by two roller pumps; fluid is recycled (cleansed, oxygenated, and heated) via a third roller pump. Continuous infant weight and airway pressure measurements allow for monitoring of driving pressures, tidal volume, functional residual capacity, respiratory mechanics, and alveolar pressure. The arrows demonstrate the flow of perfluorochemicals through the circuit.

From: Spitzer AR, et al. 1996. Special ventilatory techniques II: Liquid ventilation, nitric oxide therapy, and negative-pressure ventilation. In *Assisted Ventilation of the Neonate*, 3rd. ed., Goldsmith JP, and Karotkin EH, eds. Philadelphia: WB Saunders, 231. Reprinted by permission.

matching, air space recruitment and unfolding of pulmonary capillaries, and improved oxygenation and ventilation will decrease pulmonary vascular resistance.[20,39] When performed appropriately, studies indicate that liquid ventilation with perfluorochemicals should be able to maintain gas exchange and cardiopulmonary stability for an extended period of time in many different animal species with a wide variety of lung diseases.

Successful recovery to gas ventilation after perfluorochemical liquid ventilation has been demonstrated in animal models and some human neonates. In a sick or preterm population, this transition is associated with improved pulmonary function from preliquid ventilation values.[11,20,26,34–36] The safety, ease, and effectiveness of the conventional gas ventilation of a liquid-filled lung following liquid ventilation has led investigators to pursue partial liquid ventilation as a primary mode of liquid breathing.[16,40–42]

With this technique, a functional residual capacity (20–30 ml/kg) of perfluorochemical

FIGURE 16-2 ▲ Schematic of partial liquid ventilation: (1) conventional gas ventilation is delivered into the liquid-filled lung; (2) perflubron liquid is instilled on inspiration via a side-port of the endotracheal tube; (3) the liquid recruits potential air spaces; and (4) gas exchange occurs through the liquid medium; (5) carbon dioxide enriched gases then escape on exhalation.

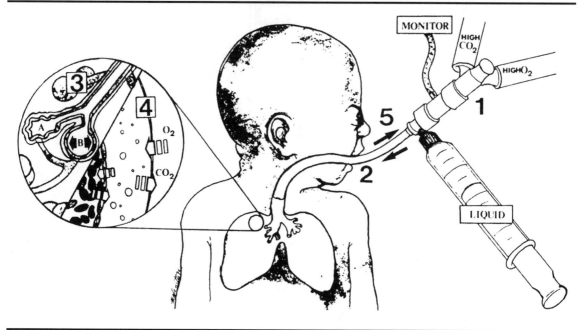

From: Spitzer AR, et al. 1996. Special ventilatory techniques II: Liquid ventilation, nitric oxide therapy, and negative-pressure ventilation. In *Assisted Ventilation of the Neonate,* 3rd. ed., Goldsmith JP, and Karotkin EH, eds. Philadelphia: WB Saunders, 234. Reprinted by permission.

liquid (not necessarily preoxygenated) is instilled into the lungs over a short period of time during gas ventilation (Figure 16-2). Conventional gas ventilation is then continued (with some adjustments in pressure and timing as necessary) with the lung expanded by the residual perfluorochemical. As the fluid evaporates out of the lungs, it can be gradually and intermittently replaced.

This technique takes advantage of some aspects of full liquid ventilation (homogeneous conditioning of the lung, volume recruitment, and lowering of surface tension, for example) without the requirement of a liquid ventilator. Studies conducted on surfactant-deficient animals demonstrate marked improvement in lung function with partial liquid ventilation as compared to conventional gas ventilation.[42]

CLINICAL APPLICATIONS IN THE NEONATE

The numerous potential clinical applications utilizing perfluorochemical liquids cross many subspecialties in medicine. Interest in adult and child therapies include imaging, cancer treatment (utilizing improved visualization, direct administration of chemotherapeutic agents, hyperoxygenation, regional heating, and agitation with ultrasound techniques), therapies for hyper/hypothermia, and treatment of primary pulmonary diseases.[20,43,44] In addition to its use in treating injured lungs, liquid ventilation could facilitate the adaptation of a healthy person to an unusual environment (space travel or diving).[11,20,45]

Because of the ongoing incidence of chronic lung disease following ventilator support in the neonate, liquid ventilation has received the most attention in neonatal therapy as a potentially attractive alternative to gas ventilation. Many potential applications in the infant capitalize on the ability of liquid ventilation to minimize surface tension and maintain gas exchange at lower driving and alveolar pressures and to facilitate drug delivery, cleansing, and lung conditioning. Animal models have demonstrated the effectiveness of liquid ventilation techniques in many different pathologic situations.[7,11,15,17,20,25–29,33,34,41,42] There are presently several protocols designed to test the safety and efficacy of partial liquid ventilation in humans.[46]

RESPIRATORY DISTRESS SYNDROME

Unfortunately for the suddenly displaced, prematurely delivered neonate, the uterine environment contains another organ, the placenta, that is no longer capable of providing the gas exchange needed for survival. Elimination of this avenue for gas exchange markedly complicates neonatal existence. Preterm animal models indicate that liquid ventilation may diminish barotrauma and decrease morbidity and mortality in infants with respiratory distress syndrome (RDS).[8,25,33,34]

To date, liquid ventilation has been studied in only a few premature human infants, most of whom have been near death at the time of treatment. In the original studies, three extremely premature infants were carefully selected for liquid breathing therapy. All three were dying of terminal lung disease, 23–28 weeks gestation, and were felt to have failed all conventional approaches to treatment. A gravity-assisted approach was used (Figure 16-3), and liquid was given in two 5-minute cycles, at a rate of three breaths per minute, separated by 15 minutes of gas ventilation.[35,36]

The infants appeared to tolerate the procedure without difficulty and showed improvement in several physiologic parameters.

FIGURE 16-3 ▲ Gravity-assisted liquid ventilation.

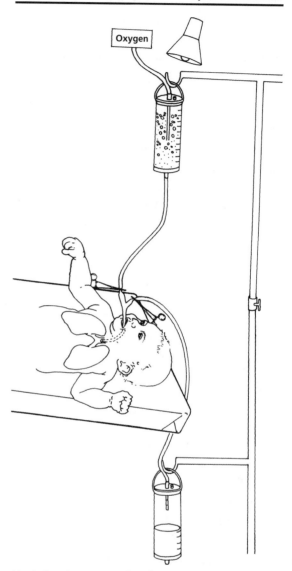

Heated and oxygenated perfluorochemical liquid is inspired and expired with gravity assistance. Driving pressures can be changed by altering the height of the reservoir. Breathing timing is altered manually, and liquid can be recycled.

Redrawn from: Greenspan JS, et al. 1990. Liquid ventilation of human preterm neonates. *Journal of Pediatrics.* 117(1 part 1): 106. Reprinted by permission.

Improvement was sustained for approximately two hours after discontinuation of liquid ventilation, after which the infants deteriorated.[35,36]

A corporate-sponsored (Alliance Pharmaceutical, San Diego) protocol for partial liquid ventilation in preterm infants is currently under way. This multicentered study is investigating the safety and efficacy of one perfluorochemical—sterile perflubron (LiquiVent)—utilized for partial liquid ventilation for up to 96 hours in preterm infants with RDS who have failed all conventional therapies. Initial results are very encouraging, and several infants have improved dramatically and progressed to nursery discharge.[46] These studies suggest the feasibility of this technique in the neonate with severe RDS.

Although the previous investigation in a "rescue" situation has stimulated much interest, additional uses for liquid ventilation of the infant with RDS are also evident. In preterm animal studies, liquid ventilation, when used early, recruits alveoli, improves oxygenation and lung mechanics, enhances cardiovascular stability, and permits the use of low inflation pressures to maintain adequate gas exchange.[34,39,40]

Perfluorochemicals might be ideally used to distend atelectatic alveoli prior to surfactant administration. A brief administration of perfluorochemical could establish lung volume in the very low birth weight infant, preparing the alveolar surface. Evidence suggests that surfactant does not get distributed effectively to atelectatic areas, which often appear immediately after birth in the child with severe lung disease. Liquid might be more effective than gas breathing in recruiting these regions of the lung for both initial and subsequent surfactant treatment. Surfactant might even be delivered with repeated liquid infusions over several minutes for optimal dispersion, after which the infant could be recovered to gas ventilation, which would then be possible at far lower levels of support.

ASPIRATION SYNDROMES, PULMONARY HYPERTENSION, AND PNEUMONIA

Initial animal protocols on the liquid-filled lung in the 1920s utilized the capability of removing pulmonary debris as a primary therapeutic modality.[9] Perfluorochemical liquid

breathing, therefore, appears to be an attractive treatment for neonates with meconium aspiration syndrome.

In the treatment of persistent pulmonary hypertension of the newborn, perfluorochemicals also appear to offer some advantages. Because increased pulmonary vascular resistance is a cardinal feature of this disease, the introduction of vasoactive substances is considered an important adjunct to treatment. With conventional drug delivery (intravascular, aerosol), the pulmonary circulation may be bypassed. Intravascular drugs may shunt through a patent foramen ovale or ductus arteriosus and fail to reach the pulmonary circulation. Aerosolized drugs, especially in the face of increased airway debris, may remain largely on the surface of the airways.

Liquid ventilation, however, may transport the desired drug to the gas-exchange regions of the lung and the pulmonary vasculature, where effectiveness would be maximal. Tolazoline, for example, has been shown to be effectively delivered to the desired location in a hypoxic animal model. Furthermore, the peripheral vasodilator effects of this drug, often a problem, were minimal.[27,28] There are currently several FDA-approved protocols that are just under way, evaluating partial liquid ventilation with perflubron in term infants, children, and adults with respiratory failure.

In addition to vasoactive drugs, delivery of other biologically active substances via liquid ventilation has been explored. As previously mentioned, effective delivery of exogenous surfactant and chemotherapeutic agents can be achieved with liquid ventilation, providing specific therapies for certain patients.[47]

Antibiotics can also be effectively administered via liquid ventilation, achieving similar blood levels and better lung tissue levels than with intravenous delivery.[29] This may be particularly beneficial in infants suffering from severe pneumonia. Liquid ventilation could remove infectious debris, recruit atelectatic regions of the lung, and effectively deliver antibiotics to regions that would receive little medication by intravenous administration.

Hence, treatments specifically tailored for pulmonary disease can be designed, with liquid ventilation serving as the vehicle. Drug delivery to the lung may become an important part of therapy with liquid breathing.

IMAGING AND TEMPERATURE CONTROL

Perfluorochemicals may be extremely valuable for use in imaging techniques of the newborn in the near future. Even in small concentrations, these substances are radiopaque and can provide excellent resolution of the small airways and parenchyma, often difficult to assess in the small neonate. [30,44] Because of the fluorine, magnetic resonance techniques can also be enhanced.

The high heat capacity of perfluorochemicals allows them to effectively heat or cool the lung—or the entire body—during liquid breathing. Because the surface area and blood supply of the lung are larger than those of the skin, the body will rapidly assume the temperature of the lung surface. Filling the lungs with a breathable liquid, therefore, could be utilized as a means to rapidly and predictably control body temperature. The value of this capacity during certain procedures (cardiothoracic) may be significant.

FUTURE CLINICAL TRIALS

Although initial studies with perfluorochemical respiration appear encouraging, many questions remain. The efficacy and safety of these substances remain to be defined in further trials. The initial human clinical trials indicated the feasibility and potential of liquid ventilation in critically ill neonates. [35,36] Initial protocols for partial liquid ventilation in preterm and term infants, as well as in adults with respiratory failure, are very encouraging.

Improvement in clinical status in terminally ill neonates has been observed, but the long-term complications of liquid ventilation in humans are unknown. In addition, although initial studies suggest that improvement can be obtained in very critically ill infants, the effect in less critically ill infants is unclear. Aside from possible reduction in mortality, might liquid ventilation permit infants to survive with less barotrauma, central nervous system dysfunction, and other morbidities? Finally, potential problems associated with longer periods of ventilation (such as secretion removal, leaks, gastrointestinal filling, and maintenance of a liquid functional residual capacity) have yet to be fully evaluated.

Future therapeutic trials will test different fluids with various delivery schemes in patients with specific diseases. Many different perfluorochemicals exist, each with specific characteristics. The properties that make one perfluorochemical superior to others for liquid breathing are not fully understood and may differ with different species and disease processes. A liquid with high density and viscosity may alter breathing strategies in some infants—particularly when small endotracheal tube sizes are utilized—because of a requirement for increased driving pressures.

The vapor pressure determines, in part, how quickly the perfluorochemical dissipates upon gas ventilation recovery. Differences in this characteristic will determine, in part, the longevity of the effect of liquid ventilation. Perfluorochemicals with the lowest surface tension may effect greater improvement in lung function upon gas recovery than those with higher surface tension. Although these issues may ultimately result in fluids "designed" for different applications, initial trials will utilize the medical-grade perfluorochemicals that have government approval.

Proposed delivery systems include partial liquid ventilation, liquid lavage techniques, and gravity- or roller-pump-driven liquid ventilators. Although roller-pump-driven ventilators appear to be the most efficacious for a wide variety of disease states in animals, they are the most cumbersome, expensive, and difficult to operate. The first trials, therefore, are utilizing a partial liquid ventilation technique so as to limit confounding variables from a new ventilator, as well as expedite FDA approval.

Finally, timing of the therapy may dramatically affect efficacy. An infant with terminal lung disease with severe acidosis, gas leak, and minimal pulmonary blood flow will respond less optimally to liquid ventilation than an infant in the earlier stages of disease. Prophylactic liquid ventilation prior to the first breath, or soon after a pulmonary insult, could prove most efficacious. Although prophylactic liquid ventilation may eventually prove to produce the most dramatic results (as evidenced by many animal studies), initial human trials will concentrate on the critically ill neonate in whom other therapies have failed. Ethical considerations, therefore, will be at the forefront in determining the exact target population for these trials.

The future of liquid ventilation technology will probably also include delivery systems that have yet to be fully developed in the animal research arena. This includes aerosolized perfluorochemical delivery, high-frequency ventilator assist of tidal liquid ventilation, and the addition of other dissolved gases or drugs to the perfluorochemical to facilitate activity. Although there is much debate on how to conduct the next phase, many different trials will be needed to define the potential therapeutic indications for perfluorochemical ventilation.

NURSING CARE

If liquid breathing proves to be safe and effective, the impact of liquid ventilation on the care of the infant will be substantial. Liquid breathing will most likely cause no pain or discomfort. The process is not unnatural: The fetus "breathes" fluid continuously during the latter portions of gestation. Although some sedation may be required, the amount should not exceed that normally utilized. Although similarities exist between partial and total liquid ventilation, the impact on nursing care is unique to each ventilation scheme.

PARTIAL LIQUID VENTILATION

The impact of partial liquid ventilation on the nursing care of an infant may appear, at first glance, to be quite limited. The infant will remain on a conventional ventilator and will have essentially no added equipment. The limited experience in human neonates thus far, however, suggests that several important issues need to be addressed during this procedure.

Prior to the initiation of partial liquid ventilation, the infant's pulmonary function and functional residual capacity may need to be measured (see Chapter 12). This will help determine the etiology of the lung dysfunction (a low pulmonary compliance suggests a high surface tension, for instance) and will determine the amount of liquid needed to fill the lung.

Depending on which perfluorochemical is utilized, a special endotracheal tube may need to be inserted because of incompatibility of the liquid with the tube's material. In addition, adequate monitoring, including access to arterial blood chemistry and on-line measurement of tidal volume, needs to be established.

During the initiation of partial liquid ventilation, a functional residual capacity of the perfluorochemical is administered via the side port of an endotracheal tube (in much the same fashion as some exogenous surfactants are given). The ideal rate of instillation has yet to be determined, but vital signs, tidal volume, and oxyhemoglobin saturation need to be closely and continuously monitored.

Particularly in critically ill infants, the transition from a gas-filled to a liquid-filled lung may be difficult. Gas trapping and nonuniform distribution of initial doses of liquid may be a problem. Stability may be facilitated by a "slow-fill" process of 1 ml/minute, gentle alterations in position, and intermittent suctioning.

Until these issues are fully addressed, careful monitoring and individualized care must be instituted. For the initial studies, the infant's lung was filled at a rate of 1 to 2 ml/minute until the measured functional residual capacity was obtained, unless significant desaturation occurred. In addition, gentle back and forth rocking of the infant while filling may be beneficial.

During this initial filling period, several infants have experienced dramatic increases in tidal volume. In order to avoid barotrauma, rapid alterations in the pressure settings of the conventional ventilator may need to be done. In one infant, a decrease in peak inflation pressure from the low 30s to 19 cm H_2O was required to maintain a desirable tidal volume. For this reason, on-line tidal volume measurements are imperative.

Once partial liquid ventilation is established, there is a diminution in the level of acuity. Alterations in pulmonary function occur more slowly, and ventilator changes can be made gradually. The infant may stabilize and require less sedation. Ongoing concerns, however, include maintenance of an adequate perfluorochemical fluid level and debris removal. Typical evaporation time of one of the perfluorochemicals, perflubron, is about 2 to 4 ml/hour. This will vary with such factors as the perfluorochemical, the endotracheal tube size, and the presence of any leak.

The determination of an adequate fluid level remains an issue of some debate. A chest radiograph will demonstrate uniform distribution, but this two-dimensional view adds little to the assessment of an adequate level of liquid. One method of determining a level is to disconnect the ventilator (remove end-distending pressure) and observe a liquid level in the endotracheal tube when looking into the mouth. If the meniscus is not seen, liquid can be added, and the fluid level is checked again. Initial trials suggest that a fluid level in the mouth may represent several milliliters more perfluorochemical than necessary.

Several infants have experienced a significant amount of pulmonary debris during partial liquid ventilation. Unlike total liquid ventilation, in which debris is removed with each breath, suctioning must be performed during partial liquid ventilation to facilitate debris removal. The debris has been found to be proteinaceous and phospholipid in nature and probably represents residual exogenous surfactant, excess endogenous surfactant, protein leakage, and cellular remnants. Failure to remove the debris can cause airway and/or endotracheal tube plugging. Plugging is best detected by sudden decreases in tidal volume measurements, which precede alterations in oxyhemoglobin saturation.

The timing of discontinuation of partial liquid ventilation has been, to date, a matter of attending to the protocol. Because the liquid evaporates from the lung, weaning the infant from partial liquid ventilation requires simply stopping additional dosing. The weaning process, therefore, takes several hours, depending on the vapor pressure of the particular liquid. Improvements in lung function have been observed beyond the first 24 hours off partial liquid ventilation. Recovered infants typically demonstrate a diminution in pulmonary compliance following gas recovery.

The decision to wean the infant from partial liquid ventilation, then, requires an understanding of the level of lung function on liquid ventilation, the potential benefit to lung function by prolonging the procedure, and the expected diminution in lung function during recovery. Until these issues are fully evaluated in clinical trials, lung function during weaning needs to be closely monitored, with partial liquid ventilation being reinitiated if significant deterioration occurs. Once again, close monitoring of tidal volume and lung function will be necessary to alter the mechanical ventilation settings during recovery and to assess tolerance.

Much has been learned about the care of the infant on partial liquid ventilation during the initial trials. Most important is the fact that animal models do not always mimic every aspect of human care, and this process and nursing protocols need to be developed systematically and cautiously.

TOTAL LIQUID VENTILATION

The human experience with total liquid ventilation is limited to the initial brief trial with a simple ventilation scheme in several very sick infants. Much of what is known about the nursing care during total liquid ventilation, therefore, is adapted from the human experience with partial liquid ventilation and the many years of animal research. Although a liquid ventilator shares some features with conventional gas ventilators, it also blends other technologies utilized in peritoneal dialysis, cardiac bypass, and ECMO.

The clinical application will require a specialized team, trained in fluid mechanics and comfortable with the procedure on animals. Attention will be directed at the fluid temperature and respiratory gas content, lung and alveolar pressures, tidal volume, and functional residual capacity. Although these concepts are familiar to the neonatal health care team, a working knowledge of these measurements and their relationship to the ventilator scheme will be required.

Other features of liquid ventilation that will require training and consideration include

responding to endotracheal tube leaks, gastrointestinal ingestion, and the importance of the height and position of the infant.

Currently available ventilator prototypes are computer-driven compact systems suitable for placement at an infant's bedside. These ventilators can be easily controlled, and they automatically monitor and adjust several parameters at once, thereby making clinical usage feasible. Following extensive testing by the FDA, the clinical application of these devices will be initiated.

SUMMARY

Liquid ventilation with oxygenated perfluorochemicals is a proven and valuable model for the study of early biologic and physiologic development. Potential therapies for liquid ventilation in the clinical arena capitalize on the unique capacity of these fluids to carry respiratory gases, eliminate interfacial surface tension at the gas-exchanging regions, deliver biologically effective drugs uniformly to the lung, and remove debris. The potential of this therapy has been demonstrated in various animal models with different disease processes; the feasibility in humans will be addressed in multicenter controlled clinical studies. These ongoing clinical trials will clarify the role of this technology over the next several years.

REFERENCES

1. Alcorn D, et al. 1977. Morphological effects of chronic tracheal ligation and drainage in the fetal lamb lung. *Journal of Anatomy* 123(3): 649–657.
2. Alcorn D, et al. 1980. Morphological effects of chronic bilateral phrenectomy or vagotomy in the fetal lamb lung. *Journal of Anatomy* 130(4): 693–695.
3. Avery ME, and Mead J. 1959. Surface properties in relation to atelectasis and hyaline membrane disease. *American Journal of Diseases of Children* 97: 517–523.
4. Clements JA. 1957. Surface tension on lung extracts. *Proceedings of the Society of Experimental Biology in Medicine* 10(1): 170–172.
5. Mead J, Whittenberger JL, and Radford EP. 1957. Surface tension as a factor in pulmonary volume-pressure hysteresis. *Journal of Applied Physiology* 10(2): 191–196.

6. Boyden EA. 1976. The programming of canalization in fetal lungs of man and monkey. *American Journal of Anatomy* 145(1): 125–131.

7. Shaffer TH, et al. 1983. Cardiopulmonary function in very preterm lambs during liquid ventilation. *Pediatric Research* 17(8): 680–684.

8. Shaffer TH, et al. 1976. Gaseous exchange and acid-base balance in premature lambs during liquid ventilation since birth. *Pediatric Research* 10(4): 227–231.

9. Winternitz MC, and Smith GH. 1920. Preliminary studies in intratracheal therapy. In *Pathology of War Gas Poisoning*. New Haven, Connecticut: Yale University Press, 144–160.

10. Clark LC, and Gollan F. 1966. Survival of mammals breathing organic liquids equilibrated with oxygen at atmosphere pressure. *Science* 152(730): 1755–1756.

11. Shaffer TH. 1987. A brief review: Liquid ventilation. *Undersea Biomedical Research* 14(2): 169–179.

12. Clark LC. 1970. Introduction. *Federation Proceedings* 29(5): 1698–1703.

13. Modell JH, et al. 1970. Effect of fluorocarbon liquid on surface tension properties of pulmonary surfactant. *Chest* 57(3): 263–265.

14. Modell JH, Calderwood HW, and Ruiz BC. 1970. Long term survival of dogs after breathing oxygenated fluorocarbon liquid. *Federation Proceedings* 29(5): 1731–1736.

15. Rufer R, and Spitzer HL. 1974. Liquid ventilation in the respiratory distress syndrome. *Chest* 66(0 supplement): S29–S30.

16. Fuhrman BP, et al. 1991. Perfluorocarbon-associated gas exchange. *Critical Care Medicine* 19(5): 712–722.

17. Schwieler GH, and Robertson B. 1976. Liquid ventilation in immature newborn rabbits. *Biology of the Neonate* 29(5–6): 343–353.

18. Matthews WH, et al. 1978. Steady-state gas exchange in normothermic, anesthetized, liquid ventilated dogs. *Undersea Biomedical Research* 5(4): 341–354.

19. Modell JH, et al. 1976. Liquid ventilation of primates. *Chest* 69(1): 79–81.

20. Shaffer TH, Wolfson MR, and Clark LC. 1992. Liquid ventilation. *Pediatric Pulmonology* 14(2): 102–109.

21. Forman D, et al. 1984. A fine structure study of the liquid-ventilated newborn rabbit. *Federation Proceedings* 43(2118): 647.

22. Wolfson MR, et al. 1992. Comparison of gas and liquid ventilation: Clinical, physiological, and histological correlates. *Journal of Applied Physiology* 72(3): 1024–1031.

23. Holaday DA, Fiserova-Bergerova V, and Modell JH. 1972. Uptake, distribution and excretion of fluorocarbon FX-80 (perfluorobutyl perfluorotetrahydrofuran) during liquid breathing in the dog. *Anesthesiology* 37(4): 387–394.

24. Goodin TH, Kaufman RJ, and Richard TJ. 1993. Comparative pulmonary toxicity of three perfluorochemicals (PFCs) in the rat and baboon. *Proceedings of the Fifth International Symposium on Blood Substitutes,* San Diego.

25. Modell JH, et al. 1970. Effect of fluorocarbon liquid on surface tension properties of pulmonary surfactant. *Chest* 57(3): 263–265.

26. Shaffer TH, et al. 1984. Liquid ventilation: Effects on pulmonary function in meconium-stained lambs. *Pediatric Research* 18(1): 49–53.

27. Wolfson MR, Greenspan JS, and Shaffer TH. 1991. Pulmonary administration of vasoactive drugs (PAD) by perfluorocarbon liquid ventilation. *Pediatric Research* 29(4): 36A.

28. Wolfson MR, and Shaffer TH. 1990. Pulmonary administration of drugs (PAD): A new approach for drug delivery using liquid ventilation. *Federation for American Society of Experimental Biology Journal* 4(4): 1105A.

29. Zelinka MA, et al. 1991. Direct administration of gentamicin during liquid ventilation of the lamb: Comparison of lung and serum levels to IV administration. *Pediatric Research* 29(4): 290A.

30. Mattrey RF. 1989. Perfluorooctylbromide: A new contrast agent for CT, sonography, and MR imaging. *American Journal of Roentgenology* 152(2): 247–252.

31. Moskowitz GD. 1970. A mechanical respirator for control of liquid breathing. *Federation Proceedings* 29(5): 1751–1752.

32. Moskowitz GD, Shaffer TH, and Dubin SE. 1975. Liquid breathing trials and animal studies with a demand-regulated liquid breathing system. *Medical Instrumentation* 9(1): 28–33.

33. Wolfson MR, et al. 1988. A new experimental approach for the study of cardiopulmonary physiology during early development. *Journal of Applied Physiology* 65(3): 1436–1443.

34. Wolfson MR, and Shaffer TH. 1990. Liquid ventilation during early development: Theory, physiologic processes and application. *Journal of Developmental Physiology* 13(1): 1–12.

35. Greenspan JS, et al. 1989. Liquid ventilation in preterm babies. *Lancet* 8671(2): 1095.

36. Greenspan JS, et al. 1990. Liquid ventilation in human preterm neonates. *Journal of Pediatrics* 117(1): 106–111.

37. Gil J, et al. 1979. Alveolar volume–surface area relation in air and liquid filled lungs fixed by vascular perfusion. *Journal of Applied Physiology* 47(5): 990–1001.

38. Lowe CA, and Shaffer TH. 1986. Pulmonary vascular resistance in the fluorocarbon-filled lung. *Journal of Applied Physiology* 60(1): 154–159.

39. Curtis SE, et al. 1991. Cardiac output during liquid (perfluorocarbon) breathing in newborn piglets. *Critical Care Medicine* 19(2): 225–230.

40. Tutuncu AS, et al. 1993. Intratracheal perfluorocarbon administration combined with mechanical ventilation in experimental respiratory distress syndrome: Dose-dependent improvement of gas exchange. *Critical Care Medicine* 21(7): 962–969.

41. Tutuncu AS, et al. 1993. Comparison of ventilatory support with intratracheal perfluorocarbon administration and conventional mechanical ventilation in animals with acute respiratory failure. *American Review of Respiratory Disease* 148(3): 785–792.

42. Leach CL, et al. 1993. Perfluorocarbon-associated gas exchange (partial liquid ventilation) in respiratory distress syndrome: A prospective, randomized, controlled study. *Critical Care Medicine* 21(9): 1270–1278.

43. Sekins KM, et al. 1990. Acoustic and physical properties of PFC liquids pertinent to ultrasound lung hyperthermia. Tenth Annual North American Hyperthermia Group. Radiation Research Society, April.

44. Liu MS, and Long DM. 1976. Biological disposition of Perfluorooctylbromide: Tracheal administration in alveolography and bronchography. *Investigative Radiology* 11(5): 479–485.

45. Sass DJ, et al. 1972. Liquid breathing: Prevention of pulmonary arterio-venous shunting during acceleration. *Journal of Applied Physiology* 32(4): 451–455.

46. Leach L, et al. 1995. Partial liquid ventilation with Liqui-Vent: A pilot safety and efficacy study in premature newborns with severe respiratory distress syndrome (RDS). *Pediatric Research* 37(4): 220A.

47. Valls-Soler A, et al. 1993. Comparison of natural surfactant and brief liquid ventilation rescue treatment in very immature lambs. *Pediatric Research* 33(4): 347A.

NOTES

Abbreviations

A	Alveolar gas	IRV	Inspiratory reserve volume
ABG	Arterial blood gas	$PaCO_2$	Partial pressure of CO_2 in arterial blood
ADS	Anatomical dead space		
C	Compliance	P_AO_2	Partial pressure of O_2 in alveolar blood
CBG	Capillary blood gas		
C_L	Lung compliance	PaO_2	Partial pressure of O_2 in arterial blood
CMV	Conventional mechanical ventilation		
		PEEP	Positive end expiratory pressure
CV	Closing volume	PIP	Peak inspiratory pressure
E	Expired gas	PVR	Pulmonary vascular resistance
ERV	Expiratory reserve volume	$\overline{Paw}$	Mean airway pressure
f	Frequency (ventilator)	Q	Volume of blood
f	Respiratory frequency	$\dot{Q}$	Volume of blood per unit time (perfusion)
FRC	Functional residual capacity		
Hgb	Hemoglobin	R	Resistance
Hgbf	Fetal hemoglobin	RQ	Respiratory quotient
HFJV	High frequency jet ventilation	RV	Residual volume
HFO	High frequency oscillation	SaO_2	Oxygen saturation of arterial blood
HFPPV	High frequency positive pressure ventilation	SVR	Systemic vascular resistance
		TLC	Total lung capacity
HFV	High frequency ventilation	V	Gas volume
I	Inspired gas	$\dot{V}$	Gas volume per unit time (ventilation)
IC	Inspiratory capacity		
IMV	Intermittent mandatory ventilation	$\dot{V}_A/\dot{Q}_C$	Ventilation-to-perfusion ratio
IPPV	Intermittent positive pressure ventilation	VC	Vital capacity
		V_T	Tidal volume

Glossary

Acidemia: An increase in the hydrogen ion concentration of the blood or a fall below normal in pH.

Acidosis: A state characterized by actual or relative decrease of alkali in body fluids in proportion to the acid content; the pH of body fluid may be normal or decreased.

Acinus, pulmonary: Respiratory bronchiole and all of its branches.

Air bronchogram: The outline of the bronchus on x-ray, visible because of diminished air in the alveolus.

Alkalemia: A decrease in H-ion concentration of the blood, or a rise in pH, irrespective of alterations in the level of bicarbonate ion.

Alkalosis: A pathophysiological disorder characterized by H-ion loss or base excess in body fluids (metabolic a.), or caused by CO_2 loss due to hyperventilation (respiratory a.).

Alveolar minute ventilation: The volume of gas moved into the alveolus per unit of time.

Alveolar-arterial oxygen gradient ($AaDO_2$): A measure of the alveolar efficiency in transporting oxygen to the pulmonary capillaries.

Amplitude: In high frequency ventilation the size of the ventilator breath or oscillation, also referred to as *delta p* (PIP – PEEP).

Anemometry: A technique for monitoring airway flow consisting of a heated filament which senses temperature changes corresponding to airway flow.

Apnea: Cessation of breathing for greater than 20 seconds accompanied by changes in color or heart rate.

Atelectasis: A collapsed or airless state in the lung.

Ball-valve obstruction: Blockage of the airway usually resulting from inhalation of particulate matter which prevents air from entering or exiting the alveolus.

Barotrauma: Injury to lung tissue resulting from pressure.

Base deficit: A reflection of the concentration of buffer or base available in the blood. A deficit reflects an excess of acid or a diminished amount of base available and is expressed as a negative number.

Base excess: Refers to either a deficit in the amount of acid present in the blood or an increased amount of base. Base excess is expressed as a positive number.

Capnogram: A graph demonstrating the concentrations of inspired and expired carbon dioxide.

Closing capacity: The lung volume at which dependent regions of the lung collapse or close to the main bronchi.

Compensation: An attempt to maintain a normal blood pH by altering the component of the blood gas that is not primarily responsible for the abnormality.

Compliance: A measurement of the elastic properties of the lung opposing a change in volume per unit of change in pressure.

Correction: An attempt to maintain a normal blood pH by altering the component of the blood gas responsible for the abnormality.

Dynamic mechanics: In a pulmonary function profile, testing during active, uninterrupted breathing.

Elastic recoil: The tendency of stretched objects to return to their resting state.

Energetics: A component of the pulmonary function profile that includes work of breathing.

Entrainment: Ability to provide additional respiratory gases during a breath without additional driving pressure.

Frequency: Breaths or cycles per minute.

Functional residual capacity (FRC): The volume of air remaining in the lung at the end of expiration.

Hertz (Hz): A unit of frequency equal to one cycle per second (60 cycles per minute).

High frequency ventilation (HFV): Ventilation provided at least four times the normal neonatal respiratory rate and at a tidal volume close to or less than anatomic dead space.

I:E ratio: The ratio of the time (in seconds) spent in inspiration compared to the time allowed for expiration.

Intrapleural pressure: Pressure within the pleural space.

Lamellar bodies: The site of surfactant synthesis and storage, lamellar bodies are located in Type II cells in the alveoli.

Laplace relationship: Describes the relationship between pressure, surface tension, and the radius of a structure. According to Laplace the pressure needed to stabilize an alveolus is directly proportional to twice the surface tension and inversely proportional to the radius of that alveoli.

Mean airway pressure (P$\overline{aw}$): The average pressure transmitted to the airways over a series of breaths.

Necrotizing tracheobronchitis: A process causing cellular death and tissue sloughing in the trachea and bronchi. The cause is unknown.

Nitric oxide: An endogenous pulmonary vasodilator.

Oxyhemoglobin dissociation curve: A graphic representation of the relationship between oxygen and hemoglobin.

Patient triggered ventilation: A system of assisted ventilation which recognizes and supports patient-initiated breaths.

Perflurochemicals: Inert liquids derived by replacing carbon bound–hydrogen atoms on organic compounds with fluorine.

pH: The negative logarithm of hydrogen ion concentration used to determine the relative acidity or alkalinity of a solution.

Phosphatidylcholine (PC): A phospholipid which comprises two-thirds of the lipid component of surfactant and is responsible for surfactant's ability to reduce lung surface tension.

Phosphatidylglycerol (PG): A phospholipid comprising eight percent of the lipid in surfactant. PG is unique to the pulmonary cells, making it a good marker for the presence of surfactant.

Pneumomediastinum: Air in the mediastinal space.

Pneumopericardium: Air in the pericardial space.

Pneumoperitoneum: Air in the peritoneum.

Pneumotachograph: A device that measures breath flow by detecting pressure drops across a fixed flow resistance.

Pneumothorax: Air in the pleural space.

Postductal: Blood flow arising from the aorta at a point distal to the ductus arteriosus.

Preductal: Blood flow from the aorta between the left ventricle and the ductus arteriosus.

Pulmonary insufficiency index: A scoring system used to calculate mortality risk based on oxygen requirement, acidosis, and time.

Pulmonary mechanics: A component of the pulmonary function profile that includes measurement of flow and pressure.

Pulse oximetry: A device utilizing a light source and photosensor to measure the amount of saturated hemoglobin in arterial blood.

Rales: An abnormal, non-musical sound usually heard during inspiration, also referred to as coarse crackles.

Resistance: Opposition to airflow resulting from friction. Resistance is proportional to the length of the airway or tube and inversely proportional to the radius of the tube.

Respiratory dead space: The volume of the anatomic passages between the external environment and the alveoli which do not function in gas exchange.

Retractions: Drawing in of the chest wall resulting from noncompliant lungs and a compliant chest wall.

Rhonchi: Deep, coarse, snoring or rattling sounds resulting from mucus plugs or debris in the bronchi.

Sail sign: A sail-shaped thymic outline seen on x-ray as the result of free air in the mediastinum.

Static mechanics: In a pulmonary function profile, testing done while briefly occluding the airway at one or more points in the respiratory cycle.

Stroke volume: The driving pressure of the piston in high frequency ventilation.

Surface tension: The force resulting from intermolecular forces at a surface.

Surfactant: A surface-active substance which reduces surface tension in the alveoli.

Tachyphylaxis: Rapid appearance of progressive decrease in response following repetitive administration of a pharmacologically or physiologically active substance.

Tidal volume: The volume of gas inspired with each breath.

Time constant: A measure of how quickly pressure generated in the proximal airway results in a 64 percent pressure change in the alveoli.

Tracheobronchomalacia: Softening of the tissues in the trachea and bronchi.

Transpulmonary pressure: Pressure across the lung from airway opening to the pleural space.

Ventilation:perfusion ratio: Expresses the relationship between alveolar ventilation and blood flow in the pulmonary capillaries.

Waveform: The shape of the delivered breath.

BIBLIOGRAPHY

McDonough JT Jr. 1994. *Stedman's Concise Medical Dictionary,* 2nd ed. Philadelphia: Williams & Wilkins.

O'Toole M. 1992. *Miller-Keane Encyclopedia and Dictionary of Medicine, Nursing and Allied Health,* 5th ed. Philadelphia: WB Saunders.

APPENDIX A ▲ Siggaard-Andersen Alignment Nomogram

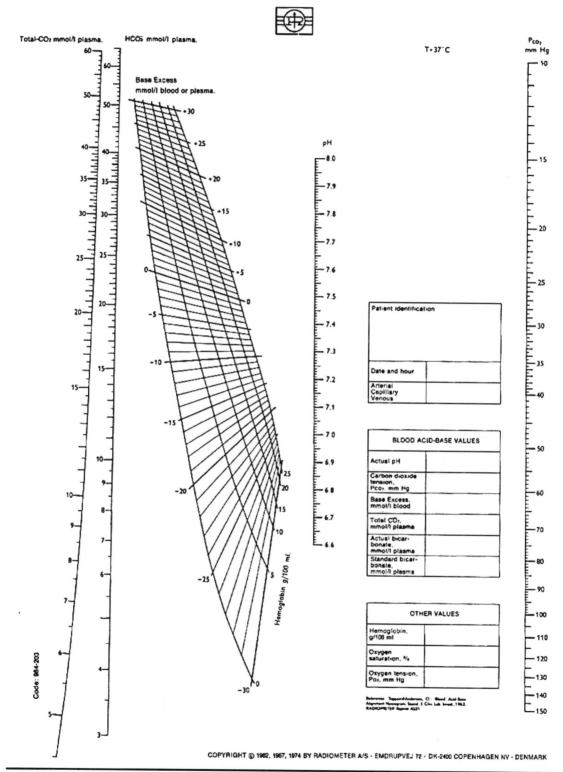

From: Siggaard-Andersen. 1963. Blood acid base alignment nomogram. *Scandinavian Journal of Clinical and Laboratory Investigation.* RADIOMETER reprint AS21. Reprinted by permission.

NOTES

Index

Acute Respiratory Care of the Neonate

TEST DIRECTIONS

1. Please fill out the answer form and include all requested information. We are unable to issue a certificate without complete information.
2. All questions and answers are developed from the information provided in the book. Select the **one best answer** and fill in the corresponding circle on the answer form.
3. Mail the answer form to: NICU INK,® 1304 Southpoint Blvd, Suite 280, Petaluma, CA 94954-6861 with a check for $50.00 (processing fee) made payable to NICU INK.® This fee is non-refundable.
4. Retain the test for your records.
5. You will be notified of your results within 6–8 weeks.
6. If you pass the test (70%) you will earn 30 contact hours (0.3 CEUs) for the course. Provider approved by the California Board of Registered Nursing, provider #CEP 6261; Florida Board to Nursing, provider #27I 1040, content code 2505; Iowa Board of Nursing, provider #189; and Alabama Board of Nursing, provider #ABNP0169.

COURSE OBJECTIVES

After reading and studying the content and taking the test the participant will be able to:
1. describe physiologic principles of the neonatal respiratory system including: embryologic development, surfactant synthesis, pulmonary and circulatory transitional events.
2. describe the pathophysiology of specific neonatal respiratory disorders including: respiratory distress syndrome, meconium aspiration, transient tachypnea of the newborn, and persistent pulmonary hypertension of the newborn.
3. differentiate various modes of neonatal ventilatory support, including: positive pressure ventilation, high-frequency jet ventilation, high-frequency oscillation, CPAP, and liquid and nitric oxide ventilation.
4. outline the general care given to infants requiring ventilatory support including: positive pressure ventilation, high-frequency jet ventilation, high-frequency oscillation, CPAP, and nitric oxide ventilation.
5. discuss the general care of infants undergoing the ECMO procedure.
6. discuss the current status of surfactant replacement therapy.
7. delineate a systematic approach for the interpretation of neonatal blood gases.
8. outline pharmacologic principles unique to the neonatal population.

---

1. The first embryonic lung structure arises from the:
   a. foregut
   b. midgut
   c. hindgut

---

2. A failure of foregut septation results in a:
   a. diaphragmatic hernia
   b. pulmonary atresia
   c. tracheoesophageal atresia

---

3. The period of lung development occurring between 5 and 17 weeks postconception is termed the:
   a. canalicular stage
   b. embryonic stage
   c. pseudoglandular stage

---

4. Branching of the pre-acinar airways is complete by:
   a. 14 weeks
   b. 16 weeks
   c. 18 weeks

---

5. The development of respiratory bronchioles begins during which stage of lung development?
   a. canalicular
   b. pseudoglandular
   c. terminal air sac

---

6. Alveoli receive their blood supply directly from:
   a. conventional arteries
   b. pre-acinar arteries
   c. supernumerary arteries

---

7. The pneumocytes most responsible for gas exchange are:
   a. granular
   b. squamous
   c. Type II

---

8. Surfactant is produced by which pneumocytes?
   a. granular
   b. squamous
   c. Type I

---

9. The majority of surfactant is composed of:
   a. lecithin
   b. glycerol
   c. lipid

---

10. Phosphatidylglycerol is a good marker for lung maturity because it is:
    a. secreted only when lungs are mature
    b. the most abundant lipid in surfactant
    c. unique to lung cells

11. Which cell structures are thought to be responsible for surfactant synthesis?
    a. lamellar bodies
    b. mitochondria
    c. rough endoplasmic reticulum

12. In its final form, surfactant is known as:
    a. ethanolamine
    b. phosphatidylcholine
    c. tubular myelin

13. Hormones implicated in the regulation of surfactant synthesis include:
    a. glucocorticoids
    b. glucagon
    c. progesterone

14. Thyroid hormones contribute to lung maturity by:
    a. depleting glycogen
    b. enhancing phosphatidylcholine production
    c. stimulating production of surfactant proteins

15. Tracheal fluid differs from amniotic fluid because tracheal fluid has higher:
    a. osmolality
    b. protein levels
    c. sodium levels

16. *In utero,* a term infant has approximately what volume of fluid in the lungs?
    a. 10–25 ml/kg
    b. 25–40 ml/kg
    c. 40–50 ml/kg

17. Loss of amniotic fluid results in which of the following lung findings?
    a. large, immature lungs
    b. reduced numbers of alveoli
    c. Type II cell deficiency

18. Following delivery, absorption of fetal lung fluid is triggered by secretion of:
    a. epinephrine
    b. glucocorticoids
    c. insulin

19. Fetal breathing movements have been reported on ultrasound as early as:
    a. 11 weeks
    b. 15 weeks
    c. 21 weeks

20. Reduction of fetal breathing movements coincides with an increase in levels of:
    a. fetal lung fluid
    b. prostaglandin E
    c. surfactant

21. *In utero,* the fetal lungs are perfused by what percentage of fetal cardiac output?
    a. 5–10
    b. 10–15
    c. 15–20

22. The average intrathoracic pressure generated by the infant's first breath is:
    a. 50 cm H_2O
    b. 60 cm H_2O
    c. 70 cm H_2O

23. By 30 minutes of age, a term newborn is expected to have a functional residual capacity of:
    a. 15–25 ml
    b. 25–35 ml
    c. 35–45 ml

24. A normal tidal volume for a term neonate is:
    a. 4–6 ml/kg
    b. 6–8 ml/kg
    c. 8–19 ml/kg

25. Chemoreceptors capable of responding to changes in H^+ levels include:
    a. aortic
    b. carotid
    c. medullary

26. The change in lung volume caused by a change in pressure is a measure of the lung's:
    a. compliance
    b. resistance
    c. time constant

27. The most significant factor affecting the lung's elastic properties is the:
    a. air-liquid interface
    b. connective tissue strength
    c. structure of the alveoli

28. Increased lung resistance is caused by an increase in:
    a. elastic recoil
    b. friction between gas molecules
    c. surface tension

29. The amount of alveolar dead space is dependent upon:
    a. alveolar size
    b. lung perfusion
    c. respiratory rate

30. The higher closing capacity seen in infants is thought to result from:
    a. decreased elastic recoil
    b. lower functional residual capacity
    c. increased airway resistance

31. The most common cause of hypoxia in the neonate is:
    a. decreased lung compliance
    b. increased airway resistance
    c. ventilation-perfusion mismatching

32. Lung perfusion is highest in which area?
    a. apex
    b. base
    c. midsection

33. A risk factor for the development of RDS is:
    a. female sex
    b. maternal hypertension
    c. second born twin

34. A factor that predisposes the infant to transient tachypnea of the newborn is:
    a. breech delivery
    b. hyperproteinemia
    c. postmaturity

35. The key to diagnosis in transient tachypnea of the newborn is:
    a. route of birth
    b. onset of symptoms
    c. radiographic pattern

36. The key pathophysiologic element in PPHN is:
    a. systemic hypotension
    b. bidirectional shunting through the foramen ovale
    c. elevated pulmonary vascular resistance

37. The presence of a right-to-left shunt may be demonstrated by comparing arterial oxygenation of blood obtained from both the:
    a. left radial and umbilical artery
    b. right radial and umbilical artery
    c. right radial and left temporal artery

38. The most distinguishing radiographic feature of RDS is the presence of:
    a. coarse infiltrates
    b. hyperinflation
    c. peripheral air bronchograms

39. The signs and symptoms of TTN mimic those of:
    a. congenital heart disease
    b. diaphragmatic hernia
    c. Group B streptococcal pneumonia

40. Risk factors for the development of neonatal pneumonia include:
    a. fetal scalp sampling
    b. multiple gestation
    c. prolonged labor

41. Presenting signs and symptoms of neonatal sepsis most commonly involve which system?
    a. cardiac
    b. central nervous
    c. gastrointestinal

42. The best indirect indicator of congenital infection during the first 8 hours of life is the presence of:
    a. bacteria in tracheal aspirates
    b. an elevated total white blood cell count
    c. white blood cells in the cerebrospinal fluid

43. Theories to explain intrauterine passage of meconium include:
    a. autonomic nervous system immaturity
    b. norepinephrine activation of peristalsis
    c. vagal stimulation from cord compression

44. Tachypnea associated with mild meconium aspiration usually resolves within:
    a. 24 hours
    b. 48 hours
    c. 72 hours

45. Apnea occurs most frequently during which state?
    a. active-alert state
    b. quiet sleep
    c. REM sleep

46. The main method of heat production in the newborn is:
    a. chemical thermogenesis
    b. involuntary shivering
    c. voluntary muscle activity

47. A small cardiac silhouette on a chest x-ray can be the result of:
    a. dehydration
    b. increased venous return
    c. a large thymic shadow

48. An opaque radiographic lung pattern will be seen with:
    a. hyperventilation
    b. pulmonary air leak
    c. pulmonary hemorrhage

49. Minimal nutritional maintenance calories are:
    a. 50 kcal/kg/day
    b. 100 kcal/kg/day
    c. 150 kcal/kg/day

50. During a normal transition following delivery, a 30 minute old infant would be expected to be:
    a. active and alert
    b. hypotonic
    c. quietly sleeping

51. Loss of body heat by an infant in a crib to nearby cold windows is an example of what type of heat loss?
    a. conductive
    b. convective
    c. radiant

52. Consequences of cold stress include:
    a. hypercapnia
    b. hypoglycemia
    c. respiratory acidosis

53. Assessment of a newborn infant reveals a barrel-shaped chest. This finding is consistent with a history of:
   a. a preterm delivery
   b. meconium at delivery
   c. suspected Group B streptococcal sepsis

54. The first scientist to describe the physiologic phenomena known as surface tension was:
   a. Boyle
   b. Pattle
   c. Laplace

55. Pressure-limited ventilators end the inspiratory phase:
   a. when a preset volume of gas is delivered
   b. after a preset time has passed
   c. when preset pressure is reached

56. Neonatal IMV ventilators use _____ to limit the amount of gas delivered during the inspiratory phase.
   a. peak inspiratory pressure (PIP)
   b. PIP and time
   c. PIP and volume

57. Lung compliance:
   a. is unaffected by disease states
   b. is the relationship of unit change in volume per unit increase in intrathoracic pressure
   c. is not related to changes in airway resistance

58. In an infant requiring IMV, unrecognized changes in lung compliance can alter:
   a. vital capacity
   b. functional residual capacity
   c. airway pressure

59. As compliance improves, chest wall excursion:
   a. decreases
   b. increases
   c. remains unchanged

60. The ventilatory parameter which plays a pivotal role in FRC and V_A during mechanical ventilation is:
   a. PEEP
   b. $P\overline{aw}$
   c. I:E ratio

61. Intermittent mandatory ventilation (IMV) differs from intermittent positive pressure ventilation (IPPV), in that IMV provides a:
   a. continuous flow of fresh gas
   b. patient-triggered breath
   c. time-limited positive pressure breath

62. Airway pressure applied with the purpose of preventing alveolar collapse is known as:
   a. continuous positive airway pressure
   b. intermittent airway pressure
   c. peak inspiratory pressure

63. A return to the smallest resting volume occurs in the lung because of which property?
   a. compliance
   b. elastic recoil
   c. surface tension

64. Commonly accepted criteria for mechanical ventilation include:
   a. $PaCO_2$ >45
   b. PaO_2 <60
   c. pH <7.25

65. Oxygen levels in the blood are most directly affected by ventilator:
   a. flow
   b. PEEP
   c. rate

66. Physiologic PEEP in an infant with normal lungs is usually:
   a. + 2
   b. + 3
   c. + 4

67. High ventilator rates may result in which of the following complications?
   a. air trapping
   b. elevated PIP
   c. loss of PEEP

68. A square wave breath is achieved by increasing which of the following ventilator settings?
   a. flow
   b. PIP
   c. rate

69. Animal studies have shown that surfactant is inactivated by:
   a. amniotic fluid
   b. bacteria
   c. blood

70. An example of an obstructive respiratory disease is:
   a. BPD
   b. pneumonia
   c. RDS

71. Hallman and Merritt suggest that infants respond better to surfactant when their initial colloid fluid loads are kept below:
   a. 10 ml/kg/day
   b. 15 ml/kg/day
   c. 20 ml/kg/day

72. In infants with PPHN, nitroprusside is used to:
   a. enhance vasoconstriction
   b. increase systemic blood pressure
   c. reduce cardiac afterload

73. Side effects of prostaglandin infusions include:
    a. decreased urinary output
    b. fever
    c. hypertension

74. Mechanical ventilation which provides a breath only during the infant's inspiratory cycle is known as:
    a. impedance pneumography
    b. intermittent positive pressure ventilation
    c. patient-triggered ventilation

75. During volume ventilation the level of PIP reached is dependent on preset:
    a. pressure limits
    b. time limits
    c. volume limits

76. What percentage of infants 500–999 grams develop PIE?
    a. 25
    b. 35
    c. 45

77. Risk factors for the development of air leak syndromes in the neonate include:
    a. hypoplastic lungs
    b. patent ductus arteriosus
    c. pneumonia

78. Radiographically, a "sail sign" is a classic feature of a pneumo_____.
    a. mediastinum
    b. pericardium
    c. thorax

79. Neonates at highest risk for bilateral pneumothoraces are those with:
    a. meconium aspiration
    b. pneumomediastinum
    c. pulmonary interstitial emphysema

80. Signs and symptoms of tracheomalacia include:
    a. coughing
    b. expiratory stridor
    c. lung hyperinflation

81. Factors placing a neonate at increased risk of pulmonary hemorrhage include:
    a. anemia
    b. fluid overload
    c. increased PIP

82. Which of the following findings is consistent with the diagnosis of a PDA in a 29 week gestational age neonate?
    a. heart rate of 110–120 bpm
    b. pulse pressure of 32 mmHg
    c. urine output of 4 ml/kg/hour

83. The dose of indomethacin recommended for closure of the PDA is:
    a. 0.1–0.3 mg/kg/dose
    b. 0.2–0.4 mg/kg/dose
    c. 0.3–0.5 mg/kg/dose

84. An infant with BPD is at risk for which of the following complications?
    a. gastroesophageal reflux
    b. hyponatremia
    c. metabolic acidosis

85. In infants with BPD, the PaO_2 should be maintained between:
    a. 40–55 torr
    b. 55–70 torr
    c. 70–90 torr

86. Which area of the retina is the last to become vascularized in the neonate?
    a. Zone I
    b. Zone II
    c. Zone III

87. In classifying ROP, a designation of plus disease refers to the:
    a. detachment of the retina
    b. presence of tortuous arterioles
    c. speed at which changes are occurring

88. Observation of fogging or condensation on the endotracheal tube indicates:
    a. the tube is in the trachea
    b. the tube is in the esophagus
    c. the tube is in the oral pharynx

89. A right main stem bronchus intubation can clinically mimic a:
    a. right pneumothorax
    b. left pneumothorax
    c. esophageal intubation

90. In suspected cases of right-to-left shunting, $TcPO_2$ readings should be taken at a preductal site such as the:
    a. upper right chest wall
    b. upper left chest wall
    c. left arm

91. The recommended negative pressure used to suction an infant's endotracheal tube is in the range of:
    a. 30–40 mmHg
    b. 75–80 mmHg
    c. 90–100 mmHg

92. Intermittent bubbling and/or fluctuation of fluid in a chest tube drainage bottle indicates:
    a. the chest tube is outside the chest wall
    b. the tube is patent and functioning
    c. an air leak in the collection tubing

93. A correctly positioned endotracheal tube should be:
    a. inserted 8 cm for a 2 kg infant
    b. three to four cm below the vocal cords
    c. visible at the aortic arch on x-ray

94. The recommended temperature of humidified gases in an oxygen hood is:
    a. 30–33°C
    b. 32–35°C
    c. 35–37°C

95. Which of the following PaO_2s is most likely to be reflected accurately by a transcutaneous oxygen monitor?
    a. 38 mmHg
    b. 84 mmHg
    c. 127 mmHg

96. Which of the following neonates is most likely to experience inaccuracies in pulse oximeter readings? The infant:
    a. under phototherapy
    b. who is febrile
    c. with adult hemoglobin levels of 75 percent

97. During end tidal CO_2 monitoring, the sharp rise at the beginning of the capnogram will be altered by a:
    a. decrease in cardiac output
    b. leak around the ET tube
    c. partially occluded ET tube

98. The theoretical basis behind the use of chest vibration is that vibrations:
    a. alter the pressure in the airways
    b. propel mucus from smaller bronchi
    c. relieve bronchospasm

99. In a term infant, postural drainage for a right middle lobe pneumonia would best be done with the infant in what position?
    a. flat, prone
    b. head down, left side lying
    c. supine

100. Each hemoglobin molecule is capable of carrying how many molecules of oxygen?
    a. 2
    b. 4
    c. 6

101. Which of following will result in a shift to left in the oxyhemoglobin dissociation curve?
    a. alkalosis
    b. hyperthermia
    c. presence of adult hemoglobin

102. To maintain acid-base balance, the kidneys excrete hydrogen ions in exchange for:
    a. chloride
    b. potassium
    c. sodium

103. To maintain a neutral pH, what ratio of acids:bases is required?
    a. 1:10
    b. 1:20
    c. 1:30

104. To compensate for metabolic acidosis the body will attempt to:
    a. acidify the urine
    b. hyperventilate
    c. increase excretion of sodium

105. An infant at risk for metabolic alkalosis is one who is:
    a. on total parenteral nutrition
    b. has diarrhea
    c. is receiving diuretics

106. To reach steady state following a ventilator change, an infant should be left undisturbed for a minimum of:
    a. 10 minutes
    b. 15 minutes
    c. 20 minutes

107. In fetal scalp sampling, what pH value is considered normal?
    a. 7.25
    b. 7.30
    c. 7.35

108. Which of the following is an acceptable position on x-ray for an umbilical arterial catheter? At the level of:
    a. T8
    b. L1
    c. L5

109. An infant with moderate RDS receiving 30 percent oxygen with a PIP of 17 and a PEEP of + 4 has an arterial blood gas with a PaO_2 value of 149. The most likely explanation for this is:
    a. heparin in the gas sample
    b. overventilation
    c. presence of an air bubble in the sample

110. Cyanosis normally becomes visible when the quantity of desaturated hemoglobin exceeds:
    a. 2 gm percent
    b. 5 gm percent
    c. 7 gm percent

111. Using the formula, how much bicarbonate would be required to correct half of the base deficit in a 2 kg infant whose deficit is −8?
    a. 2.4 mEq
    b. 4.8 mEq
    c. 9.6 mEq

Questions 112 and 113 pertain to the following question: How would you classify the following blood gas results?

112. pH 7.33, PCO_2 49, HCO_3^- 25:
    a. compensated respiratory acidosis
    b. compensated metabolic acidosis
    c. uncompensated respiratory acidosis

113. pH 7.44, PCO_2 45, HCO_3^- 30:
    a. compensated metabolic alkalosis
    b. compensated respiratory alkalosis
    c. normal blood gas

114. The major component of surfactant is:
    a. cholesterol
    b. apoprotein A
    c. phosphatidylcholine

115. Which of the following is reduced as a result of surfactant's effect on surface tension?
    a. alveolar opening pressure
    b. elastic recoil
    c. lung compliance

116. The natural surfactant Infasurf is extracted from:
    a. calf lungs
    b. human amniotic fluid
    c. pig lungs

117. The major constituent of artificial surfactants such as Exosurf is:
    a. apoproteins
    b. dipalmitoylphosphatidylcholine
    c. phosphatidylglycerol

118. Complications of surfactant replacement include:
    a. anaphylaxis
    b. apnea
    c. chest wall rigidity

119. A pulmonary hemorrhage following surfactant administration is more likely to occur in infants with which of the following conditions?
    a. patent ductus arteriosus
    b. pneumothorax
    c. sepsis

120. Repeat dosing for infants receiving Survanta should be considered at what time interval?
    a. every 2 hours
    b. every 4 hours
    c. every 6 hours

121. The recommended dose of Survanta is:
    a. 3 ml/kg
    b. 4 ml/kg
    c. 5 ml/kg

122. Which of the following nursing actions should be undertaken prior to surfactant administration?
    a. collection of a blood gas
    b. placing the infant prone
    c. suctioning the ETT

123. For infants receiving a rescue dose of surfactant what is the minimum recommended ventilator rate per minute?
    a. 35
    b. 45
    c. 55

124. Oral drugs that are poorly absorbed when the gastric pH is low include:
    a. amoxicillin
    b. phenobarbital
    c. theophylline

125. An example of a drug that requires renal tubular transport for excretion is:
    a. ampicillin
    b. gentamicin
    c. vancomycin

126. Rapid injection of a drug containing propylene glycol may result in:
    a. flushing of the skin
    b. hypotension
    c. localized vasoconstriction

127. The MICROS system of drug delivery works on the principle of:
    a. electrodiffusion
    b. retrograde flow
    c. pressure gradients

128. A potential complication of medication administration via a orogastric tube is:
    a. aspiration
    b. bezoar formation
    c. binding of the drug to the tubing

129. Disadvantages of ultrasonic nebulizers for neonatal inhalation therapy include:
    a. damage-producing inert ingredients
    b. hypoxic gas mixture administration
    c. particle size variability

130. Effects of β_2-agonists include increased production of:
    a. mucus
    b. surfactant
    c. Type I cells

131. Pulmonary effects of furosemide administration include:
    a. decreased airway resistance
    b. enhanced surfactant distribution
    c. reduced inflammation

132. Adverse effects of corticosteroids include:
    a. delayed achievement of neurodevelopmental milestones
    b. decreased linear growth
    c. inhibition of neutrophil function

133. Which of the following represents an appropriate loading dose for theophylline?
    a. 5 mg/kg
    b. 8 mg/kg
    c. 10 mg/kg

134. Local dopamine infiltrations can be treated with:
    a. heparin
    b. hyaluronidase
    c. phentolamine

135. The duration of action for vecuronium is:
    a. 30 minutes
    b. 60 minutes
    c. 120 minutes

136. What effect does the application of CPAP have on surfactant in the neonate's lung? It:
    a. decreases surfactant consumption
    b. increases surfactant production
    c. reduces surfactant distribution

137. Which of the following is recognized as an effect of CPAP application? Increased:
    a. airway resistance
    b. lung compliance
    c. tidal volume

138. When an infant is placed on CPAP, cardiac output is usually:
    a. decreased
    b. increased
    c. unchanged

139. Renal effects of CPAP include:
    a. enhanced renal blood flow
    b. increased sodium excretion
    c. stimulation of antidiuretic hormone

140. A contraindication for nasal CPAP is:
    a. cardiac disease
    b. meconium aspiration
    c. unrepaired diaphragmatic hernia

141. Which type of apnea is unresponsive to CPAP?
    a. central
    b. mixed
    c. obstructive

142. Most complications of CPAP are reported at levels that exceed:
    a. 6 cm
    b. 7 cm
    c. 8 cm

143. The minimum recommended flow for CPAP is:
    a. 5 liters/minute
    b. 6 liters/minute
    c. 7 liters/minute

144. Humidity levels for CPAP should be:
    a. 70–80 percent
    b. 80–90 percent
    c. 90–100 percent

145. Which of the following represents an acceptable temperature for inspired gases during CPAP?
    a. 35°C
    b. 37°C
    c. 39°C

146. Characteristics of a "CPAP belly" include:
    a. decreased bowel sounds
    b. soft distention
    c. visible bowel loops

147. A pneumotachograph measures respiratory flow by detecting changes in:
    a. pressure
    b. temperature
    c. voltage

148. Flow-volume loops are helpful in assessing infants with:
    a. bronchospasm
    b. meconium aspiration
    c. pneumonia

149. An advantage of the anemometer over the pneumotachograph is that the anemometer:
    a. generates no resistance
    b. has less dead space
    c. provides information on static mechanics

150. The pressure from airway opening to pleural space is referred to as:
    a. airway pressure
    b. intrapleural pressure
    c. transpulmonary pressure

151. Intrapleural pressure can be estimated by measuring:
    a. airway opening pressure
    b. esophageal pressure
    c. transpulmonary pressure

152. Lung segments that expand more slowly than others result in:
    a. altered static compliance
    b. lower dynamic compliance
    c. reduced airway compliance

173. Infants given surfactant during HFV are at increased risk for:
    a. atelectasis
    b. ET tube obstruction
    c. ventilator malfunction

174. An important factor in the etiology of necrotizing tracheobronchitis is thought to be:
    a. ET tube malposition
    b. lack of humidification
    c. sepsis

175. Decreased breath sound tone during HFJV is associated with:
    a. bronchospasm
    b. pneumothorax
    c. secretions

176. An oxygen index of 42 is predictive of a mortality risk of:
    a. 50–60 percent
    b. 60–70 percent
    c. 80–90 percent

177. Indications for ECMO include:
    a. meconium aspiration
    b. cyanotic congenital heart disease
    c. bilateral pulmonary hypoplasia

178. Contraindications for ECMO include an infant with:
    a. a birth weight of 2,100 gm
    b. a gestational age of 32 weeks
    c. presence of an atrial-septal defect

179. Final selection of an ECMO candidate is based on criteria predictive of _____ percent mortality.
    a. 50
    b. 65
    c. 80

180. Intracranial hemorrhage is a contraindication for treatment with ECMO because of:
    a. ligation of the carotid artery
    b. systemic heparinization
    c. compromised cerebral blood flow

181. The venoarterial route drains blood from the:
    a. carotid artery
    b. aortic arch
    c. right atrium

182. The venoarterial route returns blood to the:
    a. carotid artery
    b. internal jugular
    c. left ventricle

183. A major risk of venoarterial bypass is:
    a. ligation of the internal jugular vein
    b. pneumothorax
    c. air emboli

184. A limitation of venovenous double-lumen ECMO is the:
    a. decompression of the right ventricle
    b. ligation of the common carotid artery
    c. size of the catheter

185. Hypotension after initiation of ECMO is thought to be caused by:
    a. decreased ionized calcium levels
    b. hypovolemia
    c. heparin–dopamine interactions

186. The cellular blood component which demonstrates the greatest effect of exposure to a foreign surface is:
    a. white blood cells
    b. red blood cells
    c. platelets

187. An good indicator of adequate flow during venoarterial bypass is:
    a. SaO_2
    b. SvO_2
    c. PaO_2

188. One method of determining the presence of right-to-left shunting is to compare oxygen saturation measured on the left leg with that of the:
    a. left arm
    b. right arm
    c. right leg

189. In PPHN, tricuspid regurgitation is caused by increased:
    a. flow across the foramen ovale
    b. left atrial pressure
    c. right ventricular pressure

190. Cardiac lesions that present with symptoms similar to PPHN include:
    a. Epstein's anomaly
    b. tetralogy of Fallot
    c. total anomalous pulmonary venous return

191. Goals for the management of PPHN include reduction of:
    a. cardiac preload
    b. pulmonary vascular resistance
    c. systemic vascular resistance

192. For the infant with metabolic acidosis, THAM is indicated when:
    a. kidney function is inadequate
    b. hypotension is present
    c. ventilation is inadequate

153. An example of a lung disease in which time constants provide helpful information is:
    a. aspiration pneumonia
    b. respiratory distress syndrome
    c. tracheobronchomalacia

154. Helium dilution is a technique for measuring:
    a. functional residual capacity
    b. time constants
    c. work of breathing

155. Hyperextension of the neck during pulmonary function testing may result in artificially high:
    a. airway resistance
    b. functional residual capacity
    c. lung compliance

156. If sedation is required for testing an infant with chronic lung disease, the drug of choice would be:
    a. chloral hydrate
    b. morphine
    c. phenobarbital

157. When compared to pulmonary function testing done at one hour after birth in a preterm infant, testing three hours after surfactant administration would be expected to show improved:
    a. airway resistance
    b. functional residual capacity
    c. lung compliance

158. Elevated airway resistance in infants with meconium aspiration occurs because of:
    a. air trapping
    b. atelectasis
    c. debris in the airways

159. During conventional mechanical ventilation, gas moves into the alveolar region via:
    a. bulk gas flow
    b. convection
    c. passive diffusion

160. During high frequency ventilation, carbon dioxide elimination is influenced by:
    a. expiratory time
    b. mean airway pressure
    c. tidal volume

161. *Delta P* (PIP-PEEP) determines the size of a high frequency jet breath, or its:
    a. amplitude
    b. mean airway pressure
    c. percentage of inspiratory time

162. The "pendelluft" effect seen in HFV occurs because of differing:
    a. alveolar sizes
    b. airway resistance
    c. time constants

163. During HFV, the displayed pressure represents the pressure transmitted to the lung except in the presence of:
    a. atelectasis
    b. gas trapping
    c. pneumothoraces

164. The size of the jet pulses delivered to the patient is determined by the jet PIP and the:
    a. frequency
    b. inspiratory time
    c. PEEP

165. The main barrel of the Hi-Lo jet tracheal tube is used for:
    a. administration of jet pulses
    b. delivery of CMV gas
    c. pressure monitoring

166. During HFJV, rising servopressure usually indicates:
    a. improved compliance
    b. increased airway resistance
    c. tension pneumothorax

167. During HFJV, CMV breaths can be used to:
    a. decrease airway resistance
    b. increase compliance
    c. recruit atelectatic alveoli

168. An infant with pulmonary interstitial emphysema is receiving CMV with a PIP of 20. When switching this infant to HFJV what initial PIP is recommended?
    a. 14
    b. 17
    c. 20

169. In switching an infant with RDS receiving a PEEP of + 5 to HFJV, the recommended PEEP would be:
    a. + 2
    b. + 4
    c. + 6

170. Inspiratory time on the SensorMedics HFO is usually set at:
    a. 30 percent
    b. 33 percent
    c. 36 percent

171. Reducing the frequency on the SensorMedics HFO will have what effect? It will:
    a. decrease the tidal volume
    b. decrease the inspiratory time
    c. increase the tidal volume

172. When using HFOV to treat an infant with RDS, the mean airway pressure is initially set:
    a. 1–2 cm below the level on CMV
    b. at the same level as CMV
    c. 1–2 cm above CMV level

131. Pulmonary effects of furosemide administration include:
    a. decreased airway resistance
    b. enhanced surfactant distribution
    c. reduced inflammation

132. Adverse effects of corticosteroids include:
    a. delayed achievement of neurodevelopmental milestones
    b. decreased linear growth
    c. inhibition of neutrophil function

133. Which of the following represents an appropriate loading dose for theophylline?
    a. 5 mg/kg
    b. 8 mg/kg
    c. 10 mg/kg

134. Local dopamine infiltrations can be treated with:
    a. heparin
    b. hyaluronidase
    c. phentolamine

135. The duration of action for vecuronium is:
    a. 30 minutes
    b. 60 minutes
    c. 120 minutes

136. What effect does the application of CPAP have on surfactant in the neonate's lung? It:
    a. decreases surfactant consumption
    b. increases surfactant production
    c. reduces surfactant distribution

137. Which of the following is recognized as an effect of CPAP application? Increased:
    a. airway resistance
    b. lung compliance
    c. tidal volume

138. When an infant is placed on CPAP, cardiac output is usually:
    a. decreased
    b. increased
    c. unchanged

139. Renal effects of CPAP include:
    a. enhanced renal blood flow
    b. increased sodium excretion
    c. stimulation of antidiuretic hormone

140. A contraindication for nasal CPAP is:
    a. cardiac disease
    b. meconium aspiration
    c. unrepaired diaphragmatic hernia

141. Which type of apnea is unresponsive to CPAP?
    a. central
    b. mixed
    c. obstructive

142. Most complications of CPAP are reported at levels that exceed:
    a. 6 cm
    b. 7 cm
    c. 8 cm

143. The minimum recommended flow for CPAP is:
    a. 5 liters/minute
    b. 6 liters/minute
    c. 7 liters/minute

144. Humidity levels for CPAP should be:
    a. 70–80 percent
    b. 80–90 percent
    c. 90–100 percent

145. Which of the following represents an acceptable temperature for inspired gases during CPAP?
    a. 35°C
    b. 37°C
    c. 39°C

146. Characteristics of a "CPAP belly" include:
    a. decreased bowel sounds
    b. soft distention
    c. visible bowel loops

147. A pneumotachograph measures respiratory flow by detecting changes in:
    a. pressure
    b. temperature
    c. voltage

148. Flow-volume loops are helpful in assessing infants with:
    a. bronchospasm
    b. meconium aspiration
    c. pneumonia

149. An advantage of the anemometer over the pneumotachograph is that the anemometer:
    a. generates no resistance
    b. has less dead space
    c. provides information on static mechanics

150. The pressure from airway opening to pleural space is referred to as:
    a. airway pressure
    b. intrapleural pressure
    c. transpulmonary pressure

151. Intrapleural pressure can be estimated by measuring:
    a. airway opening pressure
    b. esophageal pressure
    c. transpulmonary pressure

152. Lung segments that expand more slowly than others result in:
    a. altered static compliance
    b. lower dynamic compliance
    c. reduced airway compliance

111. Using the formula, how much bicarbonate would be required to correct half of the base deficit in a 2 kg infant whose deficit is −8?
    a. 2.4 mEq
    b. 4.8 mEq
    c. 9.6 mEq

Questions 112 and 113 pertain to the following question: How would you classify the following blood gas results?

112. pH 7.33, PCO_2 49, HCO_3^- 25:
    a. compensated respiratory acidosis
    b. compensated metabolic acidosis
    c. uncompensated respiratory acidosis

113. pH 7.44, PCO_2 45, HCO_3^- 30:
    a. compensated metabolic alkalosis
    b. compensated respiratory alkalosis
    c. normal blood gas

114. The major component of surfactant is:
    a. cholesterol
    b. apoprotein A
    c. phosphatidylcholine

115. Which of the following is reduced as a result of surfactant's effect on surface tension?
    a. alveolar opening pressure
    b. elastic recoil
    c. lung compliance

116. The natural surfactant Infasurf is extracted from:
    a. calf lungs
    b. human amniotic fluid
    c. pig lungs

117. The major constituent of artificial surfactants such as Exosurf is:
    a. apoproteins
    b. dipalmitoylphosphatidylcholine
    c. phosphatidylglycerol

118. Complications of surfactant replacement include:
    a. anaphylaxis
    b. apnea
    c. chest wall rigidity

119. A pulmonary hemorrhage following surfactant administration is more likely to occur in infants with which of the following conditions?
    a. patent ductus arteriosus
    b. pneumothorax
    c. sepsis

120. Repeat dosing for infants receiving Survanta should be considered at what time interval?
    a. every 2 hours
    b. every 4 hours
    c. every 6 hours

121. The recommended dose of Survanta is:
    a. 3 ml/kg
    b. 4 ml/kg
    c. 5 ml/kg

122. Which of the following nursing actions should be undertaken prior to surfactant administration?
    a. collection of a blood gas
    b. placing the infant prone
    c. suctioning the ETT

123. For infants receiving a rescue dose of surfactant what is the minimum recommended ventilator rate per minute?
    a. 35
    b. 45
    c. 55

124. Oral drugs that are poorly absorbed when the gastric pH is low include:
    a. amoxicillin
    b. phenobarbital
    c. theophylline

125. An example of a drug that requires renal tubular transport for excretion is:
    a. ampicillin
    b. gentamicin
    c. vancomycin

126. Rapid injection of a drug containing propylene glycol may result in:
    a. flushing of the skin
    b. hypotension
    c. localized vasoconstriction

127. The MICROS system of drug delivery works on the principle of:
    a. electrodiffusion
    b. retrograde flow
    c. pressure gradients

128. A potential complication of medication administration via a orogastric tube is:
    a. aspiration
    b. bezoar formation
    c. binding of the drug to the tubing

129. Disadvantages of ultrasonic nebulizers for neonatal inhalation therapy include:
    a. damage-producing inert ingredients
    b. hypoxic gas mixture administration
    c. particle size variability

130. Effects of β_2-agonists include increased production of:
    a. mucus
    b. surfactant
    c. Type I cells

193. Nitric oxide stimulates GMP production which results in:
    a. increased cardiac output
    b. pulmonary vasodilation
    c. systemic vascular relaxation

194. A potential side effect of nitric oxide therapy is:
    a. methemoglobinemia
    b. systemic hypotension
    c. thrombocytopenia

195. During nitric oxide administration, monitoring should be done to detect the presence of:
    a. carbon monoxide
    b. cyanide
    c. nitric dioxide

196. Advantages of liquid ventilation include its ability to:
    a. decrease systemic vascular resistance
    b. increase pulmonary blood flow
    c. reduce surface tension

197. Infants with meconium aspiration may benefit from liquid ventilation because liquid has been shown to:
    a. enhance removal of pulmonary debris
    b. decrease intracardiac shunting
    c. prevent ball-valve obstruction

198. Perflurochemicals are suitable for liquid ventilation because they:
    a. dissolve adequate volumes of O_2 and CO_2
    b. are readily broken down in the lungs
    c. are water soluble

199. Perflurochemicals are mostly excreted by the:
    a. liver
    b. lungs
    c. kidneys

200. Additional benefits of perflurochemicals include the fact that they are:
    a. bacteriostatic
    b. capable of binding with vasoactive drugs
    c. nonradiopaque

201. Liquid breathing requires an increase in which of the following respiratory parameters?
    a. inspiratory time
    b. rate
    c. tidal volume

202. During liquid ventilation, adequate arterial oxygen levels can be achieved by altering the oxygen content of the liquid or the:
    a. functional residual capacity
    b. inspiratory time
    c. rate of breathing

203. Partial liquid ventilation utilizes a functional residual capacity of:
    a. 10–20 ml/kg
    b. 20–30 ml/kg
    c. 30–40 ml/kg

204. It is theorized that the effect of liquid ventilation on surfactant administration would be to:
    a. bind with the surfactant
    b. inactivate natural surfactant
    c. optimize dispersion

205. The anticipated role of liquid ventilation in the treatment of PPHN is to:
    a. deliver vasoactive drugs
    b. decrease intrapulmonary shunting
    c. enhance cardiac output

206. Current protocols call for instillation of perflurochemicals to be initiated at rates of:
    a. 1–2 ml/minute
    b. 2–3 ml/minute
    c. 3–4 ml/minute

207. Evaporation time for perflubron is:
    a. 1 ml/hour
    b. 2 ml/hour
    c. 3 ml/hour

NOTES

ANSWER FORM: Acute Respiratory Care of the Neonate, 2nd edition

Please completely fill in the circle of the **one best answer** using a dark pen.

| 1. a. ○ b. ○ c. ○ | 2. a. ○ b. ○ c. ○ | 3. a. ○ b. ○ c. ○ | 4. a. ○ b. ○ c. ○ | 5. a. ○ b. ○ c. ○ | 6. a. ○ b. ○ c. ○ | 7. a. ○ b. ○ c. ○ | 8. a. ○ b. ○ c. ○ | 9. a. ○ b. ○ c. ○ | 10. a. ○ b. ○ c. ○ |

| 11. a. ○ b. ○ c. ○ | 12. a. ○ b. ○ c. ○ | 13. a. ○ b. ○ c. ○ | 14. a. ○ b. ○ c. ○ | 15. a. ○ b. ○ c. ○ | 16. a. ○ b. ○ c. ○ | 17. a. ○ b. ○ c. ○ | 18. a. ○ b. ○ c. ○ | 19. a. ○ b. ○ c. ○ | 20. a. ○ b. ○ c. ○ |

| 21. a. ○ b. ○ c. ○ | 22. a. ○ b. ○ c. ○ | 23. a. ○ b. ○ c. ○ | 24. a. ○ b. ○ c. ○ | 25. a. ○ b. ○ c. ○ | 26. a. ○ b. ○ c. ○ | 27. a. ○ b. ○ c. ○ | 28. a. ○ b. ○ c. ○ | 29. a. ○ b. ○ c. ○ | 30. a. ○ b. ○ c. ○ |

| 31. a. ○ b. ○ c. ○ | 32. a. ○ b. ○ c. ○ | 33. a. ○ b. ○ c. ○ | 34. a. ○ b. ○ c. ○ | 35. a. ○ b. ○ c. ○ | 36. a. ○ b. ○ c. ○ | 37. a. ○ b. ○ c. ○ | 38. a. ○ b. ○ c. ○ | 39. a. ○ b. ○ c. ○ | 40. a. ○ b. ○ c. ○ |

| 41. a. ○ b. ○ | 42. a. ○ b. ○ c. ○ | 43. a. ○ b. ○ c. ○ | 44. a. ○ b. ○ c. ○ | 45. a. ○ b. ○ c. ○ | 46. a. ○ b. ○ c. ○ | 47. a. ○ b. ○ c. ○ | 48. a. ○ b. ○ c. ○ | 49. a. ○ b. ○ c. ○ | 50. a. ○ b. ○ c. ○ |

| 51. a. ○ b. ○ c. ○ | 52. a. ○ b. ○ c. ○ | 53. a. ○ b. ○ c. ○ | 54. a. ○ b. ○ c. ○ | 55. a. ○ b. ○ c. ○ | 56. a. ○ b. ○ c. ○ | 57. a. ○ b. ○ c. ○ | 58. a. ○ b. ○ c. ○ | 59. a. ○ b. ○ c. ○ | 60. a. ○ b. ○ c. ○ |

| 61 a. ○ b. ○ c. ○ | 62. a. ○ b. ○ c. ○ | 63. a. ○ b. ○ c. ○ | 64. a. ○ b. ○ c. ○ | 65. a. ○ b. ○ c. ○ | 66. a. ○ b. ○ c. ○ | 67. a. ○ b. ○ c. ○ | 68. a. ○ b. ○ c. ○ | 69. a. ○ b. ○ c. ○ | 70. a. ○ b. ○ c. ○ |

| 71. a. ○ b. ○ c. ○ | 72. a. ○ b. ○ c. ○ | 73. a. ○ b. ○ c. ○ | 74. a. ○ b. ○ c. ○ | 75. a. ○ b. ○ c. ○ | 76. a. ○ b. ○ c. ○ | 77. a. ○ b. ○ c. ○ | 78. a. ○ b. ○ c. ○ | 79. a. ○ b. ○ c. ○ | 80. a. ○ b. ○ c. ○ |

| 81. a. ○ b. ○ c. ○ | 82. a. ○ b. ○ c. ○ | 83. a. ○ b. ○ c. ○ | 84. a. ○ b. ○ c. ○ | 85. a. ○ b. ○ c. ○ | 86. a. ○ b. ○ c. ○ | 87. a. ○ b. ○ c. ○ | 88. a. ○ b. ○ c. ○ | 89. a. ○ b. ○ c. ○ | 90. a. ○ b. ○ c. ○ |

| 91. a. ○ b. ○ c. ○ | 92. a. ○ b. ○ c. ○ | 93. a. ○ b. ○ c. ○ | 94. a. ○ b. ○ c. ○ | 95. a. ○ b. ○ c. ○ | 96. a. ○ b. ○ c. ○ | 97. a. ○ b. ○ c. ○ | 98. a. ○ b. ○ c. ○ | 99. a. ○ b. ○ c. ○ | 100. a. ○ b. ○ c. ○ |

| 101. a. ○ b. ○ c. ○ | 102. a. ○ b. ○ c. ○ | 103. a. ○ b. ○ c. ○ | 104. a. ○ b. ○ c. ○ | 105. a. ○ b. ○ c. ○ | 106. a. ○ b. ○ c. ○ | 107. a. ○ b. ○ c. ○ | 108. a. ○ b. ○ c. ○ | 109. a. ○ b. ○ c. ○ | 110. a. ○ b. ○ c. ○ |

| 111. a. ○ b. ○ c. ○ | 112. a. ○ b. ○ c. ○ | 113. a. ○ b. ○ c. ○ | 114. a. ○ b. ○ c. ○ | 115. a. ○ b. ○ c. ○ | 116. a. ○ b. ○ c. ○ | 117. a. ○ b. ○ c. ○ | 118. a. ○ b. ○ c. ○ | 119. a. ○ b. ○ c. ○ | 120. a. ○ b. ○ c. ○ |

121. a. ○ b. ○ c. ○   122. a. ○ b. ○ c. ○   123. a. ○ b. ○ c. ○   124. a. ○ b. ○ c. ○   125. a. ○ b. ○ c. ○   126. a. ○ b. ○ c. ○   127. a. ○ b. ○ c. ○   128. a. ○ b. ○ c. ○   129. a. ○ b. ○ c. ○   130. a. ○ b. ○ c. ○

131. a. ○ b. ○ c. ○   132. a. ○ b. ○ c. ○   133. a. ○ b. ○ c. ○   134. a. ○ b. ○ c. ○   135. a. ○ b. ○ c. ○   136. a. ○ b. ○ c. ○   137. a. ○ b. ○ c. ○   138. a. ○ b. ○ c. ○   139. a. ○ b. ○ c. ○   140. a. ○ b. ○ c. ○

141. a. ○ b. ○ c. ○   142. a. ○ b. ○ c. ○   143. a. ○ b. ○ c. ○   144. a. ○ b. ○ c. ○   145. a. ○ b. ○ c. ○   146. a. ○ b. ○ c. ○   147. a. ○ b. ○ c. ○   148. a. ○ b. ○ c. ○   149. a. ○ b. ○ c. ○   150. a. ○ b. ○ c. ○

151. a. ○ b. ○ c. ○   152. a. ○ b. ○ c. ○   153. a. ○ b. ○ c. ○   154. a. ○ b. ○ c. ○   155. a. ○ b. ○ c. ○   156. a. ○ b. ○ c. ○   157. a. ○ b. ○ c. ○   158. a. ○ b. ○ c. ○   159. a. ○ b. ○ c. ○   160. a. ○ b. ○ c. ○

161. a. ○ b. ○ c. ○   162. a. ○ b. ○ c. ○   163. a. ○ b. ○ c. ○   164. a. ○ b. ○ c. ○   165. a. ○ b. ○ c. ○   166. a. ○ b. ○ c. ○   167. a. ○ b. ○ c. ○   168. a. ○ b. ○ c. ○   169. a. ○ b. ○ c. ○   170. a. ○ b. ○ c. ○

171. a. ○ b. ○ c. ○   172. a. ○ b. ○ c. ○   173. a. ○ b. ○ c. ○   174. a. ○ b. ○ c. ○   175. a. ○ b. ○ c. ○   176. a. ○ b. ○ c. ○   177. a. ○ b. ○ c. ○   178. a. ○ b. ○ c. ○   179. a. ○ b. ○ c. ○   180. a. ○ b. ○ c. ○

181. a. ○ b. ○ c. ○   182. a. ○ b. ○ c. ○   183. a. ○ b. ○ c. ○   184. a. ○ b. ○ c. ○   185. a. ○ b. ○ c. ○   186. a. ○ b. ○ c. ○   187. a. ○ b. ○ c. ○   188. a. ○ b. ○ c. ○   189. a. ○ b. ○ c. ○   190. a. ○ b. ○ c. ○

191. a. ○ b. ○ c. ○   192. a. ○ b. ○ c. ○   193. a. ○ b. ○ c. ○   194. a. ○ b. ○ c. ○   195. a. ○ b. ○ c. ○   196. a. ○ b. ○ c. ○   197. a. ○ b. ○ c. ○   198. a. ○ b. ○ c. ○   199. a. ○ b. ○ c. ○   200. a. ○ b. ○ c. ○

201. a. ○ b. ○ c. ○   202. a. ○ b. ○ c. ○   203. a. ○ b. ○ c. ○   204. a. ○ b. ○ c. ○   205. a. ○ b. ○ c. ○   206. a. ○ b. ○ c. ○   207. a. ○ b. ○ c. ○

Acute Respiratory Care of the Neonate
Second Edition

Name _____
Please Print

Address _____

City _____ State _____ Zip _____

Nursing License # _____ State(s) of License _____

Social Security # _____ required for Alabama participants only.

Mail with a $50.00 processing fee to
NICU INK,® 1304 Southpoint Blvd, Suite 280, Petaluma, CA 94954-6861.
Please make check payable to NICU INK.®
Foreign Participants: International Money Order drawn on U.S. Bank only. Thank you.

Other Books by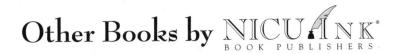

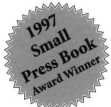

Baby Hands and Baby Feet:
Poems and Drawings from the Nursery
Nancy Kennedy and David Pegher

Chosen by AJN's panel of judges as one of the most valuable texts written in 1995, *Baby Hands and Baby Feet* is a "must read for all nurses, especially those who have been touched by experience with a high risk newborn." This book of 22 poems and 23 drawings creates "a compassionate yet realistic portrait of the day-to-day intimacies of life in an NICU." An exceptional experience you deserve to feel for yourself!

∾

Care of the 24–25 Week Gestational Age Infant:
A Small Baby Protocol, 2nd Edition
Laurie Porter Gunderson, RN, PhD, and Carole Kenner, RNC, DNS, FAAN

Newly updated and revised, this text is a valuable reference for anyone taking care of the extremely small infant. Some topics covered are thermoregulation, skin care, embryology and physiology, respiratory management, and ethics.

∾

Neonatal Infection:
Assessment, Diagnosis, and Management
Judy Wright Lott, RNC, DSN, NNP

A comprehensive, yet concise reference for neonatal staff nurses. This book covers assessment, diagnosis, and management of both congenital and neonatal infections.

∾

Physical Assessment of the Newborn:
A Comprehensive Approach to the Art of Physical Examination, 2nd Edition
Ellen P. Tappero, RNC, MN, NNP, and Mary Ellen Honeyfield, RNC, MS, NNP

This step-by-step guide, written by experts, provides a detailed approach to newborn assessment.

∾

Newborn Intensive Care
What Every Parent Needs to Know
Jeanette Zaichkin, RNC, MN

An essential reference for any parent with a sick or premature infant. Expresses in easily understandable chapters what is happening to babies in intensive care, the role of each member of the health care team, and how parents can participate in their infant's care. An exceptional book!

Other Books by NICU INK
BOOK PUBLISHERS

NAME_____

(PLEASE PRINT ALL INFORMATION)

ADDRESS _____

CITY _____STATE _____ZIP_____

PHONE (____) _____

Please enclose a check with your order. California residents add 7¼% sales tax, Sonoma County, CA residents add 7½% sales tax (applicable to books only). Orders received without correct California sales tax will not be filled. Please make your check payable to *NICU INK*®, 1304 Southpoint Blvd., Suite 280, Petaluma, CA 94954-6861. Please allow 6–8 weeks for your order to be filled. Foreign orders: International money order drawn on U.S. bank only. Please allow 8–12 weeks for surface delivery.

**To order by phone,
call toll free in the U.S. and Canada:
1(888) NICU INK or (707) 762-2646
VISA and MasterCard Accepted**

____ Newborn Intensive Care book(s) x $24.95 each = _____

____ Care of the 24–25 Week Gestational Age Infant
book(s) x $24.95 each = _____

____ Baby Hands book(s) x $17.95 each = _____

____ Neonatal Infection book(s) x $24.95 each = _____

____ Physical Assessment book(s) x $39.95 each = _____

Subtotal _____

CA residents add appropriate sales tax _____

Shipping (see below) _____

I have enclosed a total of $ _____

Shipping: Add $3.00 for the first book ordered.
Add $2.00 for each additional book ordered.
For quantity orders (six or more) or foreign orders contact
Lese Sykes for shipping charges (888) NICU INK.

Other Books by NICU INK
BOOK PUBLISHERS

NAME_____

(PLEASE PRINT ALL INFORMATION)

ADDRESS _____

CITY _____STATE _____ZIP_____

PHONE (____) _____

Please enclose a check with your order. California residents add 7¼% sales tax, Sonoma County, CA residents add 7½% sales tax (applicable to books only). Orders received without correct California sales tax will not be filled. Please make your check payable to *NICU INK*®, 1304 Southpoint Blvd., Suite 280, Petaluma, CA 94954-6861. Please allow 6–8 weeks for your order to be filled. Foreign orders: International money order drawn on U.S. bank only. Please allow 8–12 weeks for surface delivery.

**To order by phone,
call toll free in the U.S. and Canada:
1(888) NICU INK or (707) 762-2646
VISA and MasterCard Accepted**

____ Newborn Intensive Care book(s) x $24.95 each = _____

____ Care of the 24–25 Week Gestational Age Infant
book(s) x $24.95 each = _____

____ Baby Hands book(s) x $17.95 each = _____

____ Neonatal Infection book(s) x $24.95 each = _____

____ Physical Assessment book(s) x $39.95 each = _____

Subtotal _____

CA residents add appropriate sales tax _____

Shipping (see below) _____

I have enclosed a total of $ _____

Shipping: Add $3.00 for the first book ordered.
Add $2.00 for each additional book ordered.
For quantity orders (six or more) or foreign orders contact
Lese Sykes for shipping charges (888) NICU INK.

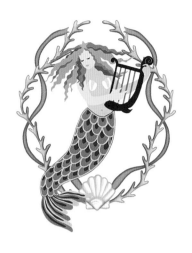

WOMEN
AND THE SEA

Hearing the Siren's Song

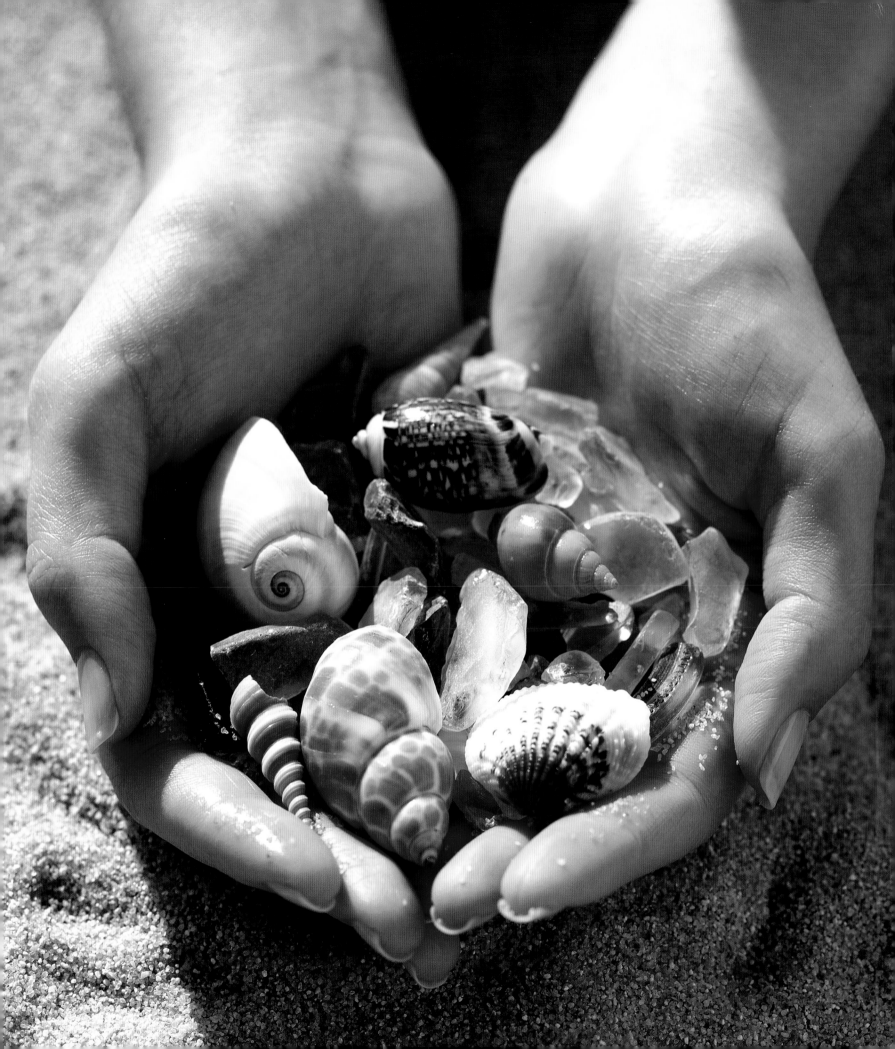

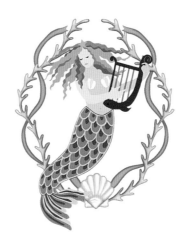

WOMEN AND THE SEA

Hearing the Siren's Song

By Claire Murray

Writer & Editor: Laurel Kornhiser
Designer: Donna Murphy

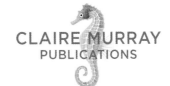

CLAIRE MURRAY
PUBLICATIONS

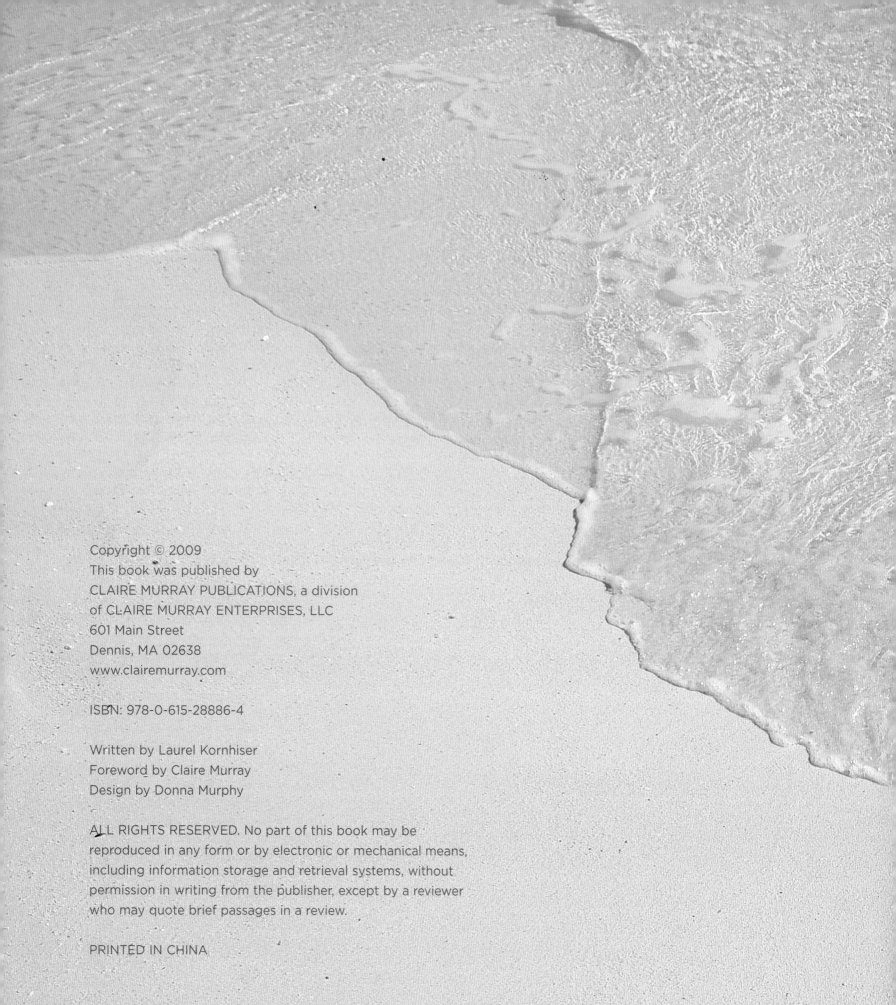

ISBN: 978-0-615-28886-4

Written by Laurel Kornhiser
Foreword by Claire Murray
Design by Donna Murphy

PRINTED IN CHINA

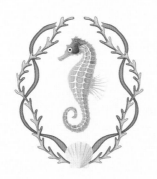

ARTIST, ENTREPRENEUR { Claire Murray }

"I was raised totally immersed in the sights
and **sounds of the seashore**;

I fell asleep to the rhythmic sound of fog horns

and awoke to the plaintive cries of the gulls."

Coast to Coast

She has hooked them all into her designs: mermaids admiring their untamed locks in the mirror; puffins gazing wide-eyed on Maine's rocky coast; clustered cottages rising to the crescendo of a church steeple overlooking Nantucket's harbor; tang, trigger, and clown fish floating among tropical coral reefs. Her nautical images multiply—scallop shells and seahorses, rainbow sailboats and three-masted schooners, historic windmills and landmark lighthouses. The images recall the many shores she has landed upon. Claire Murray is from Port Angeles, a one-time fishing village on the coast of Washington state. She studied art at the National Academy in Manhattan, "an island," she reminds us, launched her global company from her inn, Fair Gardens, on Nantucket, "another island," and now divides her time between her home on Cape Cod in Massachusetts, her retreat island in Georgian Bay, Canada, and her winter destination in Naples, Florida.

Growing up on the Olympic Peninsula, a landscape where sandy stretches share space with rock-littered coastlines and where giant logs, cast off from the nearby towering forests, stud the sand, she feels at home in places both wild and cultivated. "I was raised in one of the most beautiful places on the planet. The snow-capped Olympic Mountains literally drop to the sea. I fell asleep to the rhythmic call of foghorns and awoke to the plaintive cries of the gulls."

Sea images stimulated her receptive mind early on. She would watch her father study tidal charts and sense him leaving the house before dawn for fishing trips. "He would time his trips according to the height of the tide and the phase of the moon, hoping for the best chance of success." She would also see him engrossed in creating attractive lures. "He would sit for hours hand-crafting his own lures, painting them in an array of bright colors, then adding stripes, polka dots, and other fanciful designs." Sometimes her father, known locally as "King Fin," would take his daughter along on his thirty-six foot trawler, *The Sea Otter*. Claire remembers wildness and beauty mingling sublimely on many seafaring excursions: "We were once out in the middle of the Strait of Juan de Fuca, right off Vancouver Island, and were surrounded by a pod

For my mother...
for sharing the sea with me.

CLAIRE MURRAY

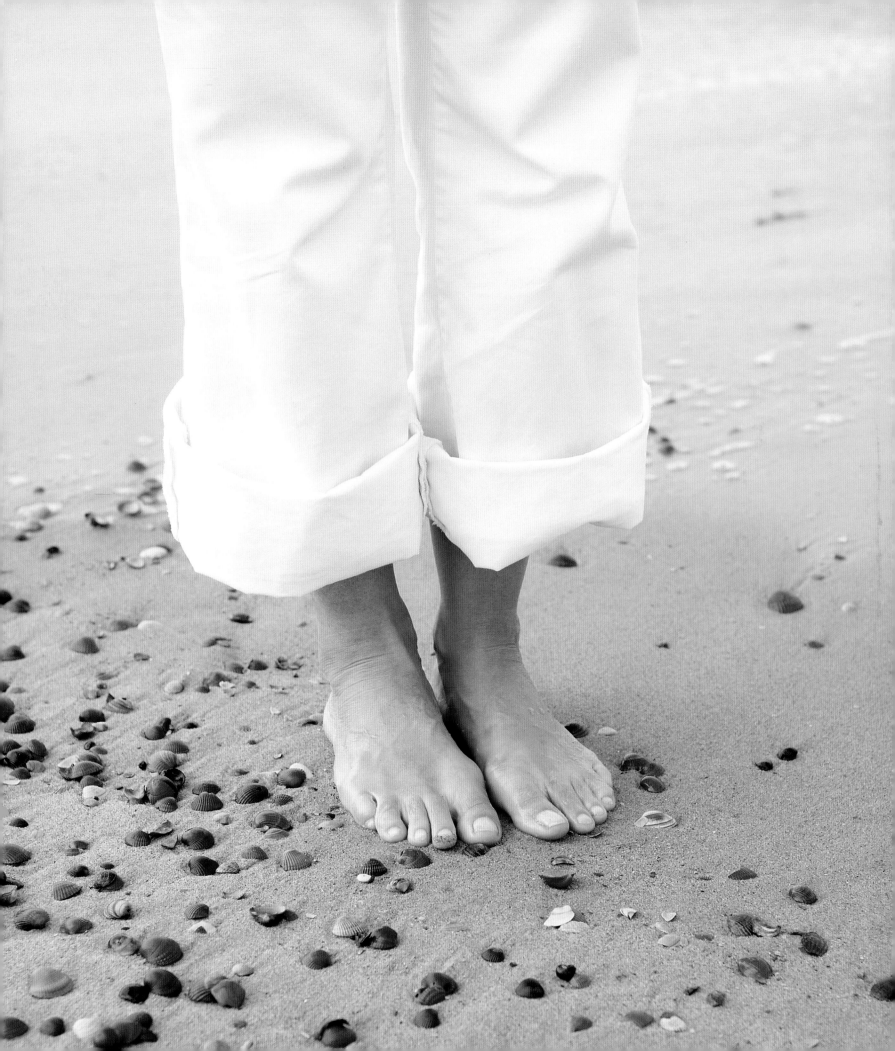

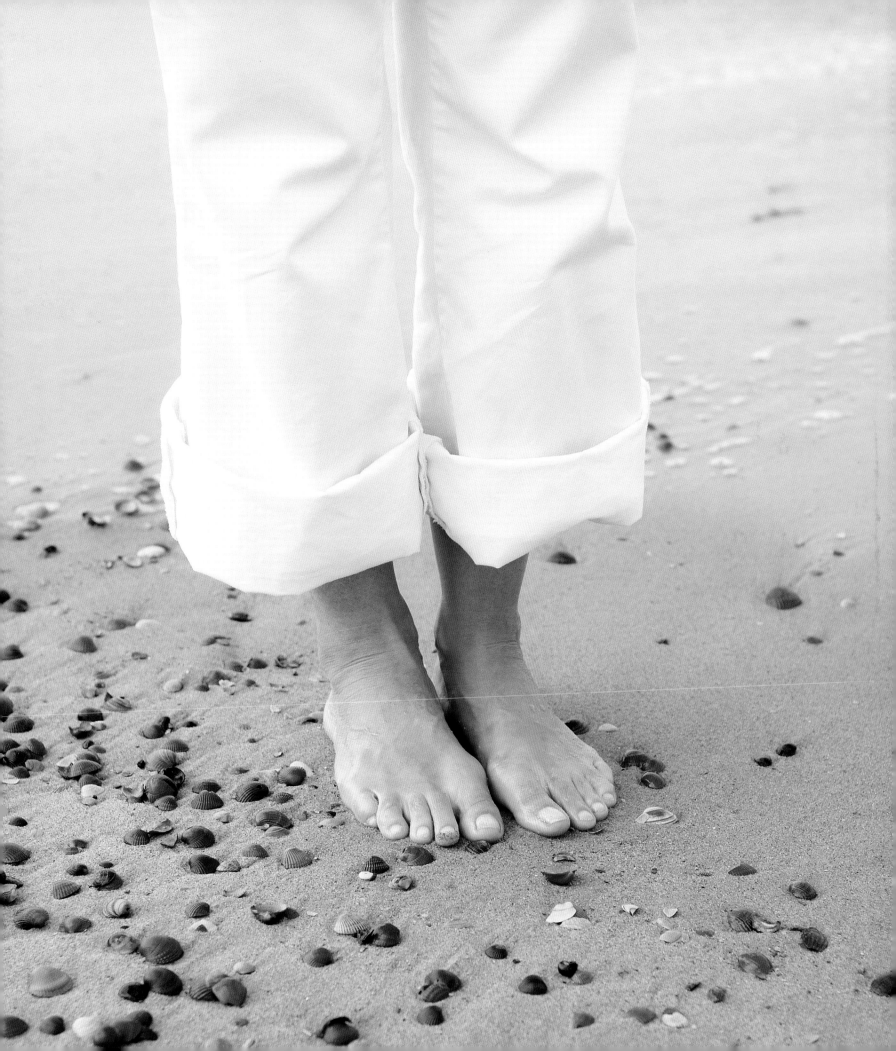

WHITE PLAINS PUBLIC LIBRARY

For my mother...
for sharing the sea with me.

CLAIRE MURRAY

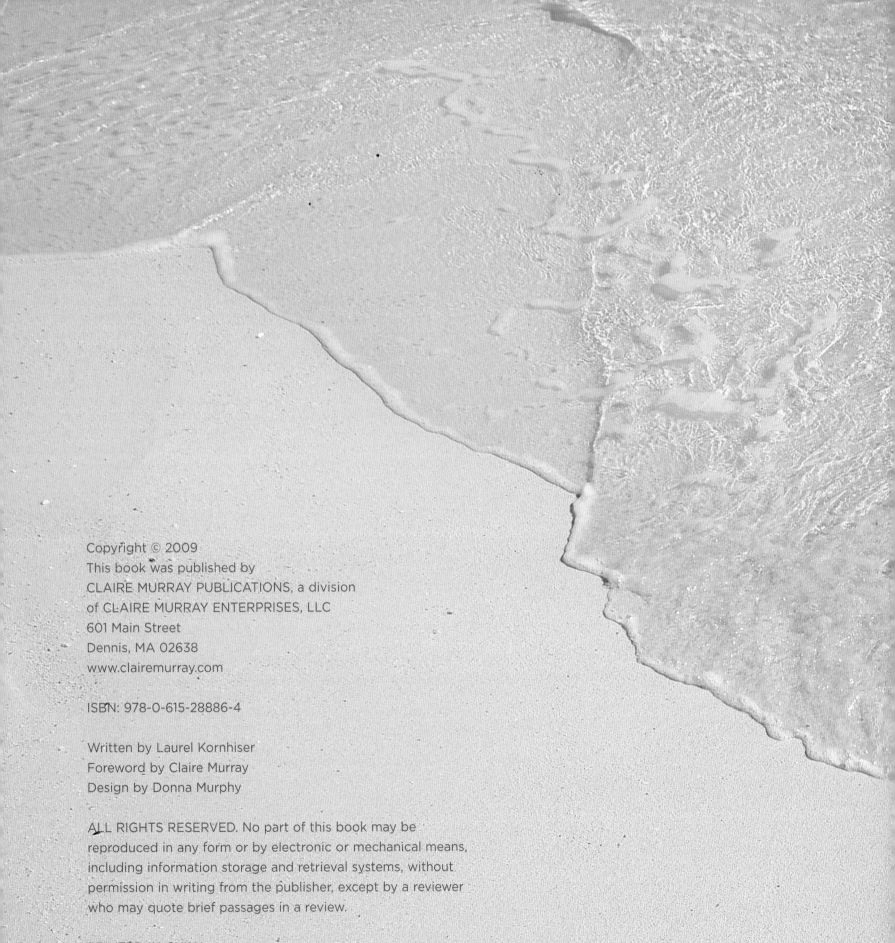

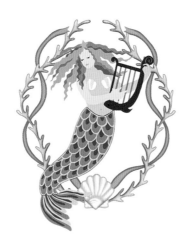

WOMEN AND THE SEA

Hearing the Siren's Song

By Claire Murray

Writer & Editor: Laurel Kornhiser
Designer: Donna Murphy

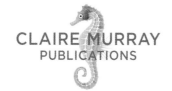

CLAIRE MURRAY
PUBLICATIONS

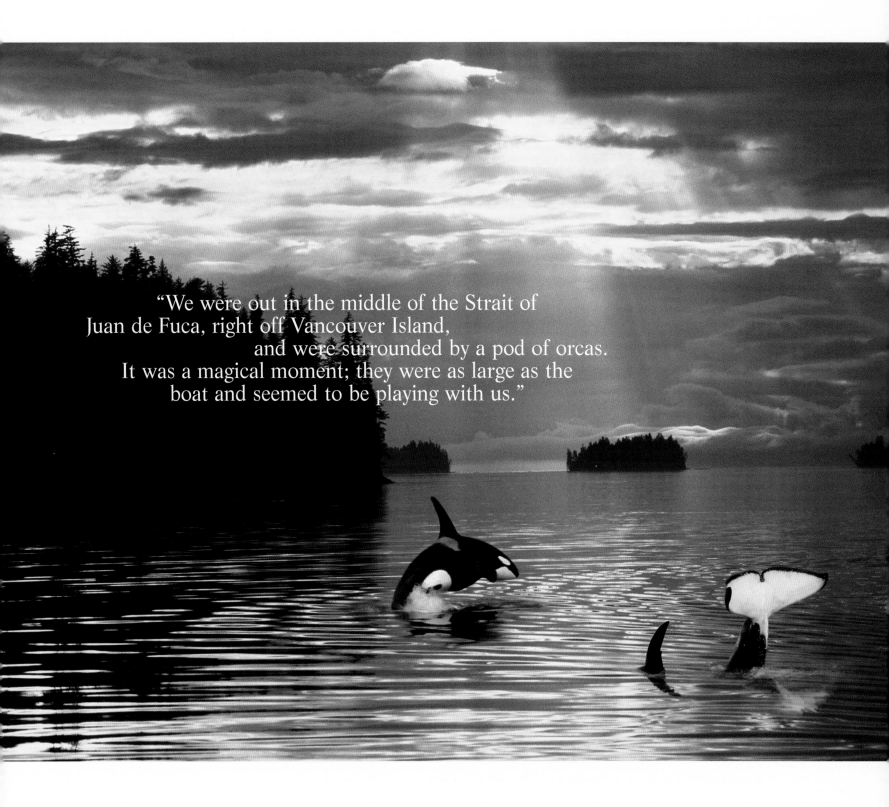

"We were out in the middle of the Strait of
Juan de Fuca, right off Vancouver Island,
and were surrounded by a pod of orcas.
It was a magical moment; they were as large as the
boat and seemed to be playing with us."

Women and the Sea

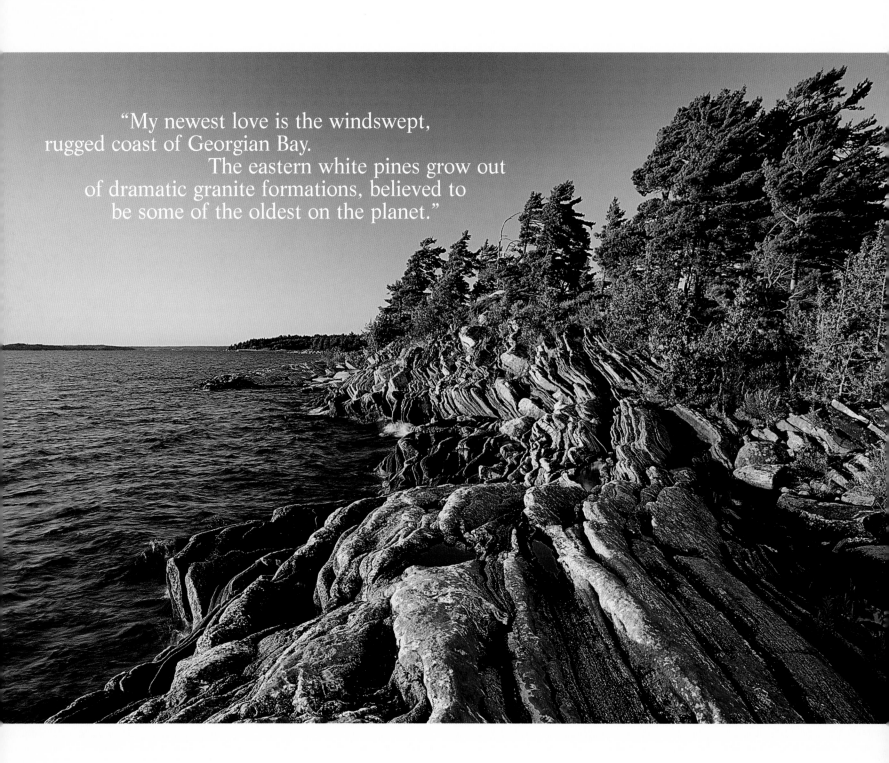

"My newest love is the windswept,
rugged coast of Georgian Bay.
The eastern white pines grow out
of dramatic granite formations, believed to
be some of the oldest on the planet."

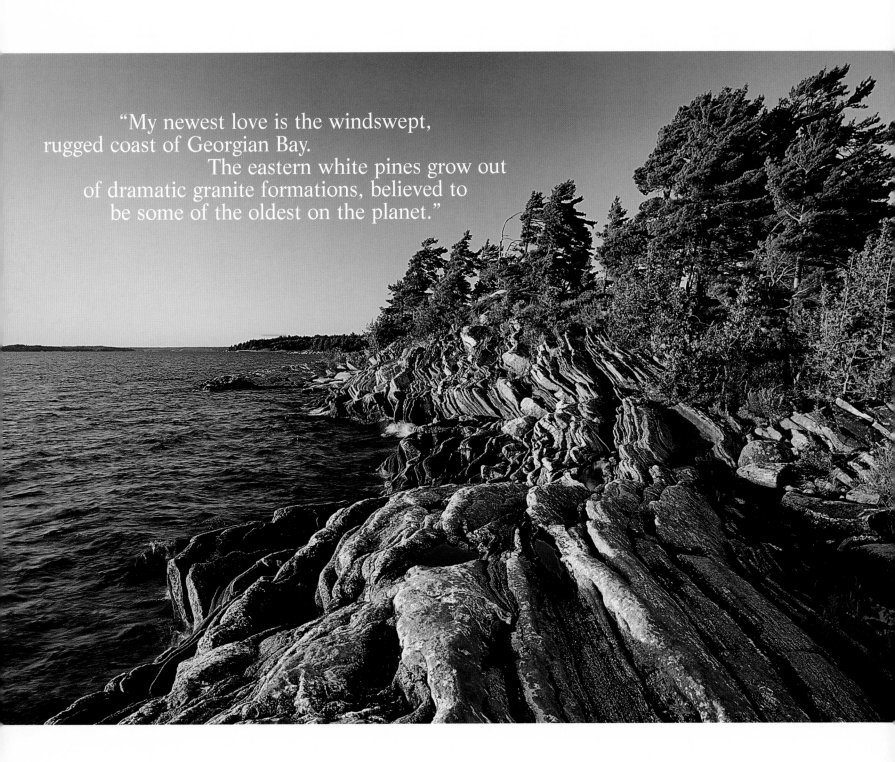

"My newest love is the windswept,
rugged coast of Georgian Bay.
The eastern white pines grow out
of dramatic granite formations, believed to
be some of the oldest on the planet."

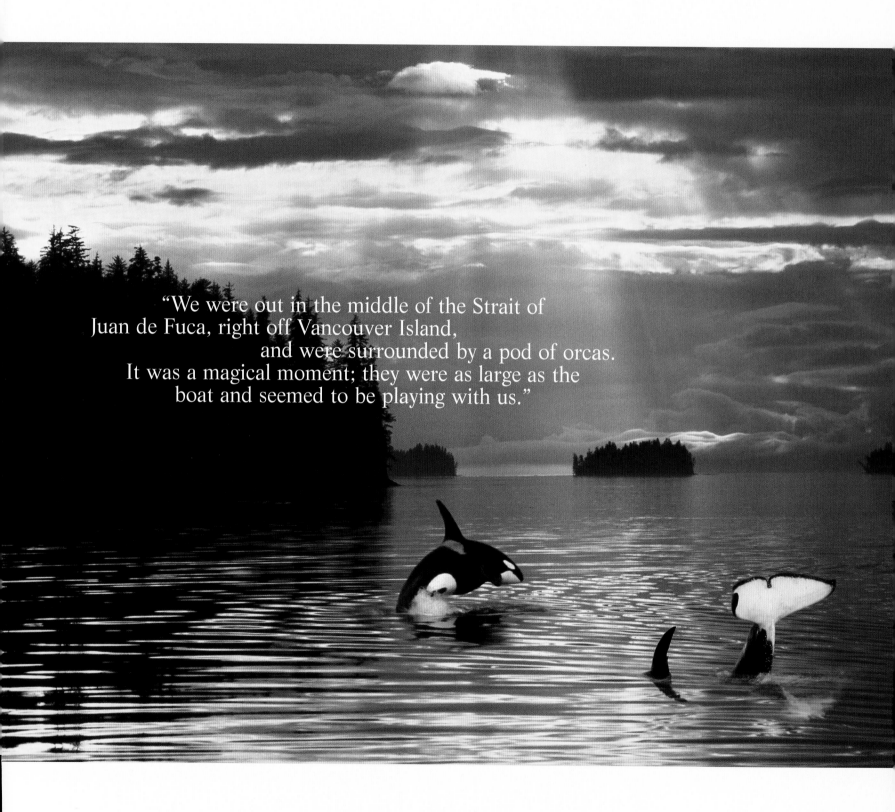

"We were out in the middle of the Strait of
Juan de Fuca, right off Vancouver Island,
and were surrounded by a pod of orcas.
It was a magical moment; they were as large as the
boat and seemed to be playing with us."

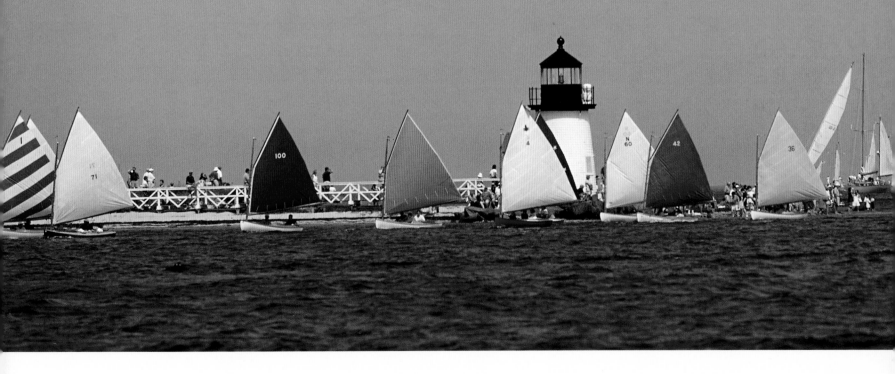

"Though known as the 'gray lady,' Nantucket
Island is awash in color—from the deep blues
of its sea and sky to its colorful Rainbow Fleet.
Its seafaring heritage has served as the inspiration
for my designs from the beginning."

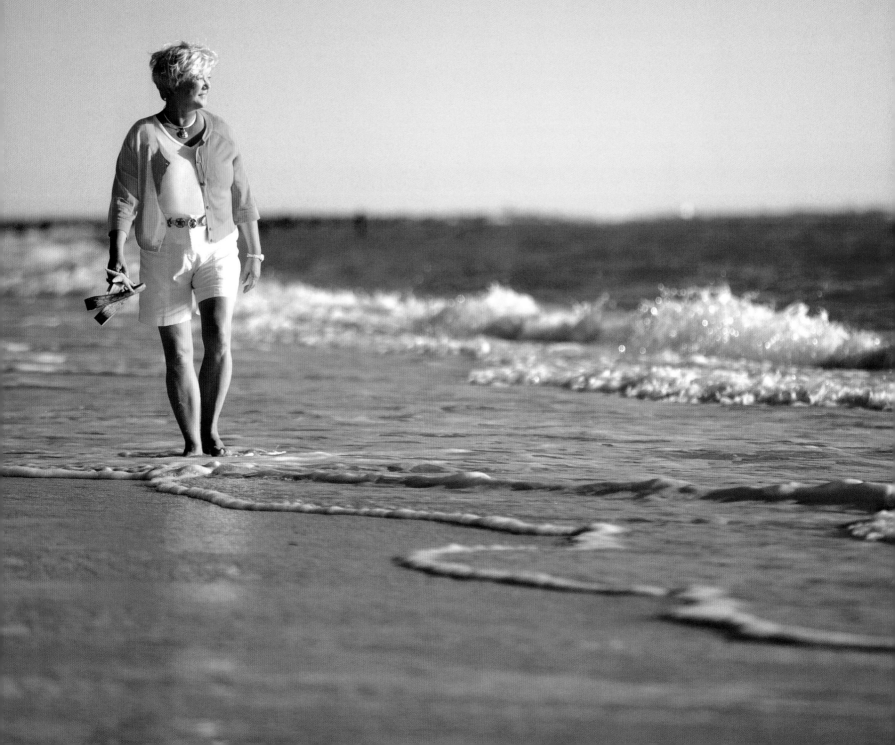

"I have been walking the beach in
the early morning hours for years,
collecting shells I plan to use for a sailor's
valentine I am making for my daughter."

of orcas, also known as killer whales. It was a magical moment; they were as large as the boat and seemed to be playing with us." Strangely, the fish were not biting. "As a young child, I did not realize that if the whales are present, the fish are not, because obviously orcas love salmon."

Poring over family photographs recently, though, she found many long-forgotten snapshots of her mother having her own adventures with the sea: "One shows her on my father's fishing boat landing a shark. In others, the sea is her backdrop, like the black and white image of her as a young woman sitting on an ancient driftwood log at the beach, the ocean behind her. With her are two children, me at the age of three and my younger brother. With the sea and all of its sights, sounds, and scents indelibly imprinted in my memory, it is no surprise that the products I design and manufacture have been influenced from the beginning by all things coastal." That her connection to the sea would spark her imagination and eventually find expression as the themes and colors of her hooked rugs and home accessories was evident early on. "My first sculpture at age fifteen was of a family of mermaids resting on the rocks." These mermaids would re-emerge as one of her first rug designs.

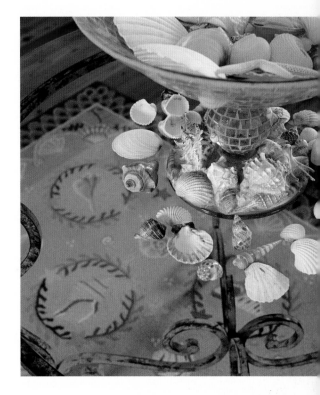

Eventually she moved to and then left the big island of Manhattan for the outpost island of Nantucket, where she would raise her daughter and run her inn. Much as the Quaker women of the island's whaling past picked up their needles to while away the long, gray days of winter while their sea captain husbands were gone, Claire discovered rug hooking. Soon women from the world over were coming to her inn to learn not only rug hooking, but quilting, stenciling, and other colonial arts. Inspired by her inn's Shake-spearean herb garden, Claire also held seminars on the lore and culinary uses of herbs. As she and her guests gathered around the fireplace, her mind

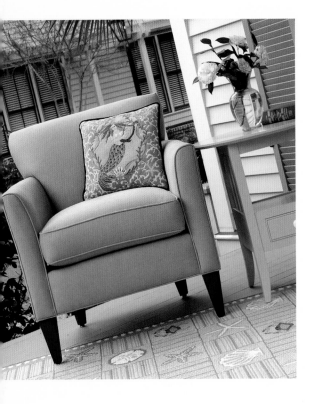

often drifted to thoughts of her nineteenth-century predecessors: "Nantucket has an incredible history of strong women of the sea; you feel it when you are there, at least I do." The island and its seafaring history continue to inspire many of Claire's hooked rug designs.

Though they may be useful, Claire's rugs are floor art. Through them, she translates the coastal places she has lived and loved. She has rendered Nantucket's cottage gardens, its whales and sailboats, and its seaside Christmas stroll. Her time spent in Georgian Bay, Canada, has spawned designs showcasing freshwater fish, loons, raccoons, and bears, and the flora of an inland sea. Florida is commemorated through designs of vibrant coral reefs, blue lagoons, and tropical shells. When there, Claire strolls the shoreline of the Gulf of Mexico, searching for materials to make another sea-inspired craft: "I have been walking the beach in the early morning hours for years, collecting shells I plan to use for a sailor's valentine I am making for my daughter."

Living in such different seaside locales has afforded Claire discriminating knowledge of their personalities: "I have wondered if other people have noticed how all of the oceans of the world have their own aura. The West Coast beaches where I spent my youth have a very strong, wild presence and a pungent scent that can be detected thirty minutes before you ever see the beach or hear the pounding surf." With the exception of the rocky coast of Maine, the East Coast has a more "genteel" disposition Claire suggests. A world traveler, Claire's journeys to the Far East, New Zealand, and Australia have convinced her even further that each body of water "has its own unique character." Though her work features forest creatures and country scenes, Claire remains permanently hooked by the endless possibilities of the water: "I love the mountains, too, but it is the sea that has shaped my life and continues to do so. The sea is my muse."

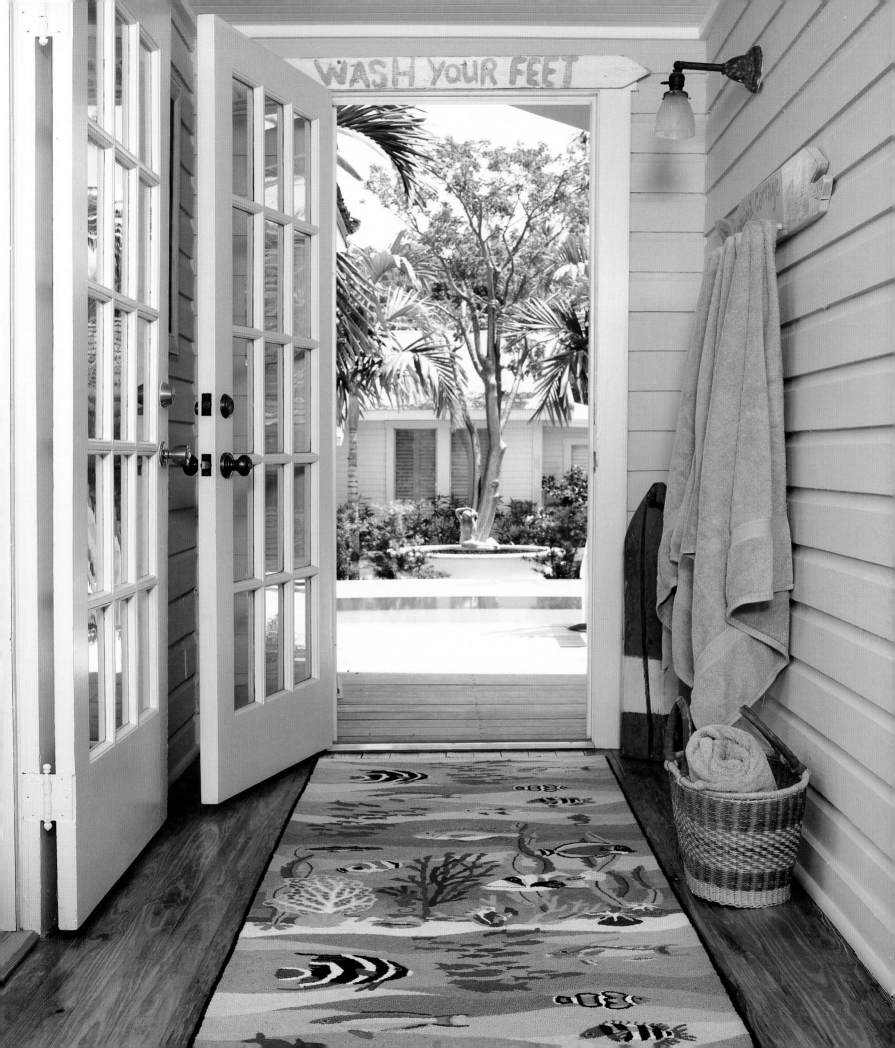

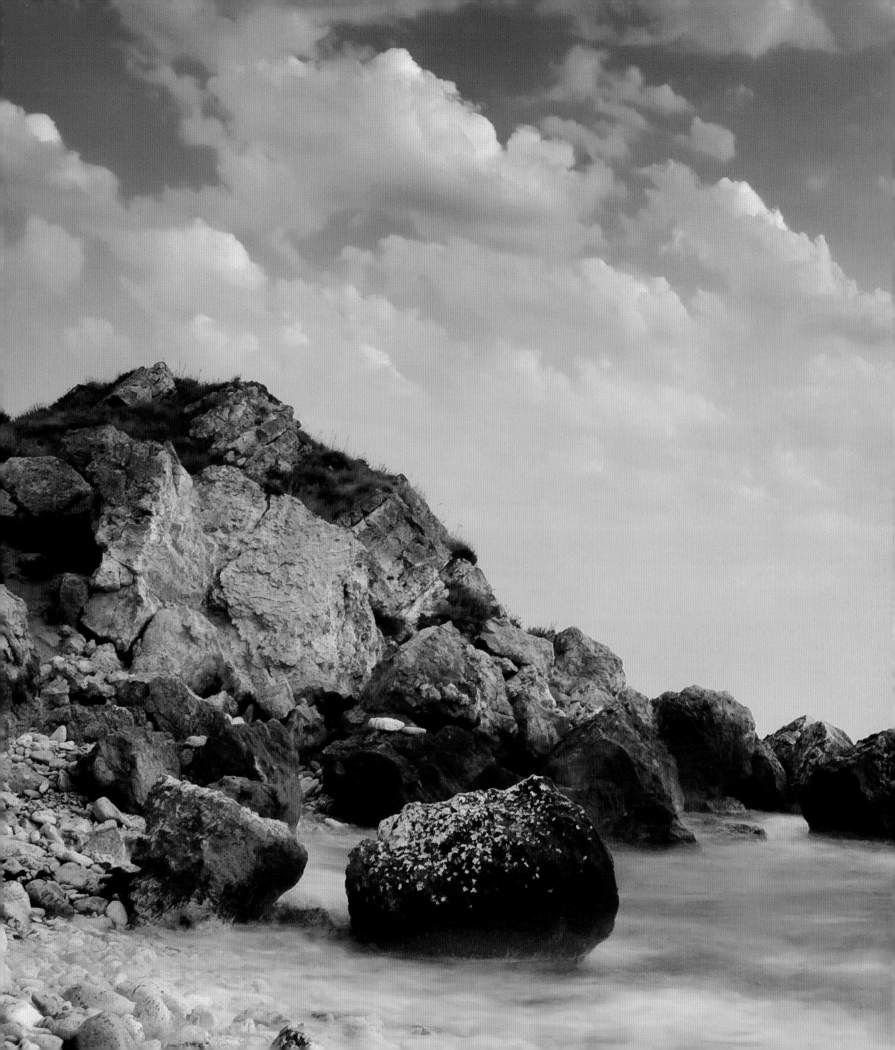

The lore of the Sea

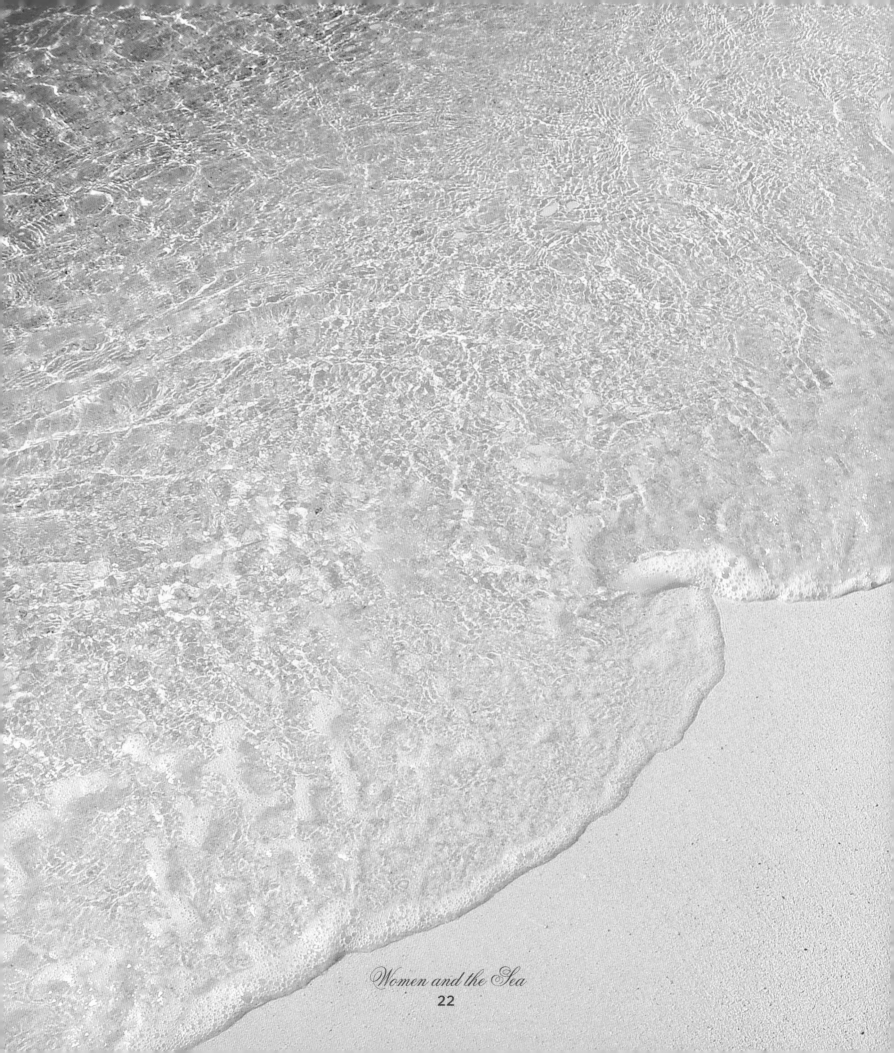

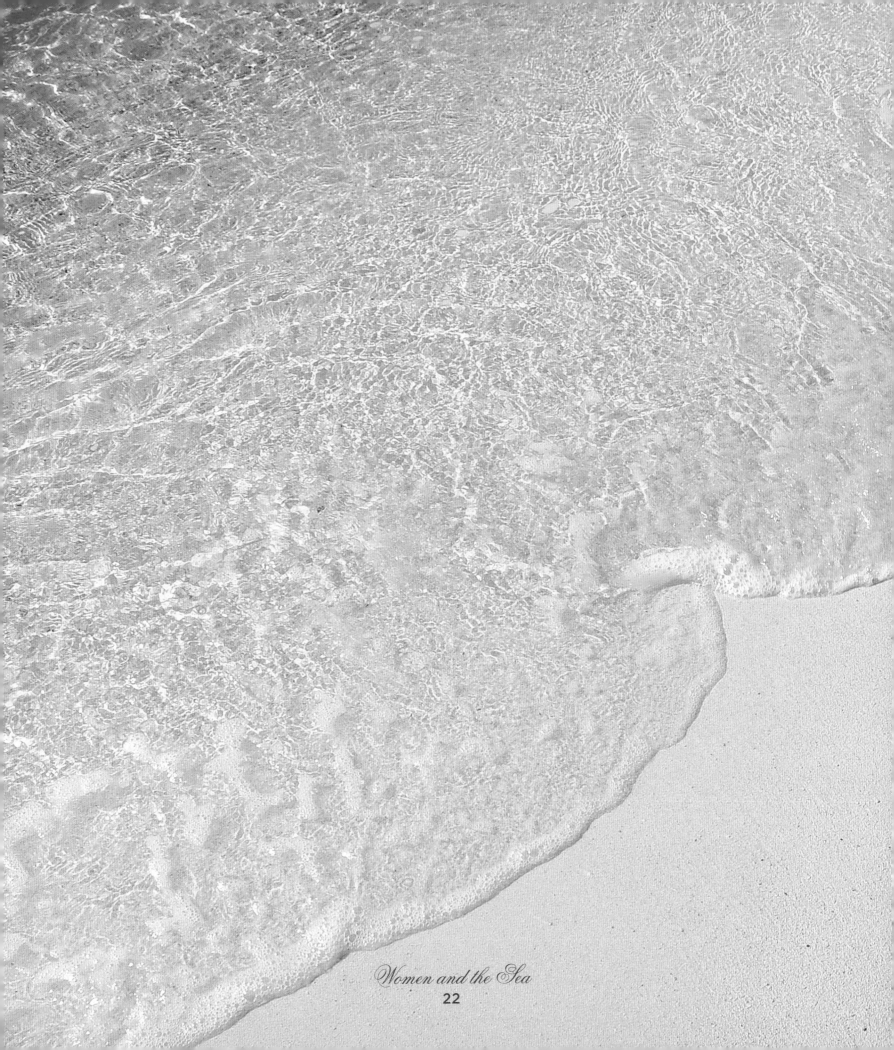

The lore of the Sea

The Lorelei

"Flows the Rhine as flowing wine,
　　Bright in its unrest,
Sweet with odors of the vine;
　　Heaven in its breast."

So the boatman Hugo sung,
　　Long, long ago,
By the Lurley-berg that hung
　　In the sunset glow.

At that fateful rock, upraised
　　From its foamy base,
Suddenly the boatman gazed
　　With a stricken face.

On its summit, wondrous fair,
　　Shining angel-wise,
Sat a maid, with golden hair
　　And beseeching eyes.

From a shoulder's rosy sphere
　　All the robe that slid,
Ripple bright and water-clear,
　　Rather show'd than hid.

As her hair her fingers through,
　　(Fingers pearly white)
Slowly pass'd, the diamond dew
　　Fell and broke in light.

But a gold harp from her feet
　　Lifted she ere long,
And its music, pulsing sweet,
　　Fed a wondrous song.

And the boatman, drifting fast,
　　Listen'd to his cost;
On the rocks before him cast!
　　In the whirlpool lost!

Then the Lorelei's luring form
　　Faded from the eye,
As a cloud fades, rosy warm,
　　In a purple sky.

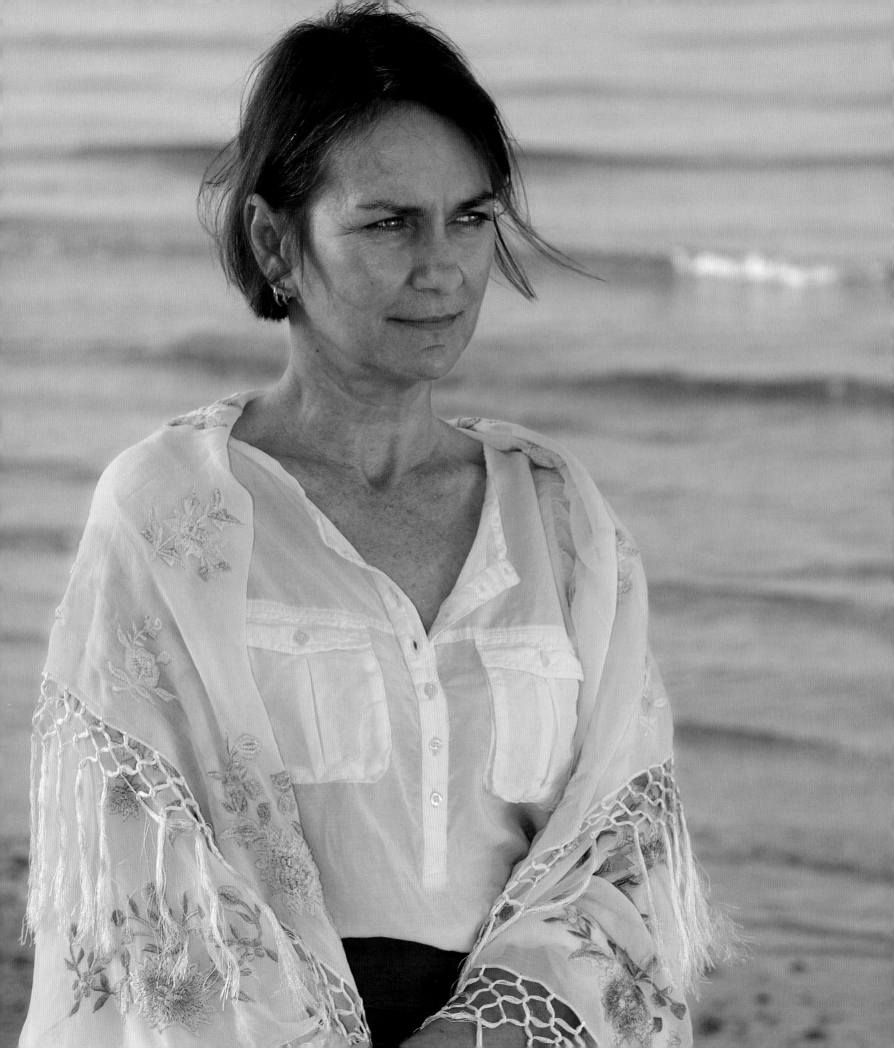

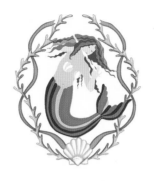

ARTIST { Christina Wyatt }

"Mermaids are the perfect woman:

beautiful, mysterious, unattainable. I am inspired

by a **sense of grace**, and mermaids

offer unlimited opportunities to express grace."

Fort Myers, Florida

The first one appeared as a ghostly image in a painting called *The Gate Keepers*. As her sisters have across centuries and cultures, the mermaid called sweetly to a receptive mind. Finding painter Christina Wyatt a willing, imaginative conduit, many more have followed, manifesting through her canvases in forms both beautiful and beguiling. Their opalescent scales shimmer, their long locks waving down their bare backs. They hold court on the ocean's floor, bright orange and yellow fish floating in attendance. They cavort with seahorses, bond with goldfish, curl and coil like moonshells, and sleep like Pisces twins on beds of sand and shells. They undulate and sway, these maidens of sea dreams. "I am inspired by a sense of grace, and mermaids offer unlimited opportunities to express grace," says their artist. "The flowing hair and swaying sea grasses—poetry emerges with each subtle movement."

Whether she is painting one of her mermaids, a medley of seashells, a gathering of beachcombers, or a pair of exotic birds in a tropical grove of bamboo, Christina glosses her work with mysticism, magic, and symbolism. A daydreamer since grade school when her teachers would complain she would rather draw than attend to lessons, she says, "I like to visually realize that place where dreams live." Her mermaids and the mesmerizing settings she places them in emerge from childhood memories of Sunday afternoons spent roaming Matheson Hammock Park in Miami, Florida, where she grew up. She and her brothers would scamper over rocks, collecting shells and outing hermit crabs. "We would run wild around this enclosed beach while our parents relaxed. I could step out of the every day and into a world of great wonderment that would occupy me for hours. It was always a pleasure to return home with a fist full of little treasures to examine and display around my room." As teens with licenses, Christina and her friends naturally gravitated toward the water, its hold on her never loosening, even when her life took her to college inland in Maine and finally to Virginia Commonwealth University where she studied art.

A dozen years ago, she returned to her native Florida. Having long pursued her art as a hobby while working "day jobs" to support herself, Christina decided a handful of years ago to paint full time and to get

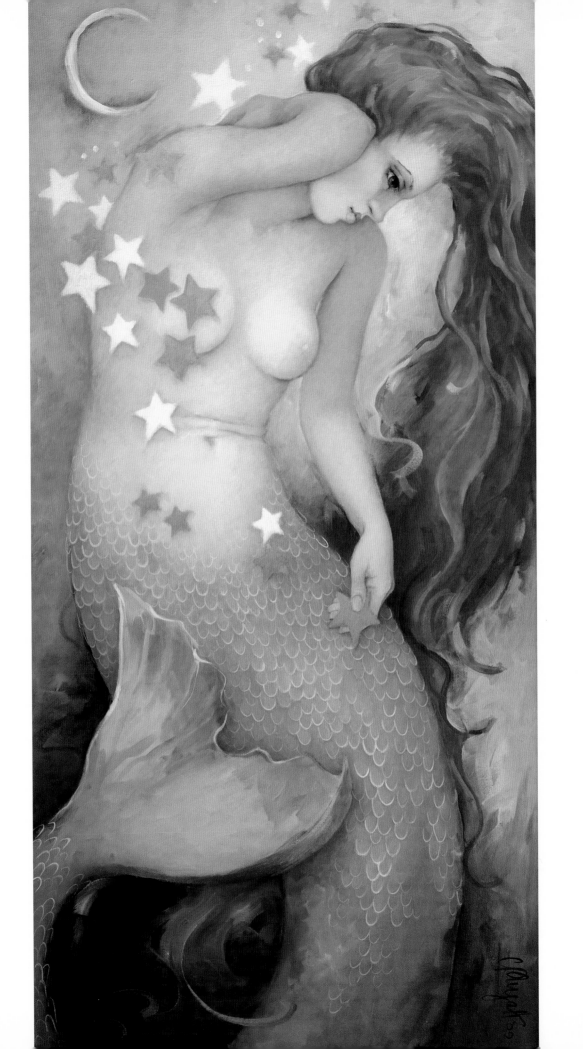

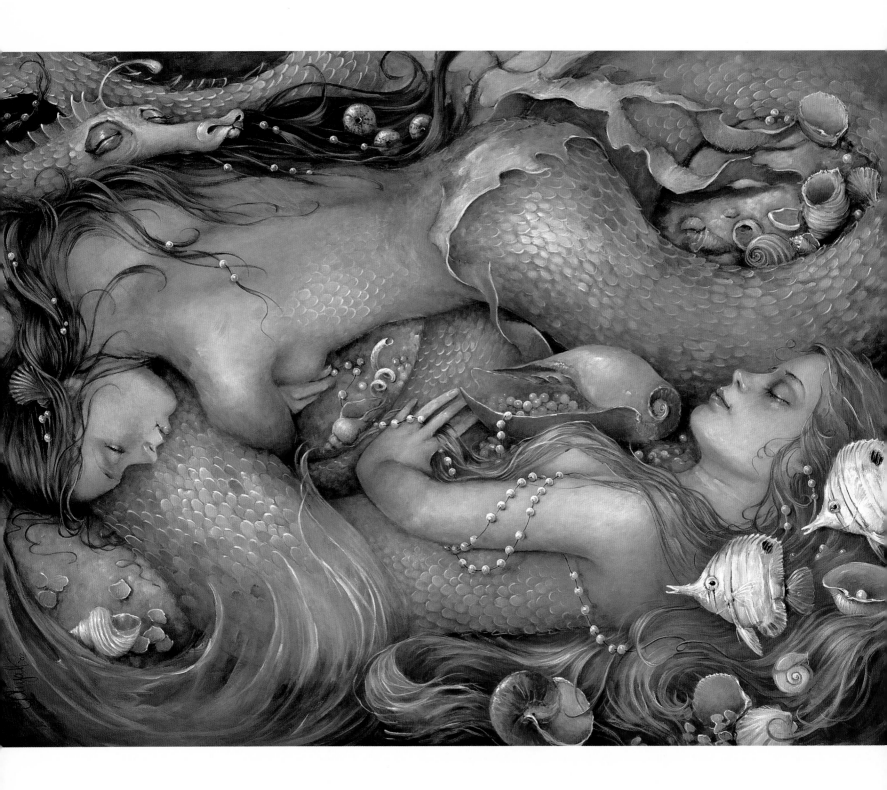

Women and the Sea

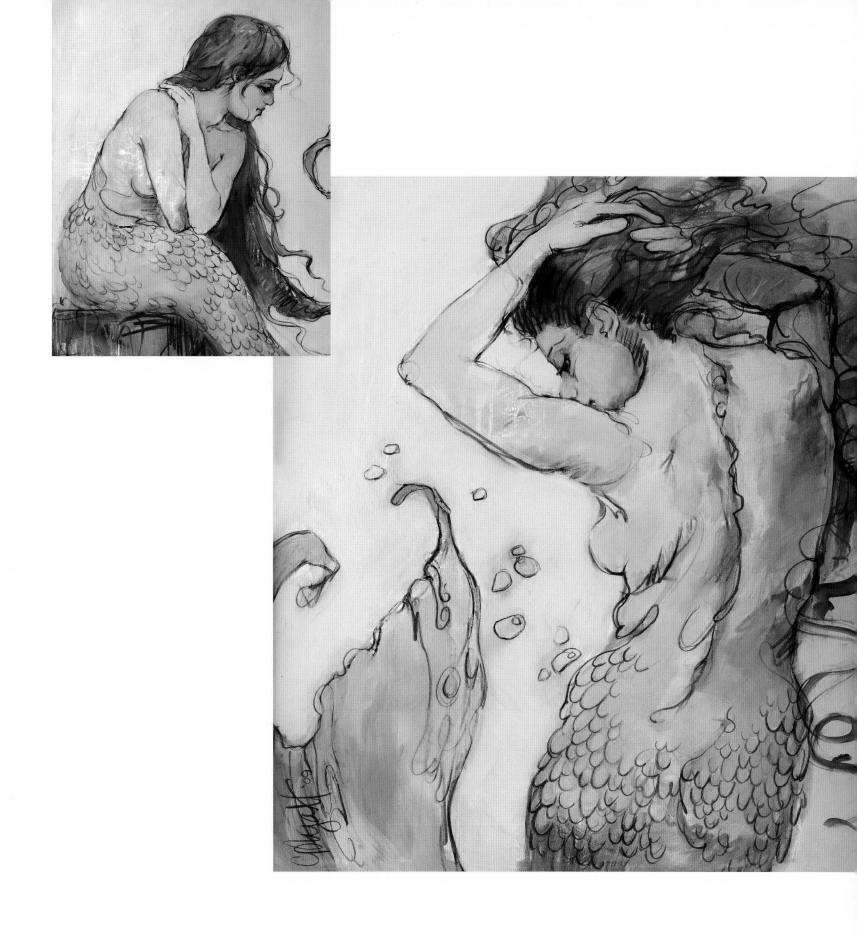

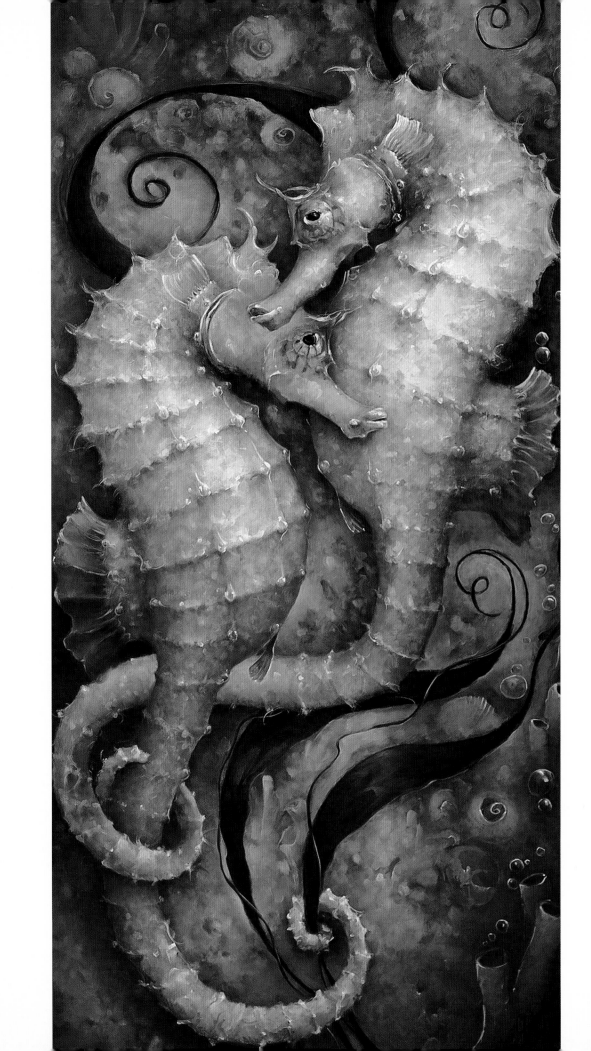

Nantucket, Massachusetts

She senses their spirit. In her mind's eye, she sees their faces—alert, calm, strong—these stalwart Quaker women of Nantucket Island's seafaring past. Shaving by painstaking shaving, their features emerge from antique teak wood. These figureheads, these protectresses of voyages, will not stand watch from the bows of ships as did their sisters of centuries past. No, these women safeguard homes while adding to them their beauty and grace.

It was to have a figurehead for her Nantucket home that Dinah Unruh put her artistic training to work and created one. In taking up her tools, she became one of only two or three people in the world who carve figureheads, a craft once in high demand as each clipper ship or square rigger left port led by one of these auspicious icons, often fashioned after a beloved wife, daughter, sister, or mother left on shore to worry and wait. Preserving this disappearing art in part fuels Dinah's passion. Creating figureheads is also a compulsion, and lest she neglect it, warnings meant for mariners remind her of her task. "The sound of a fog horn makes me crazy. I have to get to work. It's like a calling." As she carves, three or four hours will slip by—it feels like twenty minutes—and Dinah's only thought will have been of the woman who is appearing before her.

Fascinated since childhood by courageous colonial and pioneering women, she strongly feels the presence of those Nantucket Quaker wives who ran the island while their husbands were out at sea for three years at a stretch. "They were amazing women. They boost your spirit. They say, 'Yes, I can do anything because I must!'" Dinah has even coaxed friends going through hard times to experience their nurturing spirit. "They are like the wind under your wings. You feel really supported."

Before she can form one of their faces from wood, she must see her, and then she will spend three or four months refining her features. "I work and feel for the next bump, my thumb always on her. I am riveted. I am calling her forth and can feel this person coming out of the wood." Sarah Starbuck Folger was among them. The wife of a sea captain, she was the original mistress of the eighteenth-century home Dinah shares with her husband, Doug, and with shawl draped over her arms, she keeps their home light burning.

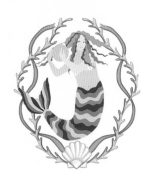

FIGUREHEAD ARTIST { Dinah Unruh }

"One woman came up to me and said of

my mermaid figurehead, 'She's land-bound and is

looking for the sea. You can see it

in her eyes.' And that's it, that's what I'm trying to say."

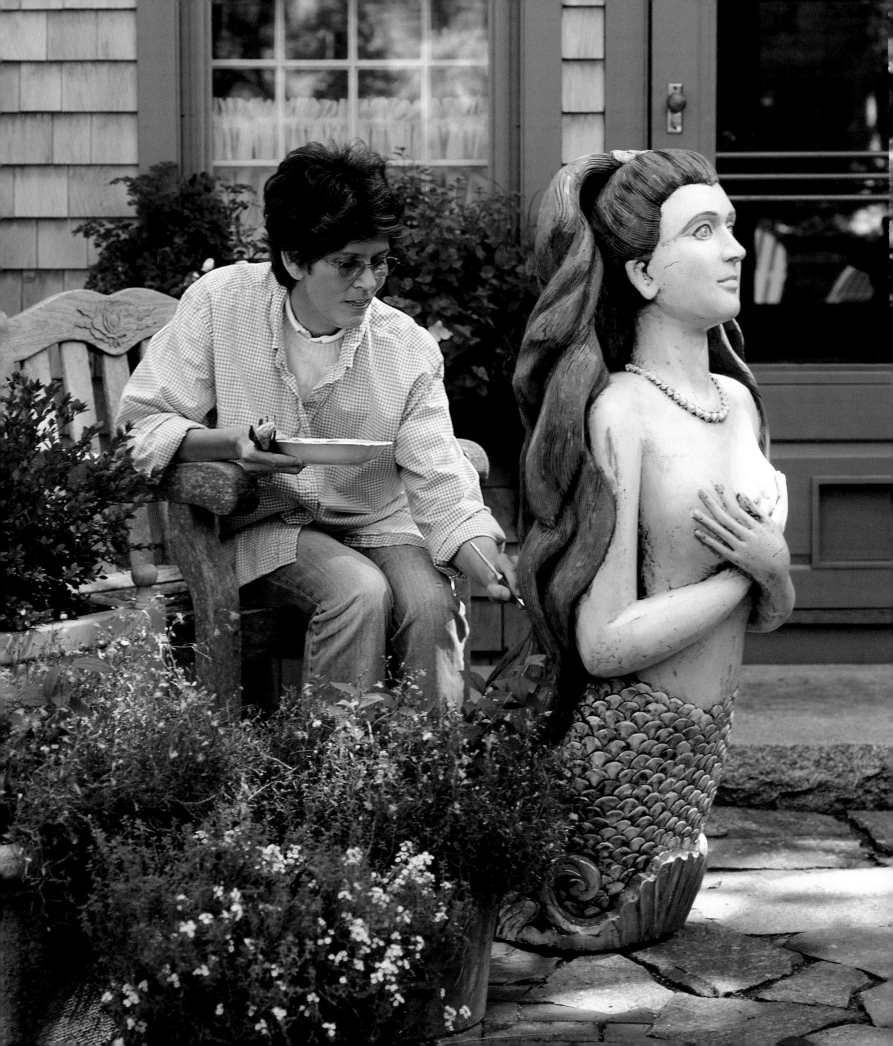

> "Till my soul is full of longing
> For secrets of the sea, And
>   the heart of the great ocean
> Sends a thrilling pulse through me."

HENRY WADSWORTH LONGFELLOW

a close-up view of the watery world she had known superficially since birth. "A few years ago, I was doing a painting of a reef, and a friend suggested I do some diving to get a better look. I discovered an astounding world I was simply in awe of. As soon as one descends from the surface of the water, everything goes silent as if a window to another world opens. Once I spent time with a moray eel while lying on my belly on the ocean floor. We each swayed back and forth with the gentle ocean rhythm while peering intensely at each other." She was struck, too, by the ocean's plant life and, she says, "by creatures you think are plants that suddenly move and run." Memories of her underwater encounters emerge in her work. "When I am creating a watery world on canvas, I remember the mysterious silence and the ocean's movement. I remember how surreal it is and how it really is another world."

A reserved woman, Christina infuses her mermaids with a quiet knowing, wise patience, and sensuous strength. "Mermaids are the perfect woman, beautiful, mysterious, unattainable. They are anything you want them to be." To represent love, she drew on two intertwined sea horses she had seen. Decorated with ribbons of seaweed, they are regal in their bearing and enwrapped with each other. In another painting, the love goddess herself, Venus, born of the ocean's foam, lounges in her silken mermaid fin, strewn with roses and shadowed by her mischievous son, Cupid. These two matchmakers, Venus and Cupid, may be at work on behalf of the mermaids as Christina is inviting a merman or two into her paintings, as in *Rendezvous*. "In it there is a mermaid and a merman along with two large seahorses all in delightful engagement with each other."

Like the narrative line of a dream, Christina never quite sees where a vision will take her. "I don't always know where a painting is going. So much of what I try to end up with in a painting comes from some place much deeper, a much more emotional place." Being surprised by what manifests has its kinship with the world hidden within the water. "The use of ocean images in my work is often symbolic. They represent to me that place where windows open to a world shrouded in timeless mystery and imagination."

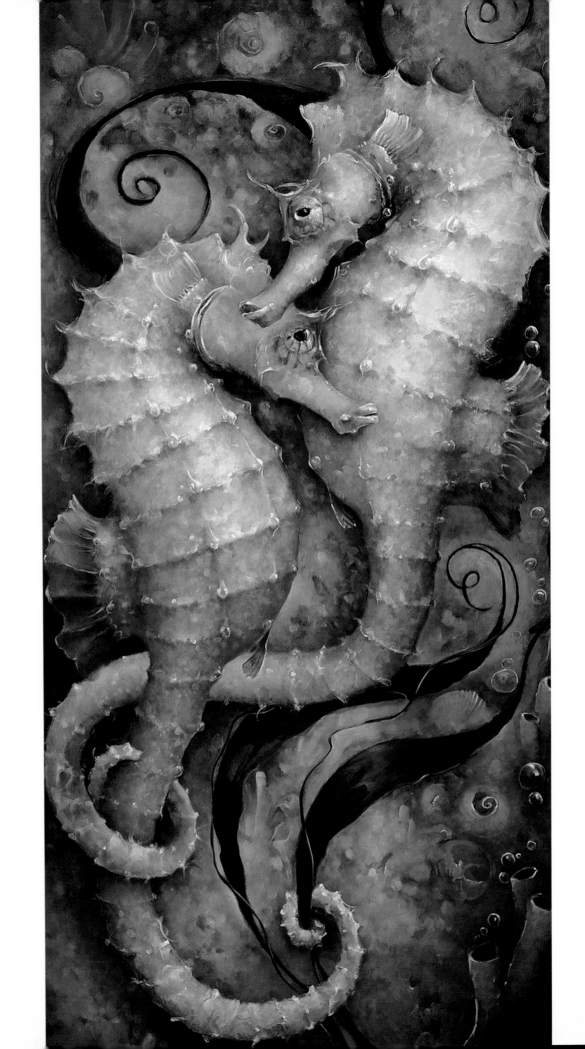

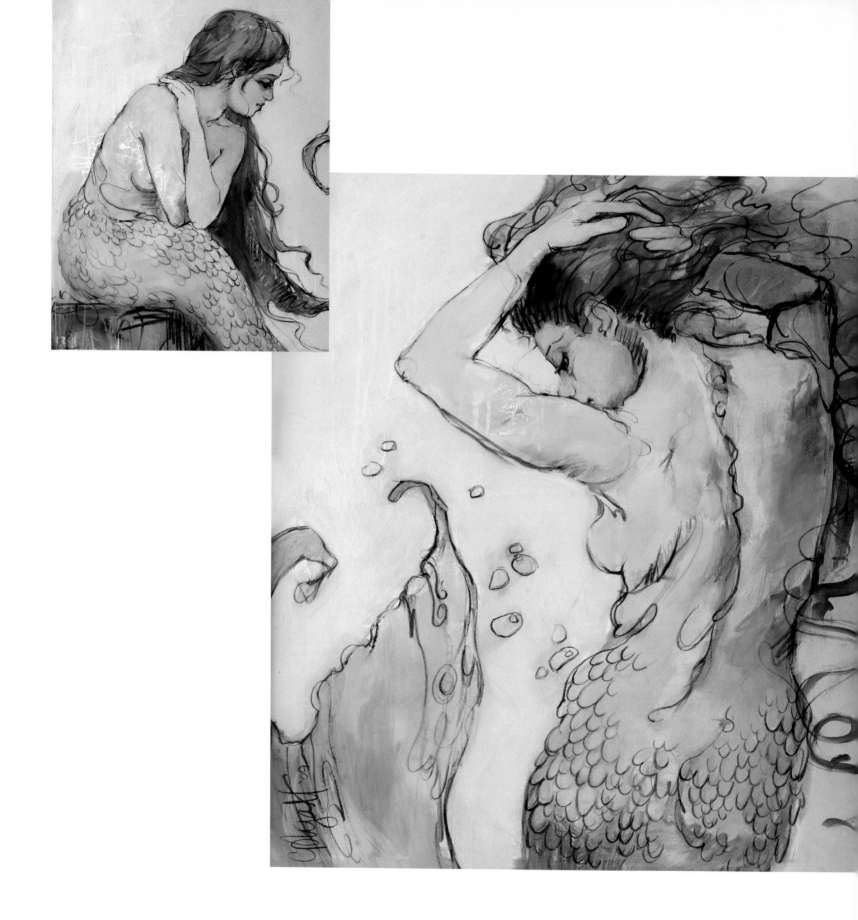

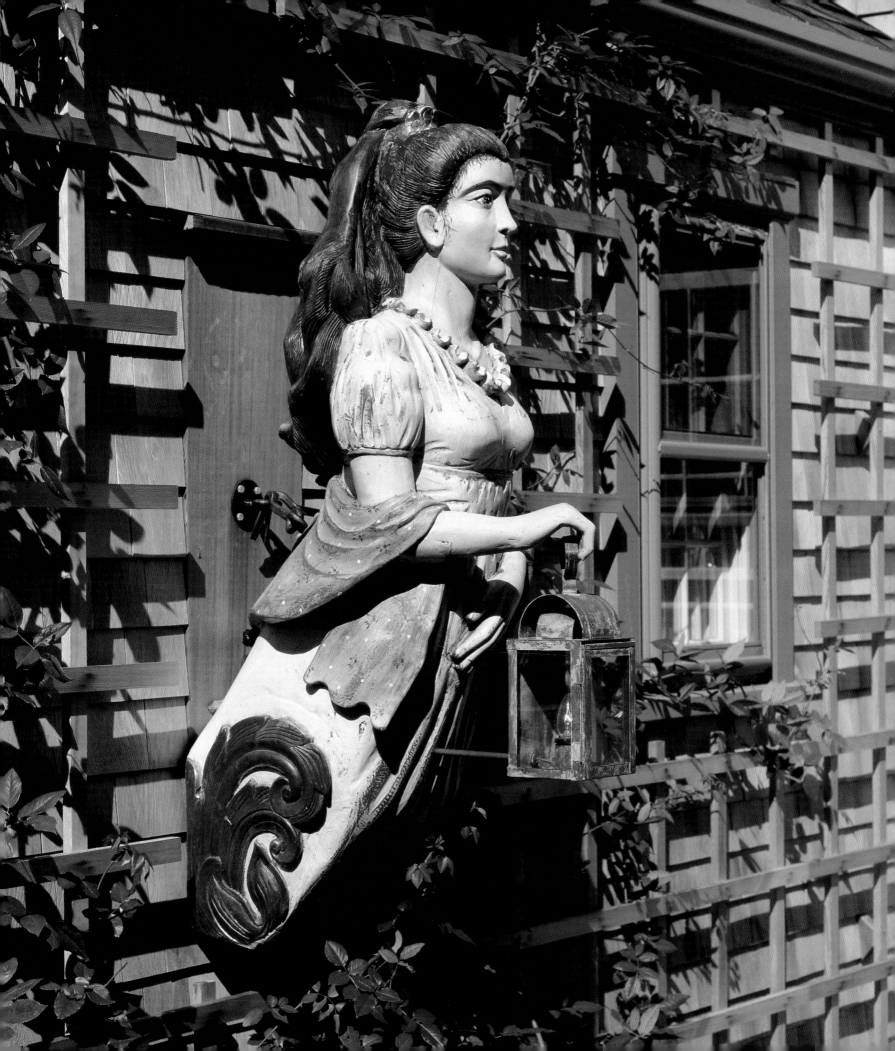

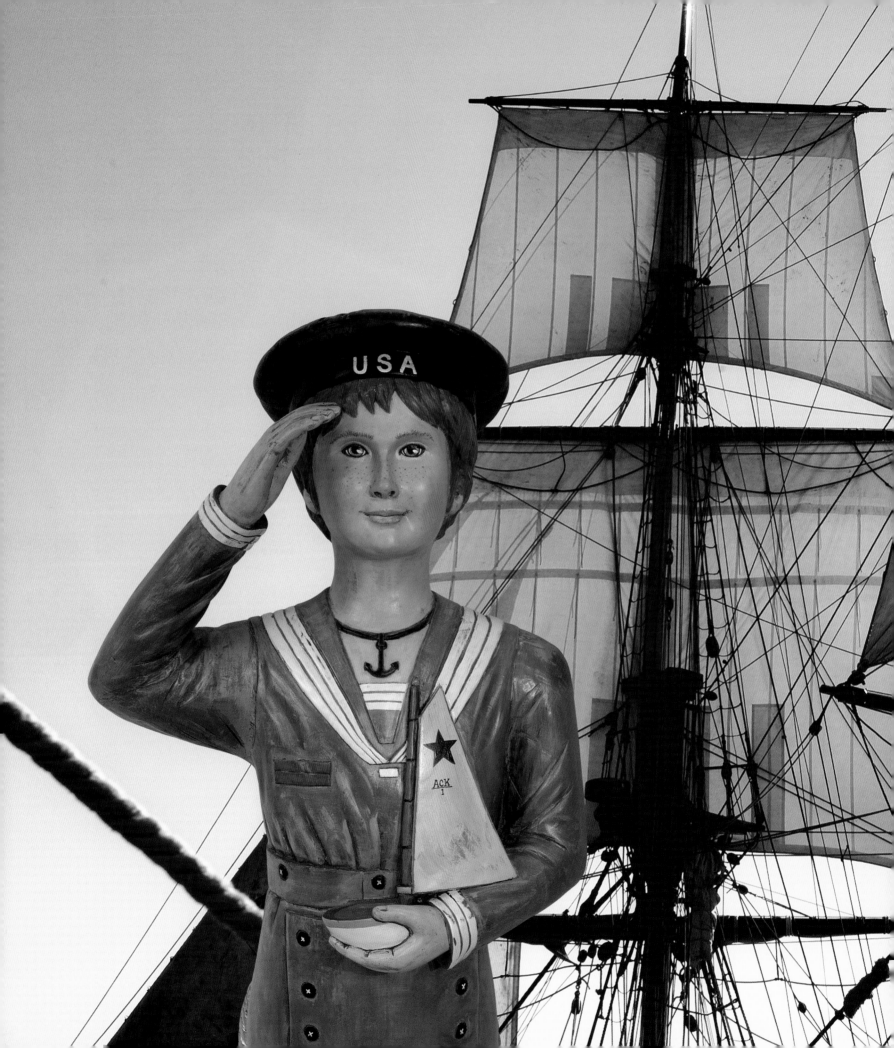

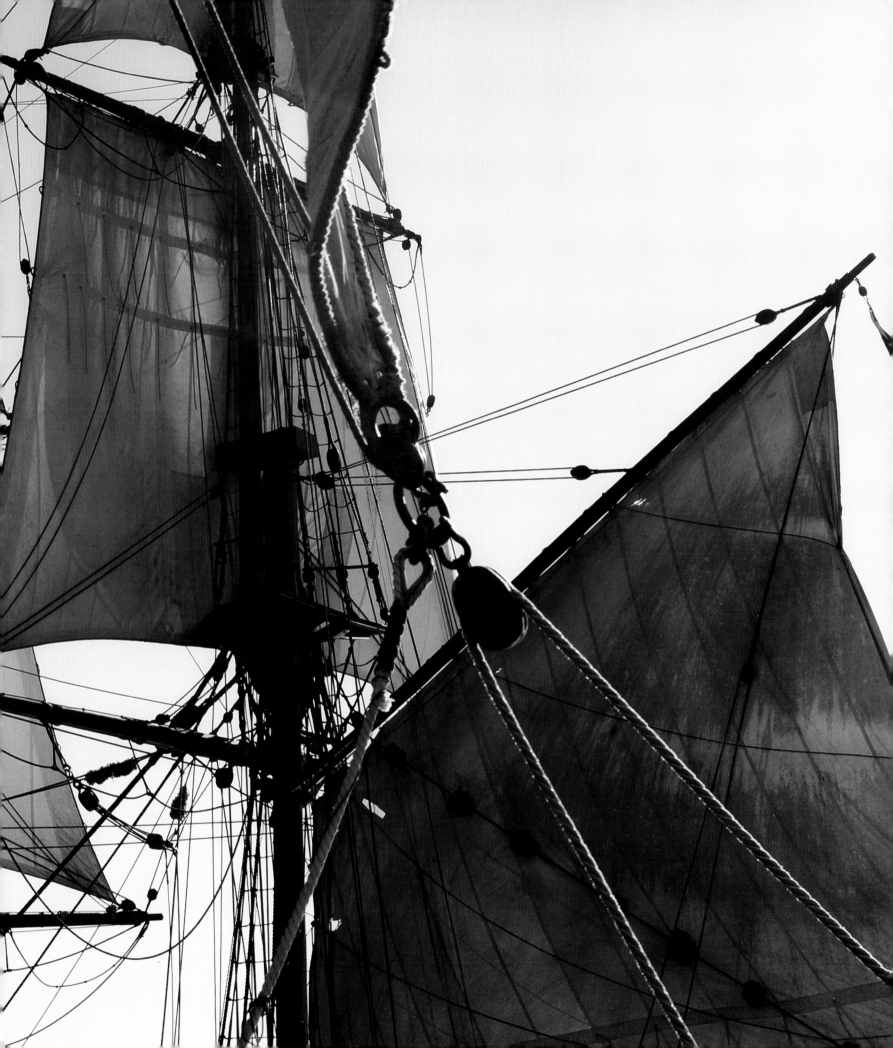

> "I have seen the sea when it is stormy and wild; when it is quiet and serene; when it is dark and moody. And in all its moods, I see myself."

MARTIN BUXBAUM

Of the nine figureheads she has carved, including a mermaid and her favorite "Lavender Maiden," only two have been male subjects, twin sailor boys recently completed. She has yet to do an adult male. "Until I 'see' him, I won't. I would only botch it up."

In making figureheads, Dinah is adding to the slim store of those that exist in the world, around 1,700 by most estimates. Ironically, many more lie on the ocean floor. Treasure seekers who encounter them while diving on wrecks in search of gold bullion must leave these beacons of hope and the ships to which they are attached alone. To Dinah, this is a crime. On rare occasions, a figurehead will wash ashore, as one mermaid did on the coast of France, its finder alerting her of the event. Dinah herself will not be diving on watery graves seeking to come face to face with these drowned maidens. Since a swim nearly turned into a tragedy when she was a young girl, she admires the ocean from the safety of land. Having grown up in Pennsylvania, Dinah's first encounter with the sea happened while she was vacationing with family on the New Jersey shore. Pulled out by a heavy undertow, she found herself struggling to get back. A lifeguard's whistle signaled all bathers to come ashore, but the call was not in response to her distress; rather, it was an alert that a shark was in the area. Fortunately a strong swimmer further out snatched and rescued her. Dinah loves the sea, but it is also a source of terror to her. She inhales its salty scent and attunes to the sound of lapping waves, but she watches in awe only from water's edge. "It is dark and deep, and I respect it enormously," she says.

Much like the captains who placed figureheads at the helm of their ships, an act born of traditions meant to mollify the sea gods and ward off ill fate, Dinah carves figures of protection. Their gaze is constant, their faces set and serene, their smiles quietly suggesting all will be well.

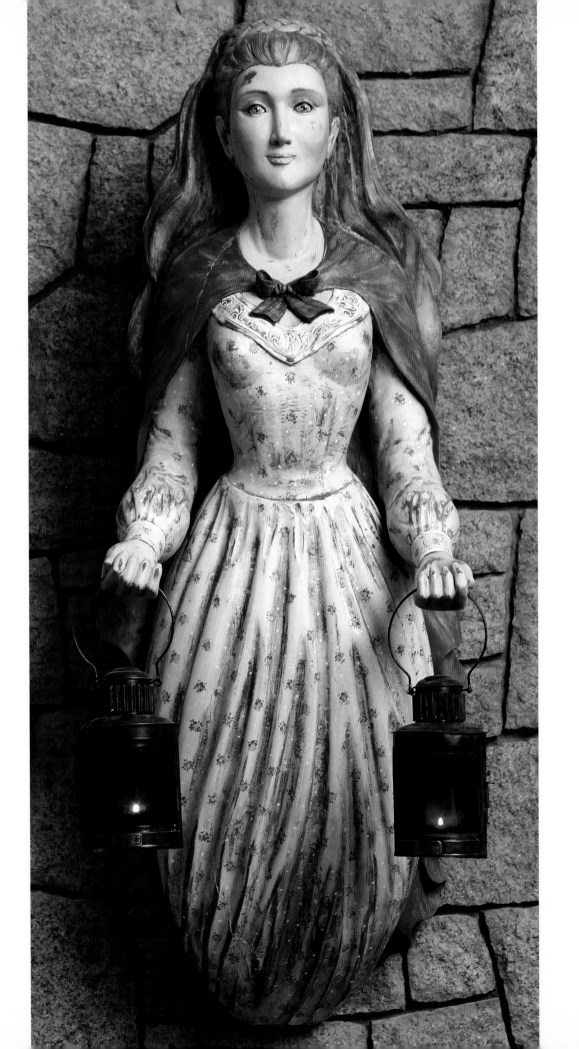

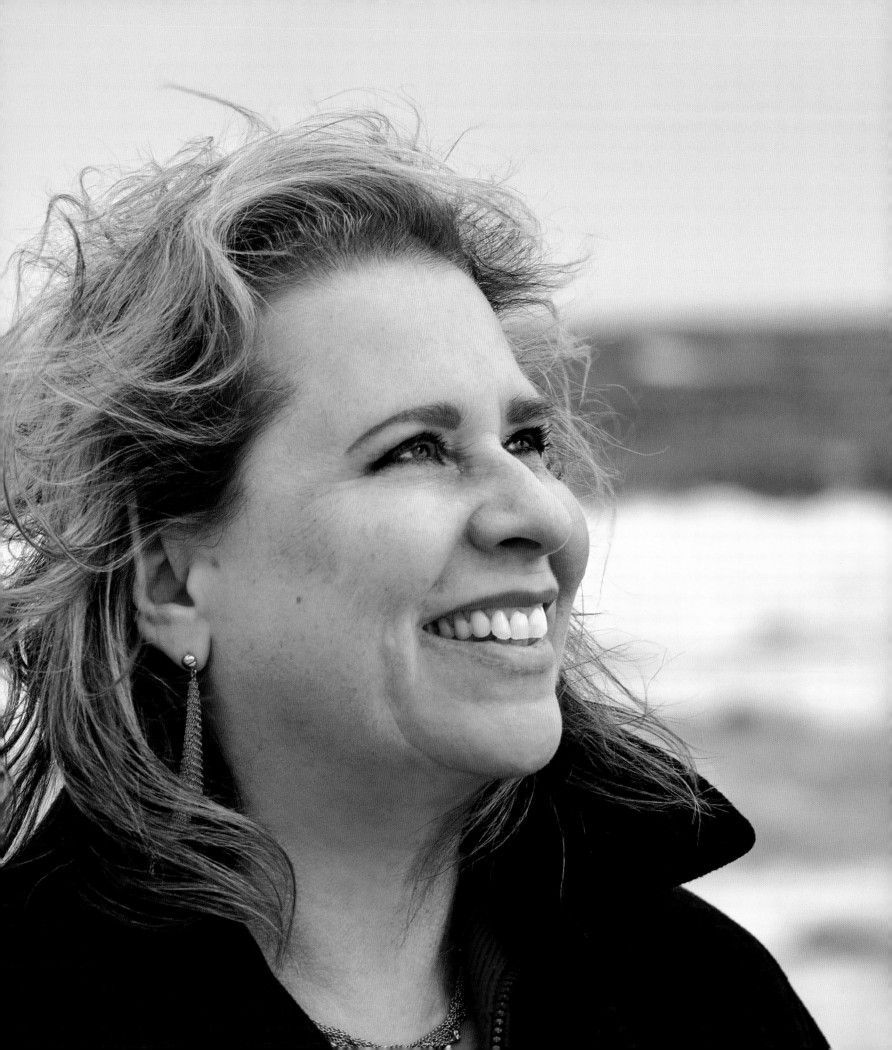

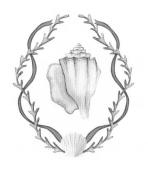

SAILOR'S VALENTINE ARTIST { Sandi Blanda }

"Every Sunday, my family went to the beach.

It didn't cost any money. It was free entertainment,

and I was never bored. I was always

looking for that perfect shell."

Plymouth, Massachusetts

The sea ceaselessly strands small sculptures along the shore—ribbed, fanned, layered, curved, curled, swirled, smooth—treasures for the taking. Nor is the ocean stingy with its colors, these shells awash in pinks, pearls, purples, sunny yellows, coral reds, butterscotch browns, pea greens, and navy blues. As she surveys the abundance before her and imagines the possible combinations that she can arrange within a wooden octagonal sailor's valentine, artist Sandi Blanda likens the experience to "opening a 120-count box of Crayola crayons."

It is no wonder, then, that after twenty-five years of creating these greetings from the sea, she continues to have "a running list a mile long" of future designs. Inspired by the seasons, by flowers, by rock music, and even colors seen in fashion advertising, her valentines bear messages that call on "Hope," capture "High Voltage" energy, promise to "Cross My Heart," admit to "Guilty Pleasures," celebrate "Autumn's Glory," and whip up a "Cyclone." "I love color and am overwhelmed by the limitless variations that appear in nature." Her approach toward her award-winning work is contemporary and three-dimensional. "From the very beginning, I knew I did not want to do reproduction work. Antique valentines are generally flat and may have only one rosette. I set out to develop a large assortment of seashell flowers, and my style developed directly from that."

Though she will not do reproduction work, she has restored over twenty antique valentines. The story of one harbors the history of many. In the mid 1800s, whaling captain Thomas H. Lawrence, of Falmouth Massachusetts, pulled into port in Barbados while on his way home from a lengthy voyage. There, at a souvenir shop, he purchased a sailor's valentine for his bride-to-be, Mercy Bassett Dimmick. If Mercy was a typical Victorian woman, she was thrilled to receive one of these ornate declarations of devotion. Bearing messages like "Think of Me" and "Forever Thine" formed in shells, antique valentines were once believed to have been crafted by the sailors themselves aboard ship. The true tale is that most made in the nineteenth century were created in Barbados as part of a cottage industry.

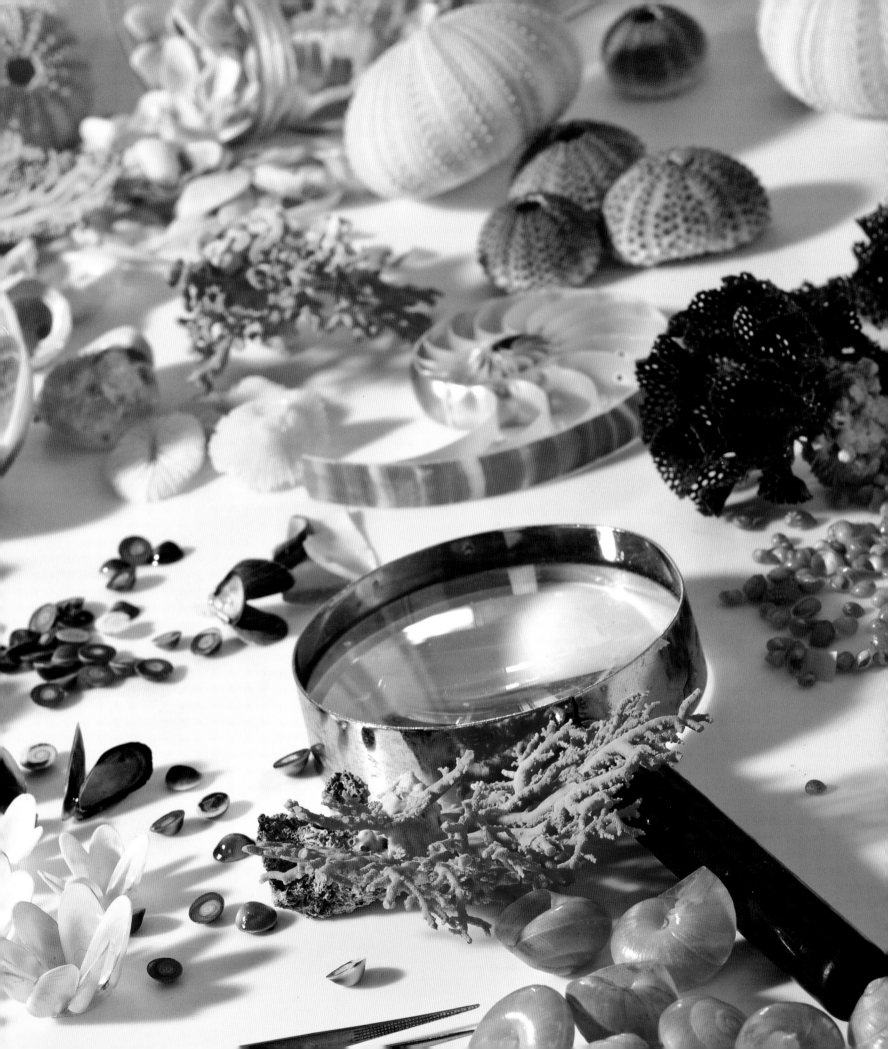

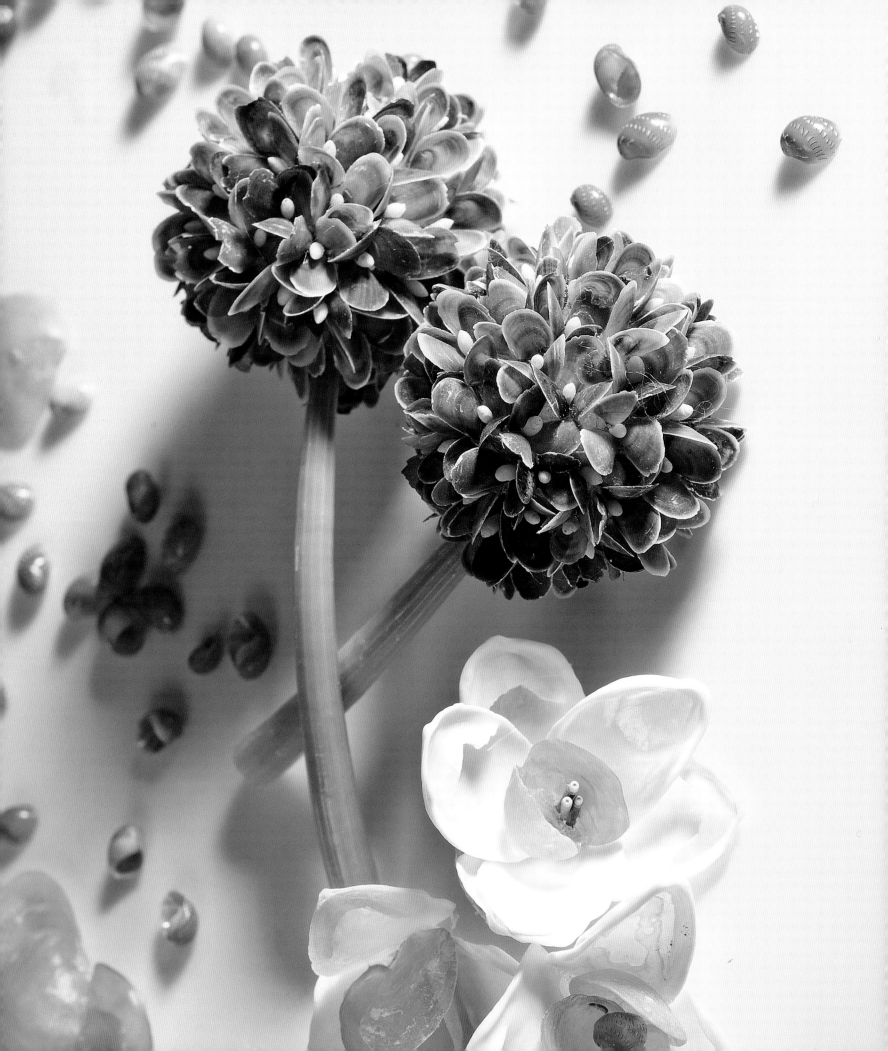

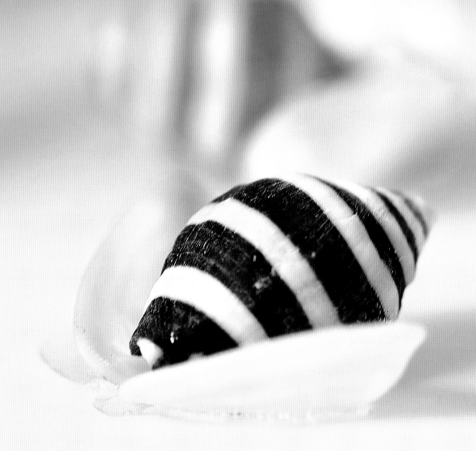

"The sea does not reward those
who are too anxious, too greedy,
or too impatient. One should
lie empty, open, choiceless as a beach—
waiting for a gift from the sea."

ANNE MORROW LINDBERGH

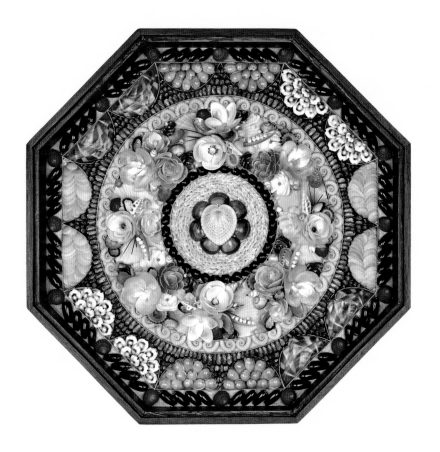

When Sandi was introduced to the valentines in 1983 by a friend, she realized she had met her creative soulmate: "I instantly fell in love. When I saw it, it turned my life around." She became obsessed, "I couldn't physically sleep. It was all consuming. I would wake up at two or three in the morning to get four or five hours of work done before everyone got up."

Today, as she sits before her table of shells, she makes notes on color combinations. Thousands of shells go into one labyrinthine piece—there they are fanned or nested to form flowers, grouped to make a geometric shape, snuggled side by side to form links like a necklace, laid along the box's inner edge as a second frame. For her supply, Sandi looks to the Caribbean, Sanibel Island, Florida, and the Philippines, but sometimes she is given or purchases shells collected by others. Unlike other sailor's valentine artists, though, Sandi will not use shells that have been dyed. "People who use dyed shells have more freedom than I do," she concedes, "but my colors have to be in nature."

As a child growing up on Long Island, Sandi and her family spent every Sunday at the beach: "I was always looking for that perfect shell. I never brought any shells home, though, because I thought they were

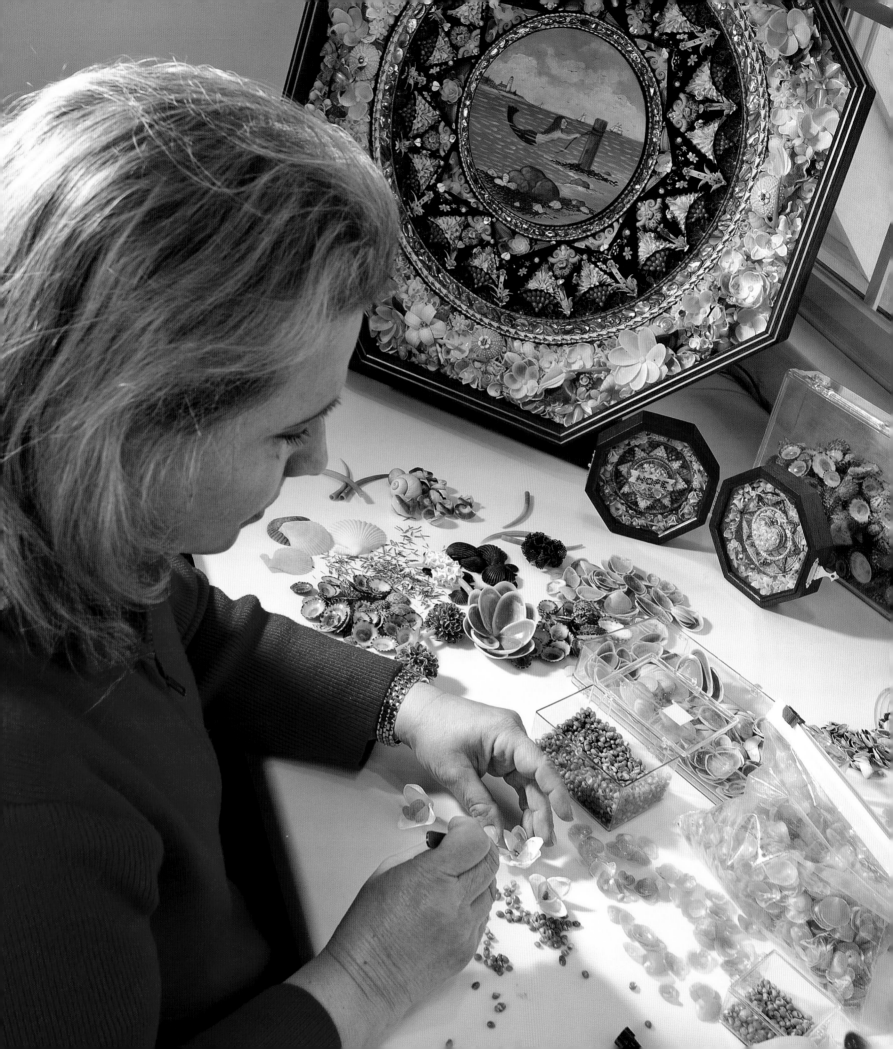

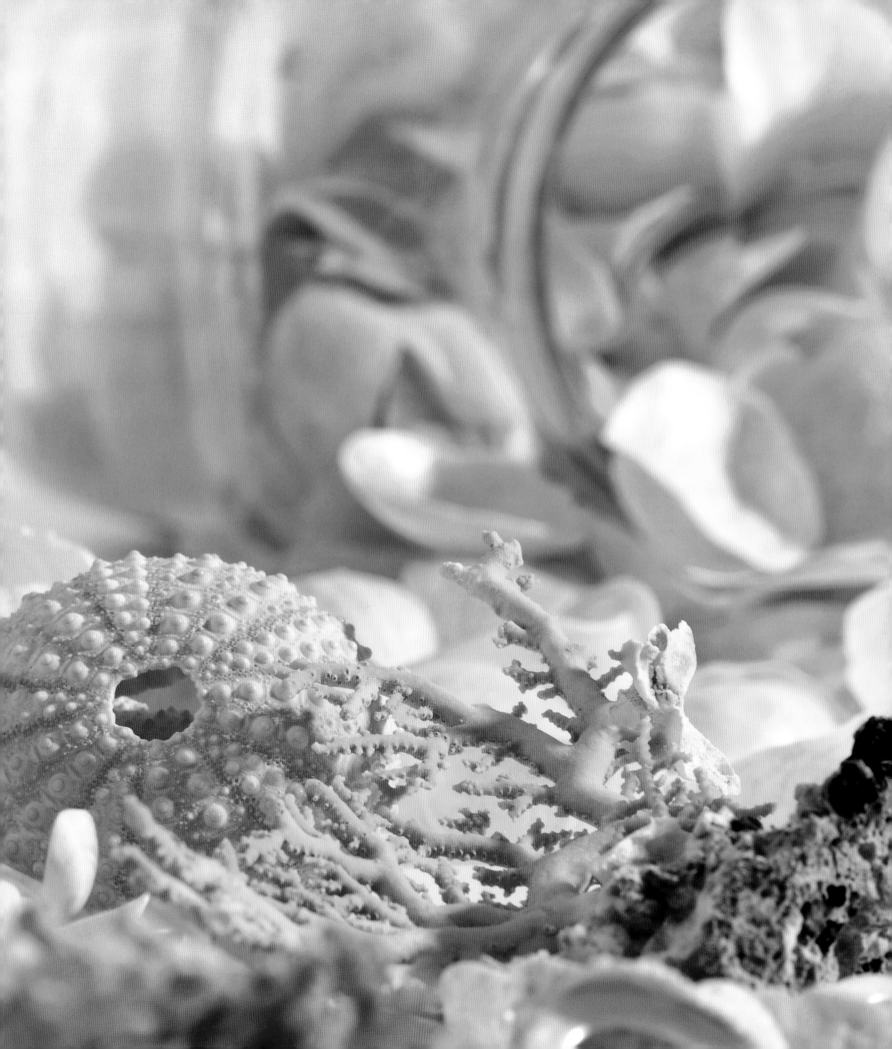

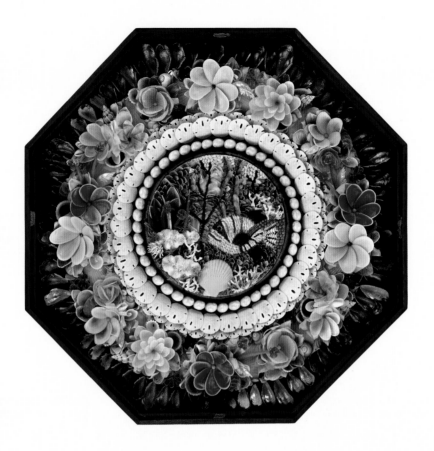

pretty awful." Her discriminating aesthetic sense likely came from her solo jaunts as a child to the city to visit art museums. She could not at that point have realized that those rejected blue mussel shells would make perfect hydrangea petals or that slipper shells and jingles are essential to daffodils. She is still searching for shells to make a peony: "I haven't found the right shells to reflect the tight, fluffy structure and delicate variations in color. There is also the additional problem of designing the flower to fit under the glass." Though she couldn't find one as a child, as an adult, she considers the Japanese Wonder Shell perfect, "Frank Lloyd Wright used it for his inspiration to design the Guggenheim Museum, and I am truly a New Yorker at heart. Sadly, it is far too large and expensive to incorporate into a sailor's valentine."

Now living in Plymouth, Massachusetts, ten minutes from the beach, she has stayed close to the water she has known all her life. "I will never live inland, and the only time I have gone to an inland place for vacation was under duress to Las Vegas. I am always near water. There is something about the light and water. Even at night, it is magical." Her relationship with the coast and with sailor's valentines has been steadfast. "I get up every morning, and I love to get to work. I can still say that after twenty-five years." That's true love.

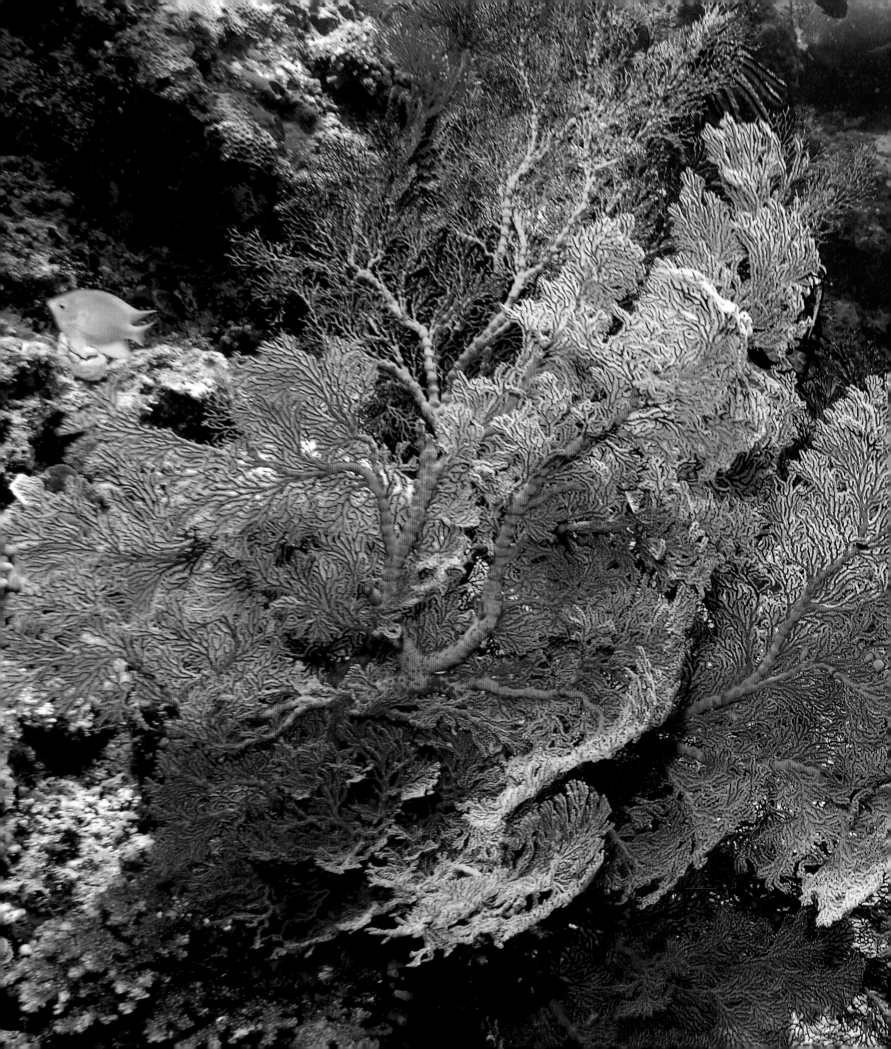

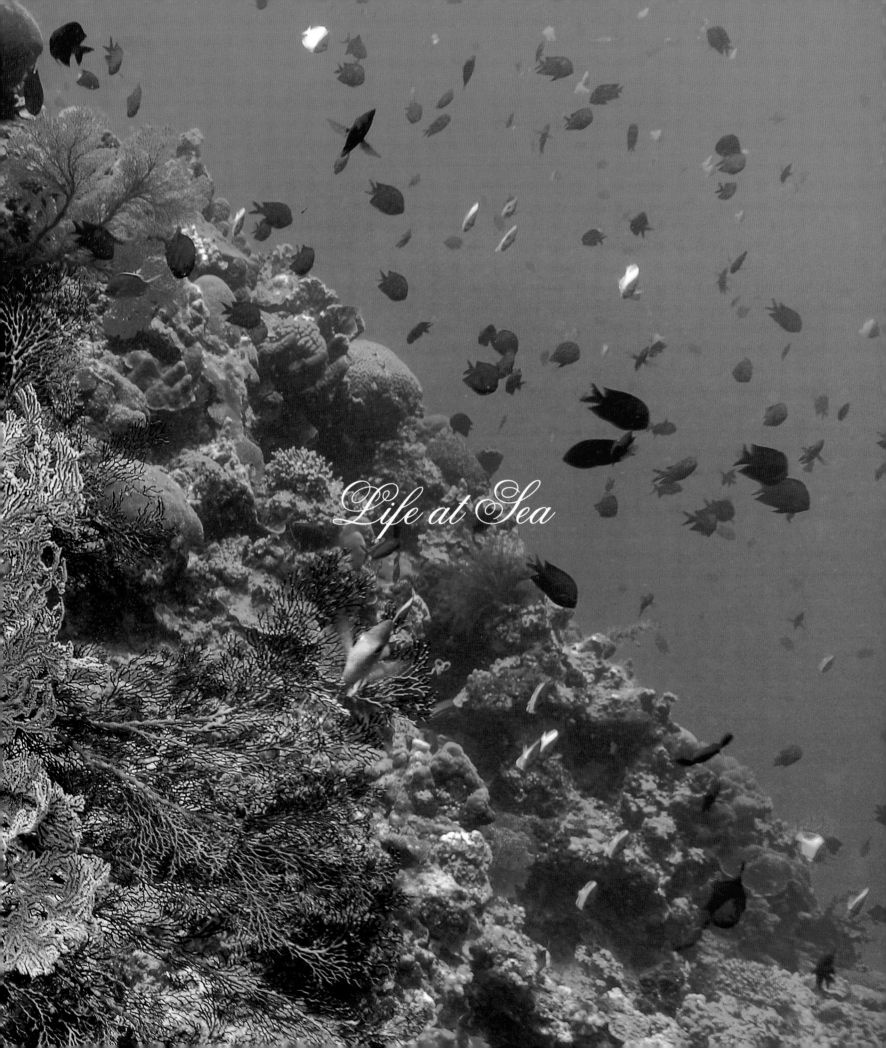

Life at Sea

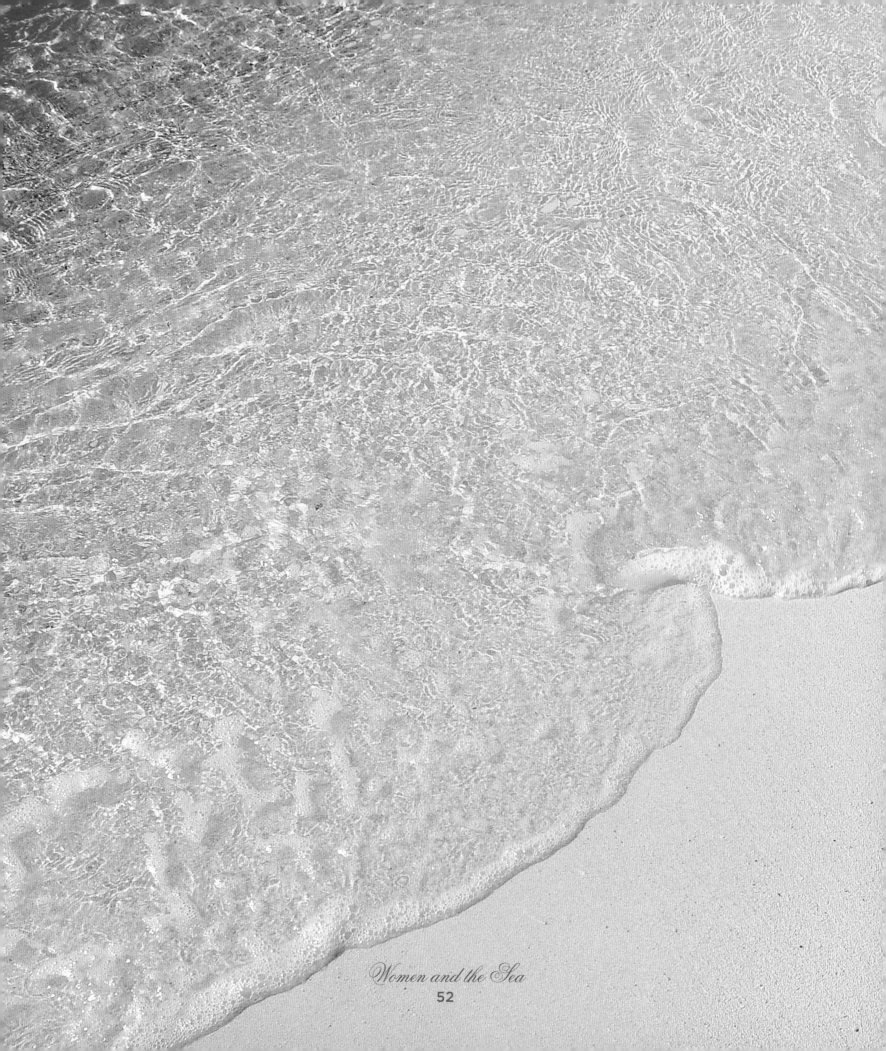

LUCY MAUD MONTGOMERY

The Sea Spirit

I smile o'er the wrinkled blue
Lo! the sea is fair,
Smooth as the flow of a maiden's hair;
And the welkin's light shines through
Into mid-sea caverns of beryl hue,
And the little waves laugh and the mermaids sing,
And the sea is a beautiful, sinuous thing!

I scowl in sullen guise
The sea grows dark and dun,
The swift clouds hide the sun
But not the bale-light in my eyes,
And the frightened wind as it flies
Ruffles the billows with stormy wing,
And the sea is a terrible, treacherous thing!

When moonlight glimmers dim
I pass in the path of the mist,
Like a pale spirit by spirits kissed,
At dawn I chant my own weird hymn,
And I dabble my hair in the sunset's rim,
And I call to the dwellers along the shore
With a voice of gramarye evermore.

And if one for love of me
Gives to my call an ear,
I will woo him and hold him dear,
And teach him the way of the sea,
And my glamor shall ever over him be;
Though he wander afar in the cities of men
He will come at last to my arms again.

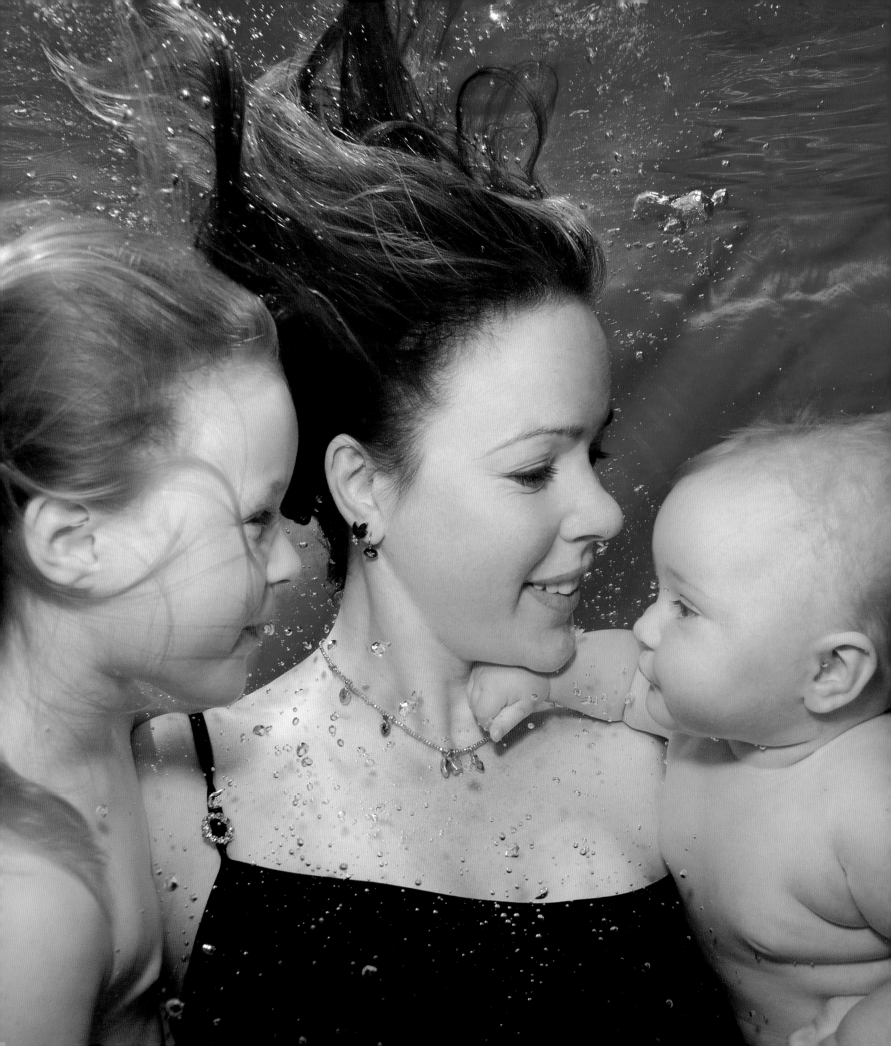

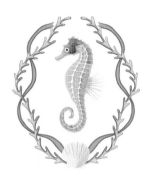

UNDERWATER PHOTOGRAPHER { Zena Holloway }

"Underwater the senses slow, and the body

takes on weightlessness. Light is altered,

and sight and sound are impeded. It really is

an alien world of deceptive calm."

London, England

The sea beguiles with its dark depths, its deep secrets, its fleeting creatures, and its treasures tenaciously trapped. For Zena Holloway, this is her working studio. With SCUBA regulator in one hand and camera in the other, this London-based underwater photographer, buoyed by waves, caught up in currents, and distracted by finned fans, shoots model mermaids, men on wires, and babies in fairy tales. Destined for the pages of magazines, television advertising, and heirloom books, her photographs capture the water's energy—its motion, its surfacing bubbles, its absorption of shafts of light, its webbing of dark pockets—all without betraying its mysteries.

Zena has made thousands of dives as a SCUBA instructor and as an award-winning photographer and so is intimately acquainted with the chimerical qualities of the sea. "Underwater the senses slow, and the body takes on weightlessness. Light is altered, and sight and sound are impeded. It really is an alien world of deceptive calm. I find it a thrilling world to work in."

Having become a certified diver at sixteen, inspired by stories of her late father's passion for "throwing on an aqualung and diving off the back of a boat," Zena says the dives themselves have become merely a means to an end. "SCUBA is just a mode of transport that allows me to experience moments that most people never have the opportunity to see." Like the Spanish galleon she saw in Uruguay. On assignment for *National Geographic*, Zena found herself exploring a mere ten meters below the surface of a murky river. There on the river's bed lay the shipwrecked remains of soldiers in heavy armor and ladies in hooped skirts pinned beneath fallen masts. Their personal artifacts joined musket balls, cannons, silver coins, and gold lions in telling the stories of the lives lost that fateful day, when only the captain and one other passenger survived. Zena photographed these precious finds, though protocol dictated they be reburied until rights to their ownership were determined. "It was the dive of fairy tales," Zena says. "And it was one of the few times I have ever breathed my tank dry to gain every last second. At one hundred eight minutes bottom time, this was the most memorable dive I have had."

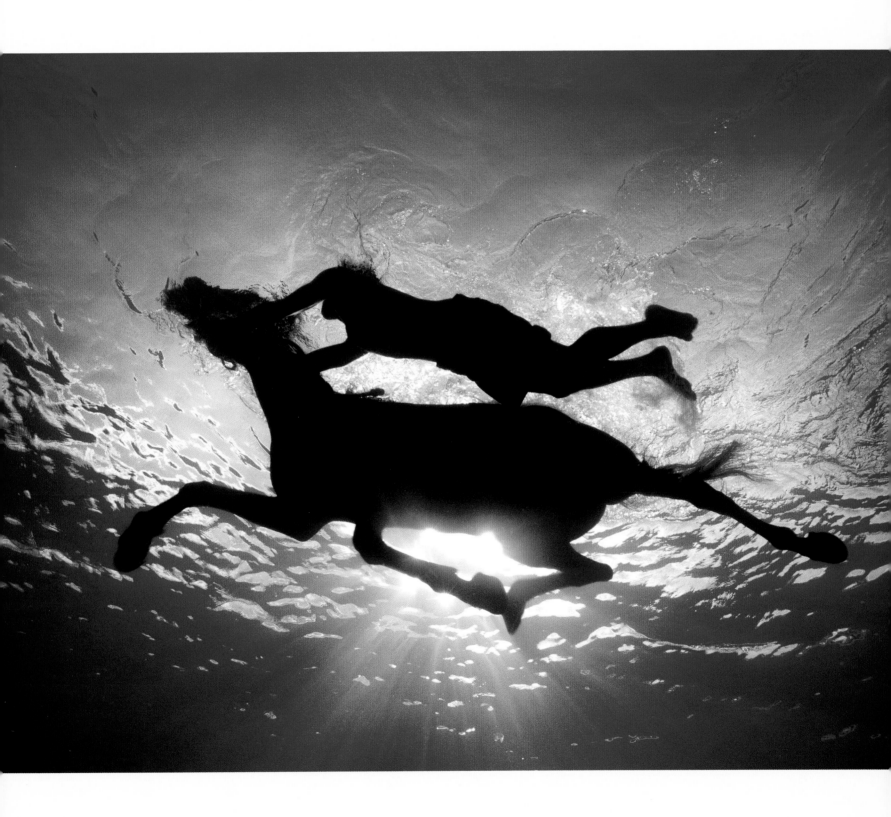

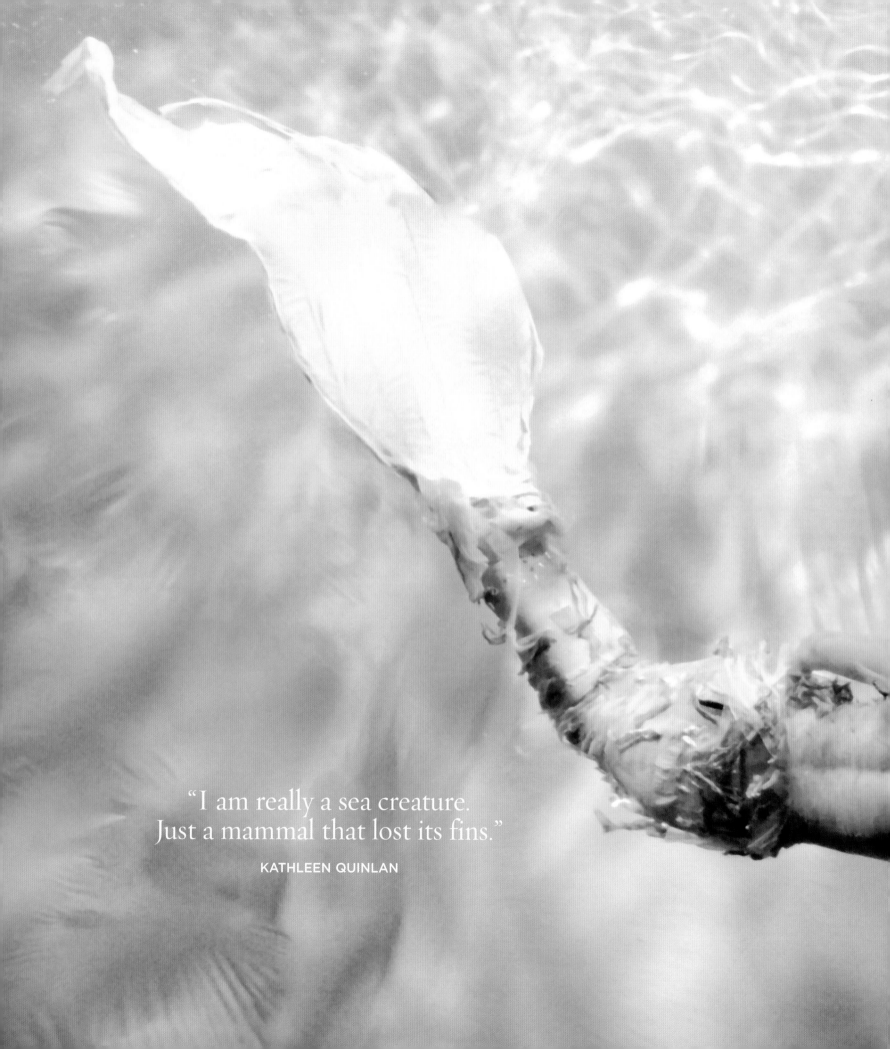

"I am really a sea creature.
Just a mammal that lost its fins."

KATHLEEN QUINLAN

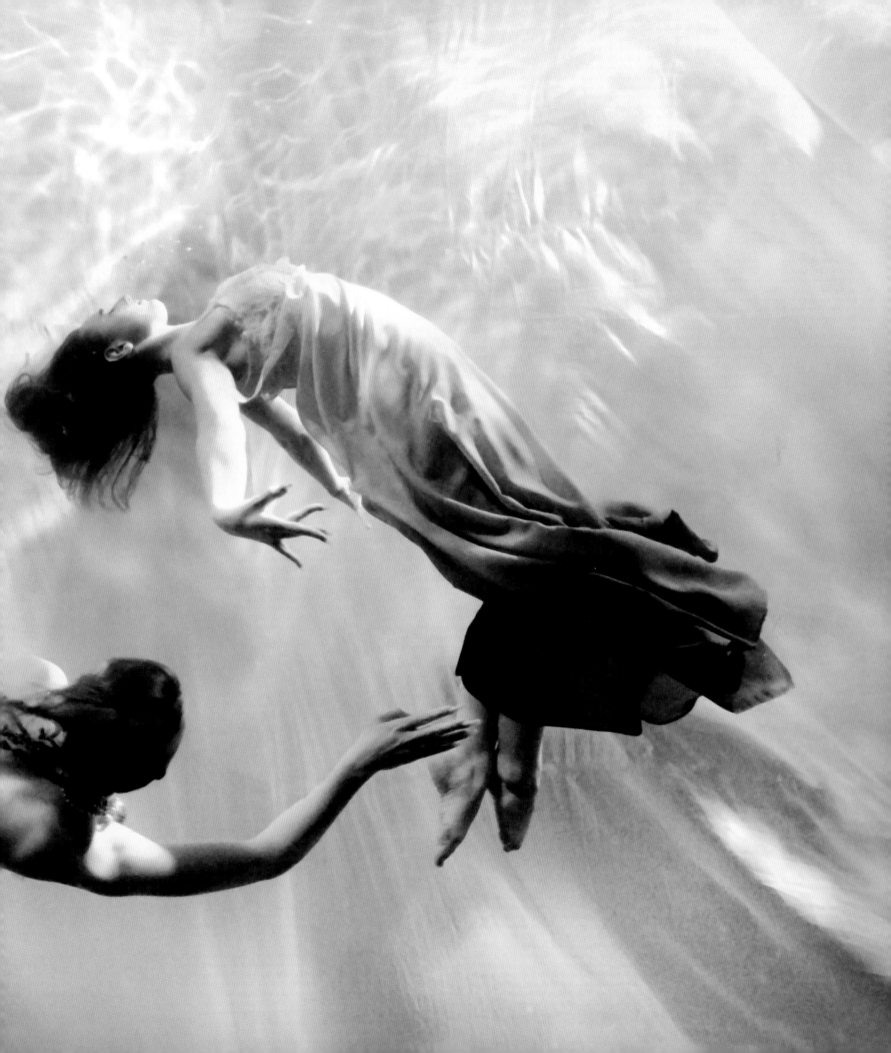

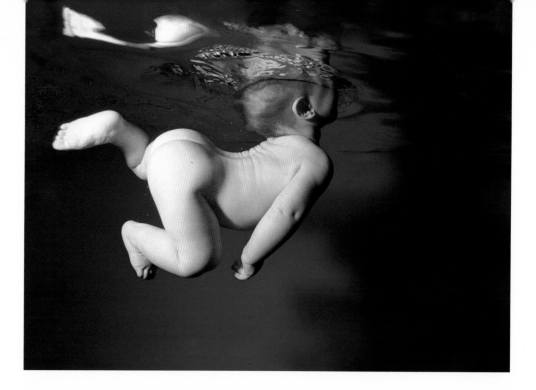

While some assignments take her to places where water preserves pieces of history, others may call for her to capture the spirit of horses frolicking in the Caribbean Sea, one of Zena's favorite shoots. "I was on location by myself for two weeks and only had access to the horses for half an hour each morning. It was tricky to get the right image, but after ten days of shooting, I finally got the shot. It was one in a million and worth all of the time I spent waiting around for the right moment." Sometimes the orchestration of a shot makes the best photograph. Sent on assignment to the Turks and Caicos by Toto, makers of bath and shower units, Zena was asked to capture mermaids under the sea. "First, it was incredible to be in a boat with two mermaids. Then in the water, they had to be tethered with fishing line. I got a shot of the two divers swimming madly away in opposite directions after tying one down, and there was the mermaid, looking gorgeous."

Naturally Zena favors the clear waters of the Caribbean and those off the coast of Egypt, where, on holiday at the age of eighteen, she first became enchanted with the underwater world and realized her creativity had found its outlet. Prior to that trip, her dives had been restricted to the waters of the United Kingdom, where she is from and lives. Those waters were cold and dark. "The only thing I could see were the ends of the instructor's fins."

Certainly being an underwater photographer has its challenges, whether shooting mermaids for a luxury bath products company or divers prodding a caged shark for an environmental organization. Waves, wind, and limited means of adding light

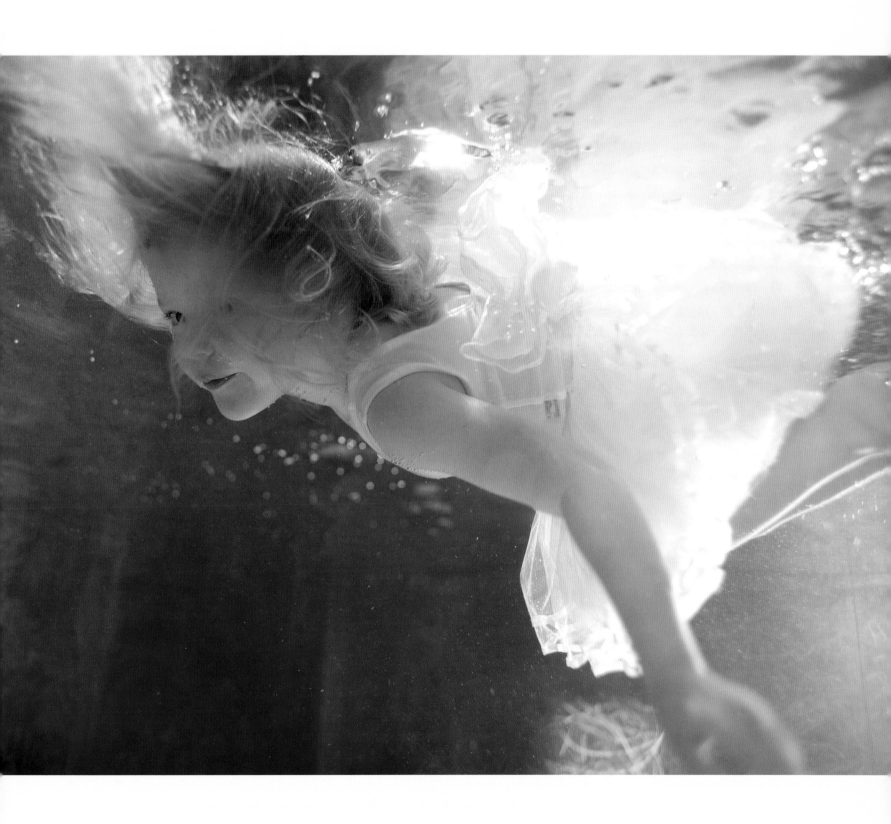

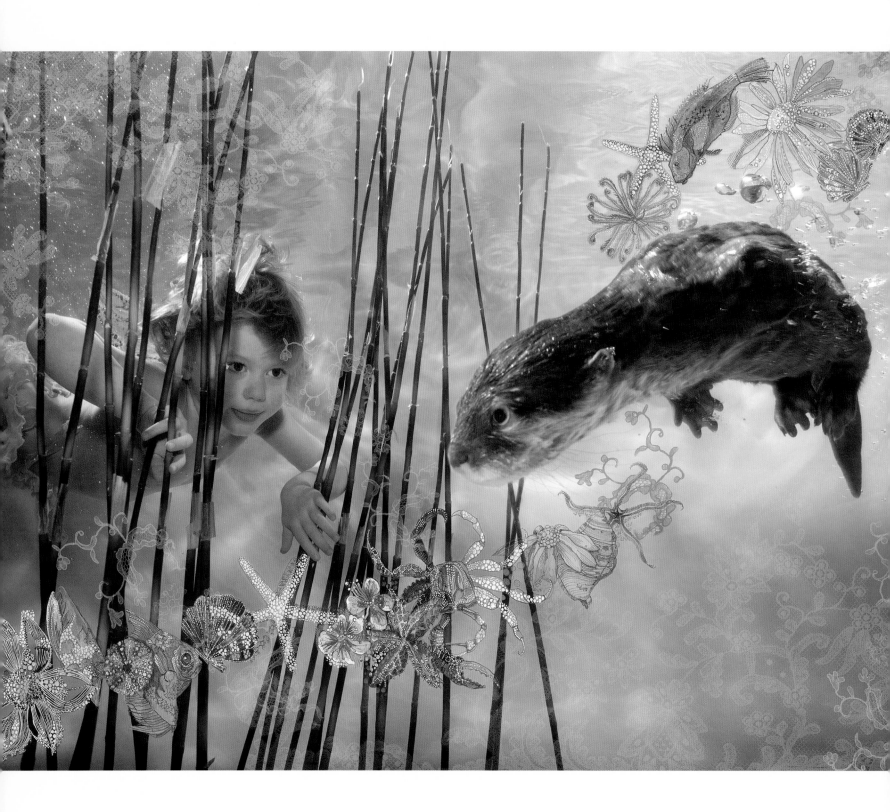

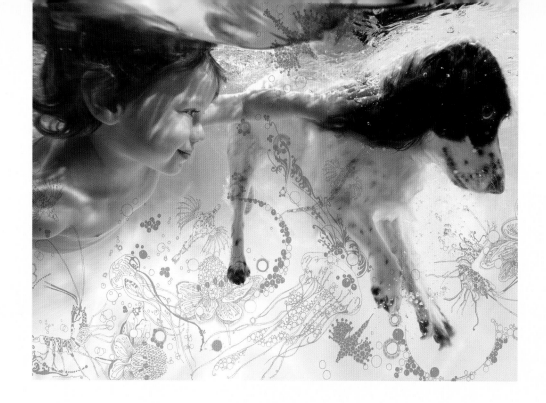

are just some of the factors. Punning pragmatically, Zena says, "You have to go with the flow, but it's fabulous. You get what you get. Sometimes you have something that swims across your lens, and you need to shoot it quickly, or it's gone." Her shoots also take place in large tanks in London, the same used for the underwater sequences in the Harry Potter and James Bond films. In either element, the water itself acts as another lens. Zena has learned to size up quickly who will photograph well under water. The ability to hold one's breath is surprisingly irrelevant, she says. She is so adept at identifying those who will clamp their mouths shut, those who will close their eyes, and those whose shoulders are so broad they will rise to the surface, that she is called upon as an underwater casting director. "You need people who can forget about the water," she says. This makes babies a natural for the medium. Shooting them for the retelling of Charles Kingsley's *The Water Babies*, was simply "easy," Zena says. Toddlers dressed like fairies look cute on dry land, but seen through a camera lens underwater, they become angelic sprites. "It's so mystical when I go underwater. It is what I see."

Like the sea, the subjects and settings it presents are infinite, and Zena looks forward to thousands more dives. "I'd love to go to Australia and all of the Pacific. I relish the challenges that working underwater throws me. I'm never one to follow the crowd, and I find that creating images beneath the surface allows me to explore uncharted territory. I love the magic of it all."

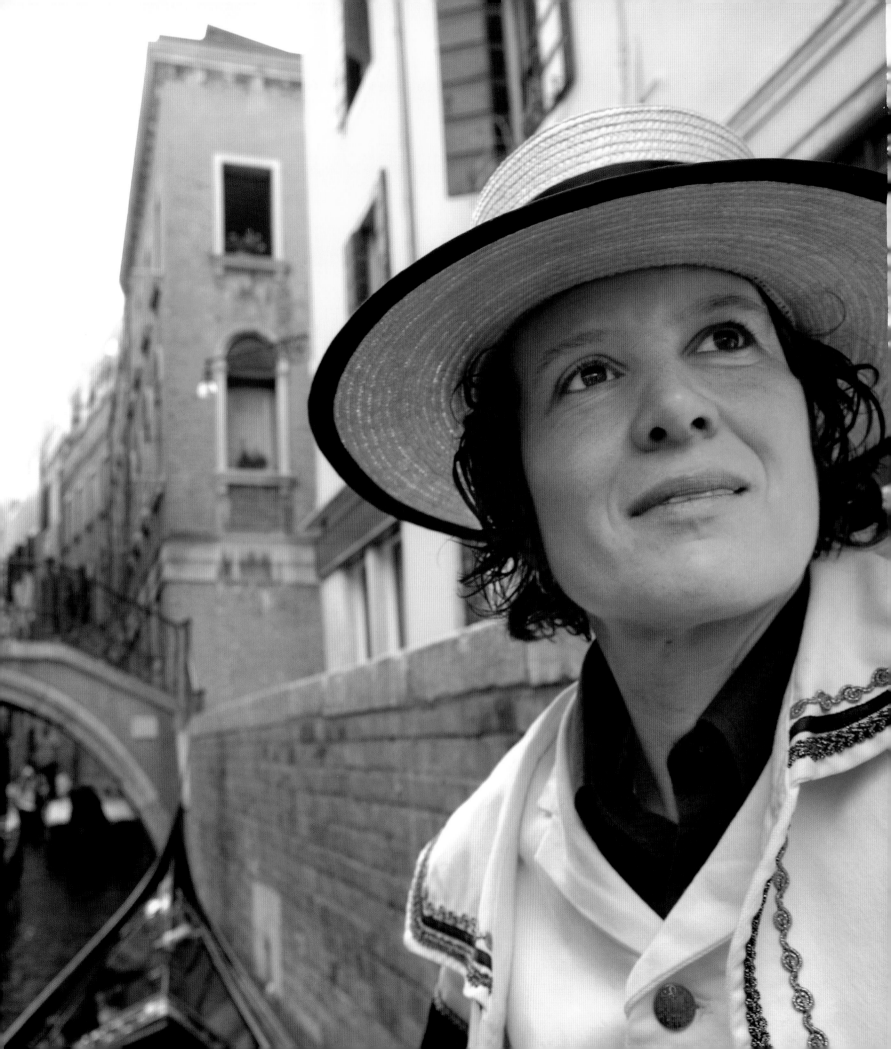

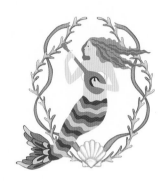

VENICE GONDOLIERA { Alexandra Hai }

"It is just magic to go around a corner in

the small canals where it seems like the palaces

move to give space to the gondola. It is like

playing an instrument in an ambience

where I can listen to the heart beat of Venice."

Venice, Italy

The sun sinks over Venice, washing its sky in amber and setting its waters aglow. *Pegaso*, named after the winged horse of Greek mythology, skims beside docks and glides under bridges, through canals, and past ancient palaces, which, if they could speak, would tell tales of intrigue and passion, triumph and tragedy. The thirty-five foot gondola pulls alongside an intimate restaurant, its honeymooner passengers disembark and disappear into the candlelight. The gondola's skipper, Alexandra Hai, has played her role, expertly rowing her restored wooden vessel and, she says, remaining quiet so she and her clients can "listen to the gondola and listen to Venice."

An archipelago city of over 100 islands, 180 canals, and 400 bridges, Venice and its sea are one. One does not outline or surround the other; they are essential features of each other. So, too, is this "City of Water" defined by its gondolas, and Alex is the first woman to have been allowed to operate one of these graceful boats, breaking beyond the boundaries that have carefully guarded a tradition of male exclusivity. For a thousand years, the coveted licenses for gondoliers have been handed from father to son. Occasionally the precious piece of paper has been purchased from a retired operator. At the height of the Renaissance, 10,000 gondoliers plied the city's waters. Today, with water buses and taxis zipping through Venice's bustling canals, there are only 465 issued licenses.

Born in Birkenfeld, Germany, Alex has also lived in her father's native Algeria as well as France. She fell in love with Venice in 1996 when she visited and rowed her first gondola. Smitten, she set out to learn the skills needed to earn the elusive license—navigating intercoastal currents, learning to maneuver the long, iconic boat smoothly around various obstacles, adjusting to the vagaries of weather, and absorbing the history of this seafaring tradition born of humble roots and intimately linked with its city.

That she dreamed of becoming a captain despite growing up far from the ocean, where she says, she had to imagine "any little 'lake' of rainwater to be her sea," is surprising. It is even more surprising given that the sea almost took her life when she was eight. "I was on vacation at Gran Canaria Beach. I went

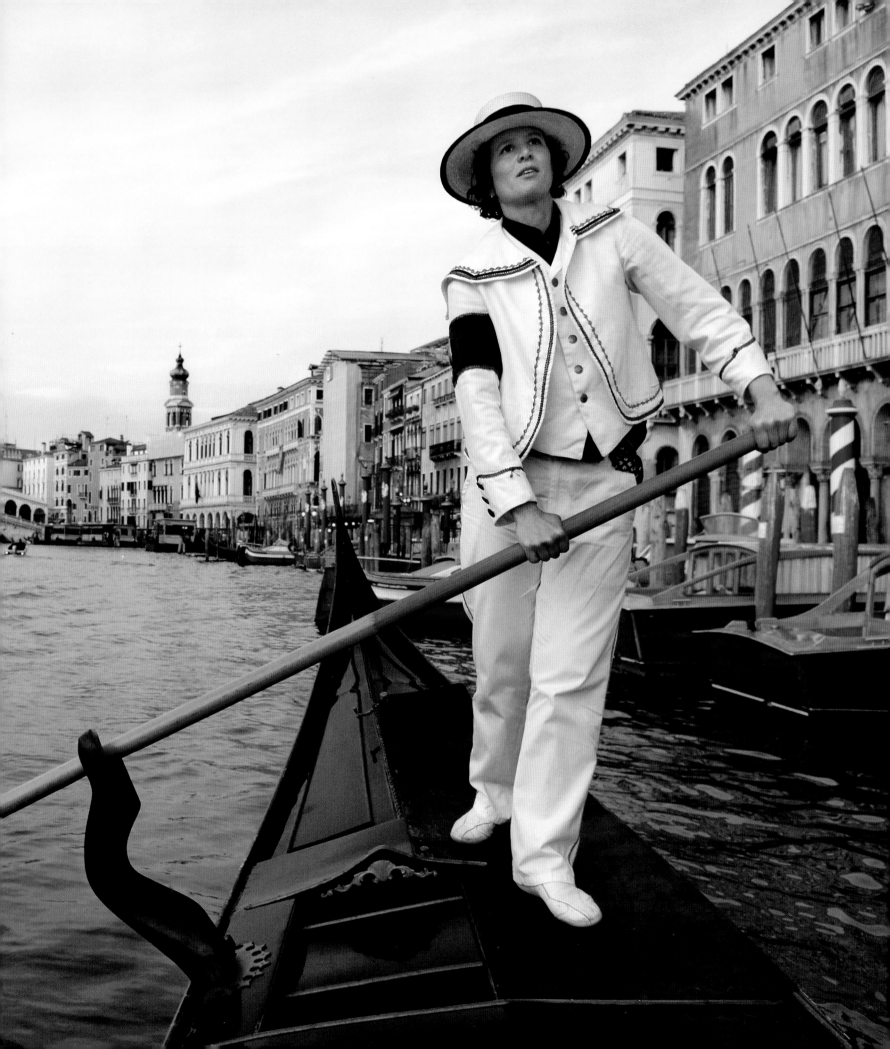

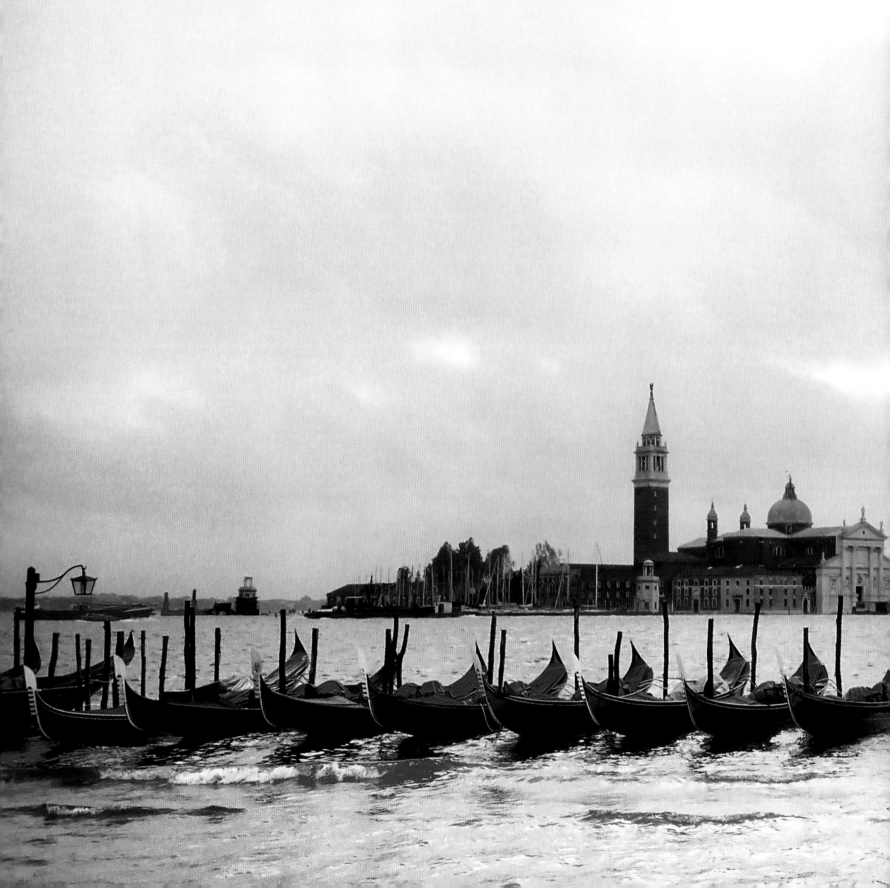

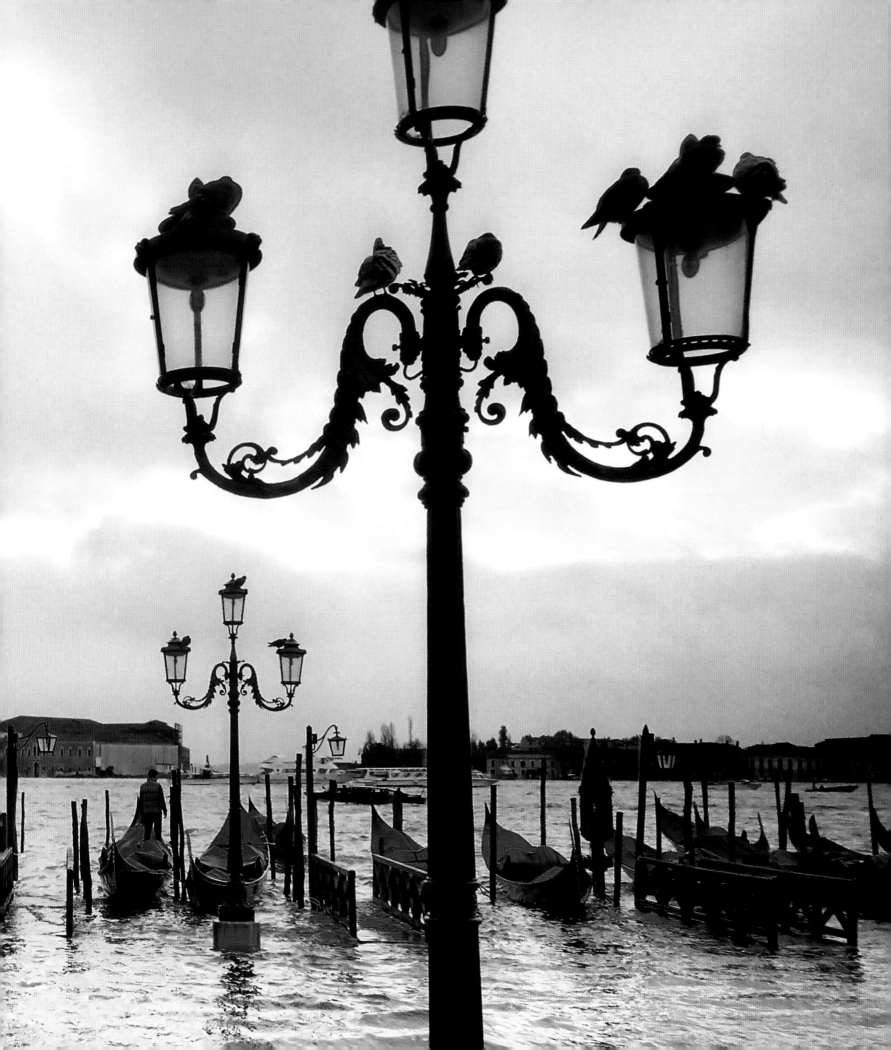

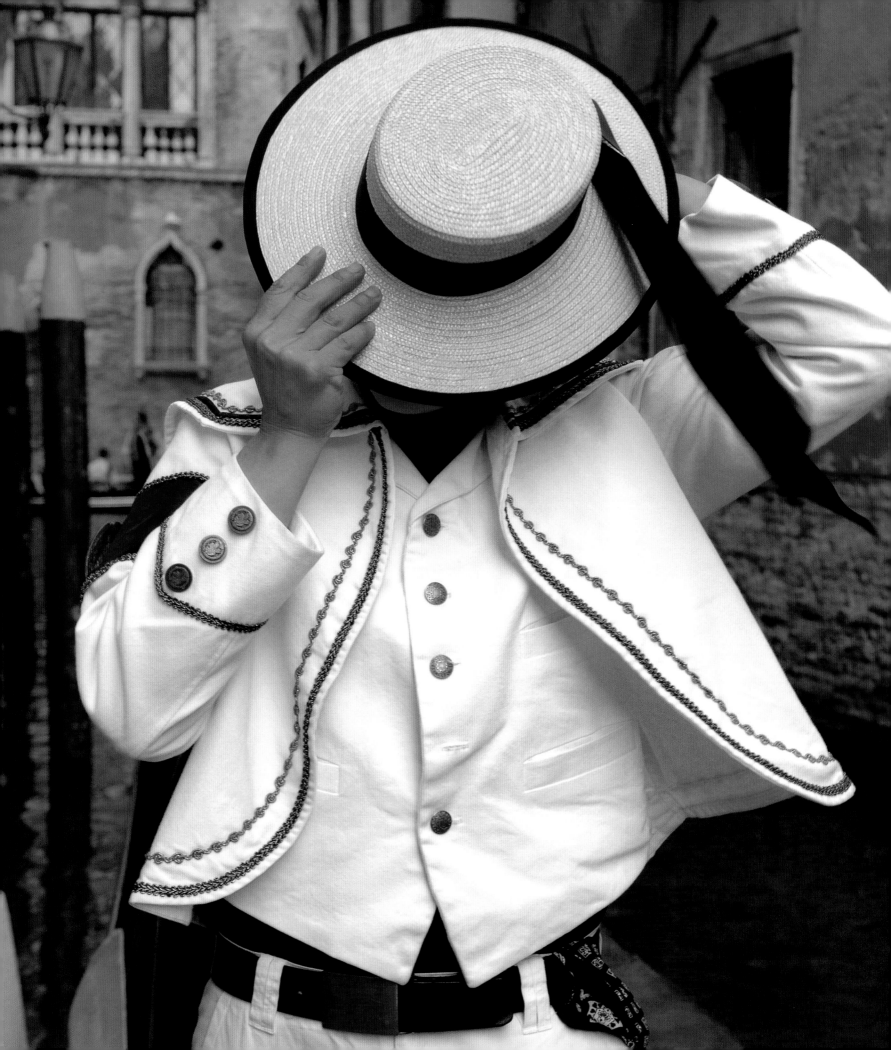

> "Voyage upon life's sea,
> To yourself be true, And,
> whatever your lot may be
> Paddle your own canoe."

SARAH BOLTON

swimming, and unwatched by my mother, I nearly drowned." Moreover, no family seafarers had set a precedent for her interest, at least "none in this lifetime," she says.

Not only has Alex forgiven and made peace with the saltwater that almost killed her, she has become one with it. When balancing on the back of her gondola, dressed in her crisp whites, working with currents and avoiding other boats, jutting buildings, and omnipresent bridges, she says, "I try to concentrate on my gondola and to have a dialogue with the elements. I try to communicate those emotions to my clients; in other words, I try to let them feel the magic of Venice."

As the private gondoliera for four Venetian hotels, she likes to take her passengers to sites off the typical tourist map. "I try to spoil my clients with a lifetime experience—the chance to have a piece of Venice, just one little moment all to themselves." While gondoliers were once members of the underprivileged class, today they channel the city's charm: "It is just magic to go around a corner in the small canals where it seems like the palaces move and give space to the gondola," Alex says.

It takes great skill and strength to maneuver the half-ton vessel, which Alex says, "grows heavier with time as it holds onto the water." When she is not working her craft and rowing through Venice's many canals, Alex, who holds an unlimited captain's license, takes to her small powerboat and explores deeper waters. If time is generous with her, she may go scuba diving, swimming alongside devil rays, giant sea flowers, and whale sharks, taking underwater photos to document her close encounters. She may even go fishing, looking to land a large tuna, or escape to the beaches of Corsica, one of her favorite islands in the Mediterranean.

If ever Venice sinks, as it has long been rumored to be doing in the wake of rising waters, or if ever she feels out of synch with the city she now loves, Alex says she would take to living aboard a galleon, calling "around the world" her home. Such visions are in keeping with the theme of her gondola: *"E la luna nassara' per sognar un altro di,"* "And the moon will be born to dreams of another day."

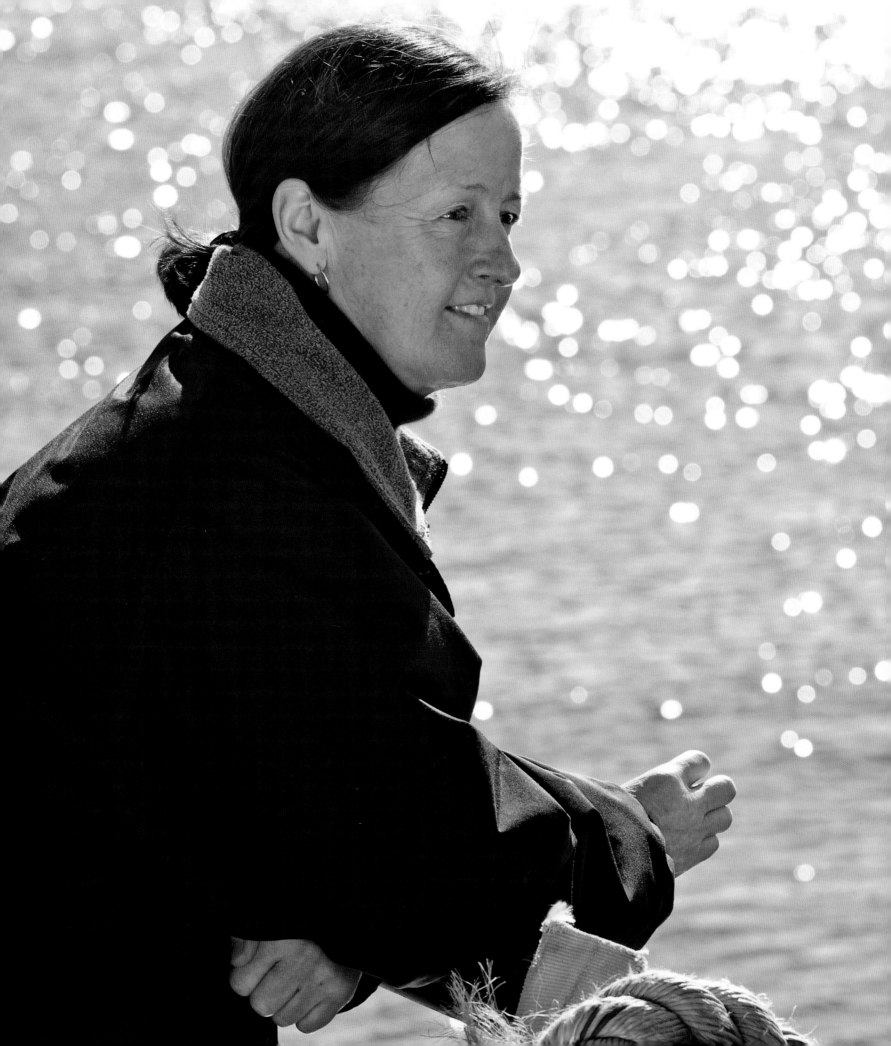

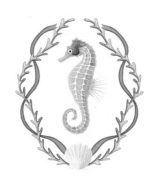

OCEANOGRAPHER { Susan Humphris }

"I love being at sea. Part of it is the remoteness. We will

be miles from anything. **It is liberating**

not being surrounded by buildings and cars."

Woods Hole, Massachusetts

She has gone where no one else has gone before. She has seen parts of our planet never before seen. Aboard *Alvin*, the only deep-diving submersible in the United States, she has traveled 12,000 feet under the ocean's surface through darkness so profound, most cannot fathom it. At first, she was searching along an underwater mountain range in the Atlantic for hot water springs scientists only suspected existed. What she found, she says, "was biologically different from anything ever described." When Dr. Susan Humphris, a senior oceanographer specializing in geochemistry at the world-renowned Woods Hole Oceanographic Institution (WHOI), goes on her underwater missions, she never knows what she will discover: "I have seen hydrothermal vents with all that hot water pouring out and the exotic communities of animals around them, like four-foot-long tubeworms or billions of shrimp."

A trip to such depths is a bit eerie. Carrying a pilot, two scientists, and equipment, quarters aboard the submersible are close and the atmosphere is a bit stuffy. Shortly after the vehicle submerges, the light disappears, leaving its passengers for the next 3,300 meters in pitch black, save for the alien creatures floating by: "While sinking, you see these beautiful fluorescent gelatinous organisms," Susan says. When they reach their destination, the crew is too busy to linger over aesthetic impressions. Instead, Susan and her fellow researcher fire up the lights, and using their limited battery power judiciously, they make observations, gather samples, record data, pack up, and ascend.

To be 12,000 feet under the sea is far from Surrey, England, where Susan spent the first thirteen years of her life. When she was a teenager, her family moved to Burnham-on-the-Sea. Ironically for this future deep-sea scientist, the family home on the Bristol Channel offered a somewhat shallow view of things. "Bristol Channel has one of the highest tide ranges in the world, so most of the day we looked at sand and mud. I learned to sail there and crewed in many races—when the tide came in!" Susan knew early on that she wanted to be a scientist, but she knew equally as well, being a lover of the outdoors, that she did not want to pursue science indoors in a laboratory. When she was in college, studying environmental science,

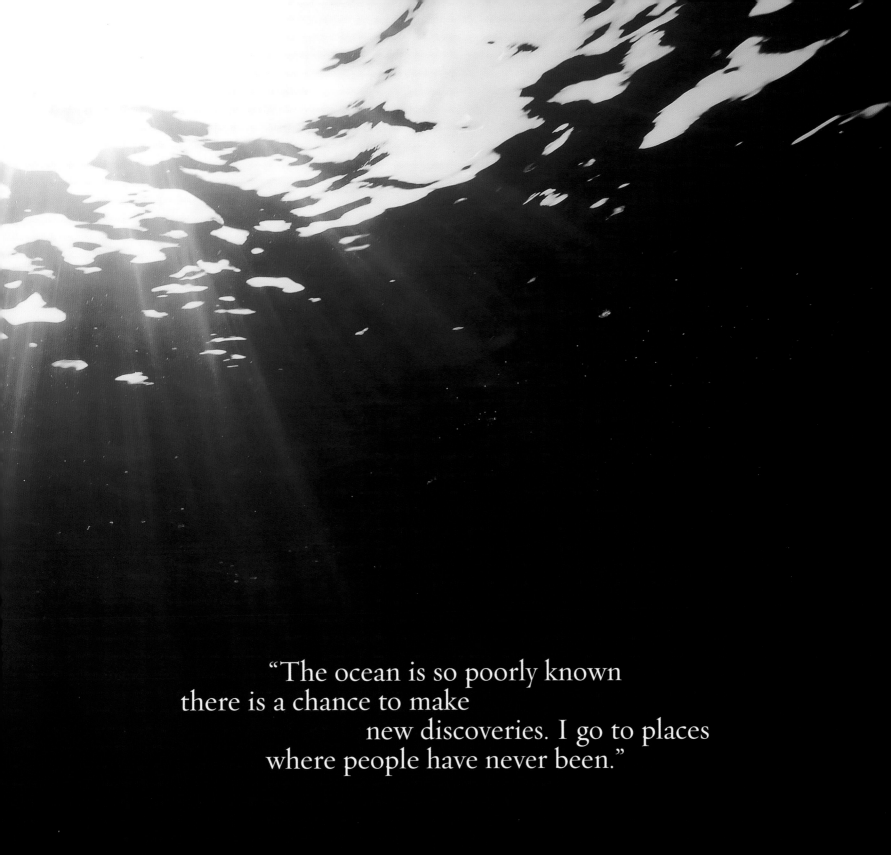

"The ocean is so poorly known
there is a chance to make
                    new discoveries. I go to places
where people have never been."

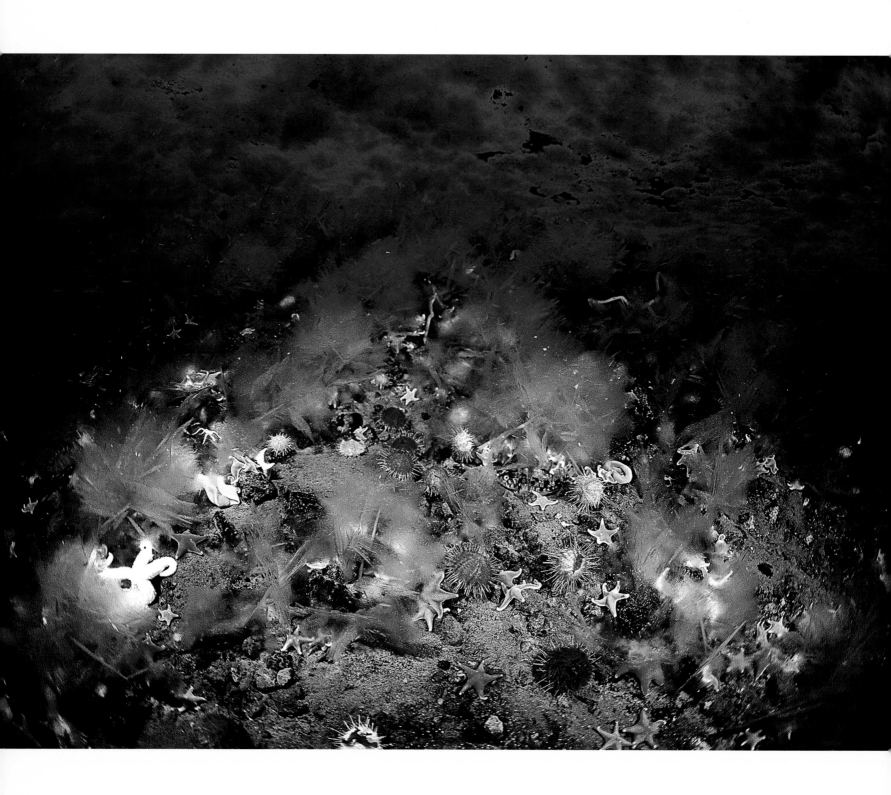

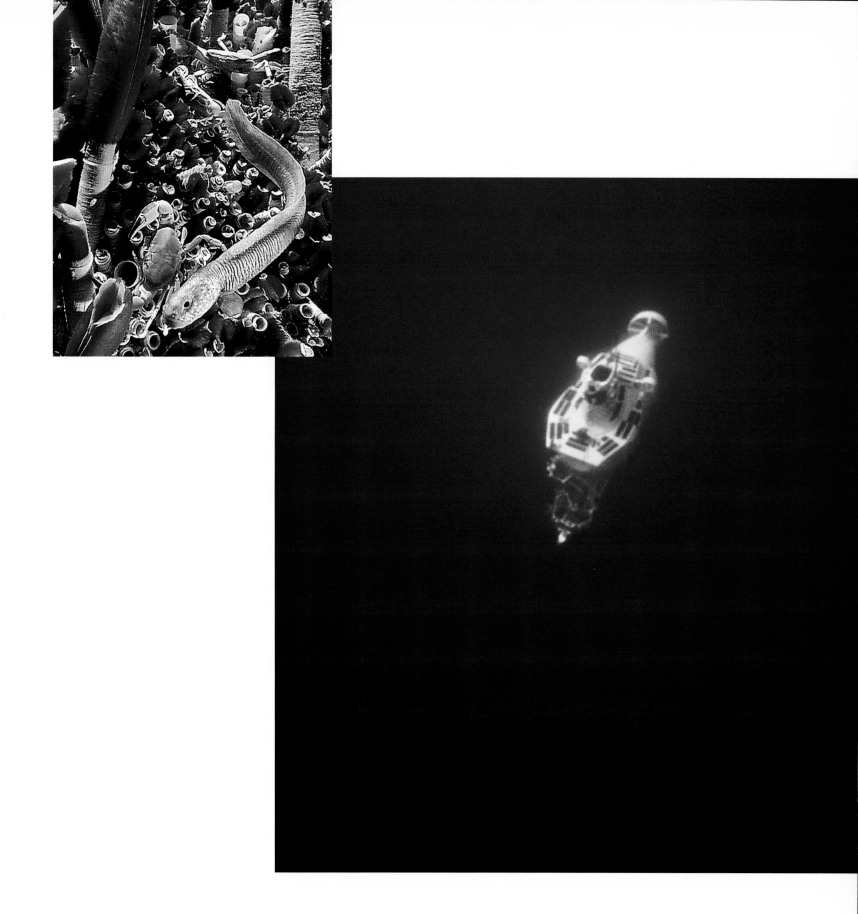

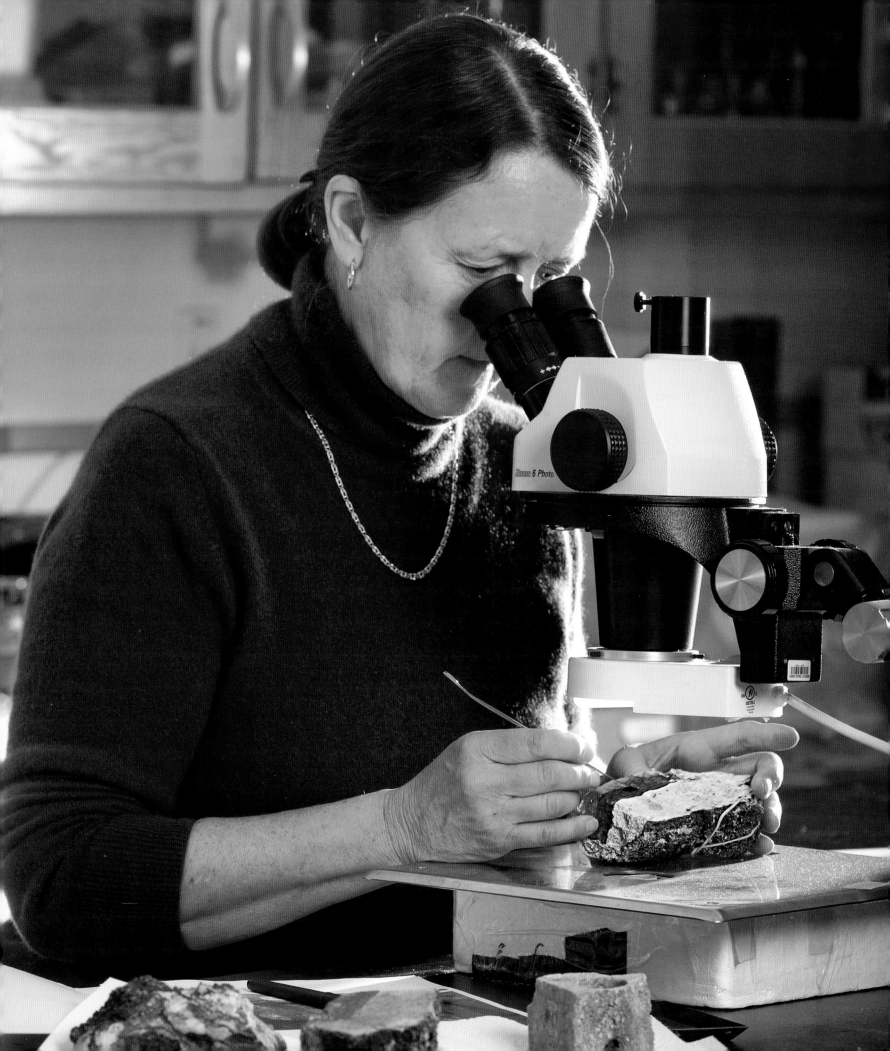

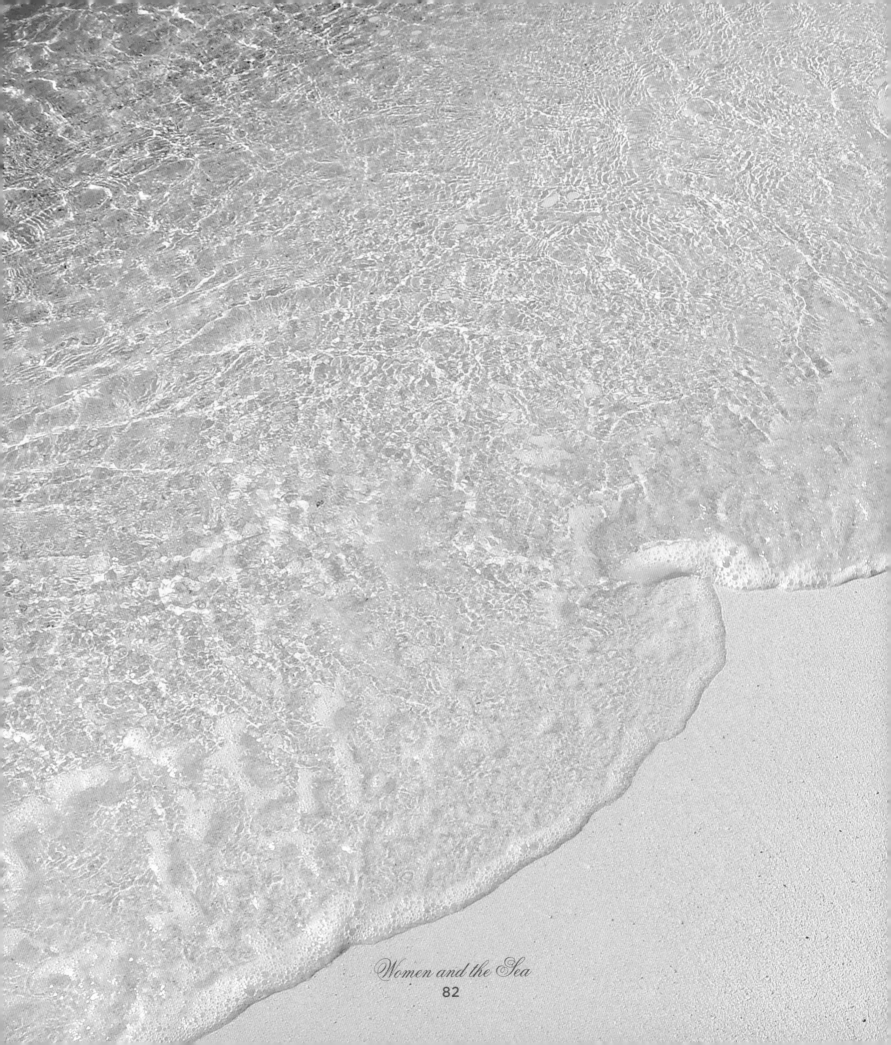

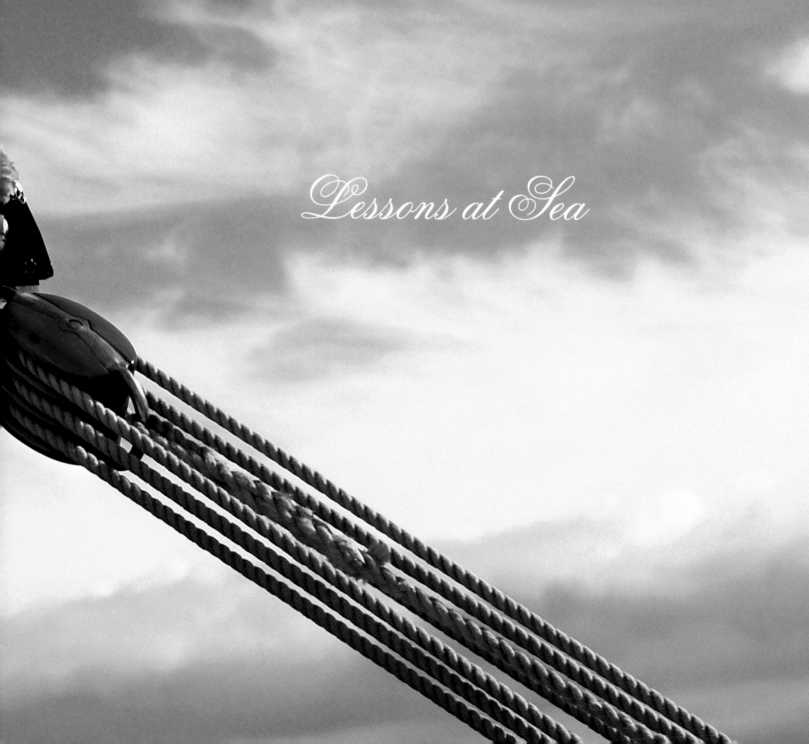

Lessons at Sea

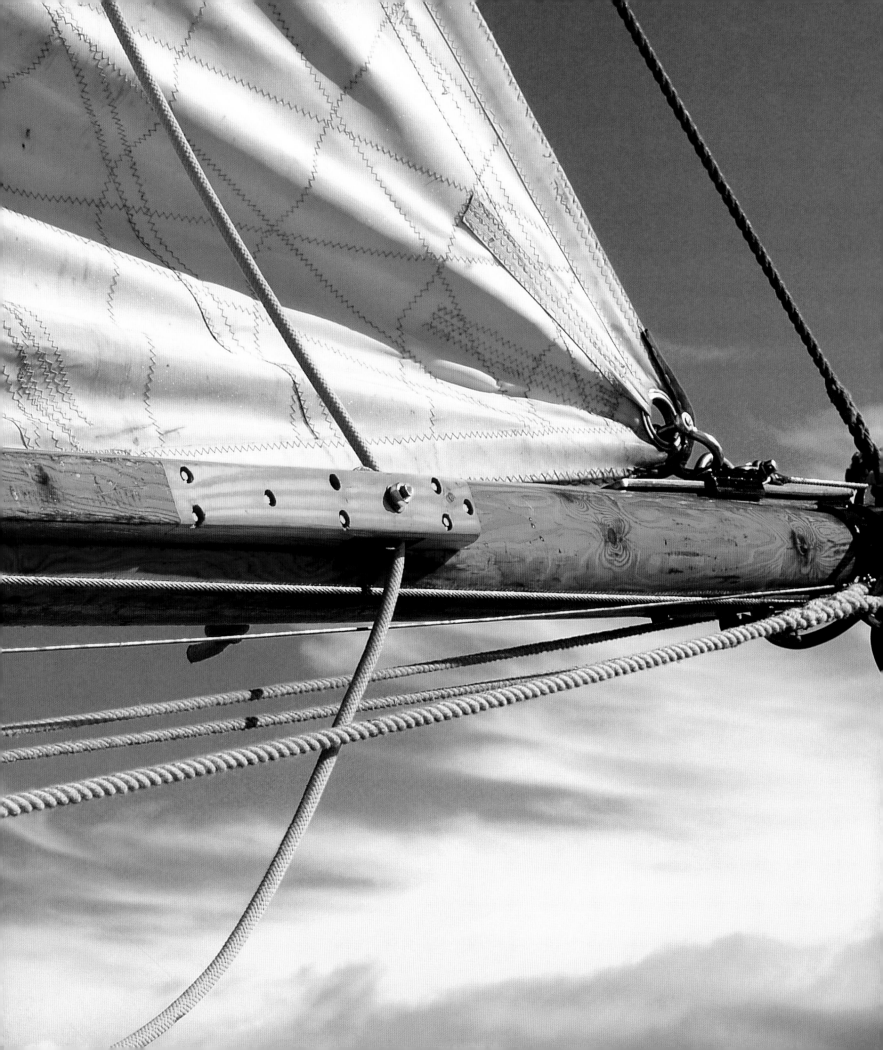

> "It is always with excitement that
> I wake in the morning wondering
> what my intuition will toss up to me,
> like gifts from the sea. I work with it
> and rely on it. It's my partner."
>
> JONAS SALK

pictures in a book sparked her interest in the path her career would follow. "In my last year I took a course in marine geochemistry. When I looked in the text and saw ships and deep submersibles, I thought this could be fun, doing something out on the ocean, applying science to the environment. I also knew that the ocean is so poorly known that there is a chance to make new discoveries."

A doctorate in hand, earned through the Joint Program between Massachusetts Institute of Technology and WHOI, Susan has for some time made regular journeys to the deep ocean and still finds that world "vast, mysterious, and unpredictable," and she loves to share what she has seen and learned with others. "I like to bring the cruises in real time to the public." As part of her outreach, she has been a guest lecturer aboard the *Queen Mary II*. "What I study is very visual. To see a black smoker, a hot spring, is incredible. I have a lot of footage from the deep ocean that I show, and it excites people." She can also speak knowingly as the ship crosses the Gulf Stream or reaches the Mid-Atlantic Ridge, describing the volcanic chain under the ship's keel.

What keeps Susan fascinated is all that is yet to be known. She would like to understand more about that volcanic chain, visit the abyssal plains, and investigate the "big, deep" trenches known to be under the ocean. "There is so much unexplored. There is so much down there that we don't know about. One of the things I like about the field is that it is a learning experience for me."

When she is not nearly two miles below the water's surface, not in her lab studying samples and analyzing data, not writing papers, attending seminars, or giving lectures, Susan can be found with her husband, a fellow scientist, sailing the waters around the mostly uninhabited Elizabeth Islands chain just off the Woods Hole coast. "Almost every weekend we are out exploring coves and little bays. I think the Elizabeth Islands are very beautiful. They're unspoiled, and I think their wildness is very appealing." It is this very quality that keeps Susan cruising far offshore for work: "I love being at sea. Part of it is the remoteness. I like the feeling of being miles from anywhere. It is so liberating not being surrounded by buildings and cars"—instead there are just a few billion shrimp, giant worms, and glowing creatures.

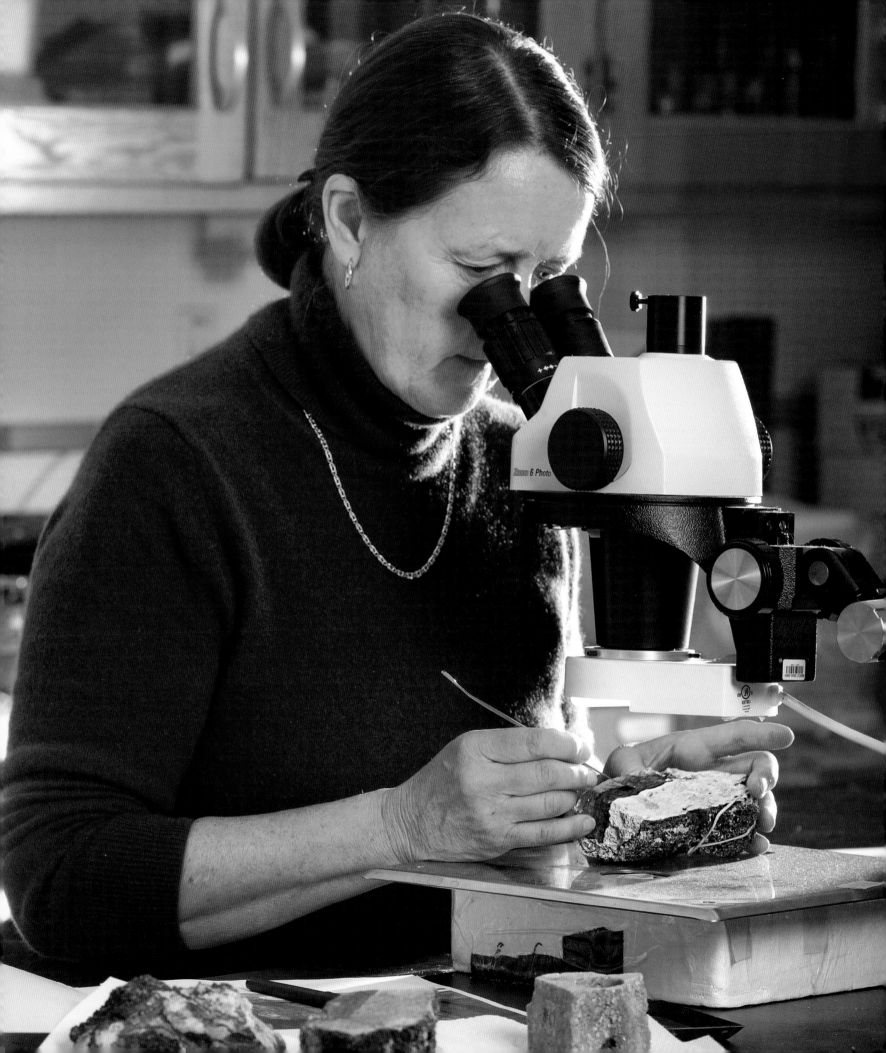

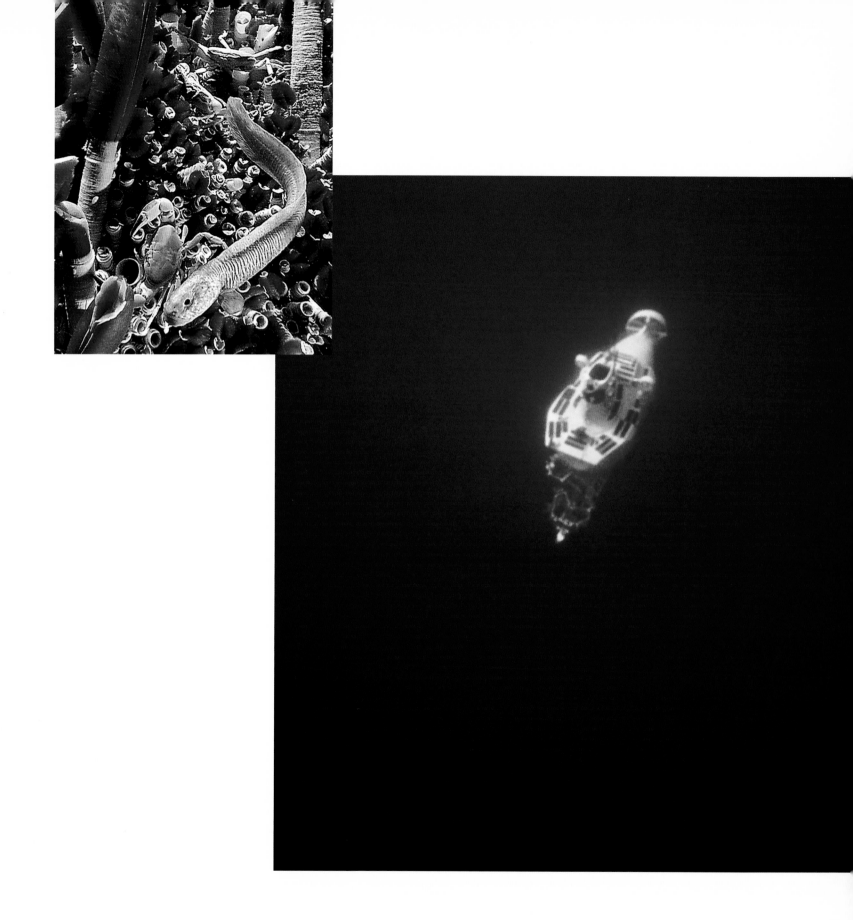

LUCY MAUD MONTGOMERY

The Sea to the Shore

Lo, I have loved thee long, long have I yearned and entreated!
Tell me how I may win thee, tell me how I must woo.
Shall I creep to thy white feet, in guise of a humble lover?
Shall I croon in mild petition, murmuring vows anew?

Shall I stretch my arms unto thee, biding thy maiden coyness,
Under the silver of morning, under the purple of night?
Taming my ancient rudeness, checking my heady clamor
Thus, is it thus I must woo thee, oh, my delight?

Nay, 'tis no way of the sea thus to be meekly suitor
I shall storm thee away with laughter wrapped in my beard of snow,
With the wildest of billows for chords I shall harp thee a song for thy bridal,
A mighty lyric of love that feared not nor would forego!

With a red-gold wedding ring, mined from the caves of sunset,
Fast shall I bind thy faith to my faith evermore,
And the stars will wait on our pleasure, the great north wind will trumpet
A thunderous marriage march for the nuptials of sea and shore.

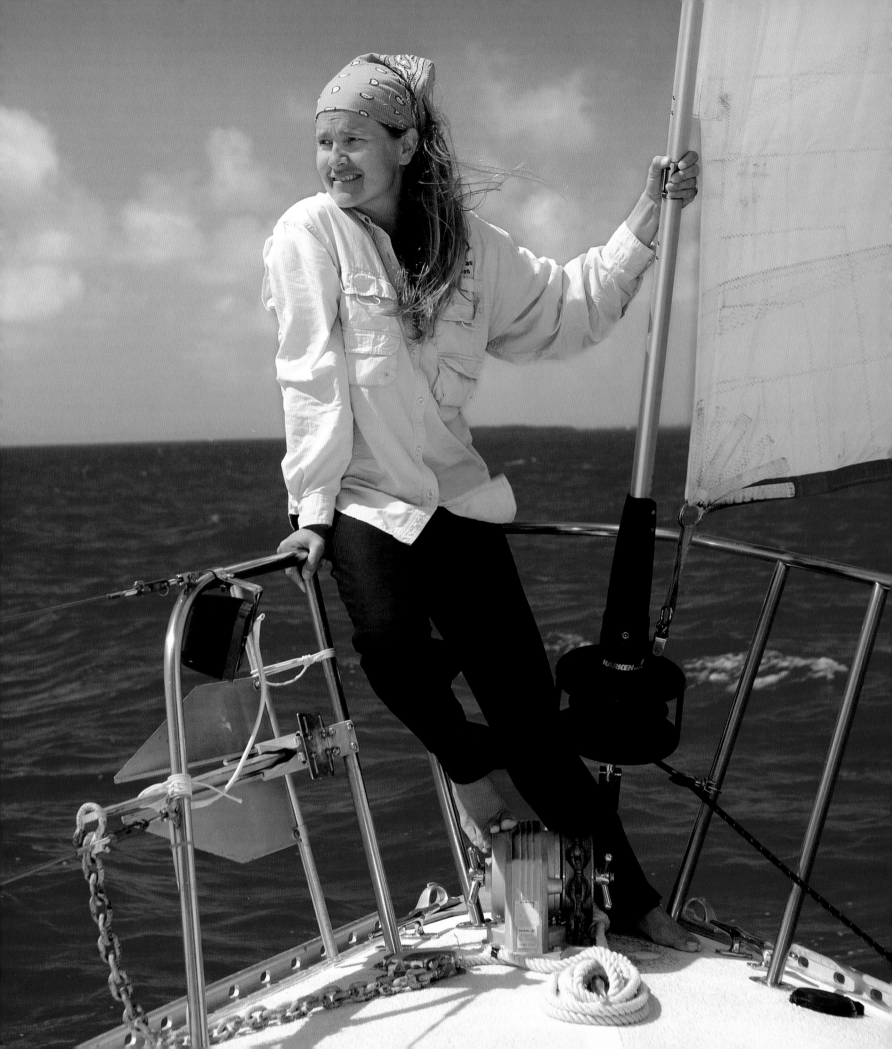

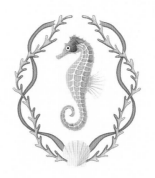

SAILING INSTRUCTOR { Jennifer MacLean }

"I love the sense of freedom I get when I get out

on the water. As soon as you get past the jetty and out to

the open sea, you forget about the small things.

The sea has a tendency to draw the big picture for us."

Tavernier, Florida

The sun's rays splinter the morning clouds, illuminating the turquoise waters of the Florida Keys. Osprey scan for their breakfast, while in a nearby mangrove, egrets and heron stir. Waves rock the *Indian Summer II*, at anchor, ready for another day of sailing. On its bow is its captain, Jennifer MacLean, moving through the warrior poses of her sun salutation yoga series. This is how she starts her workday, not fighting traffic, not stopping for a grande latte, not tucked into business attire. She is centering her spirit for another day of guiding women through the ropes of sailing. She will share her knowledge and her passion, her infectious smile and her generous good will, and at day's end, she may serenade her fellow "pirates," as she calls them, with a song or two from her acoustic guitar. These women—maybe they are doctors, nurses, writers, teachers, housewives, economists, or massage therapists in their shore life—have signed on for American Sailing Association certificate courses aboard Captain MacLean's forty-one foot cruising boat. For a handful of days, Captain Jenn will teach these women the craft of tying knots, the science of navigation, the skill of managing sails, the beauty of snorkeling coral reefs, the art of catching mahi-mahi or lobster for dinner, and the peace of being at sea.

Captain Jenn cannot imagine any other way to spend her days, as this is exactly what she envisioned when she was growing up on the St. Lawrence Seaway in Quebec, Canada. As a teenager, she dreamt of exploring the Amazon and sailing across the Atlantic. She has done both. After a stint as a crewmember aboard a trimaran in Canada, she sought warmer weather and abundantly more sailing days. She pointed her compass south and landed in the Florida Keys. There she crewed for the Boy Scouts of America aboard their eighty-foot sailboat, eventually becoming their first female captain. As gratifying as that role was and continues to be for her, she longed to entice more women into the wonders of sailing and to help them experience the confidence that comes from finessing a docking or capitalizing on a breeze. The Girl Scouts did not have a parallel program. "I kept running into people who said that it is a dangerous thing for girls to do. There are still a lot of barriers, but I decided to start a women's sailing program. I thought maybe women would like to be

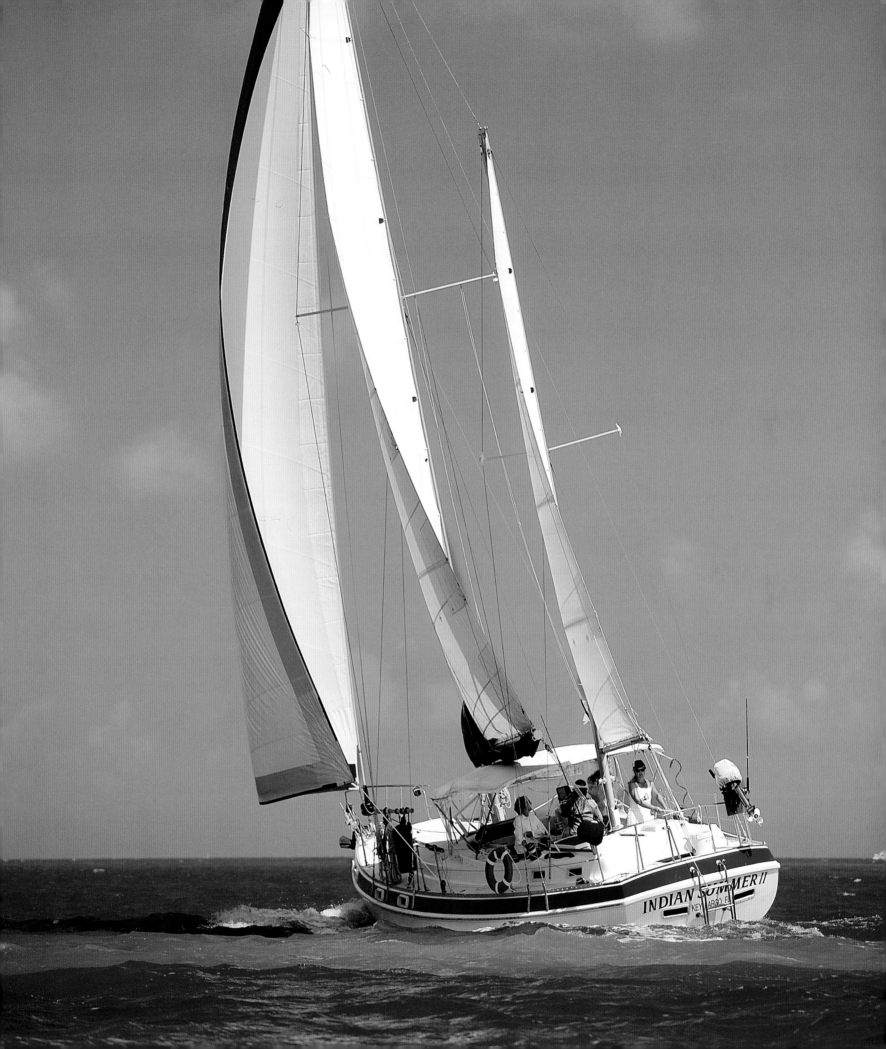

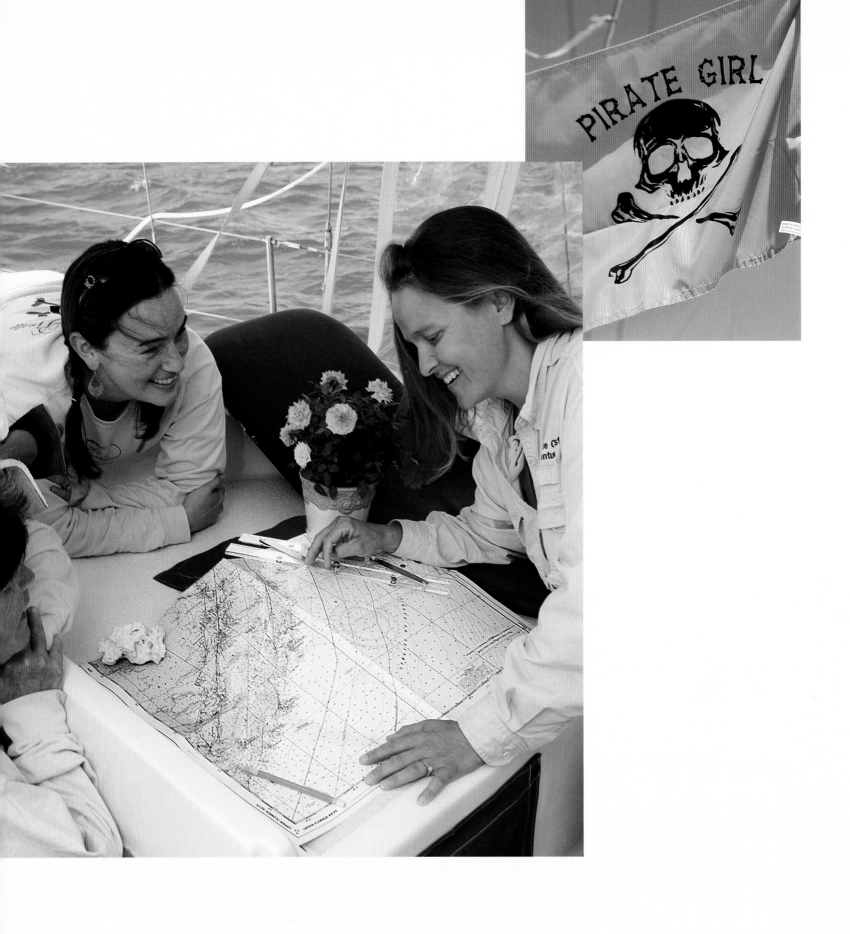

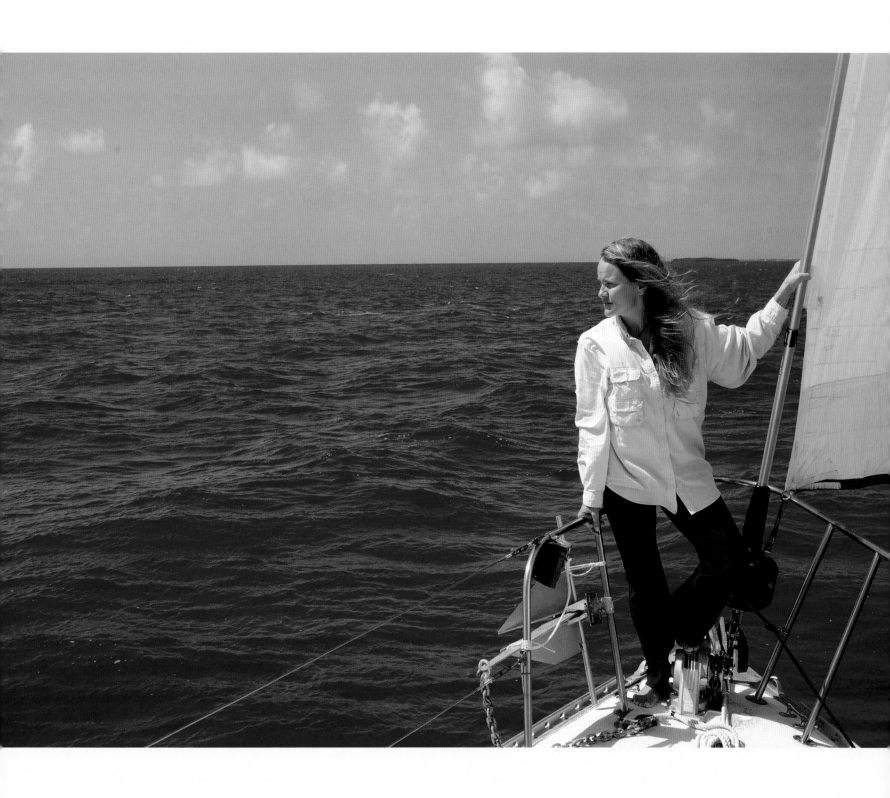

> "We are tied to the ocean.
> And when we go back to the sea,
>   whether it is to sail or to watch, we
> are going back from whence we came."

JOHN F. KENNEDY

taught by women." Thus was born Her Ladyship Sailing, the offspring of Jenn's Sunshine Coast Adventures Sailing School. While she teaches couples as well as youth groups, Her Ladyship is for women only, and they prove themselves to be naturals. "They get in a boat and get a feel for it right away. They are better at working together and can steer a straight course. When they dock a boat, they get pumped up," Jenn says.

Though she shares her expertise in all things nautical from the Keys to the Chesapeake Bay and from the Atlantic to the Pacific, what Jenn most wants to share is her love for this lifestyle, a lifestyle that runs deep in her genes, encoded by her New Brunswick ancestors who, too, made their living at sea. When the women board Captain Jenn's boat, they are asked to take off their watches and shut off their cell phones. It is time to tune into a world beyond the busyness of life. "It's the sense of freedom you get when you're on the water. As soon as you get past the jetty and to the open sea, there is water, water, water—all of the daily stuff, all of that small stuff that fills your life, feels useless." Instead, days are spent practicing sailing skills, kayaking to nearby islands, swimming in clear waters, or relaxing to the lull of lapping waves.

Days at sea are also always full of surprises. Maybe the *Indian Summer II* is being pursued by a pod of two dozen dolphin, maybe a shark accompanies the lobster chase or gigantic spotted eagle rays come along for the snorkeling. Maybe the encounter is of the human kind. One morning Captain Jenn and her crew of students spied an island filled with Cuban refugees. By making landfall, they had earned the right to enter the United States.

Jenn so savors the sailor's life that on her days off, she says, "I take the boat out and anchor it, spending the night. I sail even when I am not working." The experience for her goes beyond figuring out fickle winds, being rocked by waves, or thrilling to a stream of rainbow-colored fish sighted beneath the water's surface: "In its quietness, serenity, and beauty, the sea teaches us ways to find our centers as human beings. The sea has a tendency to draw the big picture for us and remind us not to sweat the small stuff. It is that special place that helps us remember the important things in life."

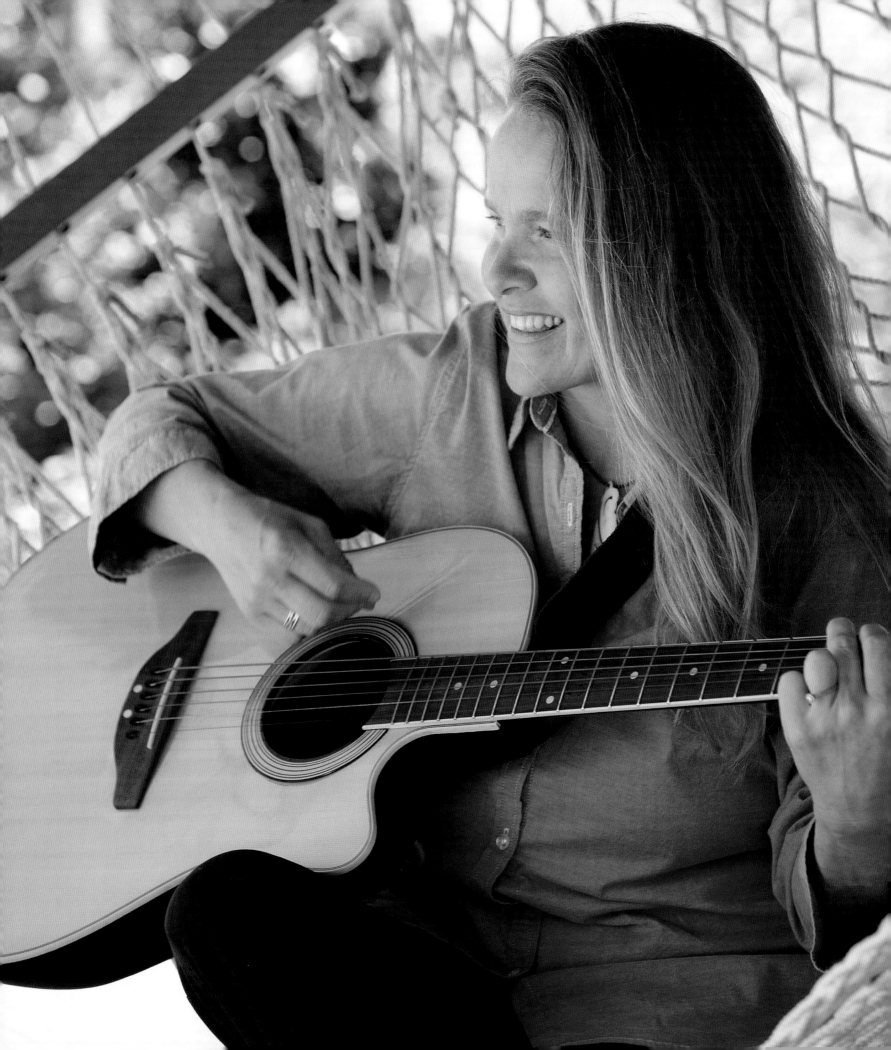

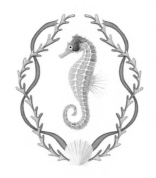

FISHIN' CHIX FOUNDER { Claudia Espenscheid }

"For me, fishing is about the sisterhood,

the bonding, spending time together, fishing for the

sake of fishing and not so much about the catching."

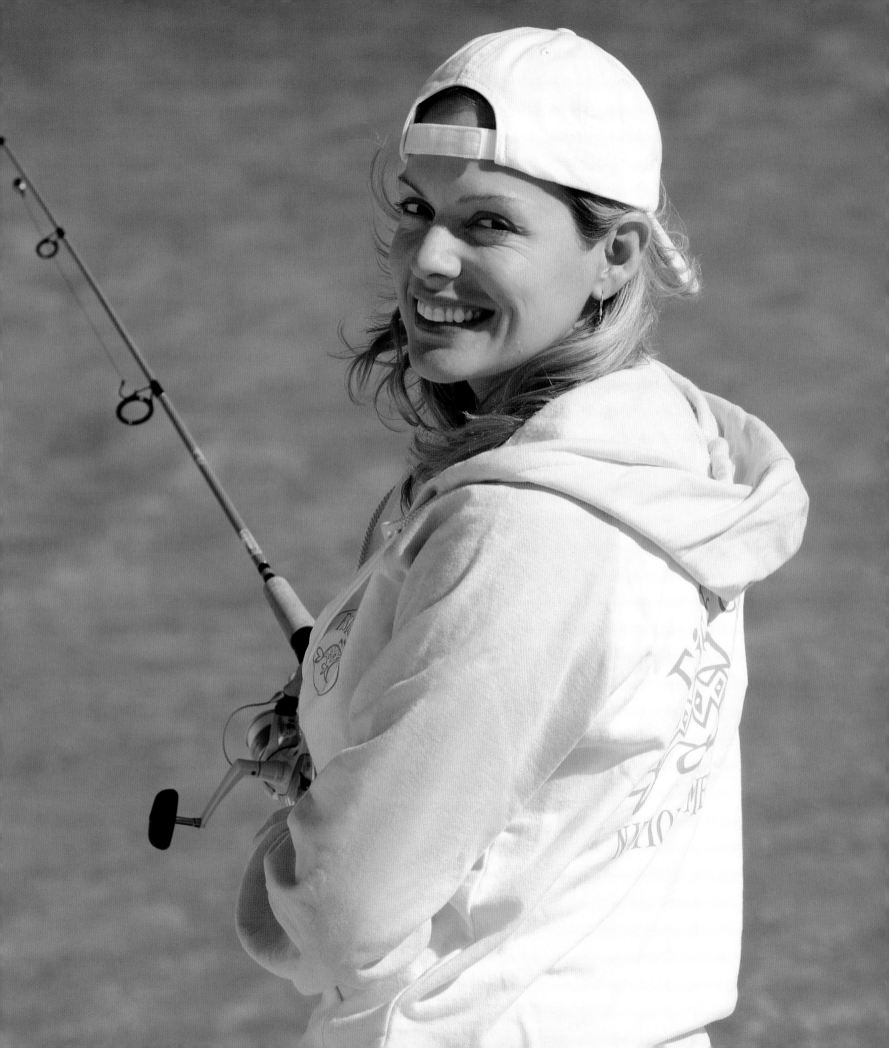

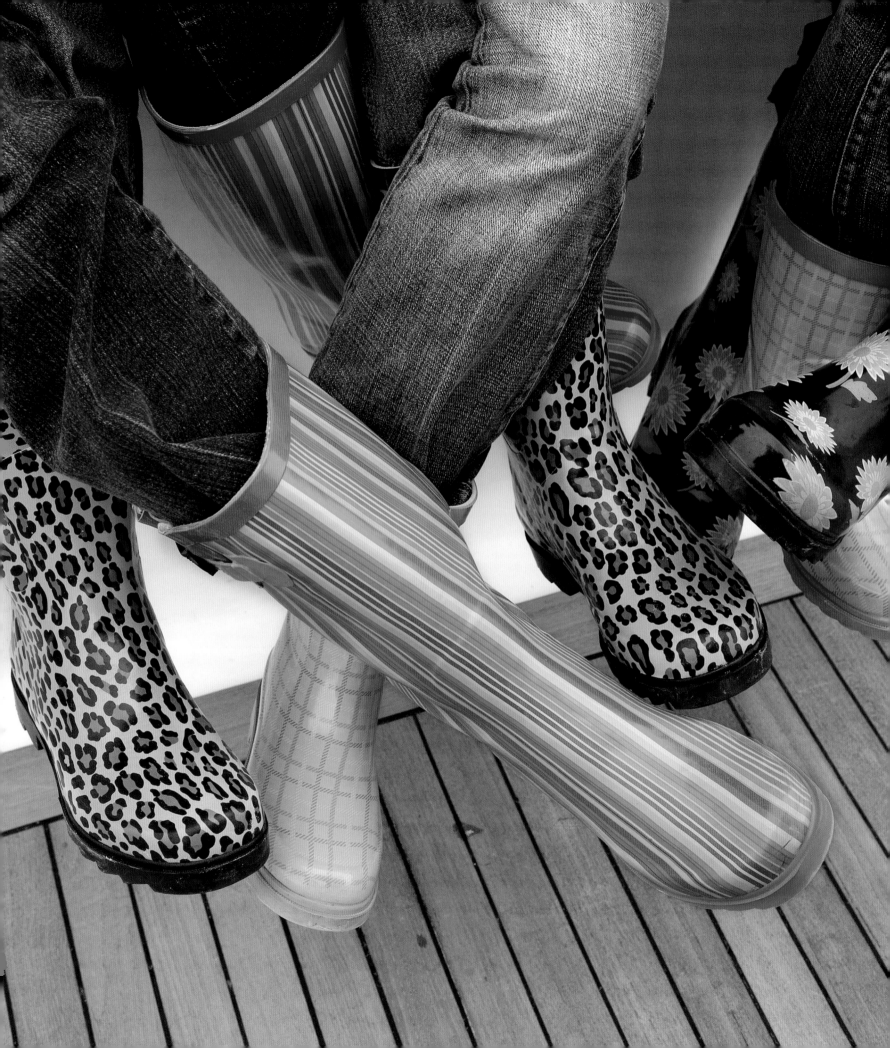

Pensacola, Florida

Maybe it was the hours spent standing on her dock, casting a wide net toward the sea, scooping back whatever it offered—mullet, speckled trout, redfish, even on one occasion a massive stingray. "Throwing the net is like Forrest Gump and the box of chocolates. You never know what you are going to get. You catch these creatures, and it is like interacting with another planet." Claudia Espenscheid's meditative gesture of openness and acceptance was at first a means of relaxing before and after stressful days spent as a financial adviser. It would become a critical life philosophy.

When Ivan the Terrible pummeled Florida's Gulf Coast in 2004, it damaged Claudia's home and destroyed her beloved dock. She had evacuated to Jacksonville at the last possible moment. When Ivan was followed by Hurricane Dennis, the storm that would crack her concrete pool and send it floating to her neighbor's house, she stayed home, confronting its force. "Maybe it wasn't smart, but as someone who loves danger and risk taking, I stayed. It was awe-inspiring, especially when you see the gigantic walls of water coming at you. Hurricanes Ivan and Dennis made me love and respect the water even more." Like a cast net, you never know what a storm might bring, and for Claudia, it brought a sea change. Eschewing long lines waiting for rationed food, ice, and water, Claudia visited her local bait shop and asked to be outfitted for fishing and for lessons on how to do it. She then invited other women to join her. Of course, adopting a new sport raises the inevitable question, what does one wear? Man-sized foul weather gear in caution yellow? Leave it to women to take a sport of mystery (the location of hot fishing spots is not revealed), of indolent quietness, of competition and bragging rights (the biggest fish, the fish that got away), and turn it into a pastime reeling with laughter and lightened up by candy-colored rubber boots and pink camouflage caps. Fishin' Chix, the club and retail outlet that Claudia formed for new female fishing devotees, has as its membership requirements, "Nice Women, Fun Loving, Like Fish." Its logo features a parti-colored fish with well-lined, pouty lips.

Fishing for food after Ivan became fishing for the exhilaration of it. "Women get unexpected excitement from fishing," Claudia says. "It is unadulterated joy. I never expected to like fishing, and other women say

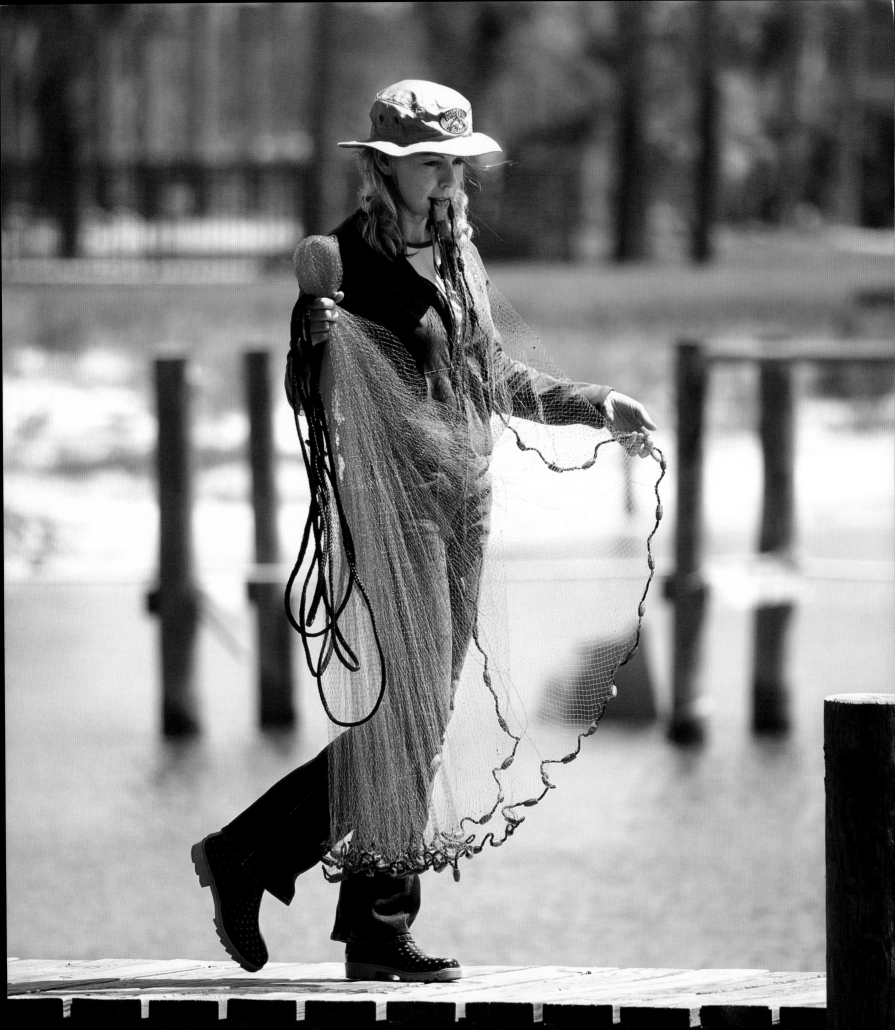

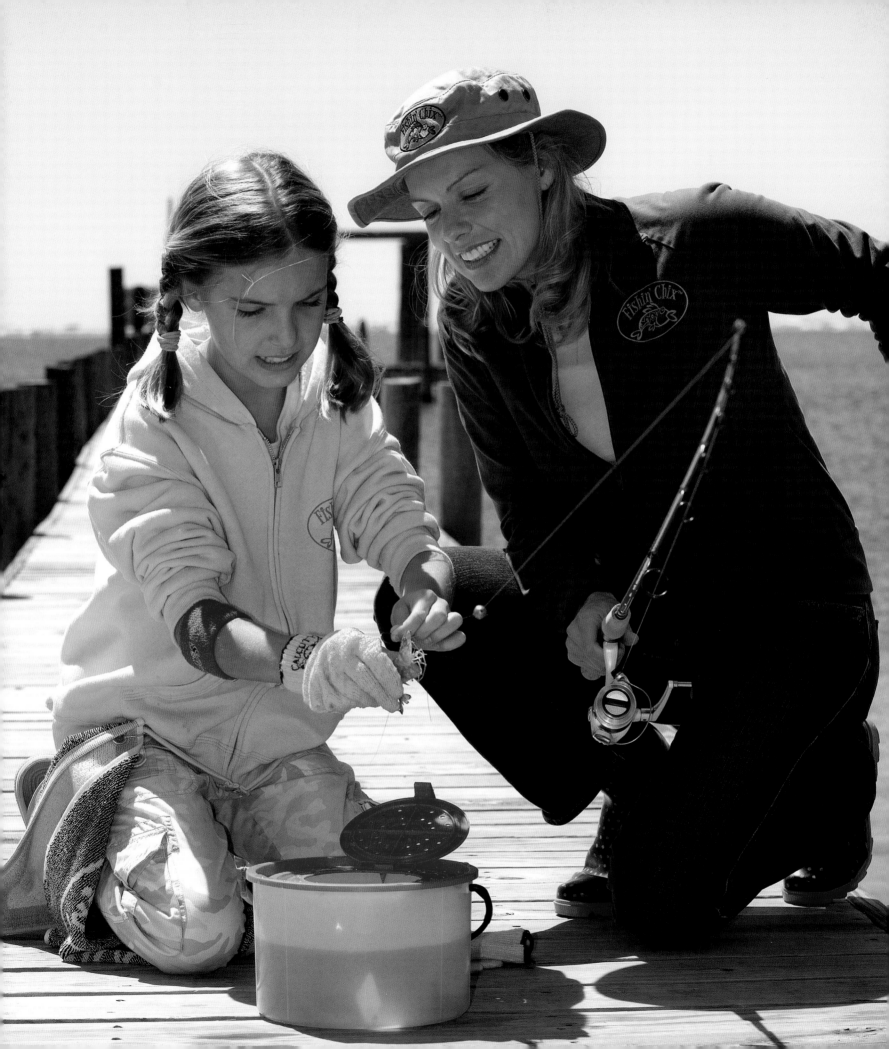

> "The fishermen know that the sea is dangerous and the storm terrible, but they have never found these dangers sufficient reason for remaining ashore."

VINCENT VAN GOGH

the same thing. Sure enough, every time they'll say, 'That's just the greatest experience in the world.'" Women are curious, they ask questions, they follow advice, and they share their amazement at what they land. "Women scream their heads off even if it's a teeny fish they have caught. It's almost as if they have reeled in a Volkswagen."

Each time Claudia introduces a new convert to the joys of fishing, whether through a mother-daughter tournament, her Pink Rubber Boots Ladies Fishing Rodeo, or an organized trip to fish for black marlin in Panama, she is renewed in her own love of the sport. "There's something about catching a fish. It makes me feel powerful. I can bring in the bacon. That is independence." Shared independence through sisterhood is even better. "It seems like on the water, men are more concerned with the size of the boat, the type of tackle, and the competitiveness that surrounds being out fishing. For the women, it's about the bonding, spending time together. We fish for the sake of fishing and for relaxation. It's not so much about the catching." Fishing is also one more way for her to connect to her daughters. "Stereotypically, it's a father/son bonding experience, but times are changing. One time I let my daughters skip school, so the three of us could go fishing together."

Claudia spent her early years in Germany, and it took moving to Florida for her seagoing genes, inherited from Viking ancestors, to surface. "I loved and still love the mountains, but it was not until I moved here when I was seventeen that my love of the water manifested." Even then, she mostly wanted to ski on top of it. "I did not have as much interaction with the water before the hurricanes. I had not fished. All I cared about was whether conditions were good for waterskiing." Now she is deeply attuned to the sea's many moods. "The water really personifies Mother Nature. Like a person, there are different personalities that emerge day to day. Sometimes it is smooth, flat, and clear like glass. When it is foggy and misty, there is so much unknown. Sometimes the mood is serene; sometimes it is angry and furious. I think it affects my moods too."

When Ivan and Dennis blew in with all of their fury, Claudia did not shrink before their wrath. Her nets and dock gone, she cast a line and caught a whole new life. No wonder she believes, "fishing is empowering."

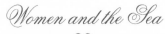

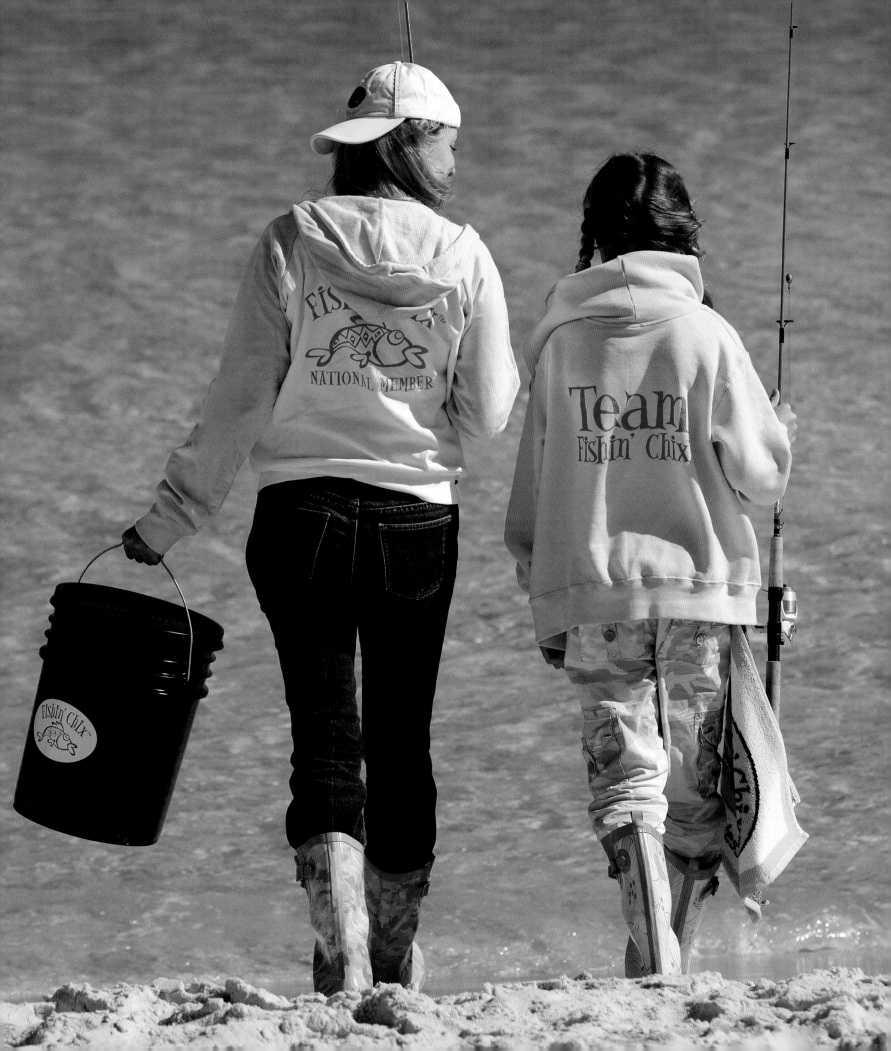

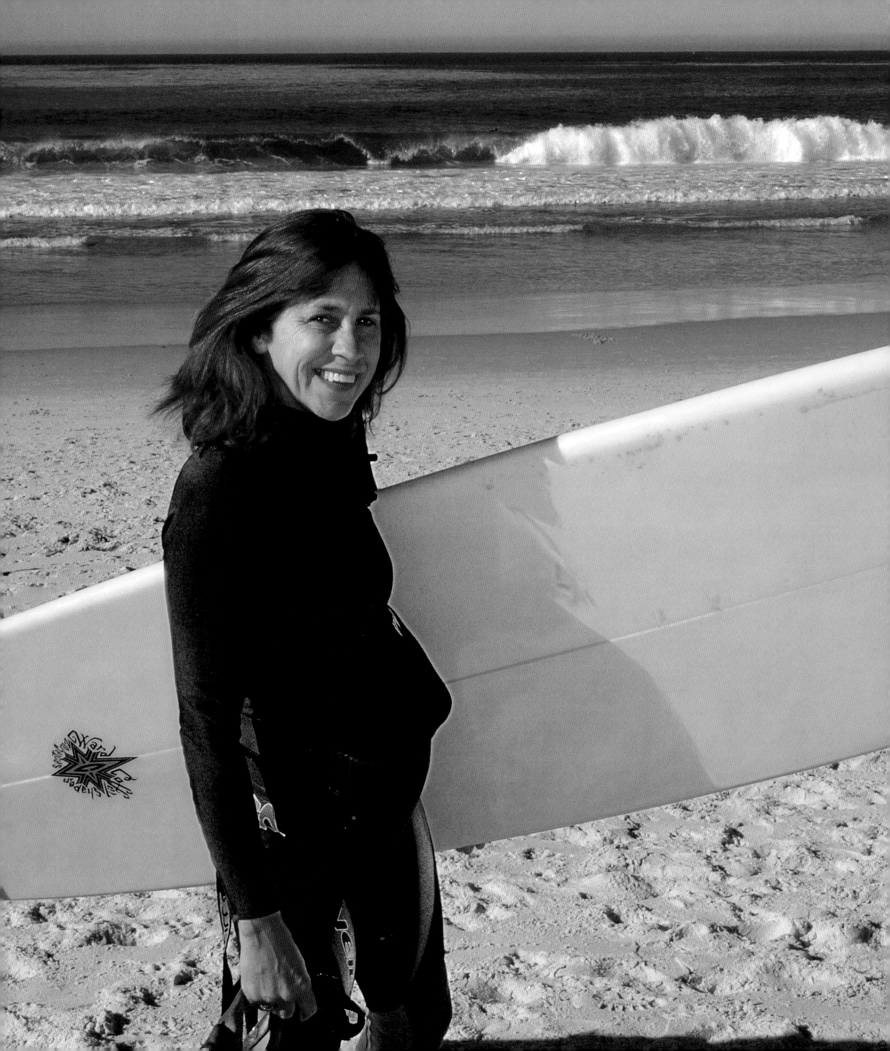

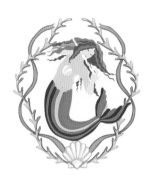

LAS OLAS SURF SAFARIS FOUNDER { Bev Sanders }

"Surfing gave me confidence I hadn't felt since
I was eleven. I started seeing things through a
sense of joy. Things don't have to be a task."

Carmel-by-the-Sea, California

Determinedly she paddles through the cobalt waters off Mexico's Pacific coast. A wave rises before her. Swinging around to face the beach, she waits to feel the surge. Standing, she balances on her flowered board, all thoughts falling away, and rides the water to shore. "There's a giggle that overcomes me. It's like a shudder, a physical rush. Some waves have actually brought tears to my eyes." When she strands on the sand, thought returns: "One more wave!" Bev Sanders calls the year she learned to surf, her forty-fourth, "the best year of my life." She was on vacation in Hawaii with her husband, Chris, when an advertisement in a phone book caught her eye. It featured a canine surfer and proclaimed, "If a dog can surf, you can too." She immediately signed up for lessons and re-experienced herself as a pre-teen. "Surfing gave me confidence I hadn't felt since I was eleven." It also reconnected her with a lightness of being she had forgotten. "I started seeing things through a sense of joy. Things don't have to be a task."

What had become a task was "going against the grain" for years to gain acceptance for women in snowboarding. Having grown up in Massachusetts, she later landed in Lake Tahoe intending to teach skiing. A skier since childhood, she was intrigued by a man drawing snowboards on a napkin. They talked, fell in love, married, and started their own company, Avalanche Snowboards. Frustrated by the glacial pace at which manufacturers and sponsors were responding to the needs and desires of women in the sport, she decided to walk away. Surfing had taught her to let go of the struggle: "I was a girl growing up between two brothers and then working in the male world of snowboarding. I had a lot of anger, but when I started surfing, I lost that anger. In surfing, you do not do well if you are trying too hard. You have to go with the flow."

To share her newfound outlook, she launched Las Olas Surf Safaris: "I set out to create something that is entirely women focused—of, by, and for women, bringing women into the sport and doing it on our own terms," she says. Those terms extend beyond surfboards with feminine appeal. They include a gentle introduction to the sport on beginner friendly waves. The women might arrive anxious, fearful, stressed, and weighed down by responsibilities, but starting each day of the safari with yoga, they begin to let go. After

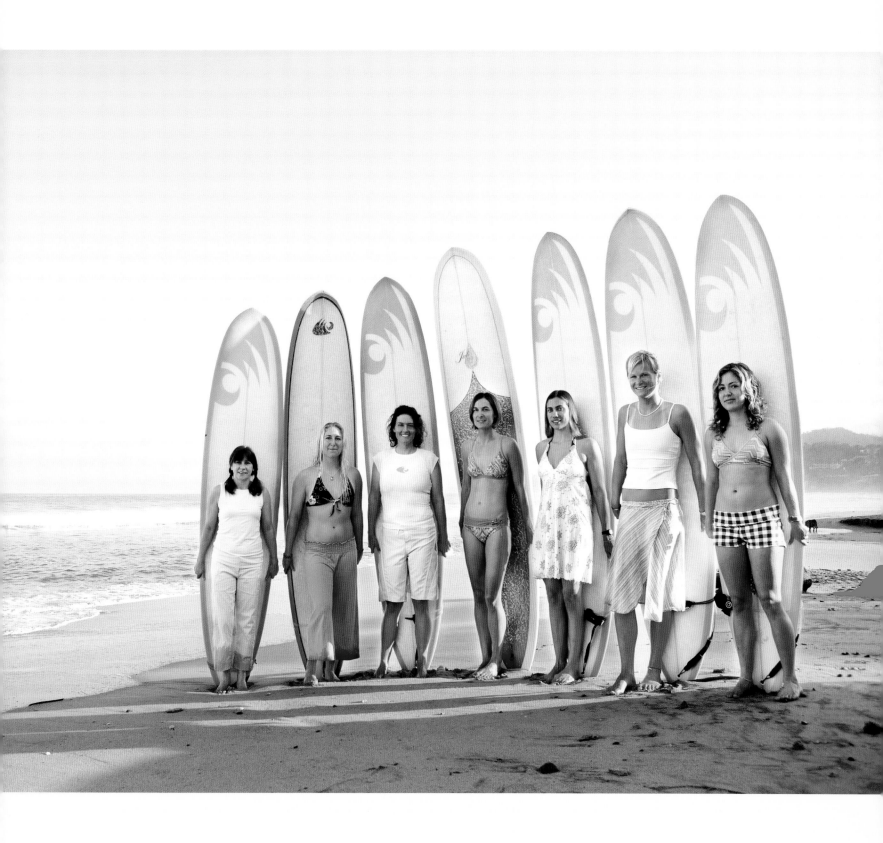

Women and the Sea

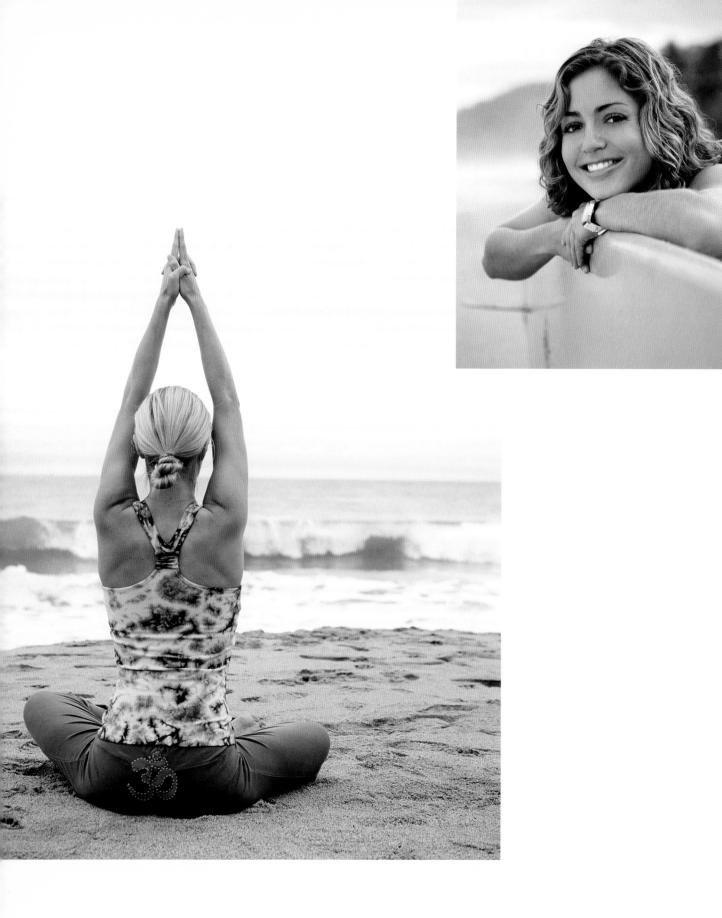

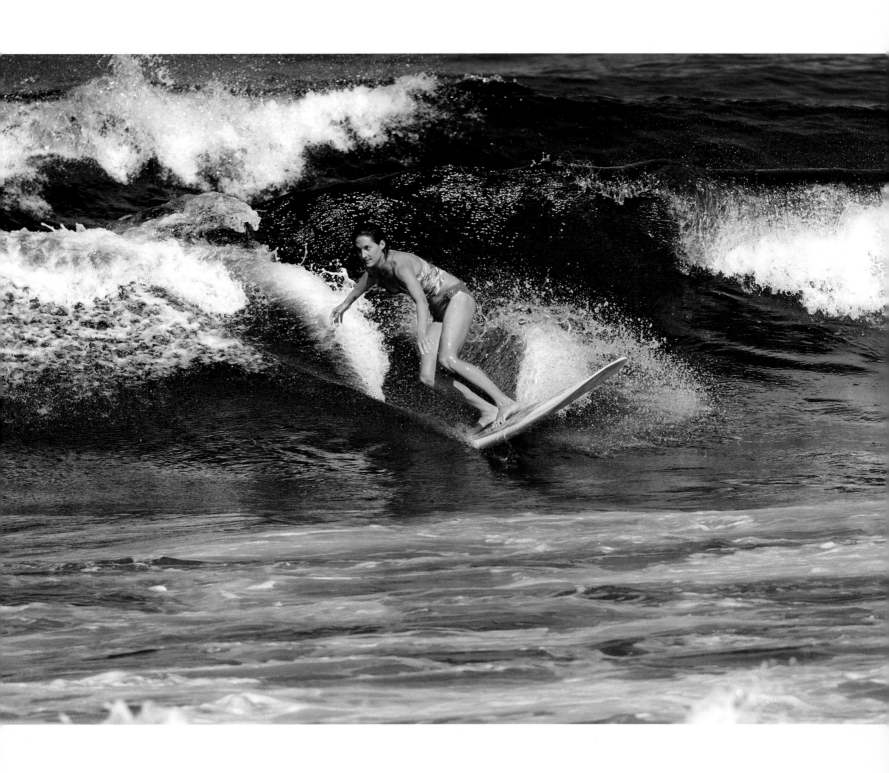

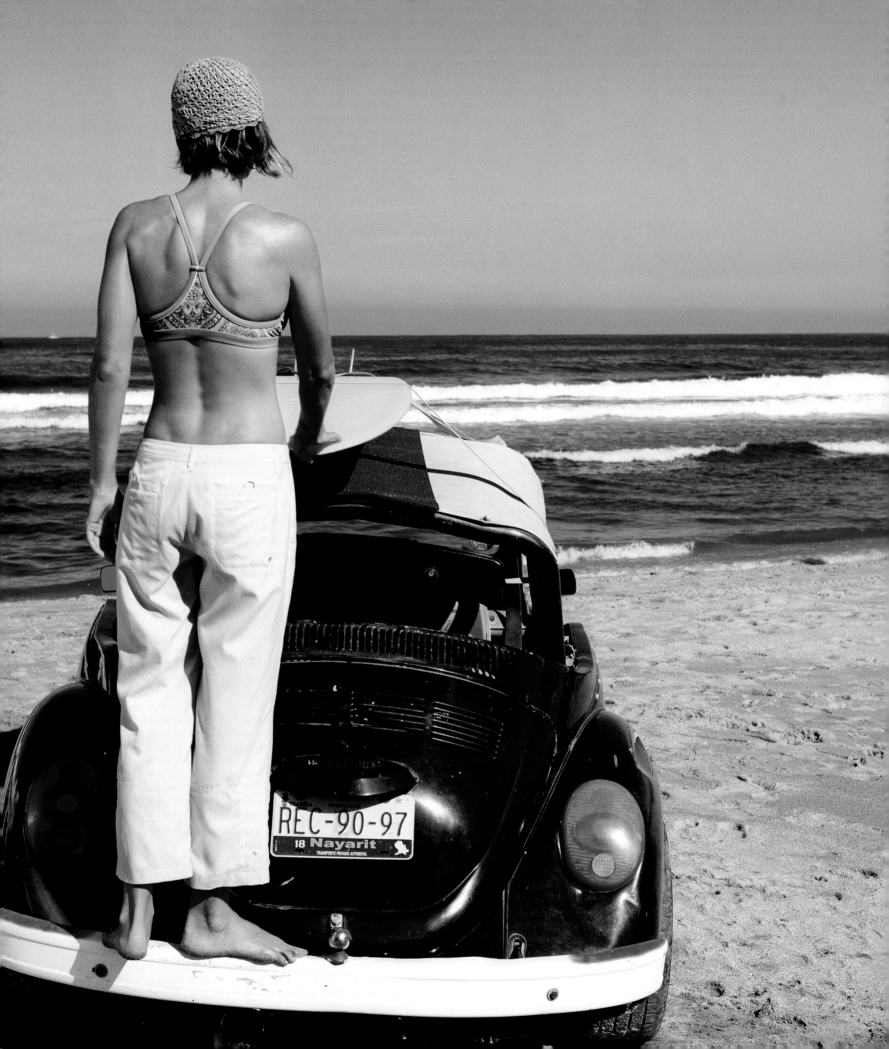

> "I must go down to the seas again,
> for the call of the running tide
>   Is a wild call and a clear call
> that may not be denied."

JOHN MASEFIELD

a tutorial under cover of a casita, the women paddle out on their stomachs, getting a feeling for their boards and for the waves. They might linger and chat for a bit. When they stand up and ride their first wave, Bev shares the excitement: "When I see people get their first wave, it brings back my first surfing experience." Over a dozen years, she has helped two thousand women experience the pure joy and natural empowerment that come from learning how to surf. Her company's motto is "We make girls out of women."

Bev's inner girl was initiated into the exhilaration of ocean play during frequent excursions to the New Hampshire coast. "I grew up inland, so when I was a kid, going to the ocean was a big treat. My father was the instigator. He put us in the car, and we'd go to Hampton Beach." Often the beach would be shrouded in fog, but no matter. Her father always assured the family it would burn off. "We would be so hopeful," Bev says, "and it would burn off. We felt like our family had the power to make the sun come out." Though she was at first intimidated by the thought of surfing, she has never been afraid of the ocean. "My dad was great at hurling me into the water. I would tumble all around. I really enjoyed it." At day's end, Bev says, "We'd all squeeze into one small hotel room." Sometimes her mother and her aunts would rent a cottage, with the fathers arriving to spend the weekend. "We didn't have much in the way of equipment, but that didn't matter."

Bev is once again traveling light. In exchanging snowboarding for surfing, her life has been freed up in more ways than one. "With snowboarding you have to have boots, boards, heavy clothes. Surfing is simple. Board and bare feet." In Carmel, California, Bev lives eight blocks from the ocean, though she can see it thanks to the elevation of her home. She walks the beach almost every day, and though occasionally the tide of her mind pulls her into deep water, she quickly resurfaces. "Once the ocean catches you, it is as if you are in a net. You can't get away. We have the exact percentage of salt in our blood that exists in the ocean. That's deep and probably worth lots of thought, but I would rather just play in the ocean. I prefer just to enjoy it." In that simple sentiment lies deep wisdom.

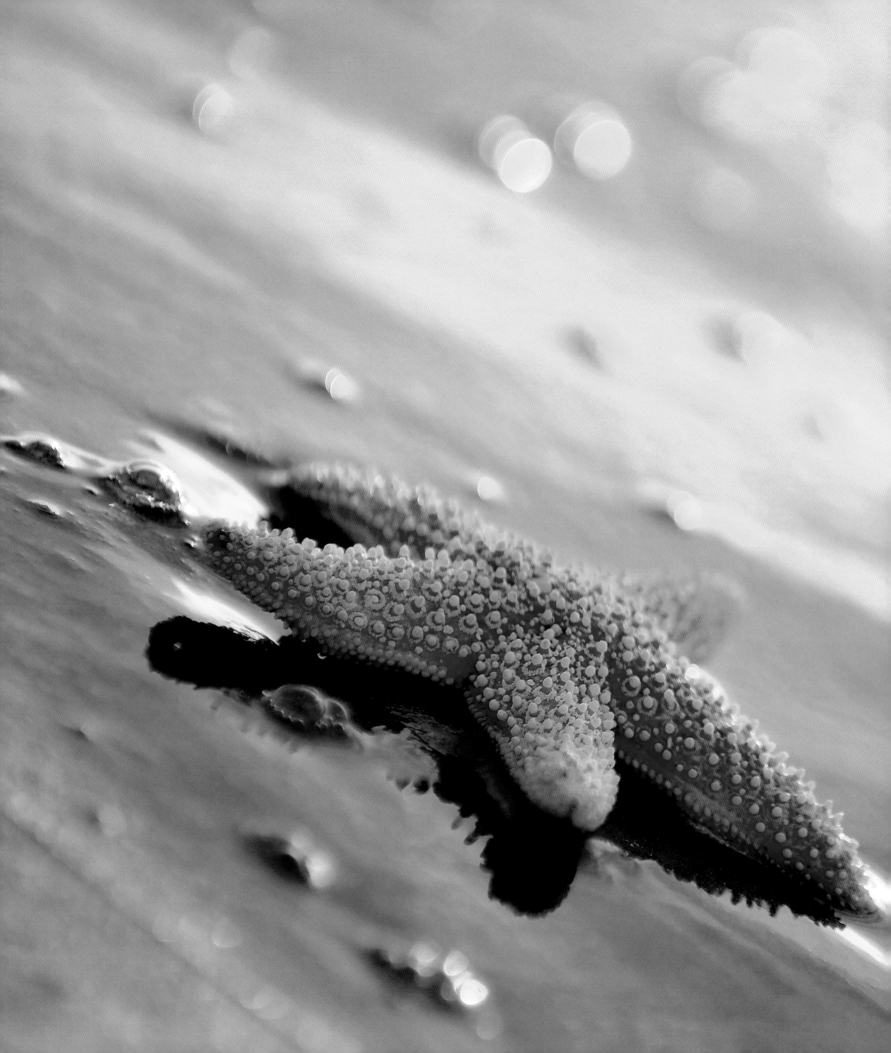

Gifts from the Sea

MARGARET CAVENDISH

The Sea-Goddess

My cabinets are oyster-shells,
In which I keep my orient pearls;
To open them I use the tide,
As keys to locks, which opens wide
The oyster shells, then out I take
Those orient pearls and crowns do make;
And modest coral I do wear,
Which blushes when it touches air.
On silver waves I sit and sing,
And then the fish lie listening:
Then sitting on a rocky stone
I comb my hair with fishes' bone;
The whilst Apollo with his beams
Doth dry my hair from watery streams.
His light doth glaze the water's face,
Make the large sea my looking-glass:
So when I swim on waters high,
I see myself as I glide by:
But when the sun begins to burn,
I back into my waters turn,
And dive unto the bottom low:
Then on my head the waters flow
In curled waves and circles round,
And thus with waters am I crowned.

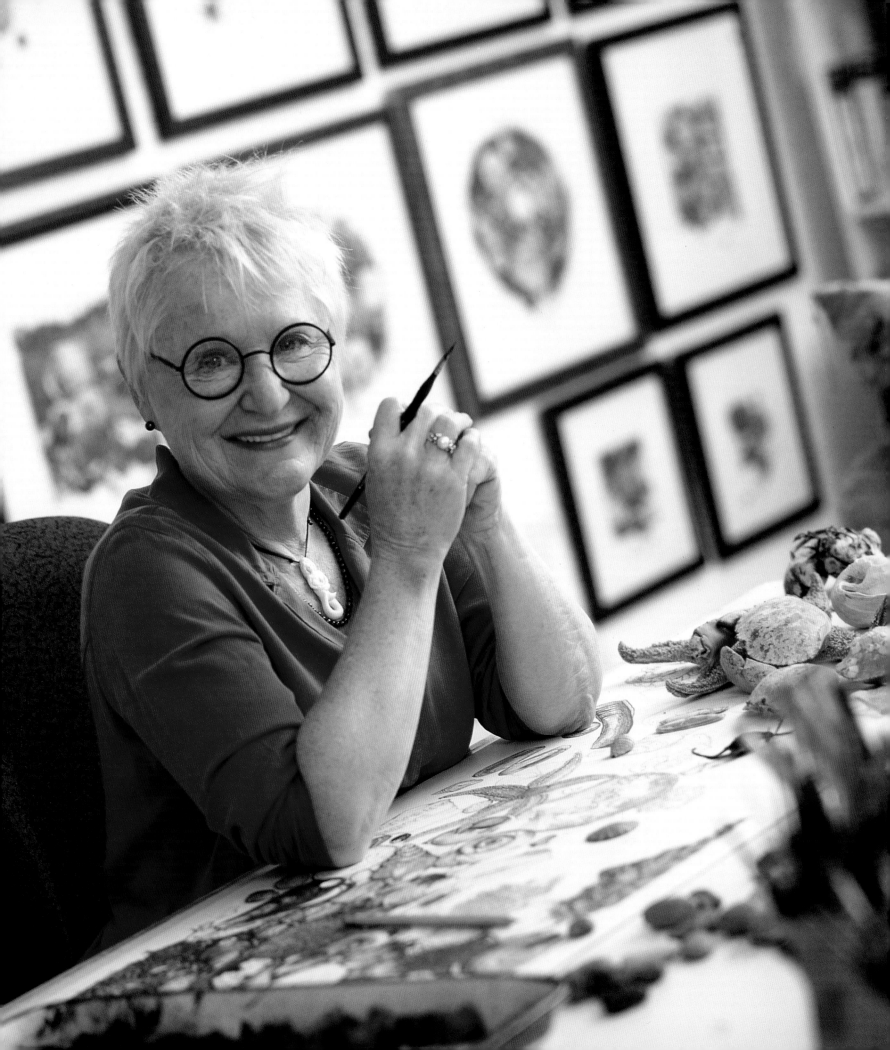

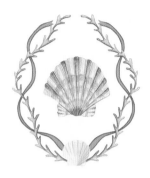

ARTIST { Mimi Gregoire Carpenter }

"Broken shells are beautiful because

you can see inside of them more; they have

more character. Tropical shells are too pretty.

I am a New England shells girl."

Biddeford, Maine

Nothing is too lowly for her notice, not the knobby seaweed, not the humble razor clam, not the ubiquitous barnacle, not the broken horseshoe crab carapace. She singles them out, and through her eyes, they reveal their poetry. Painting them as portraits, as species studies, as Bachian pieces of point and counterpoint, Mimi Gregoire Carpenter spotlights that which is often overlooked—discovered hiding in rock piles, stranded by the tide, and tangled in flotsam. She even waxes enthusiastic about little green crabs: "Even though all of the crabs are essentially the same, no two are alike. They have different, amazing patterns of yellow speckles." The "pretty" does have a place in her watercolor paintings, the blanched sand dollars, the twirled whelks, the glittering shards of beach glass, the graceful starfish, but she is just as likely to include skeleton bits and broken shells. The latter, in fact, are some of her favorites: "Broken shells are beautiful because you can see inside of them more; they have more character. They might even have little bites taken out of them. I want a shell with a little barnacle. Tropical shells are too pretty; I am a New England shells girl."

For Mimi, every walk along her favorite Goose Rocks Beach in Maine is a treasure hunt. Sometimes seagulls come to her aid, like the time she had been scouring the shore looking for urchins. A baby gull had found one but was struggling to figure out how to eat it. "The mother wouldn't eat it because she was trying to teach the other one how to crack it open. I waited and waited because I really wanted that urchin." Her patience paid off when the gull left the spiky creature behind to become a subject in one of her paintings. Sometimes a storm's surge leaves unusual characters for her work; sometimes it's low tide, depositing baseball-sized moon shells, which she scoops up before they roll like eggs back into the water. Sometimes it's mermaids. "Little mermaids drop their fairy wings," Mimi says, referring playfully to the thin, shimmery tagelus shells, believed to be left behind by mermaids and their mermen as they return to sea to become full merpeople.

Though she can sketch and then paint her beach finds from memory, Mimi takes them home and sets them out on the table in her studio, where seaweed dries on the walls and moon shells line the railing. "When

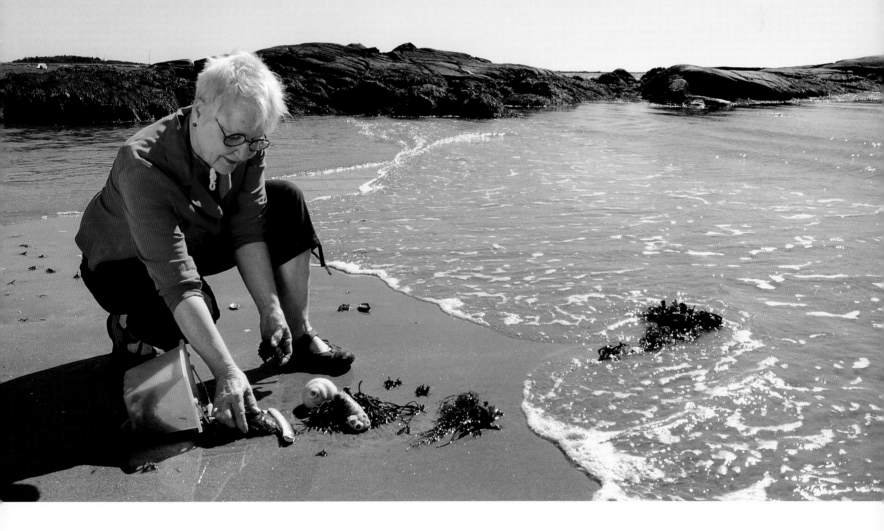

"Every time we walk along the beach
some ancient urge disturbs us so that we
find ourselves shedding shoes and garments
or scavenging among seaweed and whitened timbers
like the homesick refugees of a long war."

LOREN EISELEY

Women and the Sea

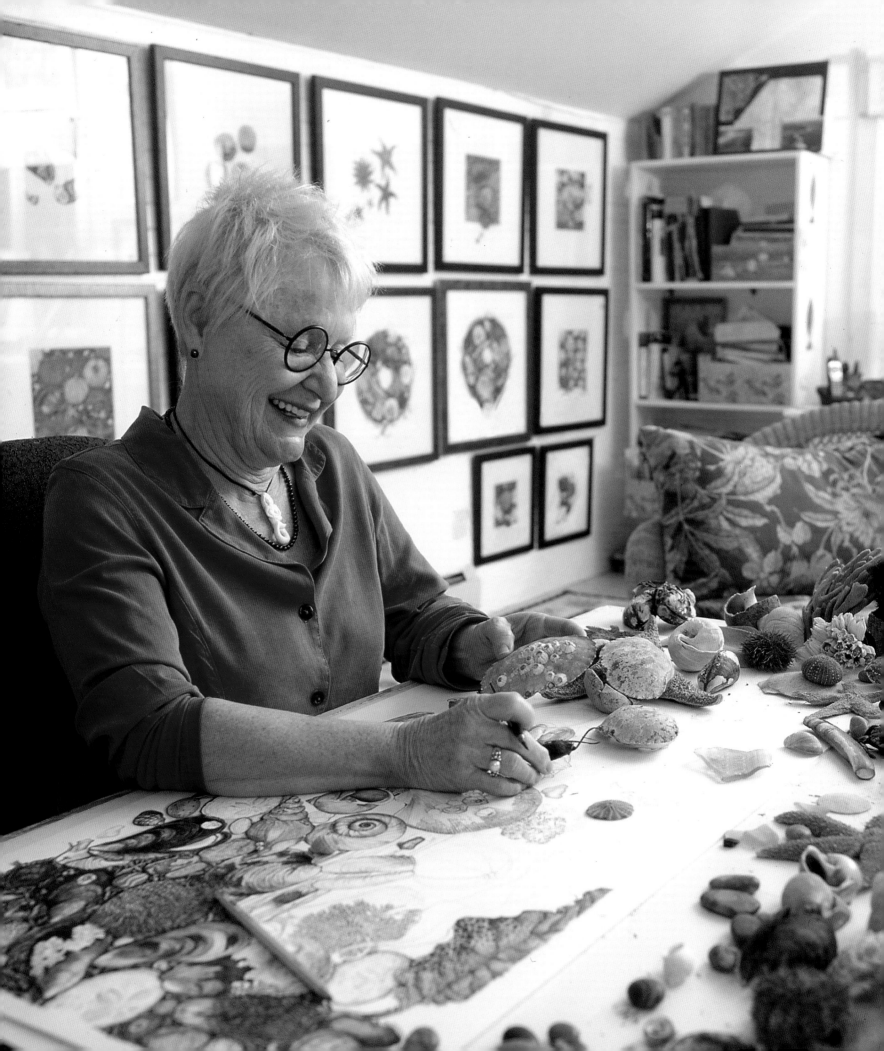

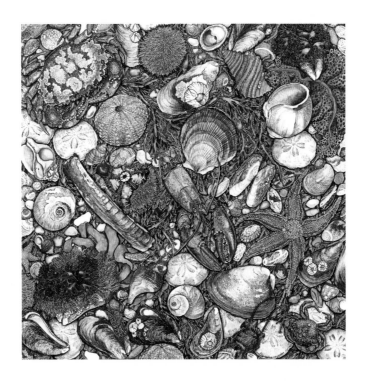

I look at them, I see their personalities. I set them up like a stage, and they're actors. Each shell has a role to play. Then the backdrop is seaweed and pebbles." Some may even become characters in the children's books she writes. If there is a childlike quality to her viewpoint, it is not surprising. Mimi fell in love with Maine's beaches as a youngster. Though she grew up and eventually went to college and worked in central Maine, family visits to the shore, especially Pemaquid, had left a deep impression. "All of the good things in my life came from Pemaquid," she says. "I have always identified happy times with water and the beach."

Mimi's life-long love affair with the Maine coast was sealed when she and her husband took a trip to Islesboro, off the coast of Camden, in the early 1970s. There she collected piles of pebbles, "precious things," better than diamonds and emeralds, she thought. She brought them back to the inland town of Oakland where she, having graduated from the University of Maine, Gorham, taught art and her husband taught English. Landlocked, the couple surrounded their plants and pool with beach pebbles and even brought in large rocks to create a cliff-like setting, all in an effort to "pretend we lived by the beach," says Mimi.

At the time, she was busy painting flowers, but her scrutiny of them proved fatal. She realized, she says, "that I was really looking for an excuse to paint their pots and the pebbles I put in them. I really wanted to paint the pebbles. Then I started adding shells, and I realized how many amazing things I had collected. I couldn't stop." She calls her original collection of beach stones her "lucky pebbles," and,

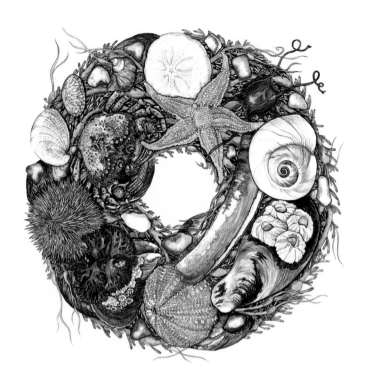

grateful for their inspiration, she keeps them safe in a "treasure chest," saying, "If there were a fire in my house, I would grab the chest first."

She so carefully depicts her subjects that scientists and marine biologists love to scrutinize her work at shows. One even tried to stump her, searching for a sea creature found on the Maine coast that she had yet to paint. After she had answered in the affirmative to several possibilities, he finally said, "I know what you don't have." As part of his work, he studied a type of worm with small tentacles. In truth, she had never seen one and traveled to his lab to be introduced. It wasn't long before she encountered one on her own. She was depicting two mussels she had just brought home: "I am painting away, and ooze comes out of the mussels, and then out of the Irish moss jumps this worm!"

The sea never ceases to surprise her with its offspring, and she wants to paint it all. She has to pry the brushes from her hands now and then just to go and lie on the beach: "Every single one of your senses is touched. The ocean smells different from any other place. Then there are the words, the rote sound of the waves, the rippling. It evens you out and calms you down. When it's foggy, the gray wraps right around you." Mimi knows scientists attribute the sea's mood-elevating effects to the ions it gives off, but for her, it is that and so much more. "For me, the ocean is the closest thing to what heaven will be like. It's the closest thing to paradise."

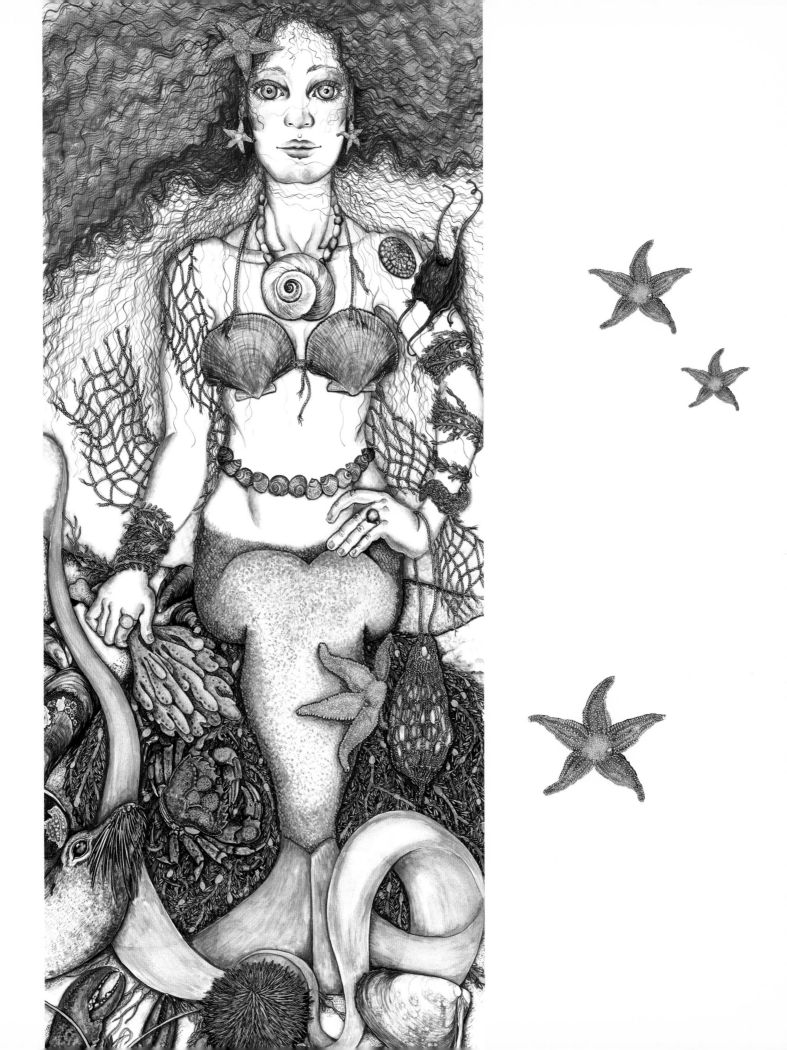

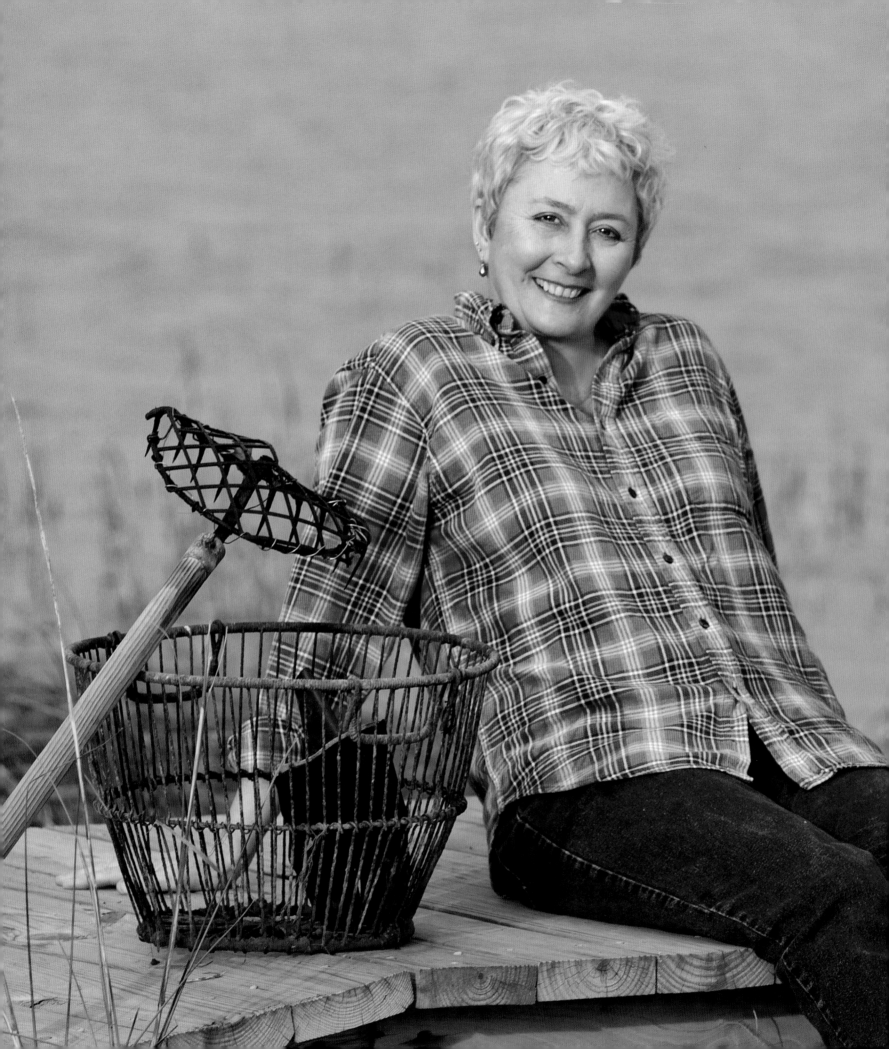

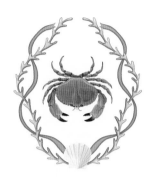

BLUE CRAB BAY CO. FOUNDER { Pamela Barefoot }

"When I close my eyes and think of the

expansive water of the Chesapeake or the ocean,

I feel freedom, a relaxing deep breath.

It is peaceful, unifying, cleansing, and ever changing."

Chesapeake Bay, Virginia

She is frequently found on the waters of the Chesapeake, the bay that inspired her Blue Crab Bay Company. She motors to barrier island beaches, picking up shells to use as adornments for the packages holding her specialty food and gift products. She paddles her kayak, dreamily watching jets draw trails, eagles and osprey glide and nosedive, heron stalk, and schools of dolphin swim. Most of all, Pamela Barefoot loves to fish the Bay. "Fishing takes my mind off everything in the world. And you never know what you'll find in the Bay—striped bass, sea trout, bluefish, flounder, croaker, spot…" Though she grew up inland, she inherited this fondness for saltwater fishing from her feisty grandmother. "She would go to the fishing piers on the coast of North Carolina. She dipped snuff, fished with bloodworms, caught spot, and wore a bonnet in public." When they were not fishing in local ponds, Pamela and her mother would trek to the coast to join her. When it came time for marrying, she chose a man who shared her passion. "My husband loved to fish, and we love to fish together. I think that still keeps us connected."

Pamela lives on a small peninsula on Virginia's eastern coast, spends her days developing and marketing products like Dune Buggies (sea salted almonds), She Crab Soup, Shore Seasonings, and Inner Ocean seaweed soaps, and spends her spare time crabbing and fishing. When she takes a vacation, she simply heads to another shore. She and her husband have fished from Deer Isle, Maine, to Playa Zancudo, Costa Rica, and have salmon fished in Alaska and sought out brown trout in Chile. They spent their twenty-fifth wedding anniversary on Elba Island, Italy, infamous as the place of Napoleon's exile, but full of small fishing villages, perfect for this celebrating couple.

It is no wonder that Pamela was not content to remain in landlocked Richmond, Virginia, where, after majoring in Psychology at Virginia Commonwealth University, she was doing public relations and taking photos for the Flowerdew Hundred Plantation archaeology project. When she and her husband moved, she scanned the coast seeking inspiration for her own business. "I had always dreamed that I was going to do my own thing." Though not a cook, she did have one specialty: clam dip. Noticing that there were few

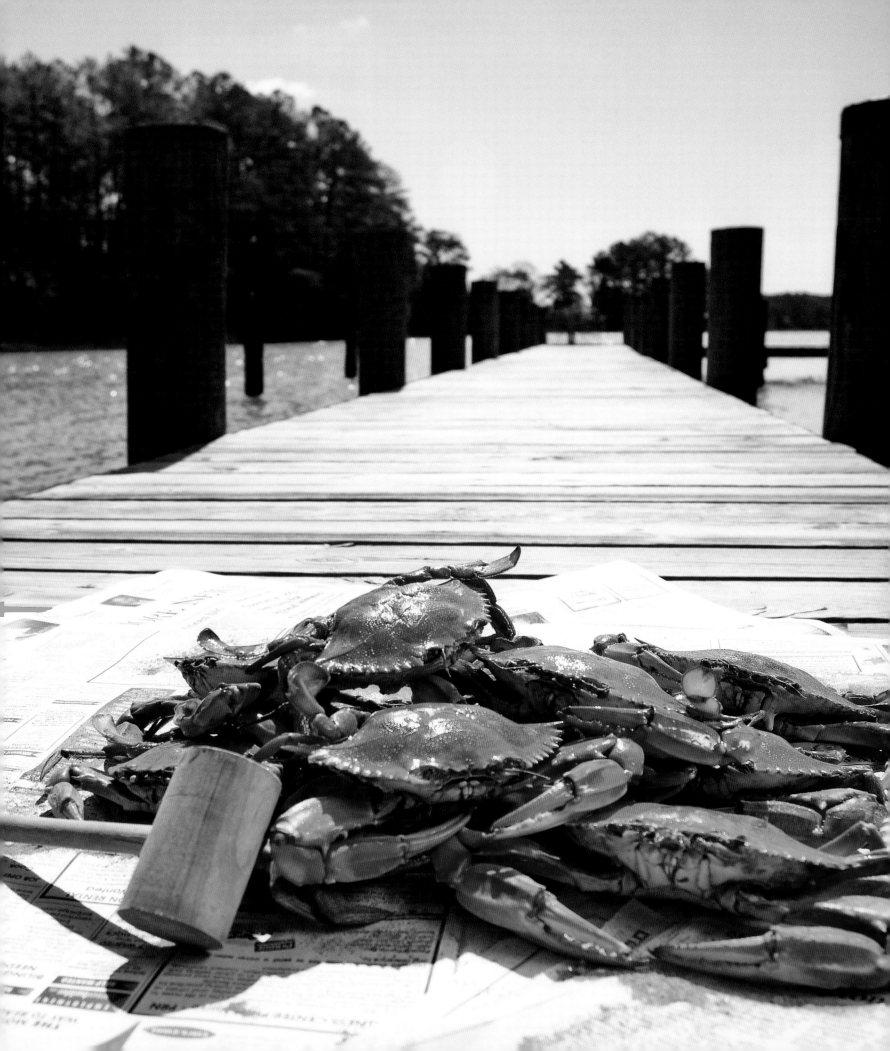

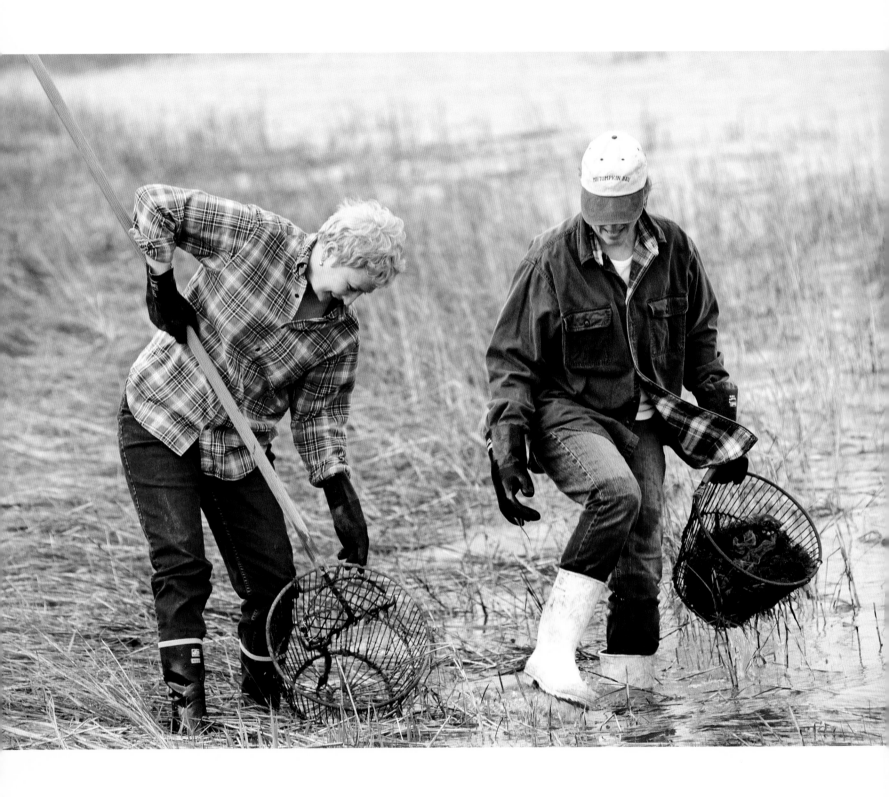

Women and the Sea
124

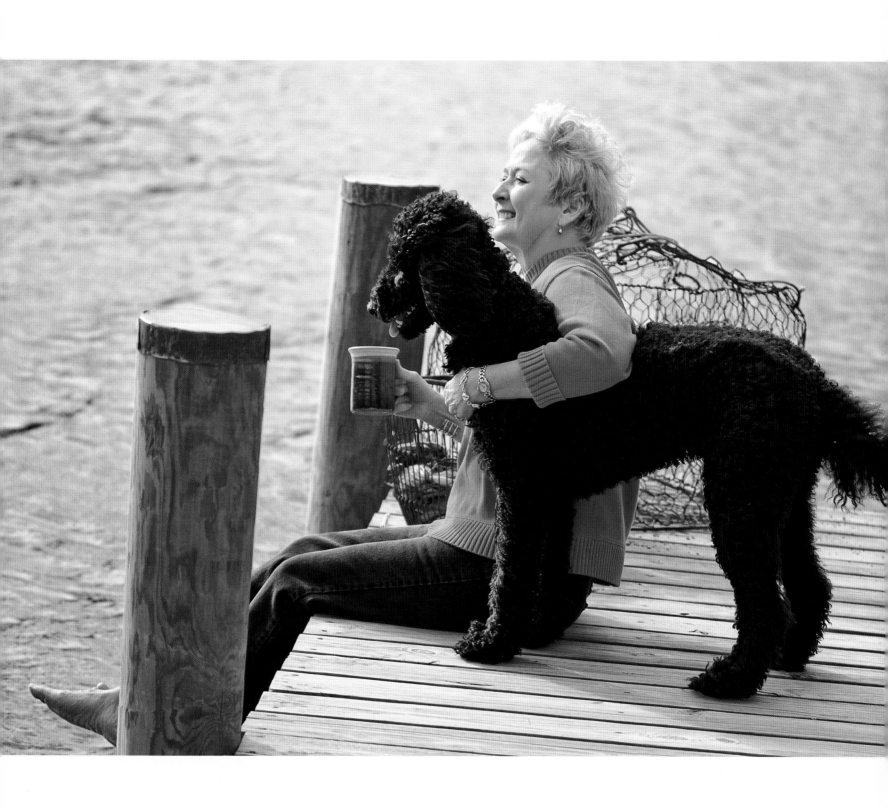

> "Those who live by the sea can
> hardly form a single thought of which
> the sea would not be part."
>
> HERMANN BROCH

regional food and gift basket businesses in the Chesapeake Bay area and not one seasoning packet for clam dip on supermarket shelves, she knew she had found her niche.

When the stress of running a successful business weighs her down, Pamela heads to her dock, and with a dog on each side acting as a spotter, she tosses out a baited line, catches some crabs, steams them right then and there, and with iPod speakers set up outside, she and her husband sit and take stock of the abundance surrounding them. "When I close my eyes and think of the expansive water of the Chesapeake or the ocean, I feel freedom, a relaxing deep breath. It is peaceful, unifying, cleansing, and ever changing. Water connects us to other continents, other islands, other people."

Life on the water has also taught her lessons, like perseverance. When fishing with her husband aboard their motorboat one summer day was yielding them nothing, Pamela told her husband that she was going to take her kayak out and bring home some fish. He said, "Good luck." A backpack filled with ice and squid bait spoke of her optimism, while the thermos of wine revealed a bit of relaxed resignation. Her cell phone hanging on a string around her neck, she called a friend to keep her company. "I went around the cove to a larger inlet, and within five minutes, I caught a three-pound croaker. It was pulling my kayak along." She caught it, tossed it in her backpack, and cast her line again. "I caught another big fish and told my friend, 'I have to go.'" Then she phoned her husband, "Jim, get your fillet knife and meet me at the dock."

Whether she is helping Jim gather seaweed for soaps, selling her products to stores across the world, or testing a new recipe to highlight the flavor of Gulf shrimp or Chesapeake Bay crabs, Pamela is intimately connected to the water. "Water is a living thing. It can be a companion. A friend of mine moved from a secluded Bayside home into our local town as she was lonely. She had divorced years earlier, and her children had grown up and moved away. I visited her in the new home in town where she was surrounded by people, and she said, 'I miss the water. I'm lonelier here than I was in my home by the water alone.' I think I would feel the same. I don't intend to live anywhere else except by the water."

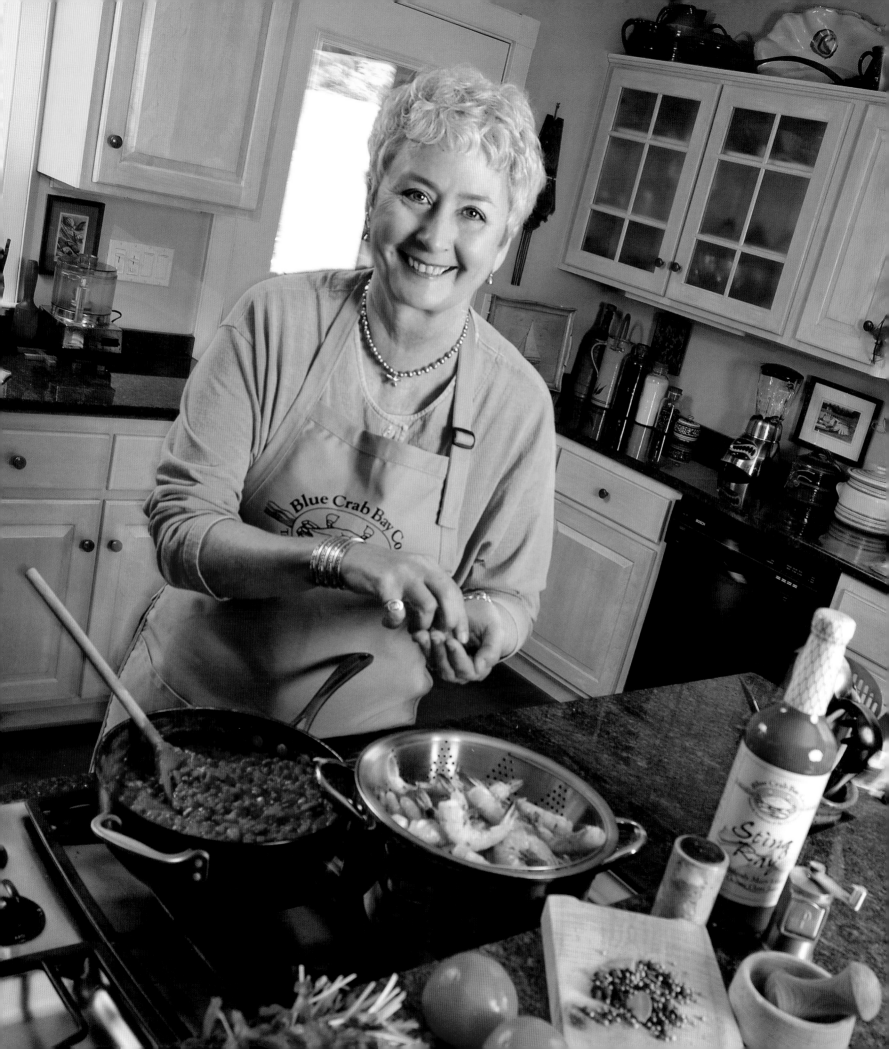

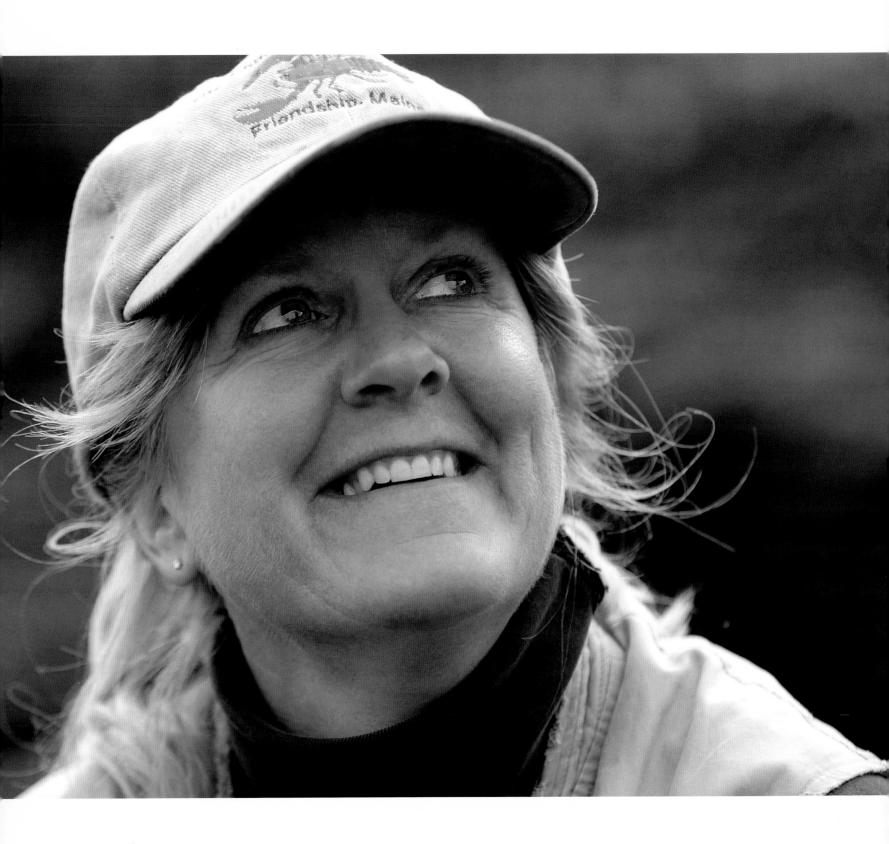

Women and the Sea

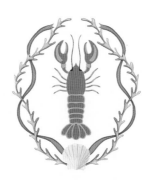

THE LOBSTER CONSERVANCY FOUNDER { Diane Cowan }

"People ask me how I can keep doing what I am doing. It's because **I never know** what I am going to find at low tide. One time I lifted a rock and there were twelve lobsters underneath it."

Friendship Long Island, Maine

It is an hour before low tide. The full moon is rising over Friendship Long Island, Maine. The night is crisp, clear, quiet. Diane Cowan, carrying forty pounds of gear, treks the three-quarters of a mile to her workplace, the intertidal mudflats of a cove. Her headlamp shining, her feet kept dry by rubber boots, her microcassette in hand, she gets to work. She notes the details of the weather, listens for owls, loons, and raccoons, measures the salinity of the water, and within a grid of squares, she overturns rocks. Finding baby lobsters that fit on the tip of a finger, she carries them over to her "favorite rock," now cushioned to soften the impact of years of sitting on hard surfaces. She scans the tiny creature for a tag, and if there is none, she takes one, smaller than a grain of rice, from a vial and attaches it using a hypodermic needle. She measures the bug-like crustacean and returns it to its nursery.

Diane Cowan, a marine biologist and founder of The Lobster Conservancy, has been performing these tasks tirelessly and training others to do the same for seventeen years. Chasing low tides, she has missed out on Christmas, New Years, and birthday celebrations. For her sacrifices, she is rewarded with spectacular sunrises and sunsets, occasional meteor showers, and the knowledge that the data she collects will help to keep lobster habitats safe and fisheries sustainable.

She also has gotten to know the sea intimately. "My favorite connection to the sea isn't the way she looks; it's the way she smells and how her scent changes with the seasons. I think I would know the time of the year on my island if you just gave me a whiff, or if you put me in a boat, and I could feel the way the boat moved through the water—that changes with the seasons too."

Over the years, she has gotten to know lobsters intimately as well. Once used as bait and fertilizer and considered junk food, lobsters are seen as solitary, cannibalistic scavengers, a reputation Diane wants to dispel. In winter, when she dives down to the six-acre lobster pound set up on the twenty-two-acre property donated to The Lobster Conservancy, she has found the shelters she created "crammed with males piled on top of each other in some male bonding ritual. They block off the entrance with rock and gravel."

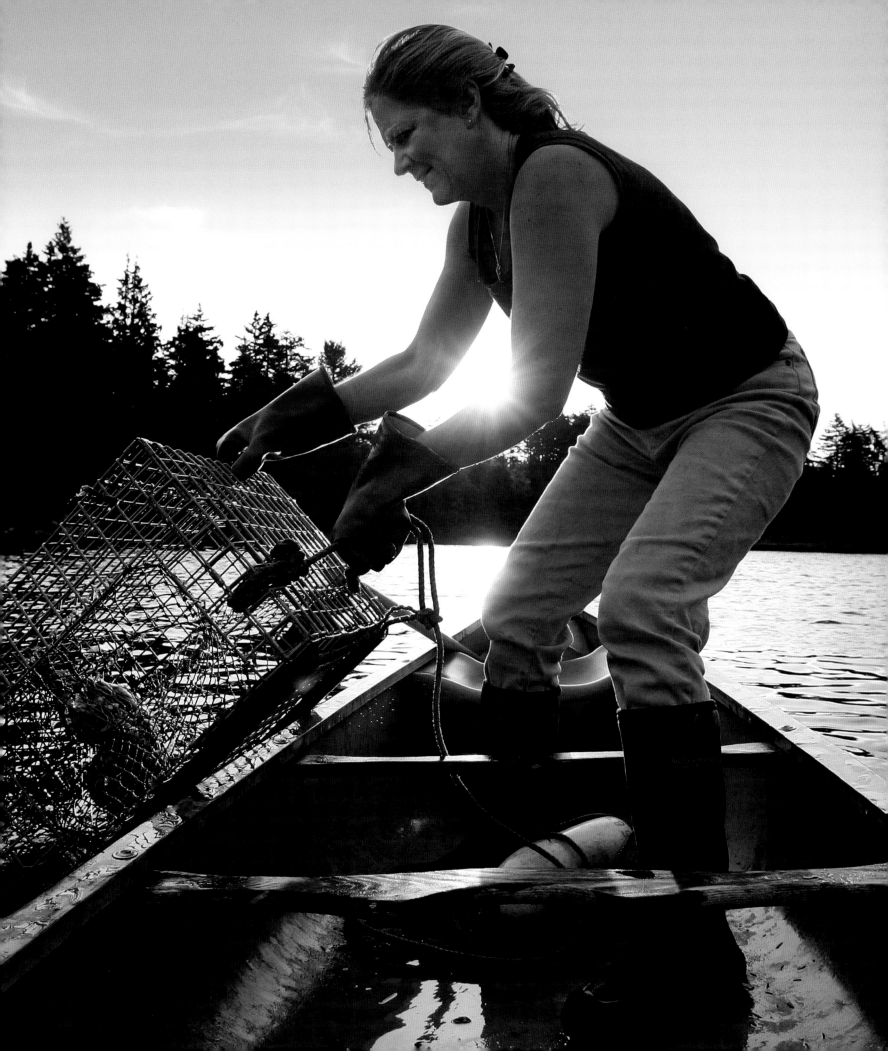

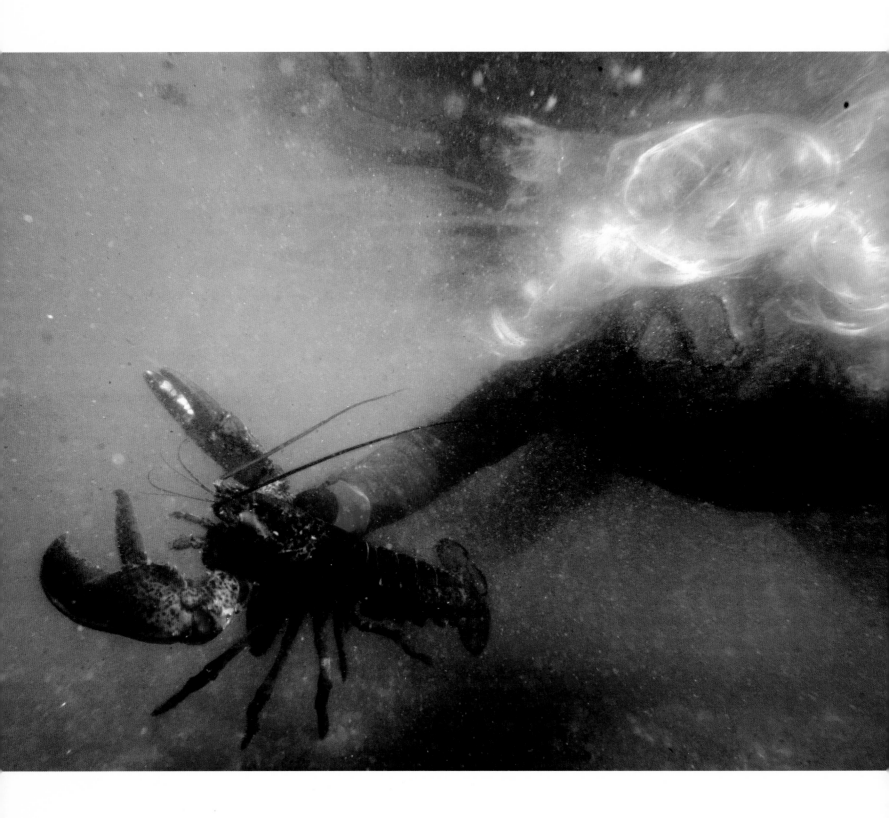

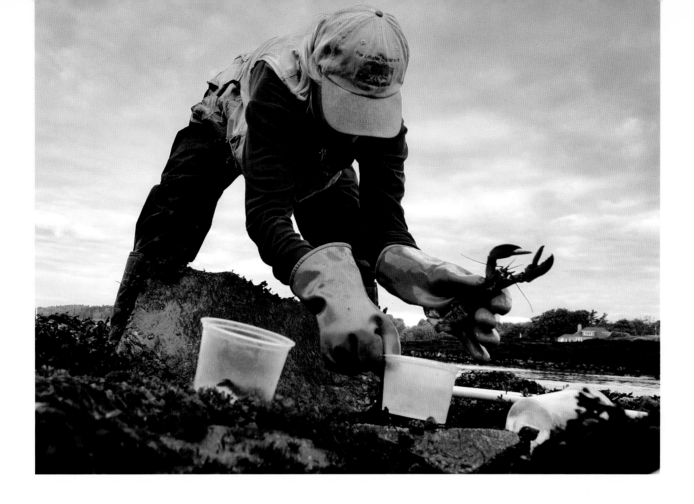

Come spring when a male's fancy turns to finding a mate, however, she says, "One male will occupy many shelters and won't let anyone near." While much of her research focuses on determining where juveniles live and how they grow, her organization's mission is to understand and disseminate knowledge of the entire lobster life cycle. "My life is so wrapped up in lobsters. I appreciate all aspects of them, and I do like to dispel the myths about them."

Diane knew from an early age that she would someday work as a marine biologist; she just did not know that her life would revolve around finding lobsters at low tide. Originally from the Midwest, she spent summers on a lake in nearby Lansing, Michigan, and it was there, she says, "I got my love of water. I played around in boats and with crayfish and water snakes."

An article in *National Geographic* turned her on to lobsters, which she immediately thought were "exotic, cool." When she filled in for a Bates College professor after earning her Ph.D. and scouted around for a research project for her undergraduate students, she "happened upon" one involving lobsters on Orrs Island, Maine. She and her students started amassing data, and "When that teaching gig was up," Diane says, "I didn't want to give up the project."

She moved to Harpswell and learned to time her life around low tides. "I couldn't have a nine to five job. Tides happen when they want to." She substitute taught, and then seeking even more flexibility, she

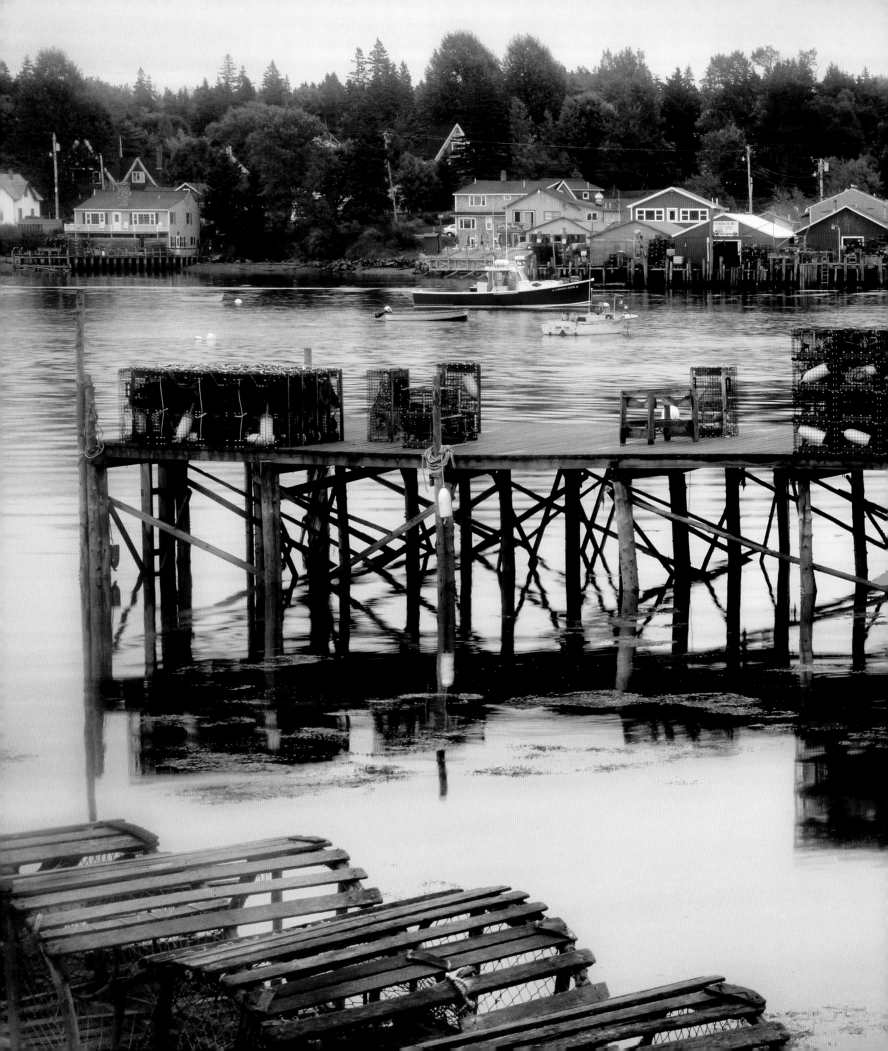

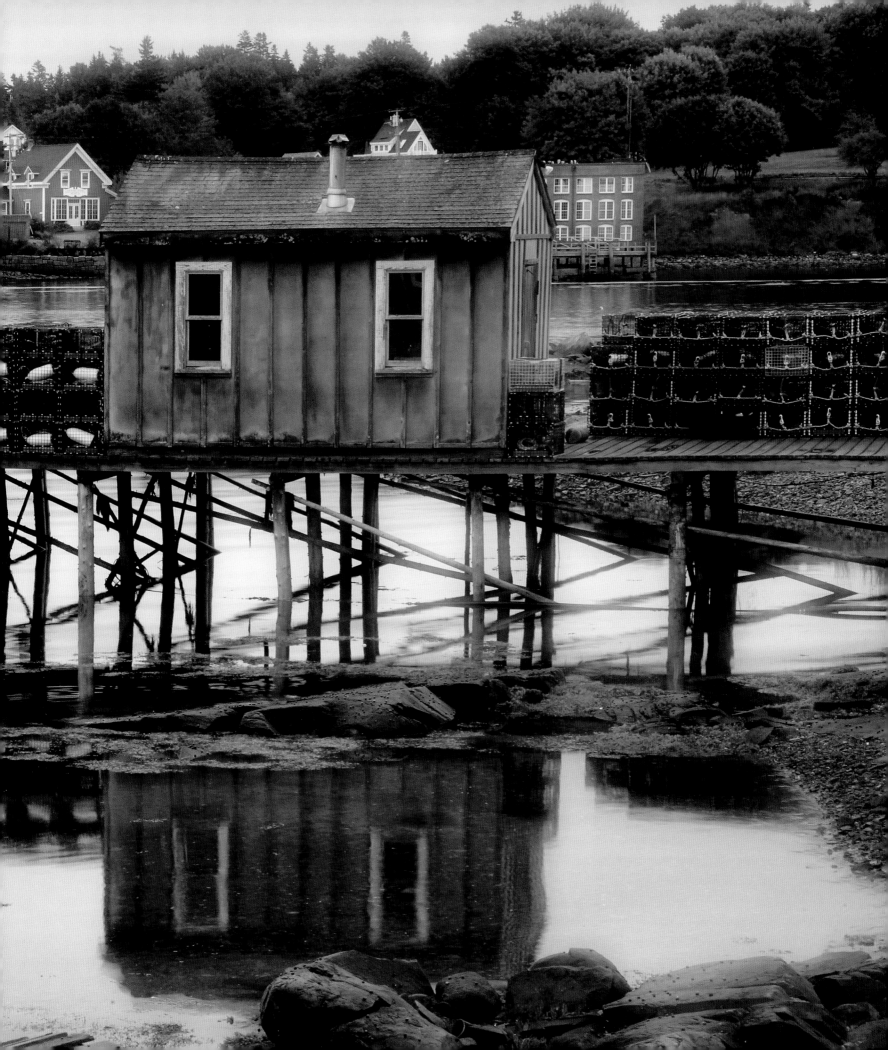

"I feel we are all islands in a common sea."

ANNE MORROW LINDBERGH

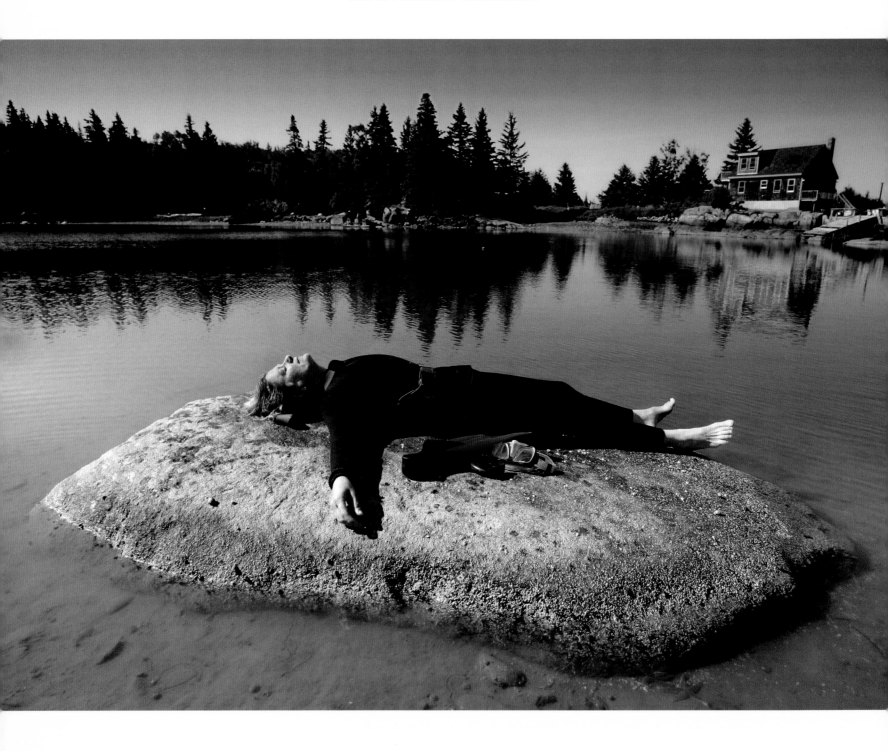

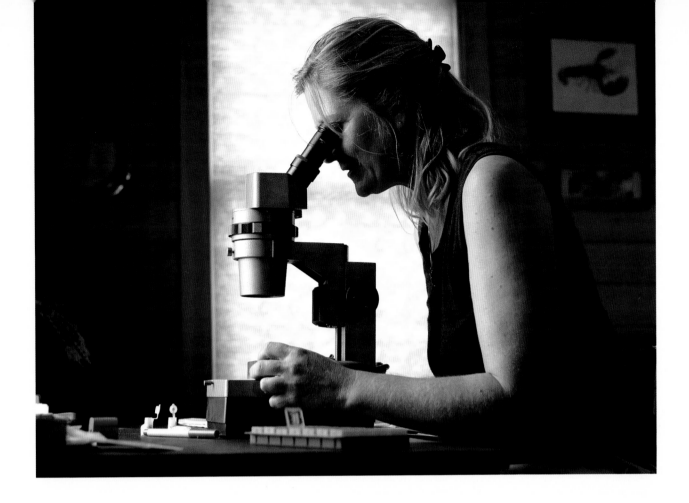

became a waitress at Cook's Lobster House. There she became acquainted with the other end of the lobster cycle. "Lobster men landed their catch at Cook's Lobster House. I had been in academics and research, but waitressing gave me insight into the industry and into the community." She got involved with the Harpswell Conservation Commission, and one thing leading to another, she established The Lobster Conservancy in 1996. In addition to working with students, Diane works with over a hundred volunteers to map and census lobster habitat, sharing the information with the scientific community and through school outreach programs.

When she is not recording or analyzing data, Diane spends her time writing about nature, including her current project about swamps, which she calls "the soul-cleansing tears of the world." She so loves writing that she considered going to the famed Iowa Writer's Workshop, but she says, "I used to be okay inland, and I considered going to Iowa, but I don't think I could live away from the shore now." Residing on a three-mile-long island in a home heated by a wood stove, using solar electricity, and having running water only six months out of the year, she has become quite self-reliant and strong, like the ocean she lives beside: "The mighty ocean awes me forever. She is full of strength, fury, quiet, calm, ever changing, ever present, and seemingly invincible—mostly she is beautiful and awesome. I feel small and insignificant in the face of the ocean, but I also feel free and at peace in her presence."

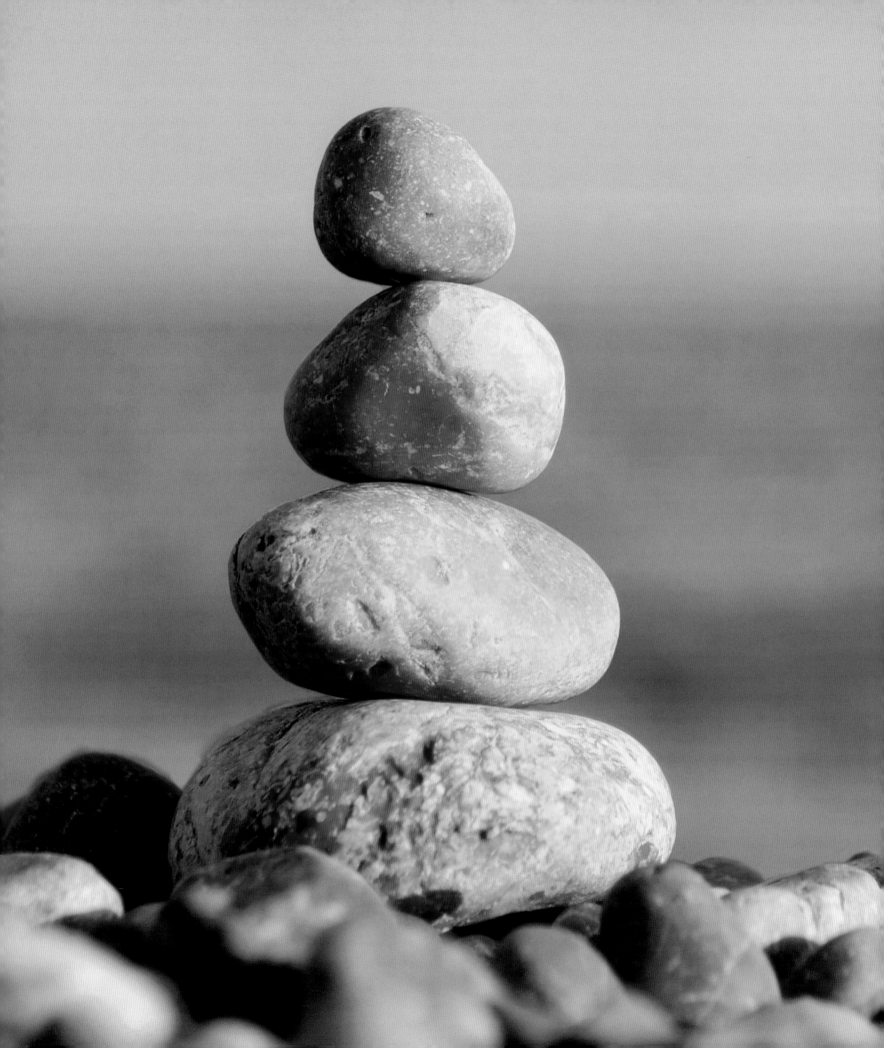

By the Sea

CHRISTINA GEORGINA ROSSETTI

By the Sea

Why does the sea moan evermore?
Shut out from heaven it makes its moan,
It frets against the boundary shore;
All earth's full rivers cannot fill
The sea, that drinking thirsteth still.

Sheer miracles of loveliness
Lie hid in its unlooked-on bed:
Anemones, salt, passionless,
Blow flower-like; just enough alive
To blow and multiply and thrive.

Shells quaint with curve, or spot, or spike,
Encrusted live things argus-eyed,
All fair alike, yet all unlike,
Are born without a pang, and die
Without a pang, and so pass by.

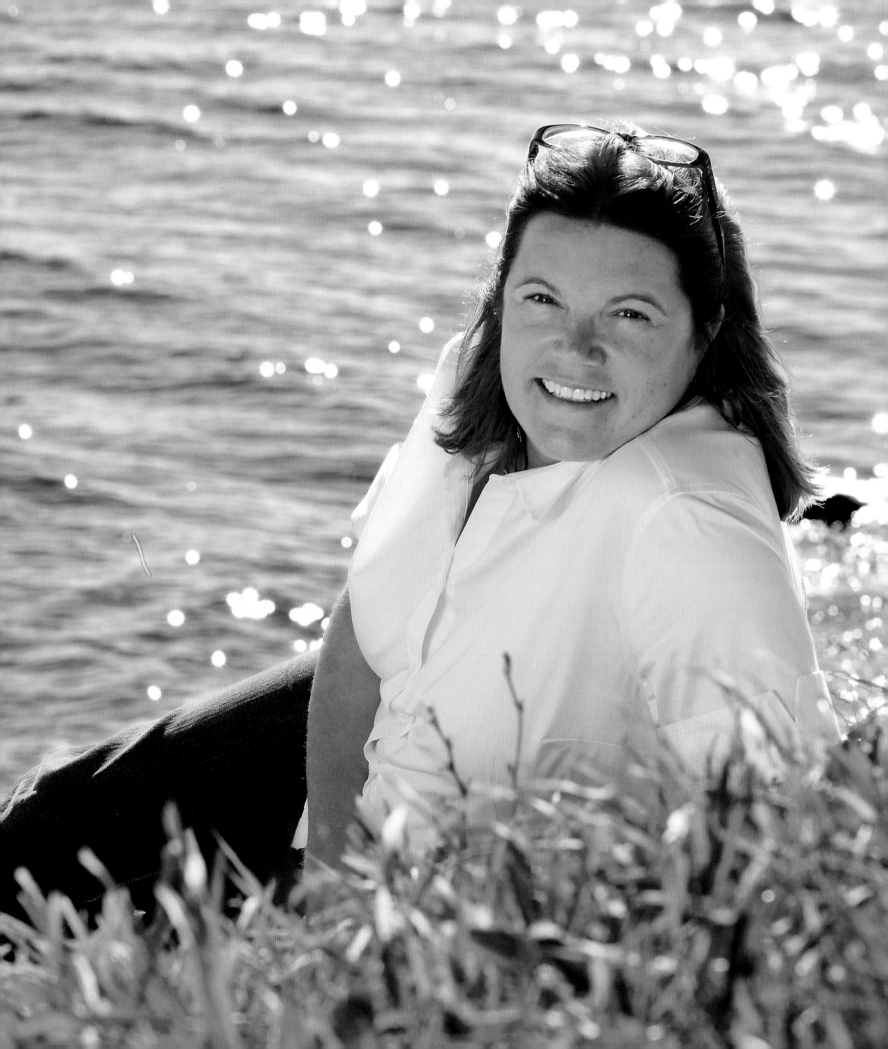

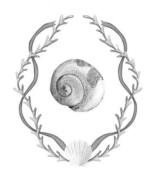

JEWELRY WEAVER { Genevieve Hunt }

"Our family spent two weeks every summer in Maryland—
a magical time that left an imprint.

Now, I comb local beaches at least once

a day if possible for new sources of inspiration."

New Bedford, Massachusetts

For the waters of Buzzards Bay in the spring before the seaweed sprouts, there is apatite. Iolite or pale blue quartz makes a fine sky at noon on a sunny July day. Ochre and dove gray freshwater pearls capture quite nicely variegated grains of beach sand. Genevieve Hunt will weave, crochet, and knit these gems into cuffs, necklaces, and pendants that evoke scenes imprinted in her mind, scenes absorbed during her daily two- to three-hour walks along the beaches near her Southeastern Massachusetts home. She'll watch the clouds accumulating as they prepare to break into storm. She'll note the swirls in the sand, carved by beach grass blades. She'll catch the changes in the water's color as the sun's angle shifts. A collector, she scans for shells, stones, and glass. Already adept at weaving and knitting her beads with silver wire, she is now teaching herself "knotless netting," an old-fashioned way of making a fisherman's net, so she can trap some of those found stones into pendants.

Her first steps along the beach are weighted with the everyday thoughts that eddy through her mind, thoughts about needed ingredients for the coming night's dinner, about a conversation had last night with her husband, or of the friends she saw at her coffee klatch that morning. Soon, though, the setting takes over. "It acts like a gate. I walk through the gate, and all of that falls away. I start thinking, 'Boy, that's a beautiful color. Look at that sand. Look at the incredible amber of that mermaid's tear.'"

Her eye is stimulated, and she starts to see these impressions forming in gems, crystals, pearls, and shells that she will transform into one-of-a-kind heirloom pieces of jewelry. "The beach is a relaxing place for me, a place I go to to work something out in my eye. I'm walking, my feet are in the water, and I look down and see how the light strikes the water. It calls me. I am centered, and I go home calm."

Though she lived inland for a time, working as an architect, when she moved to the coast of Maine years ago, she told her husband, "I can never live away from the sea again." Her love of the ocean runs deep, passed on by a father who packed the family into the car each summer, driving them from their home in Pittsburgh, Pennsylvania, to Ocean City, Maryland, where they would spend two weeks, their

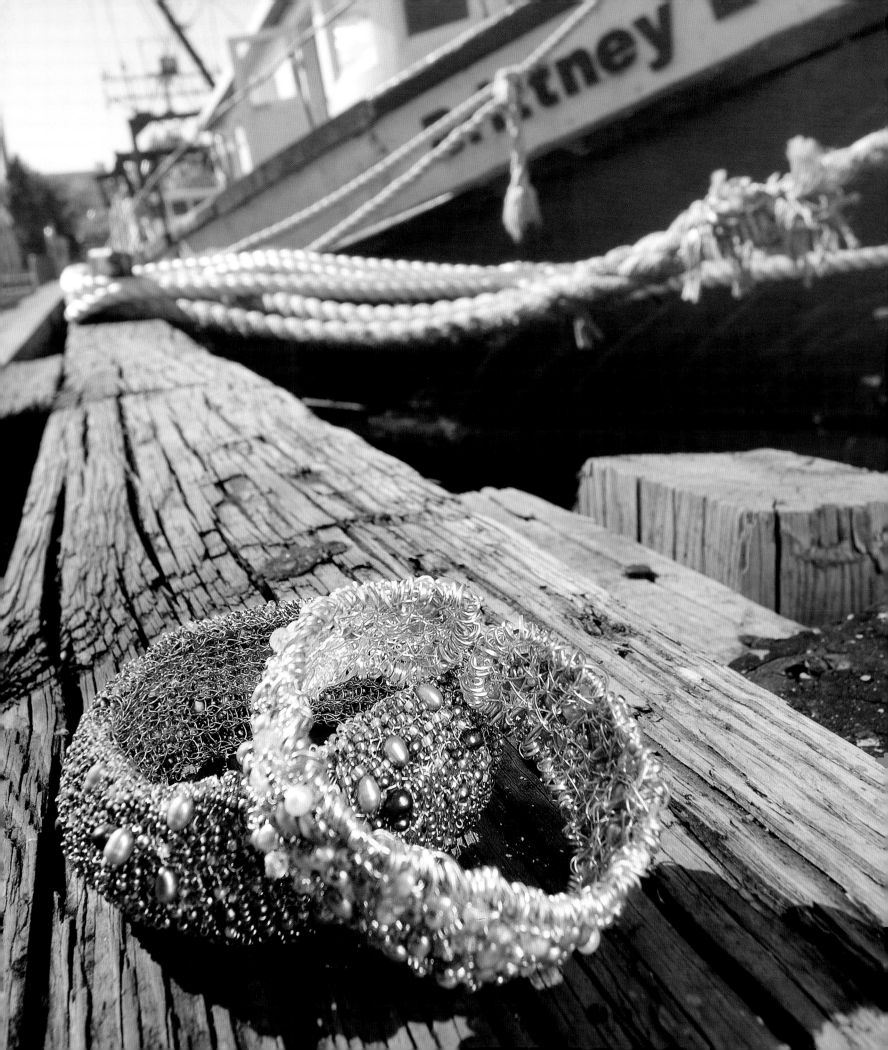

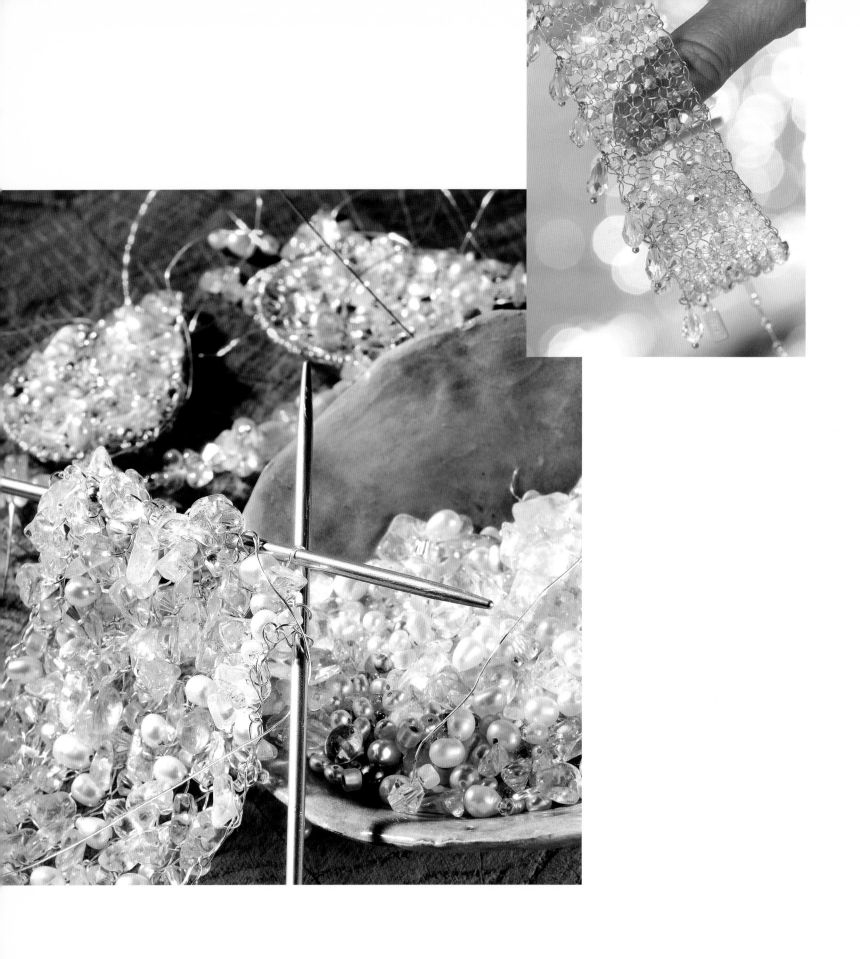

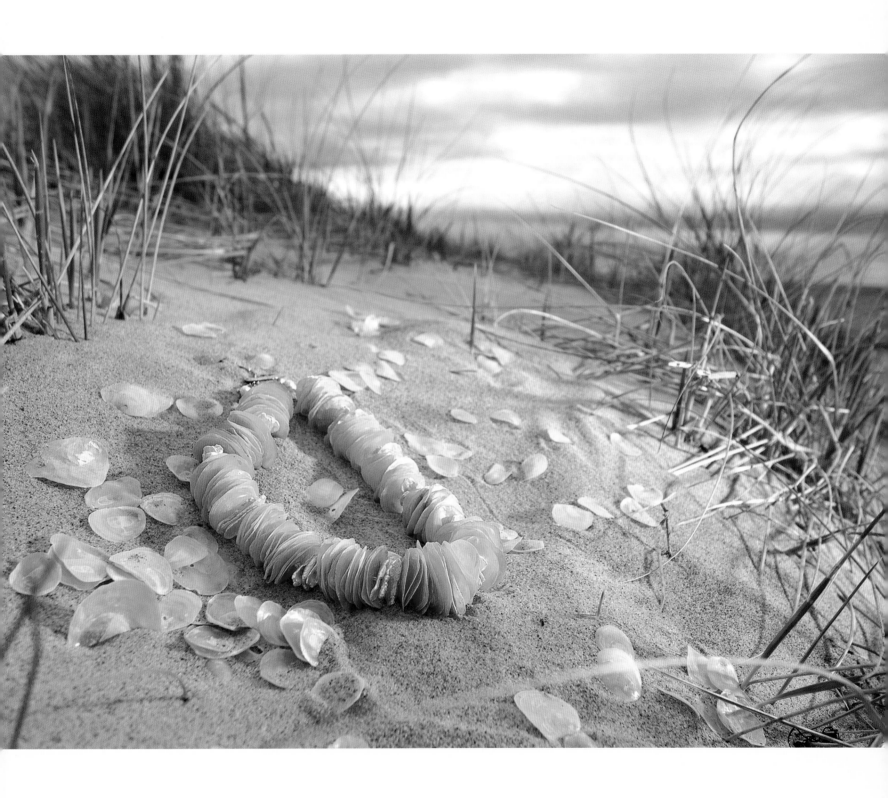

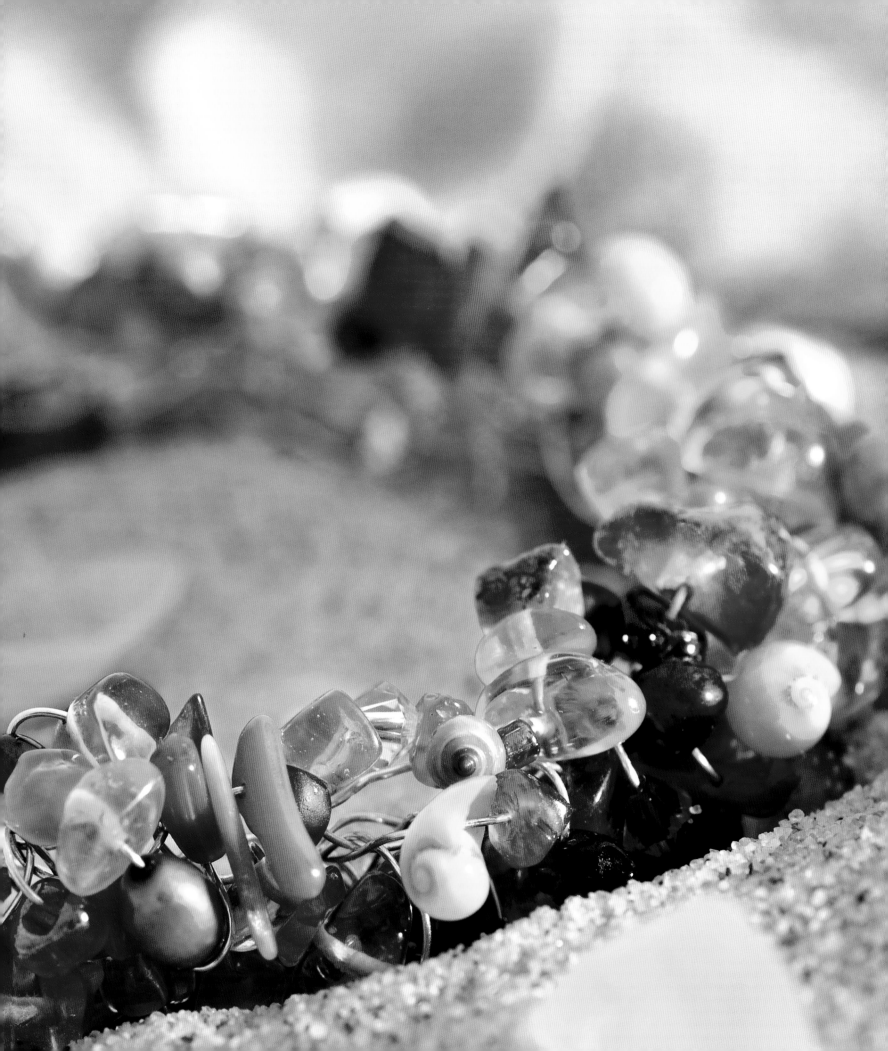

> "We cannot live only for ourselves. A thousand
> fibers connect us with our fellow men; and among
> those fibers, as sympathetic threads, our actions
> run as causes, and they come back to us as effects."

HERMAN MELVILLE

days filled with body surfing, eating French fries under the beach umbrella, and playing skee ball on the boardwalk. "I was probably three when we started going to the beach. It was a huge deal to drive over the Chesapeake Bay Bridge. Dad would roll down the window and yell, 'Smell that salt air.' He loved it, so I learned to love it."

Hawaii is her newest love. Having recently taken a vacation there, Genevieve envisions herself eventually joining the elderly ladies she envied as she watched them having a blast riding the tide on their boogie boards. Until then, she is re-creating scenes, saved as pictures on her cell phone, in jewelry. "Last night I mixed up a sunset. I put beads, crystals, and tourmaline into a bowl, and the colors looked like a sunset I saw in Hawaii."

Closer to home, Genevieve absorbs the sights of New Bedford, the fishing village where she lives. "New Bedford is a very historic, scruffy little seaside town. It is complex, rich, and tattered on the edges. Everyone's lives are touched by the sea one way or another." Her studio is in the historic district, where the city's once illustrious whaling history is celebrated. There you can still visit the iconic Seaman's Bethel, where Melville's fictional hero Ishmael heard Father Mapple preach before leaving for his fateful encounter with Moby-Dick. Around town, Genevieve registers the old-fashioned gardens, the purple flowers that emerge from a bed of hostas, the Victorian architecture. She feels the sea breeze and keeps an eye on the ever-changeable weather. She may return to her studio to work, but in the summer, she retreats to her outdoor work space: the beach. "I will sit out at the beach in my bathing suit, knitting, weaving, crocheting. I'll walk around for a while and then plop down again." When she is removed from the coast, all she needs to do is pick up a piece of her jewelry, and it all comes back. "I will look at a piece and remember when I got those shells and what a beautiful day it was, and I'll see that the clasp looks like a sand dollar. It is like a cue, and it brings me right back." Through her sparkling, complex, bewitching pieces of art, she transports their wearer as well to join her in her seaside reverie.

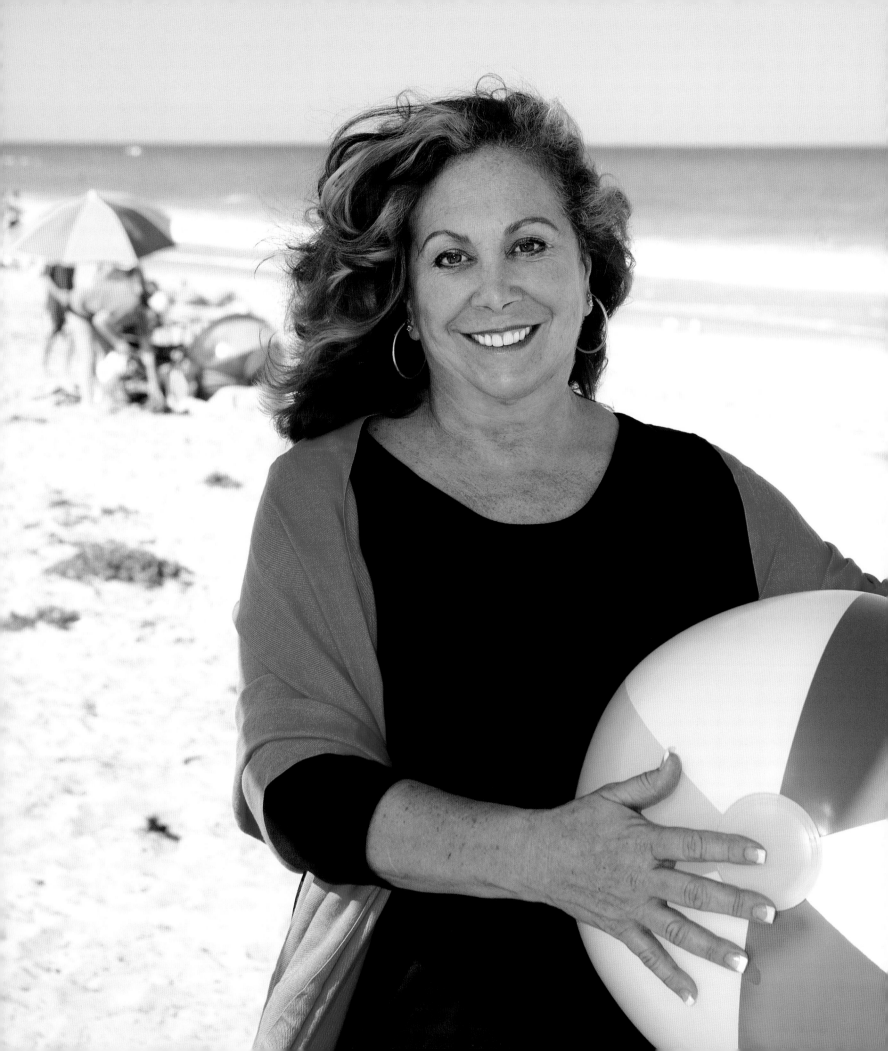

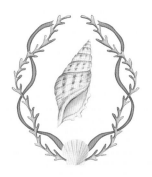

ARTIST { Beth Carver }

"Everything my girls do in my paintings, I do.

I am enamored of the beach and everything about it.

It makes you feel like **a child again.**"

Indialantic, Florida

Her women are larger-than-life, literally and figuratively. They have to be to contain all of the joy that emanates from them. They kick up their heels for an inner tube ballet, relish a double scoop ice cream cone with nary a sign of guilt, and pose with beach balls and model sailboats, laughing with child-like abandon. Painting the buoyant spirits, colorful character, and unself-conscious pleasure of these bathing beauties has become Beth Carver's life mission, a mission that came to her during a sad, solitary walk along the shore.

Only the sea knows how many people have called out to it during times of crisis or confusion, asking for direction or solace. Only individuals know how often such soul-searching has been answered; Beth is one of those individuals. Lost and distraught after watching her father die of cancer, she strolled the beach and pleaded, "Oh, God, give me something for my spirit." Then she saw a vision, a real vision, of an older woman playing in the waves. For the first time in six months, Beth laughed, sharing in the woman's lighthearted fun.

A classically trained artist who attended the Arts Students League and the National Academy of Art in New York, Beth knew then and there that she had to portray and so share the infectious spirit of women reveling in waves, in life at the beach, in each other's company. She paints them in bathing suits of turquoise, purple, and orange polka dots. Their bright swimming caps came about by default: "I was so sad about my father's passing, I couldn't make an executive decision about whether the women in the surf should have wet hair or dry, so I put them in bathing caps. They add color and shape." The impressionistic sea behind her subjects shimmers restlessly. "The sea is an energy force that I use—the color, the movement, the power. It works with my women, who are colorful and powerful."

The *joie de vivre* of these women and their depicter seems barely containable, even when the canvas involves two eight-foot by twenty-four foot triptych murals stretching across the second-floor landing of the Daytona Beach Ocean Center. *Water Music* and *Wings on the Water* show "universal women" splashing with good cheer and waving with optimism. "The women are frolicking in the water, and most of the

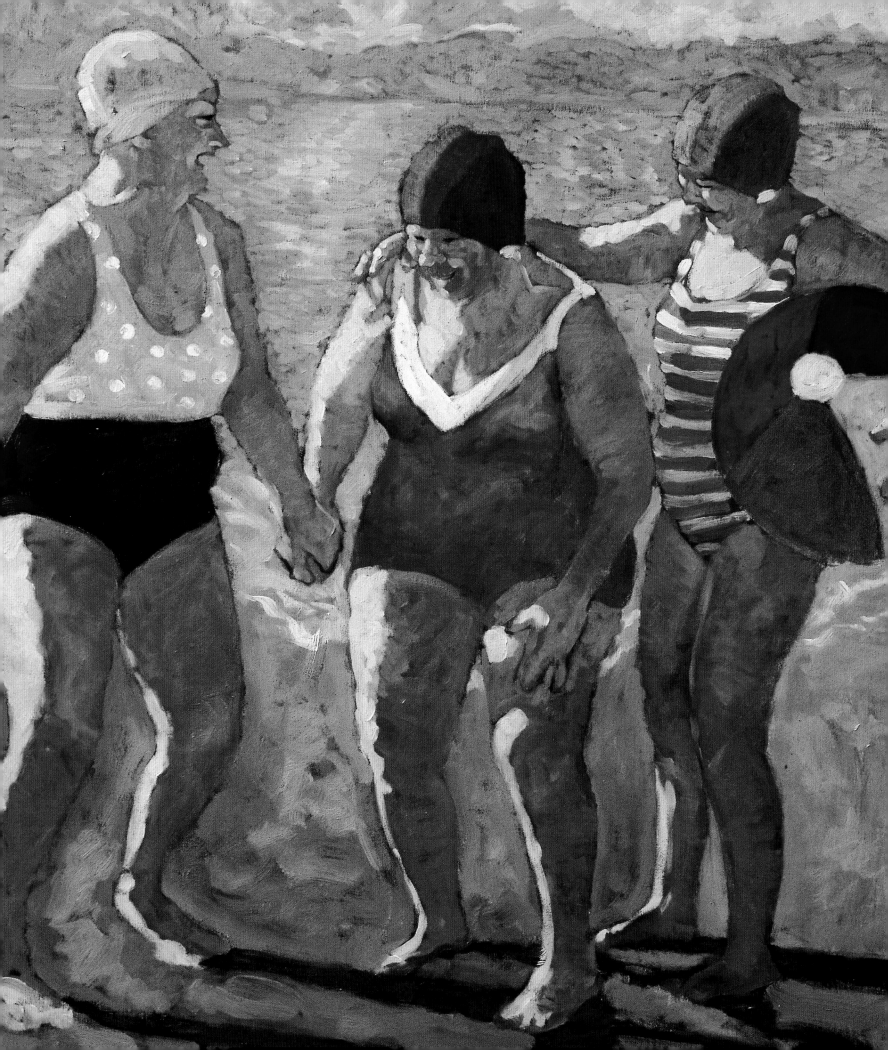

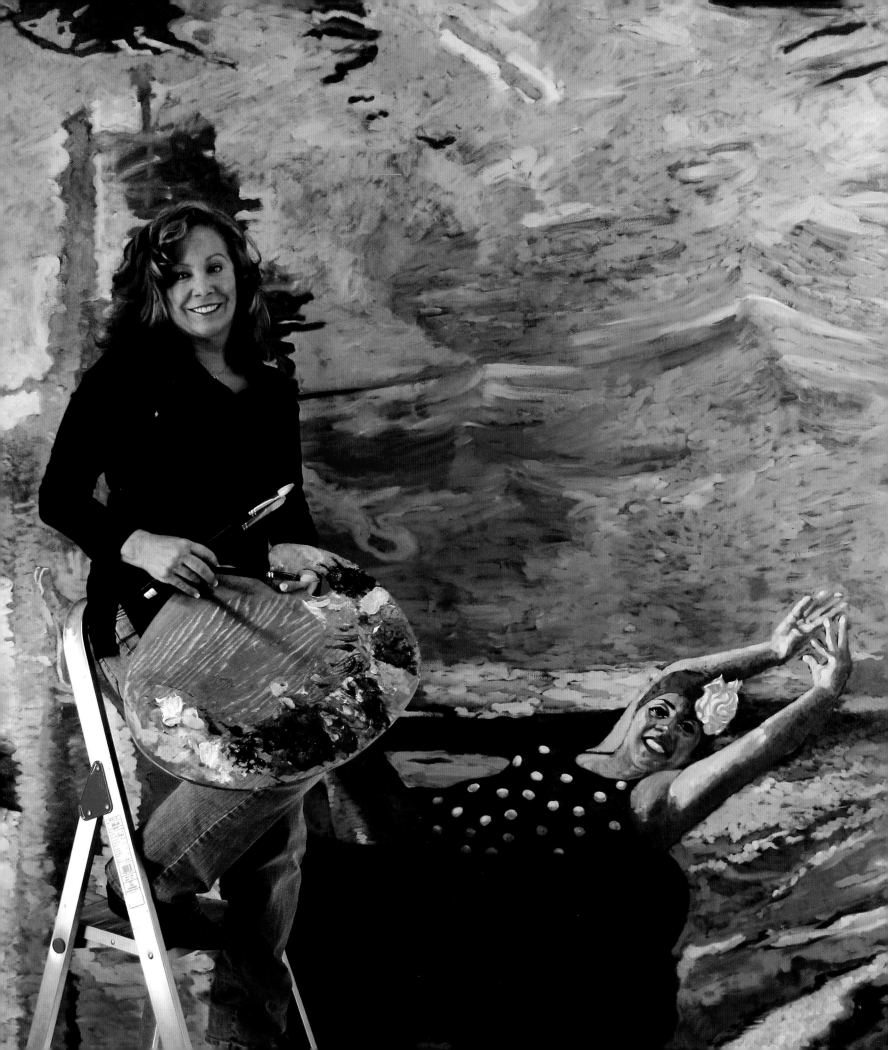

> "To me, the sea is like a person—like a child I've known for a long time. It sounds crazy, I know, but when I swim in the sea I talk to it. I never feel alone when I'm out there."

GERTRUDE EDERLE

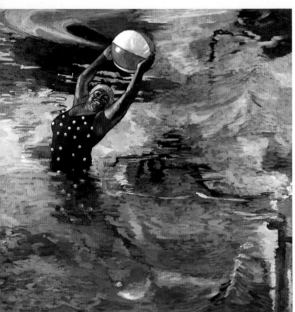 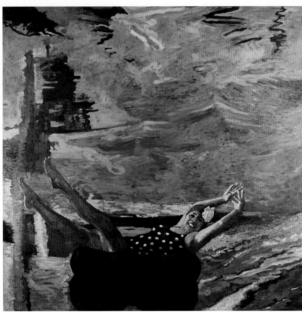 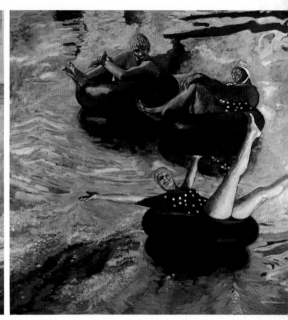

background is swelling waves. The women are on tubes, wearing bathing caps, and of course are color coordinated. They are interesting types from around the world—Asian-American, African-American, Spanish…" One mural captures the rising light of morning, the other twilight, and in both, the waves are on the brink of breaking. "You feel a little seasick," Beth says of the underlying movement. "The water and the light are alive. It is theatrical, like the women are on stage."

That Beth's moment of darkness led to work that highlights the lightness of being felt in the water makes sense. Beth grew up on the New Jersey shore. Her family owned Carver Boat Sales, and her father and grandfather were both boat builders. Her father would even build boats in the living room of the large family's cottage: "We would have to take a door off to get it out," Beth says proudly. "My mother's focus was to get us to the river or the

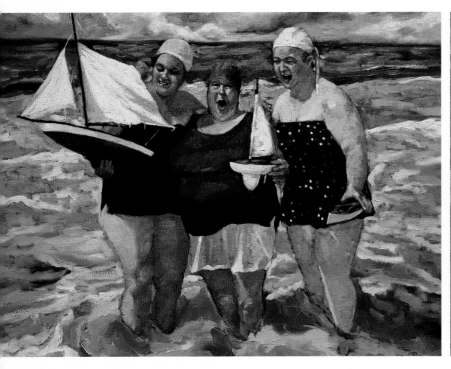 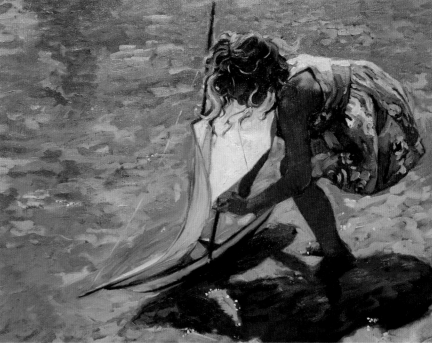

beach every day. We went crabbing and fishing. We would get up at five with our nets to look for crabs and little snappers. I thought everyone lived like that."

Now living in Florida, a block from the ocean, Beth rides her bike to the beach daily to check on surfing conditions. "It's a solitary sport, but I go with friends. I have a fun-shaped board, rounder, more stable. You get on the water and sitting on your board, sitting in the ocean, you see life all around you. Fish and dolphin swim by. If you catch a wave, it's like going on a sleigh ride." Like the ladies she paints, Beth knows how to have fun in the water. "Everything my girls do in my paintings, I do. I am enamored of the beach and everything about it. It makes you feel like a child again."

She paints six or seven days a week, but a day off is always spent at the beach. "Every time you jump in the sea, it is baptismal. The sea is alive." She likens the form her women take to the element in which she places them, "fertile with ideas and life." Those who buy her oil paintings, including the many men who respond to her Rubenesque women, "resonate with the ocean, the joy of life, getting together at the beach with family, sitting in chairs, and eating peanut butter and jelly sandwiches. My women are everyone's family. They're secure and they're joyful."

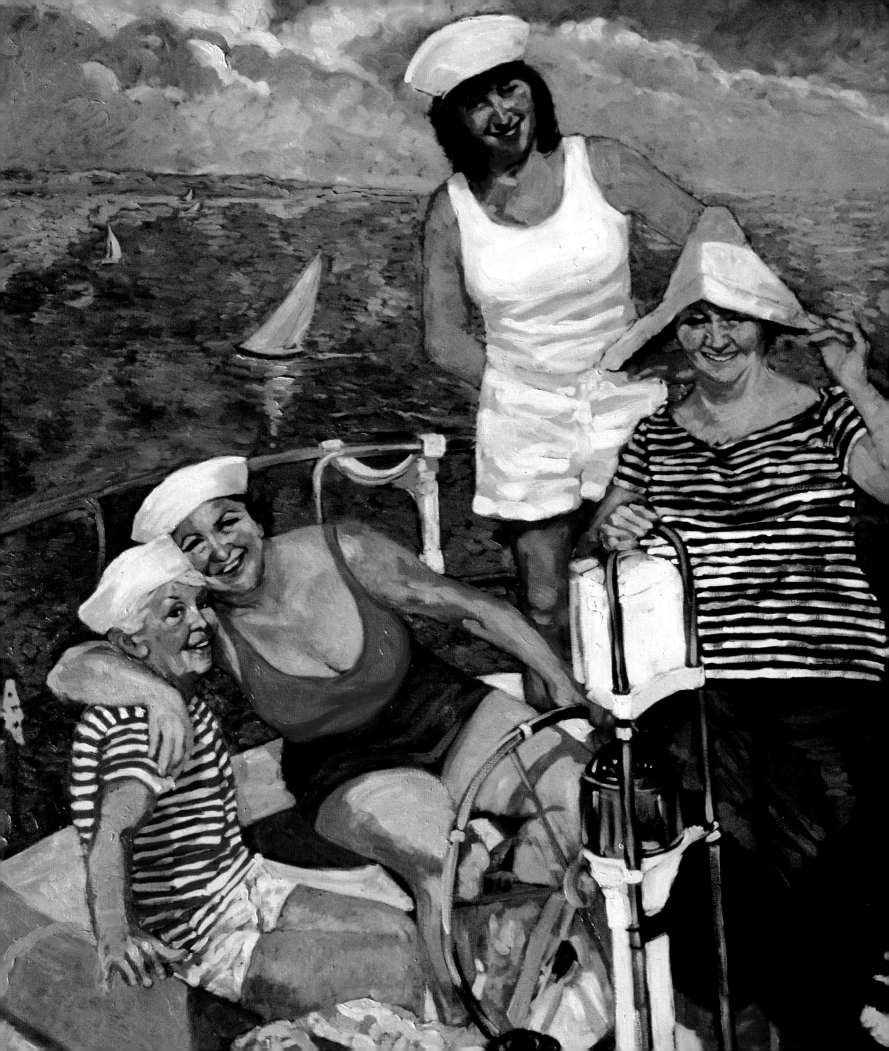

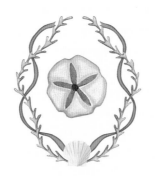

SAND SCULPTOR { Jenny Rossen }

"I only build ephemeral sand sculptures,

which after a time, return to a pile of sand.

It is like buying a bunch of flowers; you do

it for the **beauty of the moment**."

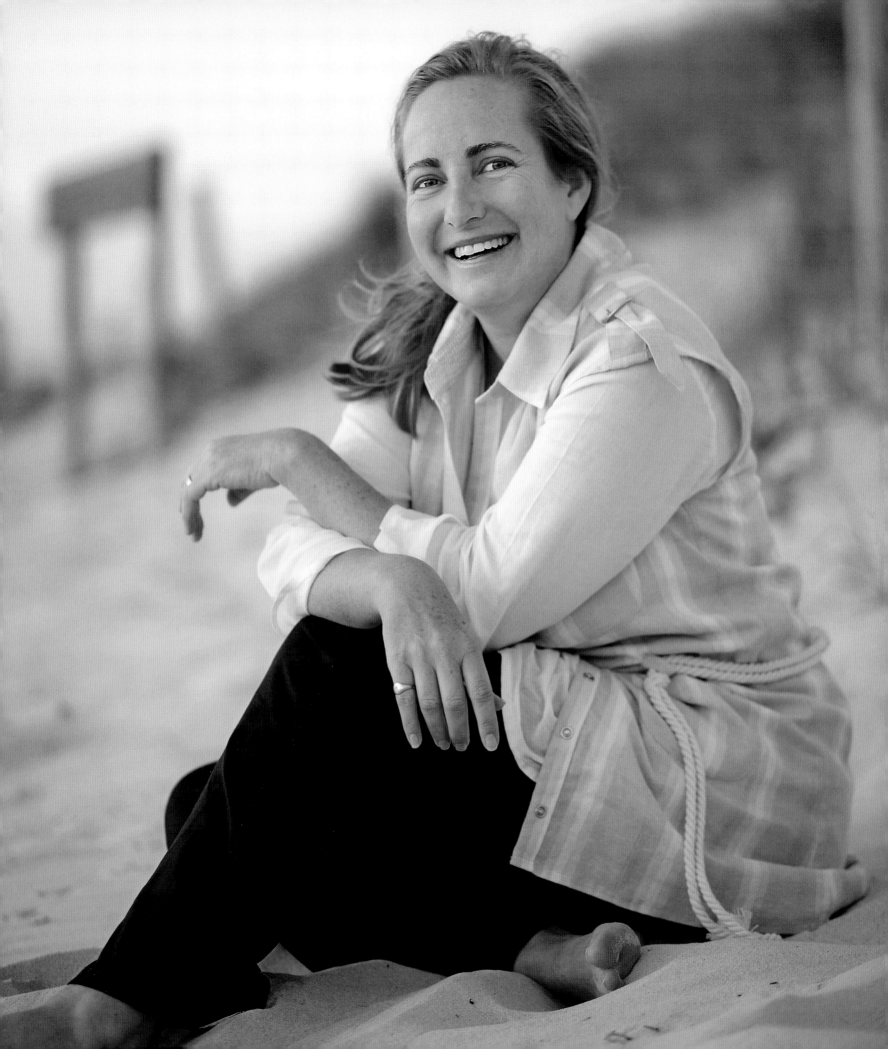

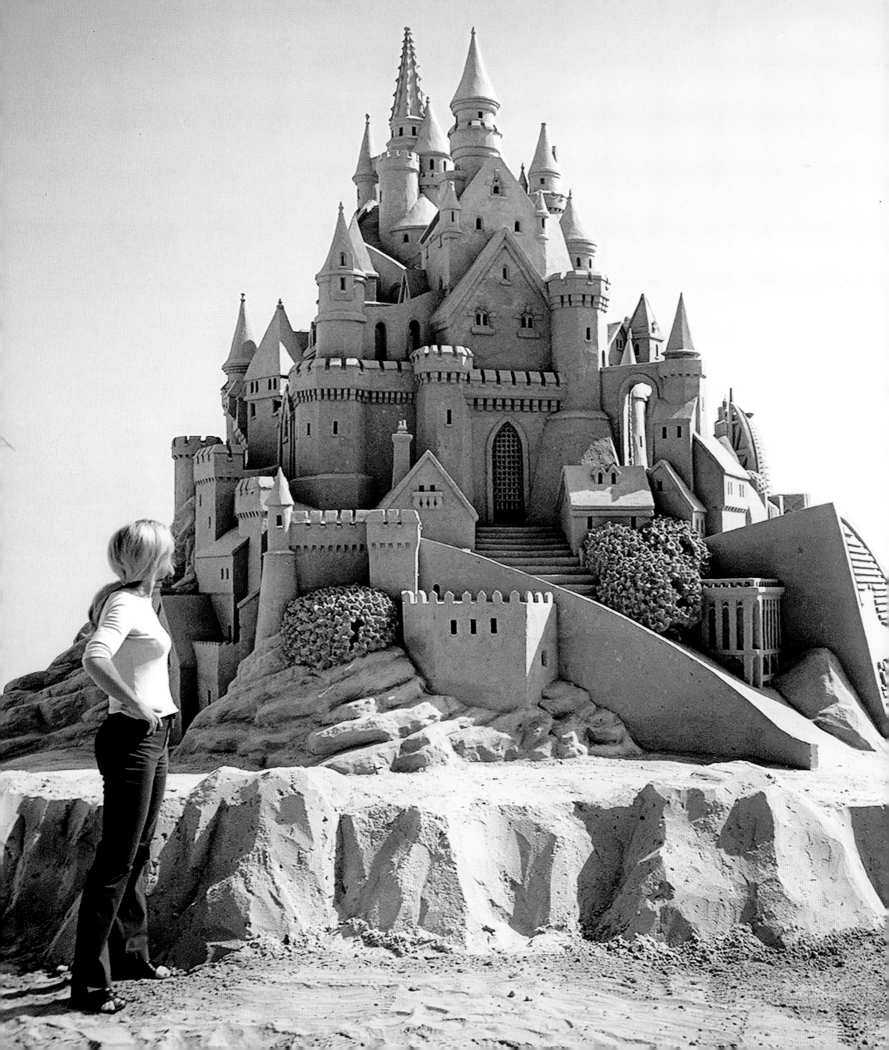

Dubai, United Arab Emirates

The sea moves with eternity but waves to ephemerality. No one understands this better than sand sculptor Jennifer Rossen. She spends days, months even, watering, packing, and shaping sand into hobbit-sized sandcastles. These fairy-tale palaces—with their carved domes, crowned towers, choir of steeples and spires—enjoy their day in the sun, inviting imaginations to visit and delight in them, and then they are gone. A trained artist, Jennifer is fine with the brief life of her creations. "I only build ephemeral sand sculptures, which after a time, return to a pile of sand. It is like buying a bunch of flowers; you do it for the beauty of the moment. No one gets sad when a song finishes. Some things just live in the present. That is what makes them magical." There is a transcendental quality to Jenny's work and life. While she creates castles, characters, flowers, and symbols for competitions, weddings, and exhibitions, knowing they will last mere days or, if indoors, a handful of years, she remains attuned to the timeless aspects of the sea: "The sea is kind of my church. The infinity that is around you, that is spiritual."

The ocean has always been there for Jenny. Each morning, her mother sent her to walk the shores of Cottlesloe Beach in her native Australia. "We lived right on the beach, and Mum used to make us go to the beach early in the morning before school. As an adolescent, I was exhausted. Now whenever I can, I go to the beach the first thing in the morning." Jenny's mother, an architect raising nine children on her own, understood well the therapeutic value of sunrise strolls. "This is what she did. She would wake up and walk the beach. It was her way of dealing with stresses." When it came time for their annual summer vacation, where would her mother take her brood? "To Rottnest Island. We'd bike around, get fish and chips, and sit on the grasses and eat."

To protect their youngest sibling from strong currents and deep waters, Jenny's brothers and sisters would surround her with a sand fortress, the ocean slowly seeping in to make a private pool for her, and there she would play. "I would make towers by dribbling wet sand. I would imagine that tiny people lived in these towers, and I would invent whole villages and lives and dramas," she recalls. Jenny, now with a child of her own, retains a bit of the sprite in her. Though she has been known to sneak into situations replete

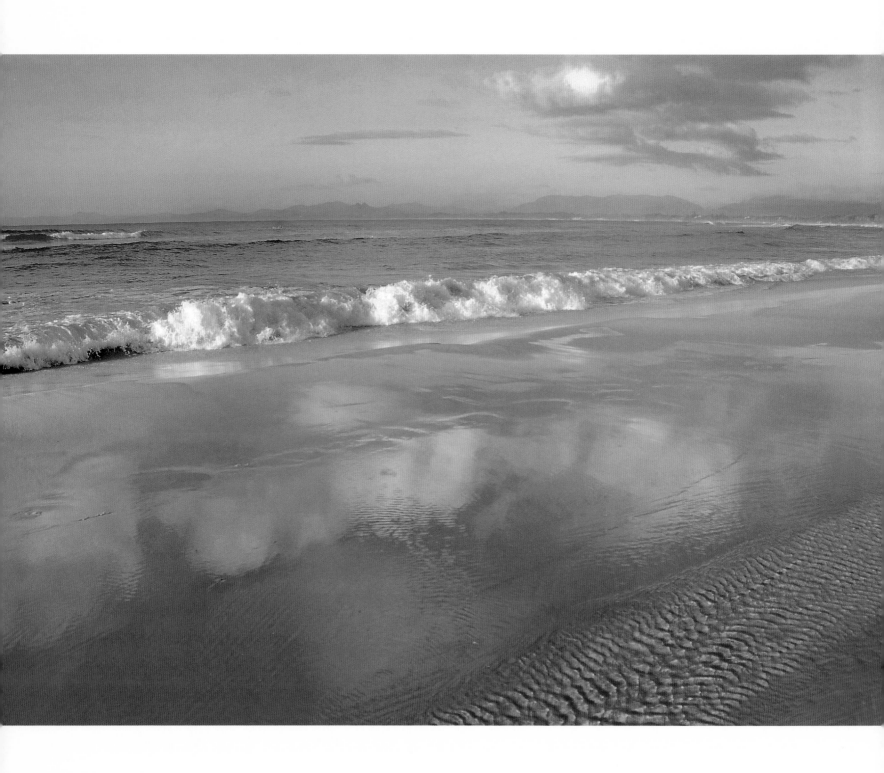

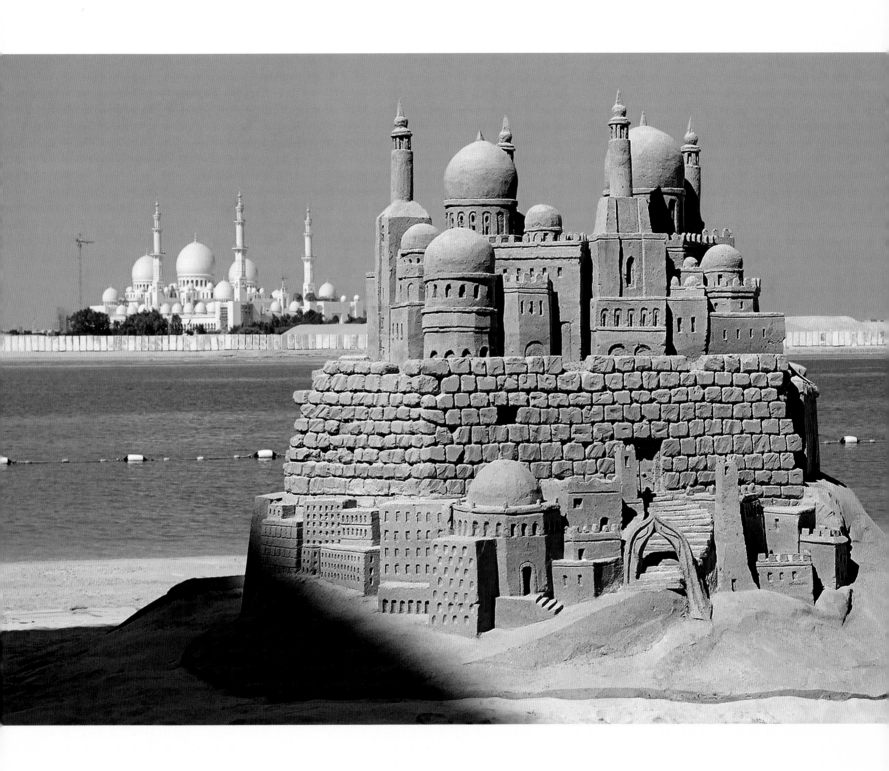

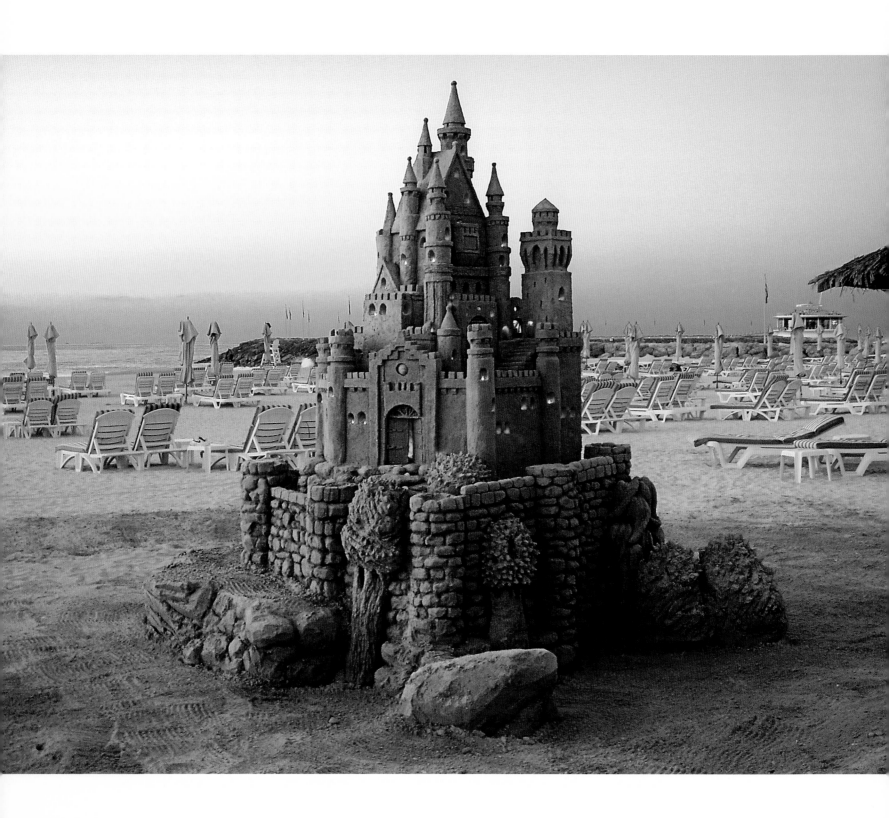

> "Countless as the sands
> of the sea are human passions."
>
> NIKOLAI GOGOL

with sand, sculpt a scene, and leave unseen, she recognizes that what she does is performance art, and she welcomes the curious children who ask in disbelief, "Are you really doing that? Is it hard?" To which she will reply, wink unseen, "It is almost impossible!" Adults amuse her when they ask if she uses molds or has the sand shipped in from elsewhere. "Tell me who will do that for me," she answers. She loves getting teenagers involved and remembers her early ventures into sand sculpture, when in college she and her friends would dig holes and illuminate them with candles, the flames dancing in the sunset seabreezes. She would also carve eternity knots or Buddhist symbols in the sand, "ground art," she calls it. Over time, she took to portraiture and published a book of locals from her hometown of Perth perched on a distressed chair, their favorite beach venue serving as their backdrop. Maybe one sat before the nudist beach, while another may have been part of the triathlon crowd training for the swimming portion of the race.

Eventually trading her paints and brushes for grains of sand and knives, she has traveled the world entering and winning competitions and fulfilling sand sculpture commissions from Canada to the United States, Australia to Dubai, where she now lives. She calls herself a "beach bum," and when told that her habit of lying in Australia's hot sun and then diving face first into its ice cube cold water is detrimental to the dewy youthfulness of her skin, she simply replied, "You have got to have your priorities right!" This life affords her enviable benefits: "The big decision of my day is whether to wear shoes or not."

Jenny has many more castles to sculpt and stories to tell through sand. "I want to make a giant sand-castle theme park of all of the places you cannot go, like the tombs of Egypt or the moon. I want to create all of these fantasy places." She likens her art to being a "magician," and part of the magic is her own amazement at what emerges as she whittles down a pile of sand. As she sculpts, she is reminded of Michelangelo's declaration: "I saw the angel in the marble and carved until I set him free." Michelangelo, of course, was working in materials solid enough to last for eons. Jenny works with remnant grains. Her creations have their moment on the stage, and then the curtain of water rises and falls, reclaiming them.

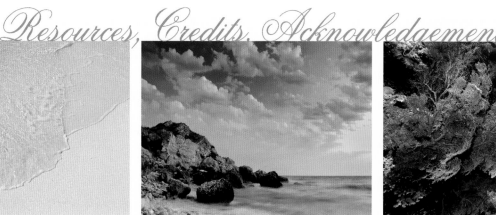

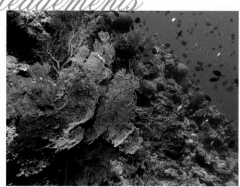

WOMEN AND THE SEA

▶ **Claire Murray**
Claire Murray Enterprises, LLC
www.clairemurray.com
800-252-4733

LORE OF THE SEA

▶ **Christina Wyatt**
www.cpwyatt.com
239-337-5050

▶ **Dinah Unruh**
Eight Bells Carving
www.eightbells.com
508-228-4495

▶ **Sandi Blanda**
email: sgblanda@aol.com
508-209-0970

LIFE AT SEA

▶ **Zena Holloway**
www.zenaholloway.com
+44 (0) 20 8993 9950

▶ **Alexandra Hai**
www.locandaartdeco.com
www.albergosansamuele.com
www.artdecoresidence.com

▶ **Susan Humphris**
Woods Hole Oceanographic Institution
www.whoi.edu
508-289-3451

| ART CREDITS | Claire Murray ▶ Pages 1, 3, 11, 25, 33, 41, 55, 65, 73, 85, 92, 101, 113, 121, 129, 143, 151, 158: *Sirens of the Sea* and *Shells* Medallions; Page 17: *Seashells Medallion* hooked rug; Page 18: *Siren's Song* needlepoint pillow; *Chesapeake Bay Geometric Shells* hooked rug; Page 19: *Coral Reef Runner*. Christina Wyatt ▶ Page 27: *Hope*; Page 28: *Ocean of Dreams*; Page 29: *Mermaid Figure Studies*; Page 30: *Love Knot*. Dinah Unruh ▶ Page 32: *Mermaid*; Page 35: *Sarah Starbuck Folger*; Page 36: *Sailor Boy*; Page 38: *Lavender Maiden*; Page 39: *The Watch*. Sandi Blanda ▶ Page 46: *Thunderbolt*; Page 47: (left) *Martha's Mermaid*, (right): *Hope*; Page 49: *Beyond the Sea*. Mimi Gregoire Carpenter ▶ Page 117: *Fruit de Mer*; Page 118: *Dockside Wreath*; Page 119: *The Mermaid and the Seal*. Beth Carver ▶ Page 153: *Glory Days*; Page 154-155: *Water Music*; Page 156: (left) *America's Cup*, (right) *Day Sailor*; Page 157: *Ship Shape.* | PHOTOGRAPHY CREDITS | Front cover, page 2: ©Masterfile; Page 5: courtesy Claire Murray; Pages 6-7: ©Masterfile; Pages 10, 16: Vanessa Rogers; Page 13: ©Alaska Stock Images/National Geographic Stock; Page 14: ©Daryl Benson/

"The voice of the sea speaks to
the soul. The touch of the sea
  is sensuous, enfolding the body
in its soft, close embrace."

KATE CHOPIN

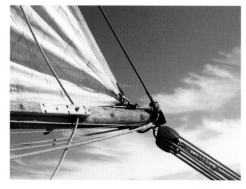 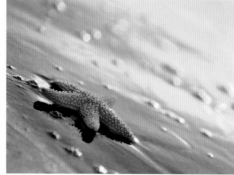 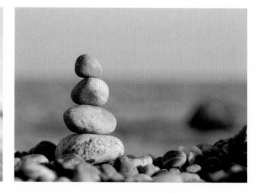

LESSONS AT SEA

▶ **Jennifer MacLean**
Her Ladyship Sailing
www.ladyshipsailing.com
305-942-9645

▶ **Claudia Espenscheid**
Fishin' Chix
www.fishinchix.com
850-916-4444

▶ **Bev Sanders**
Los Olas Surf Safaris
www.surflasolas.com
831-625-5748

GIFTS FROM THE SEA

▶ **Mimi Gregoire Carpenter**
www.artistsofmaine.com
207-284-7021

▶ **Pamela Barefoot**
Blue Crab Bay Company
www.bluecrabbay.com
800-221-2722

▶ **Diane Cowan**
The Lobster Conservancy
www.lobsters.org
207-832-8224

BY THE SEA

▶ **Genevieve Hunt**
www.genevievehunt.com
email: gennyhunt@juno.com

▶ **Beth Carver**
Beth Carver Art
www.bethcarverart.com
321-725-1526

▶ **Jenny Rossen**
www.jennyrossen.com
971 50 7549195 (Dubai)
+61 (0) 439 821 906 (Australia)

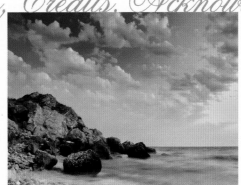

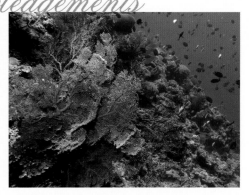

WOMEN AND THE SEA

▸ **Claire Murray**
Claire Murray Enterprises, LLC
www.clairemurray.com
800-252-4733

LORE OF THE SEA

▸ **Christina Wyatt**
www.cpwyatt.com
239-337-5050

▸ **Dinah Unruh**
Eight Bells Carving
www.eightbells.com
508-228-4495

▸ **Sandi Blanda**
email: sgblanda@aol.com
508-209-0970

LIFE AT SEA

▸ **Zena Holloway**
www.zenaholloway.com
+44 (0) 20 8993 9950

▸ **Alexandra Hai**
www.locandaartdeco.com
www.albergosansamuele.com
www.artdecoresidence.com

▸ **Susan Humphris**
Woods Hole Oceanographic Institution
www.whoi.edu
508-289-3451

| ART CREDITS | Claire Murray ▸ Pages 1, 3, 11, 25, 33, 41, 55, 65, 73, 85, 92, 101, 113, 121, 129, 143, 151, 158: *Sirens of the Sea* and *Shells* Medallions; Page 17: *Seashells Medallion* hooked rug; Page 18: *Siren's Song* needlepoint pillow; *Chesapeake Bay Geometric Shells* hooked rug; Page 19: *Coral Reef Runner*. Christina Wyatt ▸ Page 27: *Hope*; Page 28: *Ocean of Dreams*; Page 29: *Mermaid Figure Studies*; Page 30: *Love Knot*. Dinah Unruh ▸ Page 32: *Mermaid*; Page 35: *Sarah Starbuck Folger*; Page 36: *Sailor Boy*; Page 38: *Lavender Maiden*; Page 39: *The Watch*. Sandi Blanda ▸ Page 46: *Thunderbolt*; Page 47: (left) *Martha's Mermaid*, (right): *Hope*; Page 49: *Beyond the Sea*. Mimi Gregoire Carpenter ▸ Page 117: *Fruit de Mer*; Page 118: *Dockside Wreath*; Page 119: *The Mermaid and the Seal*. Beth Carver ▸ Page 153: *Glory Days*; Page 154-155: *Water Music*; Page 156: (left) *America's Cup*, (right) *Day Sailor*; Page 157: *Ship Shape*. | PHOTOGRAPHY CREDITS | Front cover, page 2: ©Masterfile; Page 5: courtesy Claire Murray; Pages 6-7: ©Masterfile; Pages 10, 16: Vanessa Rogers; Page 13: ©Alaska Stock Images/National Geographic Stock; Page 14: ©Daryl Benson/

> "Countless as the sands
> of the sea are human passions."
>
> NIKOLAI GOGOL

with sand, sculpt a scene, and leave unseen, she recognizes that what she does is performance art, and she welcomes the curious children who ask in disbelief, "Are you really doing that? Is it hard?" To which she will reply, wink unseen, "It is almost impossible!" Adults amuse her when they ask if she uses molds or has the sand shipped in from elsewhere. "Tell me who will do that for me," she answers. She loves getting teenagers involved and remembers her early ventures into sand sculpture, when in college she and her friends would dig holes and illuminate them with candles, the flames dancing in the sunset seabreezes. She would also carve eternity knots or Buddhist symbols in the sand, "ground art," she calls it. Over time, she took to portraiture and published a book of locals from her hometown of Perth perched on a distressed chair, their favorite beach venue serving as their backdrop. Maybe one sat before the nudist beach, while another may have been part of the triathlon crowd training for the swimming portion of the race.

Eventually trading her paints and brushes for grains of sand and knives, she has traveled the world entering and winning competitions and fulfilling sand sculpture commissions from Canada to the United States, Australia to Dubai, where she now lives. She calls herself a "beach bum," and when told that her habit of lying in Australia's hot sun and then diving face first into its ice cube cold water is detrimental to the dewy youthfulness of her skin, she simply replied, "You have got to have your priorities right!" This life affords her enviable benefits: "The big decision of my day is whether to wear shoes or not."

Jenny has many more castles to sculpt and stories to tell through sand. "I want to make a giant sand-castle theme park of all of the places you cannot go, like the tombs of Egypt or the moon. I want to create all of these fantasy places." She likens her art to being a "magician," and part of the magic is her own amazement at what emerges as she whittles down a pile of sand. As she sculpts, she is reminded of Michelangelo's declaration: "I saw the angel in the marble and carved until I set him free." Michelangelo, of course, was working in materials solid enough to last for eons. Jenny works with remnant grains. Her creations have their moment on the stage, and then the curtain of water rises and falls, reclaiming them.